The EAE Textbook of
Echocardiography

The EAE Textbook of
Echocardiography

Edited by

Leda Galiuto (Editor-in-Chief)

Luigi Badano

Kevin Fox

Rosa Sicari

José Luis Zamorano

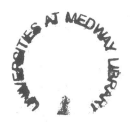

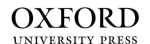
OXFORD
UNIVERSITY PRESS

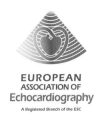
EUROPEAN
ASSOCIATION OF
Echocardiography
A Registered Branch of the ESC

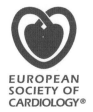
EUROPEAN
SOCIETY OF
CARDIOLOGY®

OXFORD
UNIVERSITY PRESS

Great Clarendon Street, Oxford OX2 6DP

Oxford University Press is a department of the University of Oxford.
It furthers the University's objective of excellence in research, scholarship,
and education by publishing worldwide in

Oxford New York

Auckland Cape Town Dar es Salaam Hong Kong Karachi
Kuala Lumpur Madrid Melbourne Mexico City Nairobi
New Delhi Shanghai Taipei Toronto

With offices in

Argentina Austria Brazil Chile Czech Republic France Greece
Guatemala Hungary Italy Japan Poland Portugal Singapore
South Korea Switzerland Thailand Turkey Ukraine Vietnam

Oxford is a registered trade mark of Oxford University Press
in the UK and in certain other countries

Published in the United States
by Oxford University Press Inc., New York

British Library Cataloguing-in-Publication-Data

Data available

Library of Congress Cataloging-in-Publication-Data

Data available

Typeset by Glyph International, Bangalore, India
Printed in Spain
on acid-free paper by
Grafos SA

ISBN 978-0-19-959963-9

10 9 8 7 6 5 4

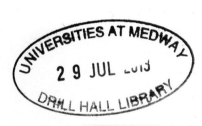

Contents

Contributors

S. Adhya
Kings College Hospital, London, UK

Río Aguilar-Torres
Cardiology Department, Hospital de Bellvitge, and
Universidad Autónoma de Barcelona, Spain

M.J. Andrade
Department of Cardiology, Hospital
Santa Cruz, Carnaxide, Portugal

Ashraf M. Anwar
Department of Cardiology, Al-Husein University
Hospital, Al-Azhar University, Cairo, Egypt

G.D. Athanassopoulos
Department of Cardiology, Onassis Cardiac Center, Greece

Luigi P. Badano
Department of Cardiac, Vascular and Thoracic
Sciences, University of Padua, Padua, Italy

H. Baumgartner
University Hospital Muenster, Germany

H. Becher
Department of Cardiology, John
Radcliffe Hospital, Oxford, UK

N. Cardim
Hospital da Luz, Lisbon, Portugal

Folkert Jan ten Cate
Thoraxcenter, Erasmus MC, Rotterdam, The Netherlands

John B. Chambers
Cardiothoracic Centre, Guy's and St
Thomas' Hospital, London, UK

Lauro Cortigiani
Division of Cardiology, Lucca Hospital, Italy

Bernard Cosyns
Cardiology Department, Universitair
Ziekenhuis, Brussels, Belgium

G.P. Diller
University Hospital Muenster,
Germany

Arturo Evangelista
Department of Cardiac Imaging, Hospital
Vall d'Hebron, Barcelona

R. Feneck
Guy's and St Thomas' Hospital, London, UK

Kevin F. Fox
Imperial College, London, UK

Frank A. Flachskampf
Uppsala University, Uppsala, Sweden

Maurizio Galderisi
Division of Cardioangiology with CCU,
Department of Clinical and Experimental Medicine,
Federico II University Hospital,
Naples, Italy

L. Galiuto
Catholic University of the Sacred Heart,
Institute of Cardiology, Rome, Italy

Madalina Garbi
North Cumbria University Hospitals NHS
Trust, Cumberland Infirmary, Carlisle, UK

Miguel Ángel García Fernández
Departamento de Medicina I, Universidad
Complutense, Madrid, Spain

José Juan Gómez de Diego
Hospital Universitario La Paz, Madrid, Spain

Alexandra Gonçalves
University Clinic San Carlos, Madrid, Spain

T. González-Alujas
Department of Cardiac Imaging, Hospital
Vall d'Hebron, Barcelona

F. Guarracino
Cardiothoracic Department, University
Hospital of Pisa, Italy

Gilbert Habib
Department of Cardiology, La Timone, Marseille, France

Andreas Hagendorff
Department of Cardiology-Angiology,
University of Leipzig, Germany

Andrea Kallmeyer
Cardiovascular Institute, San Carlos
University Hospital, Madrid, Spain

G. Karatasakis
Department of Cardiology, Onassis Cardiac Center, Greece

A. Kempny
University Hospital Muenster, Germany

Patrizio Lancellotti
Department of Cardiology, University Hospital,
Domaine Universitaire du Sart Tilman, Liège, Belgium

G. Locorotondo
Catholic University of the Sacred Heart,
Institute of Cardiology, Rome, Italy

Julien Magne
Department of Cardiology, University Hospital,
Domaine Universitaire du Sart Tilman, Liège, Belgium

Pedro Marcos-Alberca
University Clinic San Carlos, Madrid, Spain

M. Monaghan
King's College Hospital, London, UK

Sergio Mondillo
Department of Cardiology, University of Siena, Siena, Italy

Denisa Muraru
Department of Cardiac, Vascular and Thoracic
Sciences, University of Padua, Padua, Italy

Aleksandar N. Neskovic
Cardiovascular Research Center, Dedinje Cardiovascular
Institute, Belgrade University Medical School, Yugoslavia

Petros Nihoyannopoulos
National Heart and Lung Institute, UK

Kim O'Connor
Department of Cardiology, University Hospital,

Domaine Universitaire du Sart Tilman, Liège, Belgium

Bernard Paelinck
Cardiology Department, UZ Antwerp, Belgium

Mónica M. Pedro
Instituto Cardiovascular de Lisboa, Lisbon, Portugal

Eugenio Picano
Institute of Clinical Physiology, National
Research Council, Pisa, Italy

Luc A. Pierard
Department of Cardiology, University Hospital,
Domaine Universitaire du Sart Tilman, Liège, Belgium

Fausto Pinto
Department of Cardiology, University
Hospital Sta Maria, Lisbon, Portugal

B.A. Popescu
'Carol Davila' University of Medicine and Pharmacy,
Institute of Cardiovascular Diseases, Bucharest, Romania

Raphael Rosenhek
Department of Cardiology, Vienna General
Hospital, Medical University of Vienna, Austria

Christian Rost
University of Erlangen, Erlangen, Germany

R. Senior
Department of Cardiology, Northwick
Park Hospital, Harrow, UK

Peter Sogaard
Department of Cardiology, Aarhus
University Hospital, Denmark

Franck Thuny
Department of Cardiology, La Timone, Marseille, France

Jean-Louis Vanoverschelde
Divisions of Cardiology and Nuclear Medicine,
University of Louvain, Brussels, Belgium

Jens-Uwe Voigt
Department of Cardiology, Univserity
Hospital Gasthuisberg, Leuven, Belgium

José Luis Zamorano
University Clinic San Carlos, Madrid, Spain

Symbols and abbreviations

➔	cross-reference	CK	creatine kinase
🖫	additional DVD and online material	CMR	cardiac magnetic resonance
ℳ	website	CO	cardiac output
>	greater than	COPD	chronic obstructive pulmonary disease
<	less than	CRT	cardiac resynchronization therapy
2D	two-dimensional	CT	computed tomography
3D	three-dimensional	CW	continuous wave
A2C	apical two-chamber view	dB	decibel
A3C	apical three-chamber view	DBP	diastolic blood pressure
A4C	apical four-chamber view	DCM	dilated cardiomyopathy
A5C	apical five-chamber view	DTE	time of deceleration of E wave
AAA	abdominal aorta aneurysm	DVT	deep venous thrombosis
ACC	American College of Cardiology	EAE	European Association of Echocardiography
ACS	acute coronary syndromes	ECA	external carotid artery
A/D	analogue to digital	ECG	electrocardiogram/electrocardiography
AH	arterial hypertension	EDV	end diastolic velocity
AHA	American Heart Association	EF	ejection fraction
AoV	aortic valve	EMD	endomyocardial disease
AR	aortic regurgitation	EMEA	European Medicines Agency
AS	aortic stenosis	EOA	effective orifice area
ASD	atrial septal defect	EOAi	effective orifice area indexed
ASE	American Society of Echocardiography	ER	emergency room
AV	atrioventricular	EROA	effective regurgitant orifice area
AVA	aortic valve area	ESC	European Society of Cardiology
AVSD	atrioventricular septal defect	fps	frame per second
BMD	Becker muscular dystrophy	HCM	hypertrophic cardiomyopathy
bpm	beats per minute	HDDE	high-dose dobutamine echocardiography
BSA	body surface area	HF	heart failure
CABG	coronary artery bypass graft	HR	heart rate
CAD	coronary artery disease	Hz	hertz
CCA	common carotid artery	IABP	intra-aortic balloon pump
ccTGA	congenitally corrected transposition of the great arteries	ICA	internal carotid artery
		ICE	intracardiac echocardiography
CD	colour Doppler	IE	infective endocarditis
CFDS	colour-flow duplex scan	IHD	ischaemic heart disease
CFR	coronary flow reserve	IMT	intima–media thickness
CI	cardiac index	IRA	infarct-related artery

IVC	inferior vena cava		PR	pulmonary regurgitation
IVRT	isovolumic relaxation time		PRF	pulse repetition frequency
IVS	interventricular septum		PS	pulmonary stenosis
LA	left atrium/atrial		PSAX	parasternal short axis
LAP	left atrial pressure		PSS	longitudinal post-systolic shortening
LCD	liquid crystal display		PSV	peak systolic velocity
LDDE	low-dose dobutamine echocardiography		PV	pulmonary valve
LGC	lateral gain compensation		PVR	pulmonary vascular resistance
LHIS	lipomatous hypertrophy of the interatrial septum		PW	pulsed wave *or* posterior wall
LV	left ventricle/ventricular		QA	quality assurance
LVDP	left ventricular diastolic pressure		QI	quality improvement
LVEDD	left ventricular end-diastolic diameter		RA	right atrium/atrial
LVEDP	left ventricular end-diastolic pressure		RAH	renalvascular arterial hypertension
LVESD	left ventricular end-systolic diameter		RF	radiofrequency
LVFP	left ventricular filling pressure		RF%	regurgitant fraction
LVO	left ventricular opacification		RT3DE	real-time three-dimensional echocardiography
LVOT	left ventricular outflow tract		RV	right ventricle/ventricular
LVOTO	left ventricular outflow tract obstruction		RVEF	right ventricular ejection fraction
LVSP	left ventricular systolic pressure		RVFAC	right ventricular fractional area change
MBF	myocardial blood flow		RVol	regurgitant volume
MBV	myocardial blood volume		RVOT	right ventricle outflow tract
MCE	myocardial contrast echocardiography		RVOTO	RVOT obstruction
MD	microvascular damage		RVSP	right ventricular systolic pressure
MI	mechanical index		RWT	relative wall thickness
min	minute(s)		s	second(s)
MPAP	mean pulmonary arterial pressure		SAM	systolic anterior motion
MR	mitral regurgitation		SBP	systolic blood pressure
ms	millisecond(s)		SPTA	spatial peak-temporal average
MV	mitral valve		SR	strain rate
MVA	mitral valvular area		STE	speckle tracking echocardiography
MVG	myocardial velocity gradients		STEMI	ST-elevation myocardial infarction
mW	milliwatts		SV	stroke volume
NSTEMI	non-ST elevation myocardial infarction		SVC	superior vena cava
NYHA	New York Heart Association		SVR	systemic vascular resistance
PA	pulmonary artery		TAPSE	tricuspid annular systolic excursion
PADP	pulmonary artery diastolic pressure		TAVI	transcatheter valve implant
PAH	pulmonary arterial hypertension		TD	tissue Doppler
PAP	pulmonary arterial pressure		TGA	transposition of the great arteries
PASP	pulmonary artery systolic pressure		TGC	time gain compensation
PCL	primary cardiac lymphoma		TI	thermal index
PCWP	pulmonary capillary wedge pressure		TOE	transoesophageal echocardiography
PD	perfusion defect		TR	tricuspid regurgitation
PDA	patent ductus arteriosus		TS	tricuspid stenosis
PE	acute pulmonary embolism		TSI	tissue synchronicity imaging
PFO	patent foramen ovale		TTE	transthoracic echocardiography
PMC	percutaneous mitral valve commissurotomy		TV	tricuspid valve
PHT	pressure half-time		TVI	time velocity integral
PLAX	parasternal long axis		VSD	ventricular septal defect
PISA	proximal surface isovelocity area		WM	wall motion
PFE	papillary fibroelastoma		WMA	wall motion abnormality
			WMSI	wall motion score index

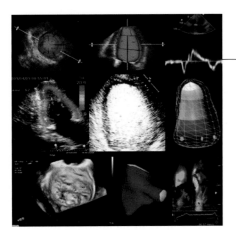

CHAPTER 1

The general principles of echocardiography

Madalina Garbi

Contents

Summary

Knowledge of basic ultrasound principles and current echocardiography technology features is essential for image interpretation and for optimal use of equipment during image acquisition and post-processing.

Echocardiography uses ultrasound waves to generate images of cardiovascular structures and to display information regarding the blood flow through these structures.

The present chapter starts by presenting the physics of ultrasound and the construction and function of instruments. Image formation, optimization, display, presentation, storage, and communication are explained. Advantages and disadvantages of available imaging modes (M-mode, 2D, 3D) are detailed and imaging artefacts are illustrated. The biological effects of ultrasound and the need for quality assurance are discussed.

Principles of ultrasound

Physics of ultrasound

Ultrasound waves are sound waves with a higher than audible frequency. The audible frequency range is 20 hertz (Hz) to 20,000Hz (20kHz). Cardiac imaging applications use an ultrasound frequency range of 1–20MHz (millions hertz) (➲ Table 1.1).

The sound wave is a longitudinal wave, consisting of cyclic pressure variation which travels inducing displacement of encountered media particles in the direction of wave propagation. The wavelength determines imaging resolution. In echocardiography, adequate resolution is obtained with wavelengths less than 1mm. The characteristics of the ultrasound wave are illustrated in ➲ Fig. 1.1.

A shorter wavelength corresponds to a higher frequency, and vice versa. The wavelength (cycle length) multiplied by frequency (cycles per second) gives the ultrasound wave propagation speed.

Propagation speed (m/s) = wavelength (mm) × frequency (MHz)   1.1

The average propagation speed in soft tissues is 1540m/s. It is higher in less compressible media (e.g. bone) and lower in more compressible media (e.g. air in the lungs).

Table 1.1 Currently used frequency range for cardiac imaging applications (including paediatric)

Transthoracic	1–8MHz
Transoesophageal	3–10MHz
Intracardiac	3–10MHz
Epicardial	4–12MHz
Intracoronary	10–20MHz

The propagation speed is used to calculate the distance of a structure and confine it in an appropriate location in the image formed.

The ultrasound is a form of energy, travelling in a beam. The energy transferred in the unit of time defines the power, measured in milliwatts (mW). The power per unit of beam cross-sectional area represents the average intensity (mW/cm²). Power and intensity are proportional with the square of the wave amplitude.

The intensity increases with power increase or cross-sectional area decrease by *focusing* the ultrasound beam. The intensity varies across the beam, being highest in the centre and lower towards the edges.

An estimate of peak intensity is given by the mechanical index (MI) calculated from the peak negative pressure (MPa) divided by the square root of transmitted frequency (MHz).

Current echocardiography uses intermittent repetitive generation of ultrasound pulses consisting of a few cycles each.

Continuous transmission is used only for continuous wave Doppler. Consequently, the ultrasound beam intensity varies with time, being zero in between pulses. The intensity varies also within each pulse, decreasing throughout the pulse length, as a result of *damping*.

Reflection and transmission of ultrasound at interfaces

Travelling through tissues, the ultrasound encounters interfaces where acoustic properties change, influencing propagation. Propagation depends also on the angle of incidence (insonation angle) with the interface. Encountering an interface, the ultrasound partially returns towards the source and is partially transmitted (➲ Fig. 1.2).

At a smooth and large interface the ultrasound obeys rules of *specular reflection*, returning towards the source with direction angle equal with the angle of incidence. Every medium has specific acoustic impedance (density × propagation speed, measured in Rayls). The impedance difference between media at an interface—acoustic impedance mismatch—influences the return signal ratio. Higher mismatch enhances reflection and lower mismatch enhances transmission. The high mismatch at air/soft tissue interfaces explains the need of using ultrasound gel as a coupling medium during examination.

At a rough interface or when encountering small structures (with dimensions in the range of the wavelength) the ultrasound

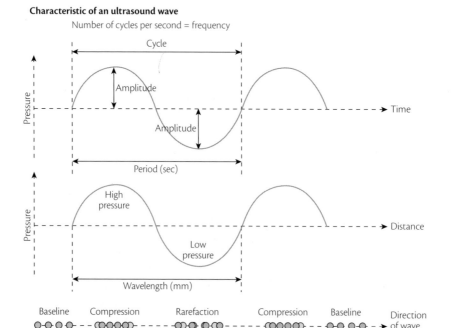

Figure 1.1 Characteristics of an ultrasound wave. Each cycle of complete pressure variation occurs over a certain length of time (period—measured in time units) and also occurs over a certain length of space (*wavelength*—measured in distance units, usually millimetres). The *frequency* is the number of complete cycles occurring in the unit of time, measured in hertz (one cycle per second). The maximal pressure variation above or below baseline represents the sound wave *amplitude*, measured in pressure units—megapascals (MPa) for ultrasound. As the wave travels, the encountered media particles are displaced, resulting in compression of the medium (increased particle density) corresponding to the high pressure wave travelling past and rarefaction of the medium (decreased particles density) corresponding to low acoustic pressure.

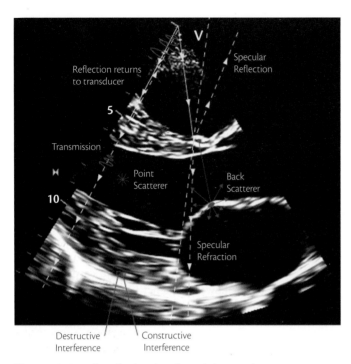

Figure 1.2 *Specular reflection:* the reflected ultrasound returns to the source in cases of perpendicular incidence, but does not return to the source in cases of an oblique incidence. Transmission of ultrasound continues in the same direction in cases of perpendicular incidence or occurs with a change in direction—refraction—in cases of oblique incidence. *Scatter reflection:* the backscatter is higher with higher ultrasound frequency and depends on scatterer size. A point scatterer sends ultrasound homogenously in all directions. The backscatter from the multitude of scatterers encountered by the ultrasound wave interfere enhancing (constructive interference) or neutralizing each other (destructive interference). This explains why the image of tissues contains *speckles* and apparent free spaces instead of having homogeneous appearance.

suffers *scattering*, returning towards the source and being transmitted in many directions (➲ Fig. 1.2). The proportion of ultrasound returning to the source (backscatter) is independent of insonation angle. Scatter reflections allow generation of an image of examined structures instead of a mirror (specular) image of the transducer.

Amplitude and intensity drop as ultrasound travels through tissues, a phenomenon named *attenuation* (measured in decibels, dB), due predominantly to *absorption* but also to *reflection* and *scattering* (➲ Fig. 1.2). Attenuation increases with travelled distance and with ultrasound frequency. It depends on a specific *attenuation coefficient*—0.5dB/cm/MHz in soft tissues. For image formation the ultrasound travels from and to the source, which doubles attenuation—1dB/cm/MHz per centimetre of depth.

Transducers

Transducer construction and characteristics

The transducers are both generators and receivers of ultrasound waves used to create echocardiographic images, based on

piezoelectric effect (conversion of electricity in ultrasound waves and the reverse, conversion of ultrasound waves in electricity).

The main component of the transducer is a piezoelectric element, which generates ultrasound waves as a result of alternating electricity-induced deformation and generates electricity as a result of the returning ultrasound waves-induced deformation. The piezoelectric properties are natural or induced by heating the material up to a specific temperature—Curie temperature—at which the molecules align in a strong electric field. Modern transducers use manufactured piezoelectric materials. Crystals, ceramics, polymers, and composites, with a range of electromechanical coupling efficiencies (ideally high) and acoustic impedances (ideally low) have been used over the years. The piezoelectric properties are lost with heating, a reason why heat-based transducer sterilization is inappropriate. Current transducers use new generation crystals with high bandwidth providing simultaneously high resolution and penetration (pure wave crystals, single crystal technology, etc.).

The transducer has a *housing case* for the piezoelectric element. Elements *backing with damping material* stops backwards propagation of waves towards the case walls, to prevent interference with waves returning from examined structures (ring-down artefact). Damping restricts the number of oscillations per pulse and their amplitude. Shorter pulse duration improves axial resolution and increases the range of generated frequencies, at the expense of sensitivity, reduced because of lower amplitude.

The generated ultrasound frequency is determined by the electric pulse frequency. The transducer nominal frequency depends on the piezoelectric element's *resonance frequency*, generated when the element thickness is half the wavelength (only tenths of millimetres, so elements break easily if dropping or banging the transducer). Damping and electrical current modulation helps generate a *broad band of frequencies* around the nominal frequency.

The piezoelectric element has much higher impedance than the tissues; direct contact would create a highly reflective interface. Materials with intermediate impedance are used to cover the element in one or more *matching layers*.

The transducer generates a main ultrasound beam, which creates diagnostic images, and accessory beams (*side lobes*) which can also create images (artefact). The beam of a basic single disc-shaped element transducer has progressively increasing width due to diffraction (deviation from initial direction) after a *natural focus* point, separating the beam in two zones. The narrow beam of the near *zone* (Fresnel field) offers better lateral resolution. Its length is proportional with ultrasound frequency and transducer aperture dimensions. The wide beam of the *far zone* (Fraunhofer field) offers reduced image resolution.

Transducer types

The first transducers were single-element transducers, which could generate and receive ultrasound waves along a single line, resulting in A-mode and M-mode imaging (for explanation of A-mode and M-mode imaging, see ➐ 'Ultrasound imaging principles'). The grey-scale M-mode had high frame rate (2000–5000 frames/second, fps), limited only by the time necessary for the waves to return from examined structures. Focusing was achieved with a concave lens or by giving curved shape to composite piezoelectric elements.

Two-dimensional (2D) imaging emerged from development of *sector scanning* necessitating beam steering—sweeping across the imaging plane. Steering prolonged imaging time, restricting frame rate, compared with single-line scanning. *Mechanical steering* was used first. The mechanical transducer had a small footprint though was inappropriate for Doppler imaging advances. *Electronic steering* was a breakthrough in transducer development (➐ Fig. 1.3A). It enabled parallel 2D and Doppler imaging advances, and in refined versions it enabled development of three-dimensional (3D) imaging. Sequential firing of elements is also used for *electronic focusing* (➐ Fig. 1.3B).

Electronic aperture variation, allowing preservation of focal beam width for a range of focus depths, is obtained by changing the fired elements number. The conventional phased array transducer is the one-dimensional (1D) transducer (➐ Fig. 1.4). Matrix array transducers are currently used (➐ Fig. 1.5). Matrix array transducers evolution established 3D imaging (➐ Figs. 1.6 and 1.7).

The received beam has electronic steering and focusing as well. Current transducers have *multiple transmission focusing* and *dynamic reception focusing*, improving resolution throughout the image depth. Dynamic reception focusing needs *dynamic aperture* to preserve focal beam width.

Complex transmission and reception focusing and the use of short intermittent pulses with multiple frequencies and damping make the current actual ultrasound beam difficult to

illustrate. Presented images (➐ Figs. 1.4–1.7) represent the beam pathway, with the transmitted beam fading away due to attenuation.

Transducer selection

Transducer selection is less of an issue with current broad-band transducers and equipment features allowing fine tuning in image optimization. A wide range of patients is scanned without changing transducer. Technology evolution resulted in a decrease in transducer size and footprint (aperture). Smaller transducers need a smaller acoustic window and are easier to handle. Aperture size reduction is limited by concomitant drop in near-field length.

Higher frequency is needed for better resolution imaging of shallow structures (e.g. heart in children and cardiac apex or coronaries in adults). Lower frequency is needed for better penetration to deeper structures (e.g. large size adults). There is a penetration–spatial resolution trade-off (for details of transducer selection, see ➐ Chapter 2, 'Principles of imaging').

Ultrasound imaging principles

Echocardiography images represent the display of returning ultrasound waves from examined structures, with location determined by their travelling time. Each returning ultrasound wave generates an electrical signal with radiofrequency (RF).

Imaging modes (advantages and limitations)

The A-mode represents a display of received signal amplitude from each depth along a scan line. The amplitude of specular

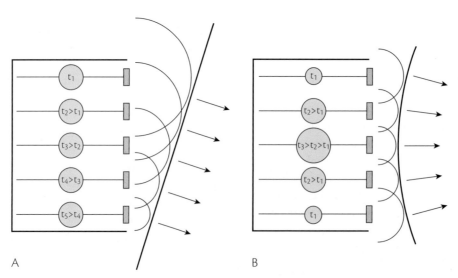

Figure 1.3 Electronic steering and focusing. A) Electronic steering: the phased array transducers consist of a series of rectangular piezoelectric elements sequentially fired (see activation time delays t1 < t2 < t3 < t4 < t5) in order to obtain ultrasound beam steering. B) Electronic focusing: see sequence of elements activation (t1 < t2 < t3) used for electronic focusing. Transmitted ultrasound beam focusing changes the length of the near zone by adjusting the depth of focus, to include the examined structure and improve resolution. The beam width is reduced to minimum in the focal area and diverges immediately after. The focal zone has maximum intensity and provides maximal lateral resolution.

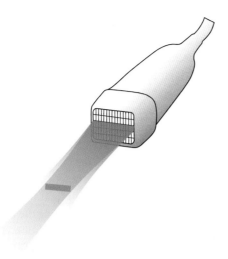

Figure 1.4 Conventional phased array transducer. The 1D transducer consists of one row of piezoelectric elements aligned in the imaging plane. This allows electronic focusing only in the imaging plane, adjusting the beam width responsible for lateral resolution. See the accessory beams (side lobes) illustrated in red.

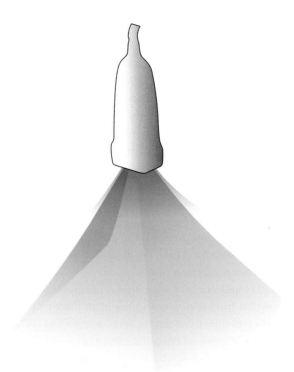

Figure 1.6 Real-time 3D imaging transducer beam. Currently, full matrix array transducers with more than 2000 elements enable second-generation real-time 3D imaging, concomitantly collecting information in sagittal, coronal, and transverse planes with a pyramidal ultrasound beam. The first 3D images were reconstructed from a series of 2D images acquired with free hand scanning or mechanically driven transducers. Later, sparse-array matrix transducers with 256 elements made possible the first generation real-time 3D transthoracic imaging with poor spatial resolution.

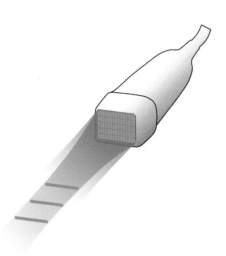

Figure 1.5 Matrix array transducer. In transducer development, the 1.5D and the 2D transducers were created by adding rows of elements in the elevation plane. This allows electronic focusing in the elevation plane as well, adjusting the beam thickness responsible for the tomographic slice thickness. The 1.5D transducer has fewer elements rows in the elevation plane and has shared electric wiring for pairs of added elements. The 2D arrays have more elements rows with separate electric wiring. Transducer advances were based on the ability to cut the elements very small, to isolate them, to fit their electric wiring in the case, and to command complex firing algorithms. The first transducers for 2D and then 3D imaging were *sparse-arrays*, concomitantly using only part of their elements. Full matrix array transducers are currently used. Side lobes of constituent elements add up in *grating lobes* of the array (illustrated in red in the image). They can be reduced by firing peripheral elements at lower amplitude—*apodization*—with continuous variation—*dynamic apodization*. They can also be reduced by cutting subelements within elements.

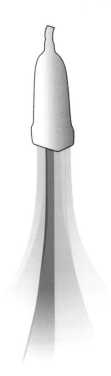

Figure 1.7 Use of 3D imaging transducer for multiplane imaging. The 3D imaging transducer can acquire and display two or three concomitant 2D tomographic images from the same cardiac cycle, using rows of transducers generating beams in two or three imaging planes.

reflections is much higher than that of scatter reflections, giving the signal a large dynamic range. Amplitude transformation in grey-scale display creates B-mode imaging—based on signal brightness. The electrical signal amplitude is analogue—proportional with the received wave pressure. Analogue to digital (A/D) conversion designates amplitude a number (from 0–255). The grey-scale display results from representing low amplitudes in black (0), high amplitudes in white (255), and intermediate amplitudes in grey. The weak scatter reflections would be almost lost at conversion without *logarithmic compression* of amplitude numeric values which restricts the dynamic range.

The M-mode—motion imaging mode—is a grey-scale display of amplitude from each depth along a scan line over time, with high temporal resolution.

The 2D image is a grey-scale display of amplitude over depth information from several scan lines in an imaging plane. The result is a real-time tomographic section providing spatial resolution at the expense of temporal resolution.

The 3D image is a colourized-scale display of amplitude over depth from several imaging planes in a pyramidal volume. The result is a real-time image with higher spatial resolution but even lower temporal resolution because of prolonged image formation time. A full volume 3D data set results from stitching together subvolumes from sequential cardiac cycles (usually four). This near-real-time mode allows high line density with relatively high frame rate (still lower than current 2D frame rate). Recently, one cardiac cycle full volume acquisition became available; these instruments achieve 2D-like frame rate in 3D when used for near-real-time imaging. The '4D' image can be colourized to display time-related tissue Doppler derived information.

Signal processing

The transducer should receive all returning waves from an ultrasound pulse before generating a new pulse, to avoid *range ambiguity artefact* (confining waves returning late from one pulse in same location with waves returning early from the next pulse). Consequently, the number of pulses per second—*pulse repetition frequency (PRF)*—depends on maximum travelling time which depends on imaging depth. For every scan line, the PRF determines the *frame rate*—number of images generated per second and stored in memory. The higher the depth, the lower the PRF so the lower the frame rate. The higher the number of scan lines, the lower the frame rate. Higher imaging sector width needs more scan lines resulting in lower frame rate. The frame rate determines the temporal resolution.

In current transducers, able to transmit and receive a range of frequencies, different PRF corresponds to different frequency:

◆ 5MHz => 71,8 PRF

◆ 4MHz => 60,9 PRF

◆ 3,3MHz => 55,8 PRF

From the image stored in memory an image display is created and presented. The number of images displayed per second defines the *refresh rate* which is smaller or equal with the frame rate. Both high frame rate and high refresh rate are needed for *real-time imaging* (rapid display of images during scanning, presenting the examined structures in motion).

Image display was first performed in a cathode-ray tube and presented on a television screen or computer monitor. The stored digital information is converted back to analogue voltages which induce a proportional strength electron beam generating a proportional brightness spot of light in the fluorescent tube. The spot moves across the tube creating the image display.

Currently both display and presentation can be performed on a flat-panel consisting of a matrix of thousands of liquid crystal display (LCD) elements, acting as electrically activated light valves which can create grey-scale or colour images.

Harmonic imaging

This imaging modality has produced a substantial improvement in 2D and M-mode image quality. Indeed, before development of harmonic imaging modality, ultrasound signals from cardiac structures were received by the transducer at the same frequency as that of emitted ultrasound wave. Such frequency is named *fundamental frequency*. When contrast agents were introduced in echocardiography, in order to enhance ultrasound signals thanks to their capability to resonate and produce frequencies higher than the fundamental one (see ➲ Chapter 7), it was discovered that also tissues are able to provide more intense signals.

As a high amplitude ultrasound wave passes through an elastic medium, it causes a high-density compression phase and a low-density refraction phase in the particles of tissue. Such particles begin to oscillate providing not only an ultrasound signal at fundamental frequency, but also some vibrations of lower amplitude and higher frequency than the original vibrations. Vibration frequencies are exact multiples of the fundamental frequency and are named *harmonics*. Harmonic amplitude is proportional to the fundamental amplitude squared. Harmonic images are created by specifically exploiting this non-linear response to the ultrasound beam.

Because harmonic generation is a cumulative process, the harmonic component of the ultrasound beam becomes progressively stronger with depth of tissue penetration. However, it results in reduction of axial resolution of the ultrasound image. Harmonic imaging places great demands on the transducer. It must be able to transmit low-frequency, but high-amplitude ultrasound pulses and receive high-frequency and low-amplitude echoes. By using the second harmonic (twice the fundamental frequency) artefactual echoes are minimized. The major advantage of harmonic imaging resides in its capability to improve the signal-to-noise ratio. Broad bandwidth transducers have enabled the use of harmonic frequencies (➲ Fig. 1.8) resulting in significant image quality improvement (➲ Fig. 1.9A,B).

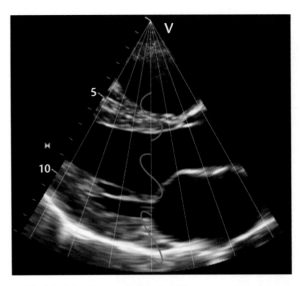

Figure 1.8 Principle of harmonic imaging. The propagation of ultrasound in tissues is non-linear, faster during higher pressure because of higher media particles compression. This results in progressive wave-shape change because of added frequencies (*harmonics*) to the transducer-generated frequency (*fundamental*). The phenomenon is more accentuated with higher ultrasound intensity and at higher depth. Harmonic imaging is obtained by filtering out the returning fundamental frequencies and receiving only the second harmonic frequency.

Image storage

In older instruments image storage was based on *video recording* or *paper printing* and later on magneto-optical disk. Video recording is still used for back-up though presently image storage is based on digital acquisition of loops or freeze frames.

Current instruments have large digital archiving memory, from which it is possible to write CD-ROM or send information to a computer workstation or an external database. Post-processing, analysis and measurements can be performed after scanning completion (off-line). The studies are easy to retrieve for comparison at follow-up, teaching, and research.

Digital memory stores numbers representing information. The image is divided in to thousands of pixels forming a matrix. Each matrix gives a 2-bit memory—stores 'black' or 'white' for each pixel. More matrixes are used for detailed shading – 8-bit memory stores 256 shades, much more that what our vision can differentiate. Echocardiography images can be stored as raw data or as compressed files following standard protocols (e.g. *AVI* for loops or *JPEG* for freeze frames).

Images can be communicated through PACS (picture archiving and communicating systems). The image communication protocol for all manufacturers is standardized in *DICOM* format (Digital Imaging and Communication in Medicine). Further communication standardization within healthcare and with manufacturers is provided by *HL7*—Health Level Seven of the ISO (International Standards Organization). For example, HL7 provides echocardiography examination report coding systems.

Image quality optimization

Echocardiography instruments have controls which allow quality optimization, operating before image storage in memory (*pre-processing*) or after image retrieval from memory in order to be displayed (*post-processing*). In other words pre-processing determines the quality of image formation, operating on the transmitted and received ultrasound. Post-processing determines the quality of image display on the screen, operating before display or even off line, on stored images. The names of the controls are manufacturer dependent and so is their level of interference in image quality and the ability to post-process off-line acquired images. Changes and improvements are rapidly occurring. Understanding the principles, we can use the specific controls of each instrument accordingly.

The instrument controls can change:

1. Ultrasound frequency: enabling us to select the appropriate frequency for the examination performed without changing transducer. For example, shallow structures, like the cardiac apex in apical views are better examined with higher frequencies. Better penetration at higher depth in an overweight patient is achieved with lower frequencies. Higher frequency gives higher resolution but lower penetration.

2. Depth: allowing maximal display of the area of interest on the screen. The higher the depth, the lower the PRF so the lower the frame rate. (See: "Signal processing" section).

3. Power output: the amount of energy emitted by the transducer. The output power is measured in percentages of the maximum power or in decibels. Output power reduction results in lower amplitude of returning waves and therefore weaker signal. Output power increase enhances the amplitude of returning ultrasound signal, but excessive increase raises concerns regarding biological effects (See "Biological effects of ultrasound and safety").

4. Focus level: the ultrasound beam can be focused to optimize resolution at a specific distance from the transducer. Structures proximal to the focus level are better visualised.

5. Angle or sector width: allows a change in the area swept by the ultrasound beam. Reducing it, we reduce the beam steering time and consequently the imaging time, achieving a higher frame rate.

6. Tilt: lateral orientation of the image sector, facilitates exploration of peripheral structures with better axial resolution.

7. Gain: changes overall amplification of the electrical signal induced by the returning ultrasound waves, similar to the volume control in an audio system.

8. Time gain compensation (TGC): allows differential adjustment of gain along the length of the ultrasound beam, to compensate for the longer time taken by waves returning from higher depth to reach the transducer. Due to attenuation, signals returning from progressively higher depth (later)

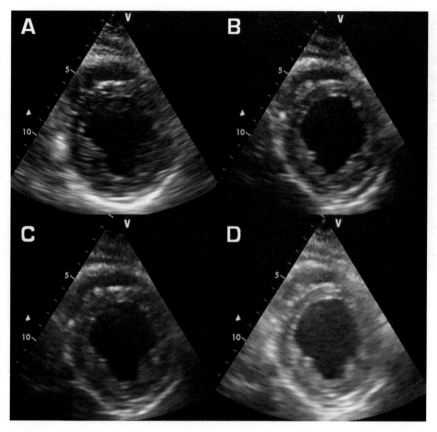

Figure 1.9 Image quality optimization. A) and B) Harmonic imaging effect on image quality: see fundamental image (A) and harmonic image (B). Relying on the high intensity central part of the beam, harmonic imaging *improves lateral resolution* and *reduces lateral lobes artefacts*. Relying on signal from higher depth, harmonic imaging *reduces near field artefact*. Because attenuation of returning waves is higher for higher depth though, the mid field has the best image quality. Relying on longer ultrasound pulses, harmonic imaging *reduces axial resolution*. The pulse inversion harmonic imaging technique uses shorter pulses in pairs which cancel each other's fundamental frequencies. This technique *improves axial resolution* but it *reduces temporal resolution* instead, having a lower frame rate. C) Compress control effect: image (C) is image (B) with maximum compress. 'Compression' increase reduces heterogeneity of grey-scale image display, reducing differences in signal strength by amplifying more the weak signals. D) Dynamic range control effect: image (D) is image (B) with maximum dynamic range. The 'dynamic range' is the range of signal strengths which can be processed—from the weaker detected signal to the stronger not inducing saturation signal. Increasing the dynamic range we increase the displayed number of shades of grey in the display; decreasing it we obtain a more black and white image.

are progressively weaker. The TGC provides a series of controls which should be set to give gradually higher amplification to signal returning from higher depth to compensate for attenuation.

9. Lateral gain compensation (LGC): allows higher amplification of the weaker lateral signal.

10. Reject: sets a strength threshold for a signal to be detected, excluding weaker signal (noise).

11. Freeze: during real time scanning or off-line, it allows the operator to stop the moving heart display and to select a single frame of interest in order to perform measurements or print.

12. Zoom: it can enlarge a particular area of interest within the displayed image.

13. Dynamic range and compress: see ➲ 'Imaging modes' and ➲ Fig. 1,9 C, D captions.

14. Edge enhancement: improves border delineation enabling more accurate measurements and better visualisation of

the endocardium for systolic function and regional wall motion assessment.

A range of ready made grey scale or colourised scale (B colour) settings are also available for post-processing image optimization, some having a better contrast resolution and some having a more smooth appearance. The smooth appearance is obtained with *pixel interpolation* and *persistence*. With pixel interpolation smoothening is achieved by feeling in the gaps with grey scale pixels, progressively more with higher depth because the scan lines progressively diverge. Persistence makes moving image smooth by practically adding frames which are an average of previous and next. Colourization improves contrast resolution. Shades of orange are widely popular for both 2D and 3D imaging.

Post-processing abilities are refined in 3D imaging, allowing colourization, shading, smoothening, contrast resolution optimization, and 3D adjustment of gain to improve the perception of perspective. Post-processing includes rendering and cropping of the full volume pyramid and changes of the angle of display.

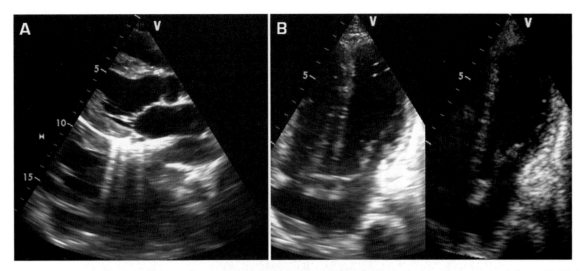

Figure 1.10 Mirror image and refraction artefacts. A) Mirror image artefact: a second image (reflection) of the same structure is formed behind a strong reflector. The second image is weaker than the first. In the example, effort was made to enhance the mirror image for illustration purposes. A whole second parasternal long axis view of the heart is formed behind a highly reflective pericardium. B) Refraction artefact: a second image of the same object positioned lateral to the real image is formed by the refracted waves. In the example (left image), a whole second interventricular septum appears to be present. By changing settings (increasing frequency and changing technique—harmonic imaging instead of pulse inversion) and slightly angulating the transducer, the artefact was resolved (right image).

Artefacts and pitfalls of imaging

Echocardiography can create images of structures in a wrong place, distorted images (in size, shape, and brightness), images of false structures, or it can miss structures in the shadow of other structures. These artefacts are due to ultrasound physics or operator interference. Some artefacts can be avoided by changing transducer position/angulation or imaging settings/technique. Artefacts are less frequent with current technology.

The *near-field clutter* is an artefact due to the high amplitude of oscillations obscuring structures present in the near field. It is reduced by harmonic imaging. Artefact recognition is crucial for image interpretations. To facilitate recognition, they have been illustrated with examples and described in the figure captions (see ➲ Figs. 1.10–1.14).

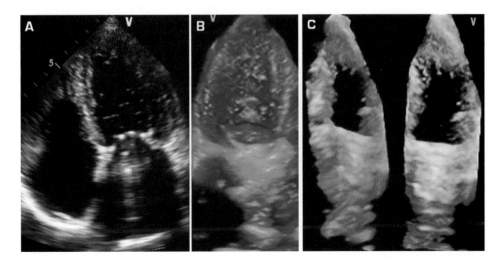

Figure 1. 11 Reverberation artefacts. A) Reverberation artefact: reverberations are multiple reflections produced by a strong reflector, giving a series of gradually weaker parallel images of the same structure behind the first. When they consist of a series of short lines near each other, they can take the form of a *comet tail*. In the example, in 2D, the prosthetic mitral valve creates reverberations which almost take the form of two comet tails. B) Reverberation artefact: reverberation artefact is generated in 3D imaging as well. They can be bigger and more obscuring of normal structures than in 2D. In the example, the 3D image belongs to the same patient, during the same study as (A). It is possible to observe a multiple parallel disc-like appearance of the reverberation with tornado shape. C) Reverberation artefact: this is another example of 3D reverberation artefact from mechanical mitral valve prosthesis, giving multiple parallel plate-like appearance when cropped and displayed to be seen from two angles.

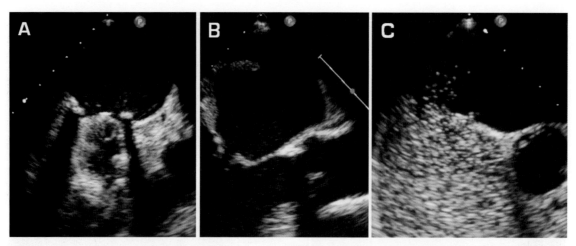

Figure 1.12 Reverberation and shadowing artefact. A) Reverberation and shadowing artefact: behind a highly reflective structure, the normal structures can be obscured not only by reverberations, but also by shadowing—absent image due to weak ultrasound transmission. In this example, in transoesophageal echocardiography (TOE), there are reverberations from a prosthetic mitral valve and also shadowing behind the valve ring. B) Shadowing artefact: The example shows shadowing artefact on TOE, produced by the ring of tissue aortic valve prosthesis. C) Shadowing artefact: the example shows an agitated saline study for interatrial septum assessment. There is a shadow in the right lower part of the image, produced by small calcium chunk in the interatrial septum and by the aortic valve which could be confused with bubbles wash-out by left-to-right flow through small interatrial communication.

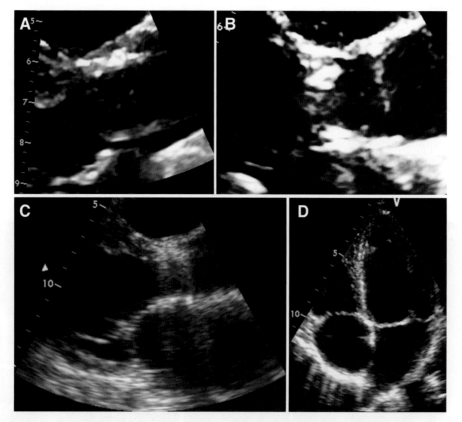

Figure 1.13 Reverberation and side lobe artefact. A) Side lobe artefact: the side lobe (grating lobe) artefact is an image created by a weak accessory beam. It can produce a misleading image of a highly reflective structure. In the example, the prosthetic aortic valve ring seems to be continued by an ascending aorta graft, which is not true. The image of the prosthetic ring is made look longer by the combination of true image and side lobe artefact. The image was 'optimized' to accentuate artefact for illustration purposes. B) Comet tail: the example shows a small comet tail produced by a calcified plaque in the aortic root, giving the appearance of a line in the aortic root perpendicular to the anterior wall of the aorta, which could be misdiagnosed as dissection. C) Reverberations and side lobe artefact: the example shows reverberations produced by prosthetic aortic valve and prolongation of the image of the anterior aspect of the valve ring by side lobe artefact. D) Enhancement and reverberations artefact: enhancement artefact is the accentuation of the brightness of a reflector behind a structure with low attenuation. It usually creates increased brightness of the distal aspect of structures which have a cavity. In the example, the distal aspect the right atrial wall appears brighter. There are also reverberations like multiple comet tails.

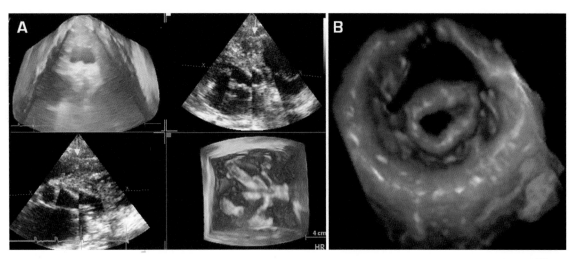

Figure 1.14 Stitching and drop-out artefact. A) Stitching artefact. if volume 3D is acquired from four cardiac cycles stitched together, stitching artefact may appear, if the cardiac cycles are unequal (atrial fibrillation or ectopic arrhythmia), or because of motion due to breathing or unstable operator hand. The example shows stitching artefact in 3D pyramidal volume. On the 2D images, the separate volumes delineation is very clear (artefact enhanced for illustration purposes). B) Drop-out artefact: the 3D images have to be acquired at higher gain than 2D images, to allow for a more extensive post-processing (which can reveal information hidden by exaggerate gain but cannot display an image if there are gaps of information). In the example, there is apparent tissue gap in the anterior wall, due to both low gain acquisition, and post-processing (cropping and reducing the gain to visualize the highly reflective stenosed mitral valve).

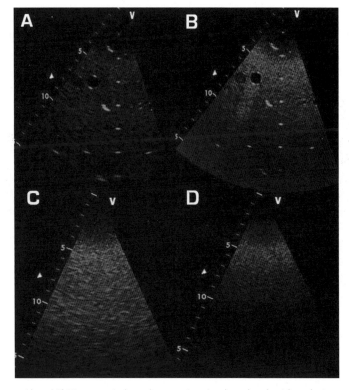

Figure 1.15 Performance measurement. A) and B) Tissue equivalent phantom imaging: lateral and axial resolution, contrast resolution, and penetration can be assessed. In the example, (A) represents fundamental imaging and (B) represents harmonic imaging. We can appreciate from the dimensions of the bright echoes the poor lateral resolution of fundamental imaging (long echo) compared with harmonic imaging (short echo). This can be appreciated also from the images of the cystic structures (hazy lateral walls in fundamental imaging). There is drop in axial resolution (the echoes are thick for their length in harmonic imaging). The improved contrast resolution with harmonic imaging can be appreciated from the image of the far lateral left cystic structure. C) and D) Penetration assessment: (C) is an image obtained with lower frequency–high penetration throughout the image field though low resolution suggested by the coarse appearance of speckles. (D) is an image obtained with higher frequency–low penetration, about two-thirds of the image field though high resolution suggested by the fine appearance of speckles.

Biological effects of ultrasound and safety

Ultrasound interacts with tissues, being a compression wave (MI-dependent mechanical effects) and having its energy absorbed (thermal index, TI, dependent heating effects).

The exposure is proportional with pressure amplitude, power, and intensity. We increase it by increasing power, MI, and with focusing. The intensity of spatial peak-temporal average (SPTA) describes exposure to intermittent, damped, and attenuated ultrasound pulses. SPTA is higher for Doppler imaging.

Biological effects are investigated with cell cultures, plant, and animal experiments. There is no evidence of risk; nevertheless rationalization is advised. Manufacturers have to comply with safety requirements for instruments output, by restricting and displaying the MI and TI (index value 1). Final responsibility remains with the operator.

Heating depends on tissue density and heat loss with blood flow. The soft tissue TI is the output power divided by the power producing more than a 1°C temperature rise. TI is higher for Doppler imaging.

Cavitation is tissue gas bubbles volume oscillation with pressure variation, similar to contrast microbubbles. It can induce disruption at very high MI. MI is higher for 2D/3D imaging.

Quality assurance and ultrasound instruments

A programme of instrument performance and safety testing every 6 months is recommended, for early identification of alterations (e.g. transducer elements breakdown) and maintenance planning.

Performance is tested on tissue-equivalent phantoms and test objects. Axial, lateral, and contrast resolution, penetration, and calibration are assessed (➲ Fig. 1.15).

Safety is tested with hydrophones, measuring acoustic output. Pressure amplitude, period, and pulse duration are determined. Frequency, pulse repetition frequency, power, and intensity are derived.

Personal perspective

Over more than half a century, echocardiography has had a spectacular evolution. With the intuitive nature of imaging and the ability to visualize function, echocardiography became a daily revelation promoting the evolution of cardiology. At present, real-time 3D echocardiography is the only real-time volumetric scanning method available for cardiac assessment; cardiac computed tomography and cardiac magnetic resonance are based on offline reconstruction. Tissue Doppler imaging-based techniques offer the highest cardiac imaging temporal resolution. Doppler imaging-based techniques offer non-invasive haemodynamic evaluations.

The challenge for maximal exploitation of echocardiography potential arises from the demand of clinical, image interpretation, and technical skills at the same time. A good understanding of current technology achievements and limitations is needed. The present chapter was written with the intention to facilitate this understanding, providing an illustrated and up-to-date account. The EAE Core Syllabus was strictly followed, for the benefit of the reader preparing for accreditation.[1]

Future advances will be parallel with computer technology advances and miniaturization. Techniques and applications will continue to emerge at the boundary between clinical practice and technical developments. A periodical update of the Core Syllabus and subsequently of this textbook will be necessary.

Reference

1 Education Committee of the European Association of Echocardiography 2009–1010. *EAE Core Syllabus A learning framework for the continuous medical education of the echocardiographers.* 2009. Available at: &8 http://www.escardio.org/communities/EAE/education/Documents/EAE-Core-Syllabus.pdf

Further reading

Armstrong WF, Ryan T. *Feigenbaum's Echocardiography*, 7th edn. Philadelphia, PA: Lippincott Williams and Wilkins; 2009.

Evangelista A, Flachskamp F, Lancellotti P, Badano L, Aguilar R, Monaghan M, *et al.*; on behalf of the European Association of Echocardiography. European Association of Echocardiography recommendations for standardization of performance, digital storage and reporting of echocardiographic studies. *Eur J Echocardiogr*, 2008; **9**(4):438–48.

Kremkau FW. *Diagnostic Ultrasound Principles and Instruments*, 7th edn. Philadelphia, PA: Saunders Elsevier; 2006.

Nihoyannopoulos P, Kisslo J (eds). *Echocardiography*. London: Springer; 2009.

Otto CM. *Textbook of Clinical Echocardiography*, 4th edn. Philadelphia, PA: Saunders Elsevier; 2009.

Sutherland GR, Hatle L, Claus P, D'hooge J, Bijnens BH (eds). *Doppler Myocardial Imaging*. Hasselt: BSWK; 2006.

Turner SP, Monaghan MJ, Tissue harmonic imaging for standard left ventricular measurements: Fundamentally flawed? *Eur J Echocardiogr* 2006; 7: 9–15.

➲   For additional multimedia materials please visit the online version of the book (http://escecho.oxfordmedicine.com).

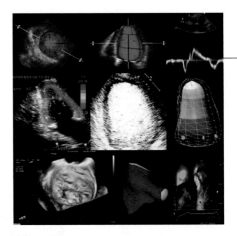

CHAPTER 2

Transthoracic echocardiography

Miguel Ángel García Fernández and
José Juan Gómez de Diego

Contents

Summary

The echocardiogram is an extremely useful and versatile technique that enables collection of all relevant information on morphology and function of the heart in a wide range of clinical situations.

Echocardiography has been pivotal in the development of modern cardiology and is an indispensable tool to effectively manage cardiological patients.

The echocardiogram is a highly operator-dependent technique in which the skills of the operator in achieving optimized images and adapting the study to the possible findings is simply fundamental.[1] In this chapter we will review the technical aspects involved in achieving the images required for a standard echocardiographic examination.

Principles of imaging

Selection of the transducer

Ultrasound systems are equipped with an array of transducers with different characteristics. Probes used in echocardiography are phased-array transducers capable of performing M-mode, two-dimensional (2D), and Doppler imaging.

From a practical point of view, the most important characteristics of the transducers are footprint and frequency. Footprint is the area of the transducer that is going to be in contact with the skin of the patient. It should be small enough to fit in the space between the ribs.

The frequency of the transducer should be carefully selected in order to have a good balance between resolution and penetration of ultrasound. As a rule, a higher frequency of ultrasound provides better resolution and more detailed images, but at the cost of having greater attenuation with substantially less penetration in depth. In large patients, a probe with a lower frequency (2–2.5MHz transducer) should be used in order to have an adequate penetration, allowing a scan of up to 20 cm in depth. In other patients, depending on their size and chest characteristics, higher frequencies (3–5MHz transducers) can be used with good resolution and penetration. In children or newborns, penetration is not an issue and high frequency (7–7.5MHz) probes are used to get high-resolution images. Second harmonic is a useful tool to improve 2D imaging quality. It allows low frequency (e.g. 1.8MHz) ultrasound transmission which provides a better ultrasound penetration, a higher frequency signal (in our example 3.6MHz) reception, and an improved image quality.

Lower frequency transducers are more suitable for Doppler technique because high-velocity flows require lower frequencies.

Patient position

To perform an echocardiographic examination the sonographer can be seated on the left or on the right side of the patient, depending on standards of practice or personal preference. However, it is useful to develop skills to work from both sides of the patient, in order to be prepared in cases where patient situation or the room does not permit a choice.

Echocardiographic examination is usually performed with the patient in left lateral decubitus position, with the left hand under the head (Fig. 2.1). By tilting the patient to the left, the heart comes nearer to the chest wall and by raising the left arm the space between the ribs widens. Both measures allow easier positioning of the transducer and improve the ultrasound beam access. Left lateral decubitus position is used to obtain images in the parasternal and apical windows. The left tilt degree required of the patient is very variable; in some cases images are

obtained with a steep tilting of the patient towards the left whereas in other cases supine position could be the best option.

To get specific views, additional positioning of the patient will be required.[2,3] Subcostal images are obtained by placing the patient in supine position. Asking the patient to flex their knees in order to relax abdominal muscles will give more room to maneuver the transducer. For suprasternal views the transducer should be placed in the suprasternal notch, with the patient in supine position. Placing a pillow under the patient's shoulders may be necessary to hyperextend the neck and thus to provide more room for the transducer. In some special cases, right lateral decubitus position shall be required as well.

Transducer position: the echocardiographic windows

Ultrasound cannot pass through air or bone. This is the reason why there are in fact only a few points that can be used to scan the heart with an ultrasound beam. These points are called *windows* (Fig. 2.2). A specific orientation of the transducer in a specific access point gives a specific imaging pattern called echocardiographic *view*.

The standard transducer locations useful to scan the heart are the parasternal, the apical, the suprasternal, and the subcostal windows. 2D, M-mode, and Doppler imaging from different windows should be obtained to get data of cardiac structures

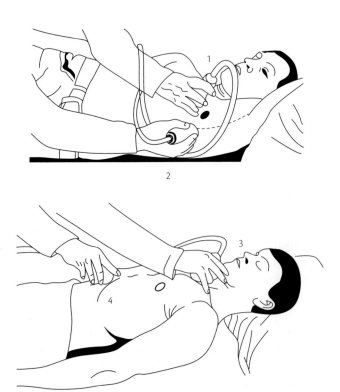

Figure 2.1 Transthoracic transducer standard positions to obtain different echo views. Parasternal (position 1) and apical planes (position 2) are obtained with the patient in left lateral decubitus position. Suprasternal (position 3) and subcostal views are usually obtained with the patient in supine position (position 4). Reproduced from Zamorano JL, Bax JJ, Rademakers FE, and Knuuti J (eds) (2010) The ESC Textbook of Cardiovascular Imaging, with kind permission from Springer Science + Business Media.

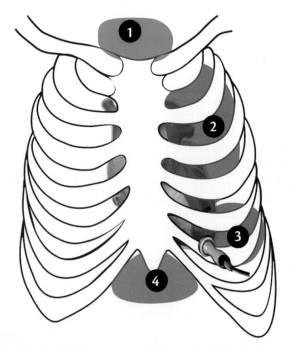

Figure 2.2 Anatomical structures and echocardiographic windows. Anatomical structures and echocardiographic windows to obtain parasternal views (position 2), apical views (position 3), suprasternal views (position 1), and subcostal views (position 4). Reproduced from Zamorano JL, Bax JJ, Rademakers FE, and Knuuti J (eds) (2010) The ESC Textbook of Cardiovascular Imaging, with kind permission from Springer Science + Business Media.

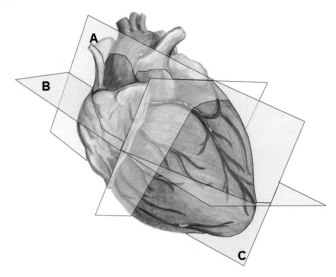

Figure 2.3 Image planes used in transthoracic echocardiography. A = long axis; B = short axis; C = four-chamber. Reproduced from Zamorano JL, Bax JJ, Rademakers FE, and Knuuti J (eds) (2010) The ESC Textbook of Cardiovascular Imaging, with kind permission from Springer Science + Business Media.

from different points of view (⊃ Fig. 2.3). This information will be integrated by the operator in a coherent model of the patient's heart anatomy and function. Usually parasternal and apical windows are the most useful windows in adults because they provide most of the required images. A subcostal approach is useful in paediatric patients but it can also be the best option where scanning patients with a low diaphragm or bad acoustic window due to respiratory diseases.[4,5] Finally, the suprasternal approach is usually used as a complementary view to study the base of the heart and great vessels.[6] The right parasternal window can be used also in specific cases to study aortic valve flow.[7,8]

It is important to bear in mind that standard transducer positions are merely informative. The best probe position is variable in each patient and some exploration with the transducer is often required to find the best location to obtain optimal images. There are even clinical situations like dextrocardia or pneumothorax where any standard approach proves ineffective. In those cases, there can be non-standard or unexpected acoustic windows that can be used to scan the heart.

2D echocardiography

2D echocardiography is based on ultrasound scanning of a series of lines steered to cover a 90-degree arc. It provides real-time and high resolution tomographic views of the heart, which are useful in obtaining anatomical and functional information.

2D echocardiography is the basis of the echocardiographic examination. Firstly, it is usually the initial imaging mode chosen for each study view as it allows an overall evaluation of structures of interest in the plane. Secondly, 2D echocardiography is

also very useful as it provides a reference map to guide other imaging modes like M-mode or Doppler.

Most echo laboratories follow the American Society of Echocardiography (ASE) recommendations[9] for image orientation, with the transducer position at the top of the image. That means that 'superficial' or 'anterior' structures will be visualized in the 'upper' part of the image, whereas 'deeper' or 'posterior' structures will be displayed in the 'lower' part of the image. Lateral structures are displayed on the right side of the screen and medial structures on the left side. Short-axis views should be considered as if the sonographer were looking from the apex towards the heart base and long views as if he/she were looking at the heart from the left side. The ASE recommendations are followed in all the figures on this chapter.

Parasternal long-axis view

The parasternal long-axis (PLAX) view (⊃ Fig. 2.4; ▣ 2.1) is obtained with the patient in left lateral decubitus position and the transducer placed in the left third or fourth intercostal space near the sternum.[2,10] This view is particularly interesting since many structures are oriented perpendicularly to the ultrasound beam. This orientation provides better spatial resolution and imaging detail; therefore this view is the best plane to measure the dimensions of the left ventricle.

The *right ventricle* (RV) is the closest structure to the transducer and it is shown as the upper structure in the image. It has an irregular shape due to the complex morphology of the RV. The *left ventricle* (LV) is found below the RV in the left area of the image. This plane allows visualization of the anterior septum (up) and the inferolateral wall (classically called posterior wall, PP, down). It is important to notice that in PLAX view the true LV apex is usually not seen; the apparent apex is, in fact, the result of an oblique angulation through the anterolateral wall. The *aortic root* is the structure below the RV on the right side of the image. It is usually easy to see the sinuses of Valsalva, the sinotubular junction, and the most proximal part of the ascending aorta. In most cases, moving the transducer to an upper intercostal space results in a focused image of a longer part of the ascending aorta.

The *LV outflow tract* (LVOT) and the *aortic valve* (AoV) are the communication between the LV and the aorta. The AoV in systole is usually visualized as two thin linear images parallel to the walls of the ascending thoracic aorta. In this view, the upper aortic cusp corresponds to the *right coronary cusp* and the lower one to the *non-coronary cusp*. A linear echodense image can be visualized in the middle of the aortic root in diastole when both cusps join together in the AoV closure. It is easy to distinguish the *mitral valve* (MV) just below the AoV. *Anterior and posterior leaflets of the MV* are linear, thin, and dense structures with a wide movement over cardiac cycle. The anterior leaflet is in close continuity with the non-coronary AoV cusp. Both leaflets are attached by many *tendinous chords* to *papillary muscles*. The *left atrium* (LA) is seen in the lower right region of the image.

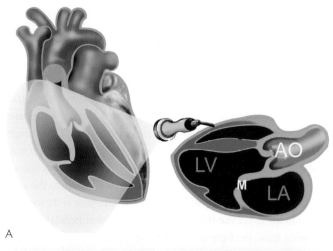

A

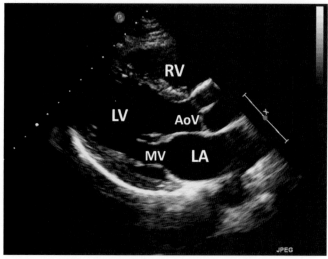

B

Figure 2.4 Parasternal long-axis view. A) Schematic anatomical section. B) 2D echocardiographic anatomy of the view. AoV, aortic valve; LA, left atrium; LV, left ventricle; MV, mitral valve; RV, right ventricle. 2.4 A) Reproduced from Zamorano JL, Bax JJ, Rademakers FE, and Knuuti J (eds) (2010) The ESC Textbook of Cardiovascular Imaging, with kind permission from Springer Science + Business Media.

The *coronary sinus* can be visualized as an echo-free structure at atrioventricular groove level that follows the motion of the atrioventricular ring. The *pericardium* sometimes can be identified at the lower edge of the LA and LV. In some cases it is possible to visualize the *descending thoracic aorta* in section as a rounded structure immediately posterior to the LA and external to the pericardium.

Parasternal right ventricle views

Parasternal RV inflow view

The parasternal *RV inflow view* (also called long-axis view of the RV) (➲ Fig. 2.5; ▣ 2.2) is obtained from PLAX view by tilting the transducer inferomedially. One particular advantage of this plane is that tricuspid regurgitation jets are usually well aligned for accurate Doppler evaluation, which is useful for

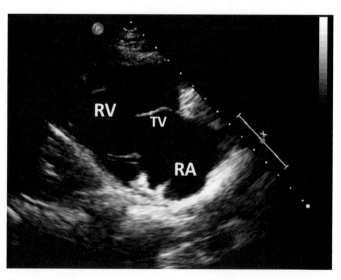

Figure 2.5 Right ventricular inflow view. 2D echocardiographic anatomy of the ventricle inflow view. RA right atrium; RV right ventricle; TV tricuspid valve.

pulmonary pressure calculations (see ➲ Chapter 5, 'Study of the intracardiac pressures'). This plane gives a detailed image of *right atrium* (RA) in the lower part of the image, the *inflow tract of RV* in the upper part of it, and the *septal and anterior leaflets of the tricuspid valve* (TV) in between. The RV is usually heavily trabeculated and sometimes it is possible to identify the *moderator band*. The *coronary sinus* is seen joining the RA wall near the tricuspid annulus. The orifice of the *inferior vena cava* (IVC) and the *Eustachian valve* can be also visualized joining the RA wall below the coronary sinus.

Parasternal RV outflow view

The parasternal *RV outflow view* (➲ Fig. 2.6; ▣ 2.3) is another variation of PLAX view that is obtained by angulating the transducer laterally. This view, which can be very difficult to obtain in adults, gives a detailed view of the *RV outflow tract* (RVOT),

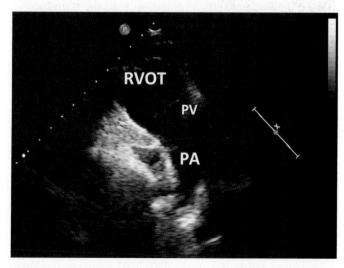

Figure 2.6 Right ventricular outflow view. 2D echocardiographic anatomy of the right ventricle outflow view. PA, pulmonary artery; PV, pulmonic valve; RVOT, right ventricle outflow tract.

the *pulmonary valve* (PV), and the proximal main *pulmonary artery* (PA).

Parasternal short-axis views

The parasternal short-axis (PSAX) view is obtained with a 90-degree clockwise rotation of the transducer from the PLAX view. Different views are made possible from the base to the apex of the heart by tilting and slightly repositioning the transducer.

PSAX view at the level of aortic valve

The PSAX view *at the level of the AoV* (➲ Fig. 2.7; 🔳 2.4) is the most basal plane. The *AoV*, located anterior to the LA and

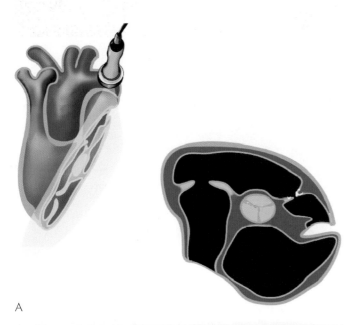

A

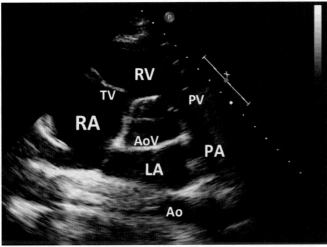

B

Figure 2.7 Parasternal short-axis view at aortic valve level. A) Schematic anatomical section. B) 2D echocardiographic anatomy of the view. Ao, descending aorta; AoV, aortic valve; LA, left atrium; PA, pulmonic artery; PV, pulmonic valve; RA, right atrium; RV, right ventricle; TV, tricuspid valve. 2.7 A) Reproduced from Zamorano JL, Bax JJ, Rademakers FE, and Knuuti J (eds) (2010) The ESC Textbook of Cardiovascular Imaging, with kind permission from Springer Science + Business Media.

posterior to the RV, is clearly seen in the central region of the image with its three leaflets in a characteristic Y-shaped configuration. The central location of the AoV in this view is very useful to understand how quickly diseases of the aortic annulus can spread over the rest of the cardiac structures. The rule to identify the cusps is to remember that *non-coronary cusp* is in continuity with interatrial septum and that the *right coronary cusp* is the nearest to the RV; the *left coronary cusp* is the third one. It is possible to see in aged people a small nodular thickening in the middle part of the free edge of the cusps called '*nodules of Arantius*'. Sometimes it is possible to visualize in this view the origins of the *coronary arteries*, with the left main coronary artery at 4 o'clock position in the aortic annulus and the right coronary artery at 11 o'clock position. The *RVOT* is wrapped anterior to the AoV; the *PV* can be visualized rightward and anterior to the AoV. The main *PA* curves around the aorta on the right of the image and it is easy to follow it to its two principal branches (*right and left pulmonary arteries*). The *TV* is visualized to the left of the AoV; in this view septal and anterior leaflets are visible. The *LA* is seen posterior to the AoV and separated from the *RA* by the *atrial septum*. The *left appendage* can be visualized in some cases attached to the lateral wall of the LA. This imaging plane is very useful to study AoV congenital anomalies and diseases of the aortic root. Although interatrial septal defects can also be assessed in this view, they are more easily detected in apical four-chamber and subcostal imaging.

PSAX view at the level of mitral valve

The PSAX view at *MV level* (➲ Fig. 2.8; 🔳 2.5) is obtained with an inferior and rightward tilting of the transducer. This view is defined by the imaging of the *MV leaflets* as two parallel thin structures, with the *anterior leaflet* in upper position and the *posterior leaflet* in the lower portion of the image. The LV is visualized in circular cross-section. The RV (anterior, lateral, and posterior segments) can be identified in the left anterior portion of the image and separated from the LV by the *interventricular septum* (IVS).

PSAX view at the level of papillary muscles

The PSAX view *at papillary muscle level* (➲ Fig. 2.9; 🔳 2.6) is obtained by tilting the transducer more apically. The MV is not more visible and it is possible to visualize a mid-ventricular circular cross-section of the LV and the *anterolateral* and *posteromedial papillary muscles* inside the ventricular cavity at 3 and 8 o'clock positions, respectively.

PSAX view at the apical level

By tilting the transducer, in some cases it is possible to have a *PSAX apical view* (➲ Fig. 2.10; 🔳 2.7) which provides a more apical cross-section visualization of the LV. See in the figures the different segments of the LV that can be observed in the PSAX view at mitral, papillary muscle, and apical levels.

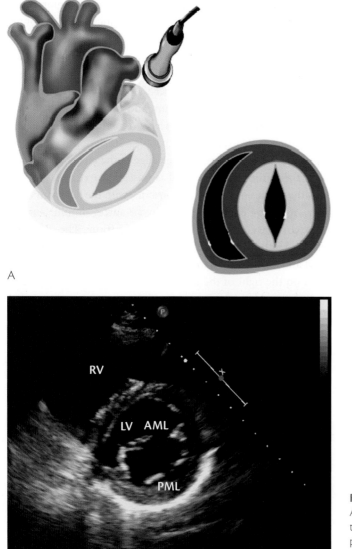

Figure 2.8 Parasternal short-axis view at mitral valve level. A) Schematic anatomical section. B) 2D echocardiographic anatomy of the view. AML, anterior mitral leaflet; LV, left ventricle; PML, posterior mitral leaflet; RV, right ventricle.

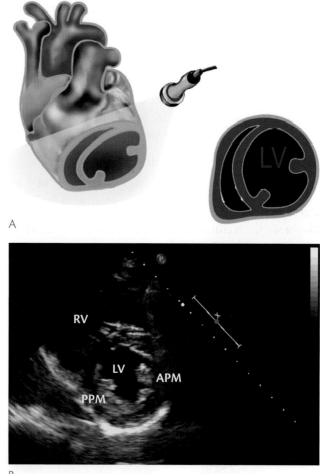

Figure 2.9 Parasternal short-axis view at papillary muscles level. A) Schematic anatomical section. B) 2D echocardiographic anatomy of the view. APM anterior papillary muscle; LV left ventricle; PPM posterior papillary muscle; RV right ventricle. 2.9 A) Reproduced from Zamorano JL, Bax JJ, Rademakers FE, and Knuuti J (eds) (2010) The ESC Textbook of Cardiovascular Imaging, with kind permission from Springer Science + Business Media.

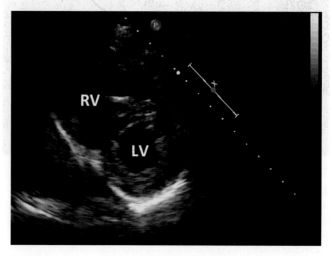

Figure 2.10 Parasternal short-axis view at apical level. 2D echocardiographic anatomy of the view. LV left ventricle; RV right ventricle.

Apical views

Apical imaging planes are obtained with the patient in left lateral decubitus position, with the transducer placed in the fifth intercostal space in the median axillary line.

The most challenging (and important!) point in apical imaging is to obtain images of the true LV apex, that can be easily foreshortened. The true apex usually has a thin wall and a slightly tapered shape. If the apex displayed in the image has a rounded shape and the same thickness than left ventricle walls there is a good probability it is, in fact, a false image due to an oblique orientation of ultrasound beam. The transducer should thus be replaced; moving it to a lower intercostal space or to a more lateral position can be a good solution. As a general rule, to be sure the true apex has been visualized, the transducer has to be placed in the lowest intercostal place and in the most lateral position in which a good image of the heart is obtained.

Apical four-chamber view

The initial view from the apical window is the *apical four-chamber view* (A4C) (◆ Fig. 2.11; ▣ 2.8). This image includes the main four chambers of the heart, ventricles, the atria, the interventricular and interatrial septa, MV and TV, and the crux of the heart. Ventricles are in the upper zone and the atria in the lower zone of the image, the left cavities are displayed in the right part of the image, and the right cavities on the left.

Where studying the crux of the heart, it is necessary to check that the TV is located slightly *more apically* than the MV. This precaution is crucial to diagnose some important congenital malformations like Ebstein disease and is of paramount

importance in identifying ventricular chambers in complex congenital malformation cases. When properly done, A4C view gives a long-axis view of the *LV* in a plane perpendicular to both PSAX and PLAX views. The anterolateral wall, the apex, and the inferior septum are displayed in the plane. The *RV* is on the left of the image, with a characteristic triangular shape and a size a third smaller than the left ventricle. The *TV* is also on the left side of the image. This view shows the septal leaflet medially and the anterior leaflet laterally. On the other side, the anterior mitral leaflet is attached to the septum and the posterior leaflet joins the lateral atrioventricular ring. Both atria and the entire atrial septum can be seen with a slight anterior repositioning of the transducer. Pulmonary veins can be visualized entering to the posterior and deep wall of the LA. In some patients it is also possible to see a transversal cross-section of the descending thoracic aorta lateral to the LA.

Apical five-chamber view

When the transducer is moved with a slight anterior angulation from A4C position, the AoV and the aortic root appear in the place previously occupied by the crux of the heart. This view is called apical *five-chambers view* (A5C) (◆ Fig. 2.12; ▣ 2.9). This is the best plane to study the LVOT and AoV flows. It allows also to visualize more anterior portions of the LV septum and inferolateral wall. An opposite angulation of the transducer with a posterior angulation provides a view without specific name in which more posterior portions of the LV and the coronary sinus can be seen.

Apical two-chamber view

From the A4C view position, a 60°–90° counterclockwise rotation of the transducer should be done to obtain the apical *two-chamber view* (A2C) (◆ Fig. 2.13, ▣ 2.10). A2C shows the anterior (on the right of the image) and inferior (on the left)

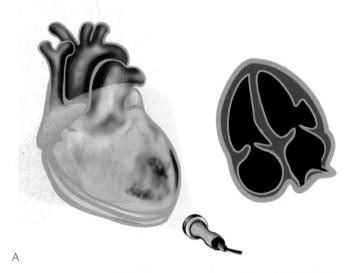

A

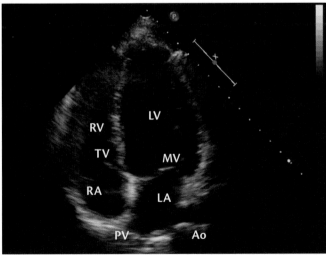

B

Figure 2.11 Apical four-chamber view. A) Schematic anatomical section. B) 2D echocardiographic anatomy of the view. Ao, descending aorta; LA, left atrium; LV, left ventricle; MV, mitral valve; PV, pulmonary vein; RA, right atrium; RV, right ventricle; TV, tricuspid valve. 2.11 A) Reproduced from Zamorano JL, Bax JJ, Rademakers FE, and Knuuti J (eds) (2010) The ESC Textbook of Cardiovascular Imaging, with kind permission from Springer Science + Business Media.

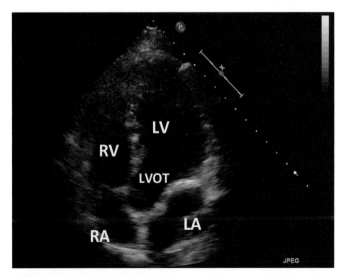

Figure 2.12 Apical five-chamber view. 2D cho anatomy of apical five chambers view (*see also* ▣ 2.12). LV, left ventricle; LVOT, left ventricle outflow tract; MV, mitral valve; RA, right atrium; RV, right ventricle.

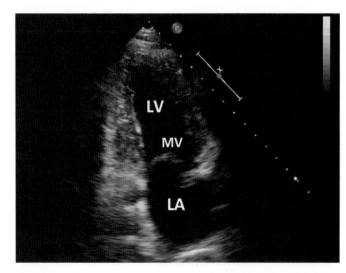

Figure 2.13 Apical two-chamber view. 2D echocardiographic anatomy of apical two-chamber view. LA, left atrium; LV, left ventricle; MV, mitral valve.

walls of the LV and (again) the apex. A2C is also useful to study the LA and the MV. Both A2C and A4C are almost orthogonal views of the LV that are widely used to assess global (using Simpson's method) and regional LV function.

Apical long-axis or three-chamber view

Finally, an image similar to PLAX view is obtained by rotating the probe another 60°. This view is called *apical long-axis view* or, more commonly, *apical three-chamber view* (A3C) (➲ Fig. 2.14; ▣ 2.11). The main difference is that in A3C the anterior portion of septal apex is seen, whereas there is no apical segment of the inferolateral wall. However, MV and AoV in A3C view are visualized at a greater image depth and with poorer resolution.

Subcostal views

Subcostal images are obtained with the patient in supine position. In some cases it is easier to accommodate the transducer when the patient flexes their knees because it helps to relax the abdominal muscles.

Subcostal four-chamber view

The *subcostal four-chamber view* (➲ Fig. 2.15; ▣ 2.12) is obtained by placing the transducer in the centre of the epigastrium and by tilting downwards pointing to the patient's left shoulder. The image is similar to A4C but with a different orientation in which interatrial and interventricular septa lie more perpendicular to the ultrasound beam. This orientation makes this view especially useful to study defects at the level of the atrial septum. The *liver* is found in the upper region of the image, while below there are the *RV* with its free wall and the apex oriented to the right, the *TV*, and the *RA*. The *LV* is visualized in the lower and right zone of the image and, in this view, as in A4C, septal inferior and lateral walls are visible. However, in subcostal view it is more difficult to visualize the true apex. A slight tilting of the transducer results in a five-chamber view that allows visualization of the *LVOT* and the *AoV*.

Subcostal short-axis view

A 90° counterclockwise rotation of the transducer from the subcostal four-chamber view gives a series of *short-axis views* very similar to those obtained in PSAX view (➲Figs. 2.16 and 2.17; ▣ 2.13). Subcostal SAX view allows evaluation and measurements of the LV that are comparable to those of parasternal and could be more suitable for the study of the RV. Subcostal views are a good alternative to image patients when poor quality images are obtained in parasternal window.

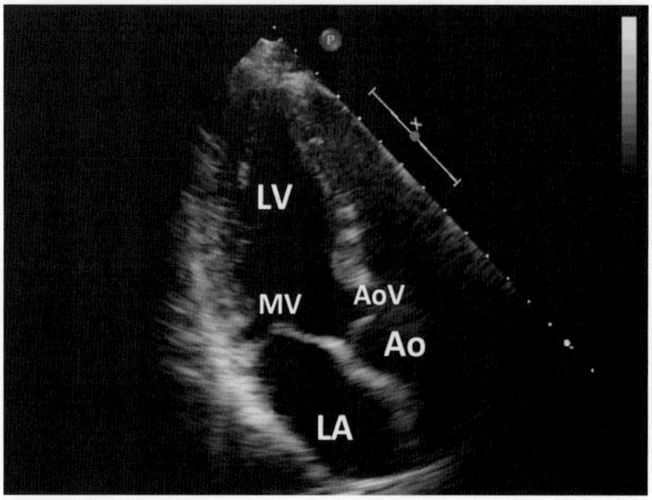

Figure 2.14 Apical long-axis or three-chamber view. 2D echocardiographic anatomy of apical three-chamber view. Ao, aortic root; AoV, aortic valve; LA, left atrium; LV, left ventricle; MV, mitral valve.

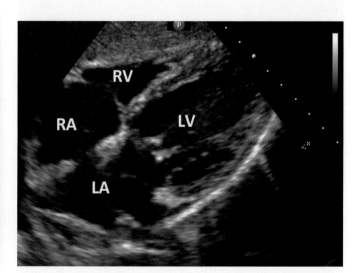

Figure 2.15 Subcostal four-chamber view. 2D echocardiographic anatomy of subcostal four-chamber view. RA, right atrium; RV, right ventricle; LA left atrium; LV, left ventricle.

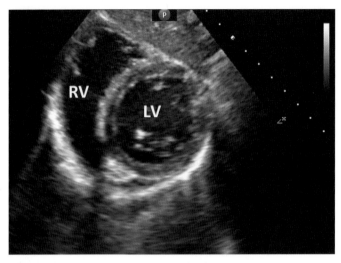

Figure 2.16 Subcostal short-axis view. 2D echocardiographic anatomy of subcostal short axis view at mitral valve level. LV, left ventricle; RV, right ventricle.

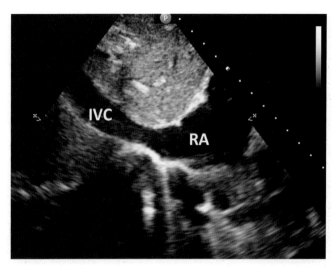

Figure 2.18 Subcostal inferior vena cava view. 2D echocardiographic anatomy of subcostal inferior vena cava view. IVC, inferior vena cava; RA, right atrium.

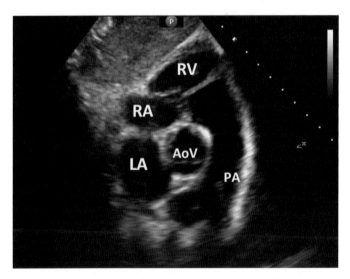

Figure 2.17 Subcostal short-axis view at aortic valve level. 2D echocardiographic anatomy of subcostal short axis view at aortic valve level. AoV, aortic valve; LA, left atrium; PA, pulmonary artery; RA, right atrium; RV, right ventricle.

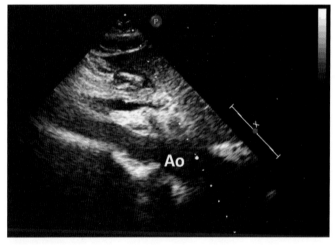

Figure 2.19 Subcostal abdominal aorta view. 2D echocardiographic anatomy of subcostal abdominal aorta view. Ao, aorta.

Suprasternal views

Suprasternal images are obtained with the transducer placed in the patient's suprasternal notch. They are mainly used to study the aorta.

Subcostal inferior vena cava view

The rotation of the transducer from subcostal four-chamber view gives a long-axis view of the IVC joining the RA (➲ Fig. 2.18; ▤ 2.14). This view is useful to measure the *IVC* and to study its changes of size with respiration, and thus for the RA pressure estimation (see ➲ Chapter 11, 'Assessment of right ventricular haemodynamics'). The *liver* and *suprahepatic* can be also visualized. In some patients, a very prominent Eustachian valve can be seen in the junction of the IVC and the RA. Further rotation of the transducer to a fully vertical position gives a long-axis view of the abdominal aorta (➲ Fig. 2.19; ▤ 2.15).

Suprasternal long-axis view

The *suprasternal long-axis view* (➲ Fig. 2.20; ▤ 2.16) is obtained with the long axis of the transducer oriented parallel to the trachea. The *ascending aorta* and the *aortic arch* with the origins of the *right brachiocephalic*, the *left common carotid*, and *subclavian* arteries can be seen in the left region of the image and the *descending thoracic aorta* is visualized in the right region. The *right pulmonary artery* and the *LA* can be seen beneath the aortic arch.

Suprasternal short-axis view

A 90-degree counterclockwise rotation of the transducer from a suprasternal long-axis view gives a *short-axis view* (➲ Fig. 2.21).

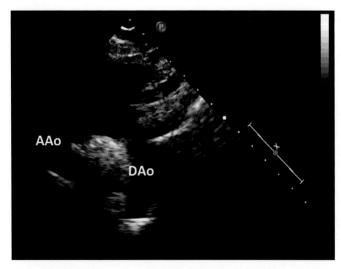

Figure 2.20 Suprasternal long-axis view. 2D echocardiofraphic anatomy of suprasternal long axis view. AAo, ascending aorta; DAo, descending aorta.

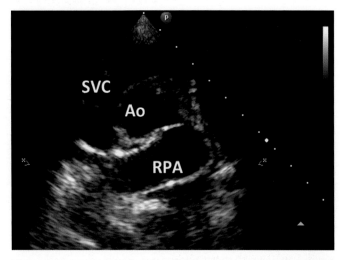

Figure 2.21 Suprasternal short-axis view. 2D echocardiographic anatomy of suprasternal short axis view. Ao, aorta; RPA, right pulmonary artery; SVC, superior vena cava.

The transverse cross-section of the *aortic arch* is in the upper region of the image, with a long axis of the right PA located below. A section of the LA and the outflow orifice of the right pulmonary veins can be observed in the lower zone of the image. Further clockwise rotation of the transducer allows visualization of the superior vena cava on the right side of the aorta.

Other imaging planes

It can be necessary to use less standardized echocardiographic windows than those formerly described to assess specific structures. A right parasternal window may be useful in some patients to assess the proximal aorta and the AoV flow. Right mirror windows and a right lateral decubitus position may be useful in cases of dextrocardia.

Regional left ventricle evaluation

Every different echocardiographic plane shows an image of a different region of the left ventricle. When combined constructively all these views allow a comprehensive evaluation of every left ventricular segment. This approach is very relevant on a clinical basis because the finding of regional contraction anomalies is the hallmark of coronary heart disease (for assessment of regional LV function see ➲ Chapter 8).

M-mode echocardiography

M-mode echocardiography was introduced into clinical practice at the beginning of the 1960s. It has been the mainstay for echocardiographic examinations for more than 20 years, but nowadays it has been largely replaced by echo 2D.

M-mode is still an important part of the echocardiographic study. In M-mode all computational resources of the system are focused on the scanning of a simple echo line. This allows the highest sample rating of more than 2000 times per second, very far away from the 40–80 frames per second in echo 2D. This high sample rate is linked to a very high spatial and temporal resolution. This is the reason why M-mode is very useful to track the movement of thin or fast-moving structures like the valves or the endocardium and to measure structures and cavities.

The major limitation of M-mode is that accurate studies are achieved only when the ultrasound beam is perpendicular to the structure of interest. Non-perpendicular orientation of the beam is linked to a slight deformation of the structure in the M-mode tracing and a bias in measurements. The problem of the orientation of the M-mode is now easily solved by using the 2D imaging as a guide to find a correct position for the M-mode sampling line. Some modern echo systems can even compute an out-of-beam orientation for the M-mode sampling line. This approach is called *anatomical M-mode* and allows the sonographer to put the M-mode sampling line in the best perpendicular orientation guided by the anatomy in echo 2D. However, this technique is largely based on data interpolation and gives less detailed M-mode tracings.

Aortic root, aortic valve, and left atrium

With the guide of the 2D PLAX view it is easy to put the M-mode sampling line over the aortic root at AoV leaflets level.

This M-mode tracing (➲ Fig. 2.22) typically shows the aortic root walls as two echodense parallel lines that move together in systole and back in diastole. The LA is posterior to aortic root. Its size shows phasic changes with cardiac cycle, increasing in atrial diastole (ventricular systole, from QRS to T wave in electrocardiogram, ECG) due to auricular filling and decreasing again in atrial systole (ventricular diastole) with LA emptying. Movement of the aortic root is due to these changes of size of

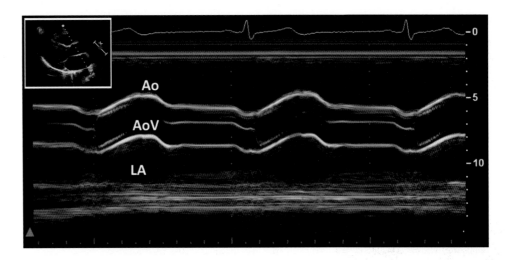

Figure 2.22 M-mode tracing of the aortic valve plane. It is possible to see aortic leaflets as a box in systole an as a thin line in diastole. Ao, aorta; AoV, aortic valve; LA, left atrium. The small inbox shows how the 2D image was used to guide the position of the M-mode sampling line.

the LA and is related to the volume of blood passing through the atrium. Increased aortic root movement is seen in hyperdynamic states and in mitral regurgitation whereas it is decreased in low output states.

AoV movement can be nicely studied. The AoV leaflets are seen together in diastole as a thin line half way between both aortic root walls. In systole, this thin line suddenly splits into two parallel lines that move near the aortic root walls in a typical box-like appearance. It is easy to measure in this M-mode tracing the pre-ejection (the time between the beginning of the QRS in the ECG and the AoV opening) and ejection (time in which the AoV is open) times.

Mitral valve

The 2D PLAX view is useful again to guide the M-mode sampling line over the MV. The echo beam in this orientation passes through the anterior RV wall, the RV chamber, the IVS, the anterior and posterior MV leaflets, the posterior LV wall, and the pericardium (➲ Fig. 2.23).

The leaflets of the MV are seen as echodense lines between the LV walls. The closed MV is seen in systole with both leaflets joined together in a thin line in the middle of the cavity. In early diastole, the MV opening and the fast early filling phase are linked to a wide and quick separation of the MV leaflets. The maximum anterior movement of the anterior leaflet is called the *E point*. In the diastasis phase of diastole both leaflets are parallel near the middle of the cavity. The atrial contraction causes a new flow movement that leads to a late diastolic peak in the leaflets' movement tracing called *A point*. After atrial contraction, both leaflets join together in the middle of the cavity in the *C point*. The point in which the leaflets start their separation is also called the *D point*.

In the normal ventricle, the trace from A point to mitral closure in C point is linear. In the case of an elevated LV end-diastolic pressure (LVEDP), an A–C shoulder or *B bump* can be seen.

Left and right ventricles

LV sizes are measured in PLAX view at papillary muscles level, by two ways; both need to use 2D imaging. The first uses M-mode by deriving the optimal position from 2D imaging; the second is represented by measurement of LV diameters

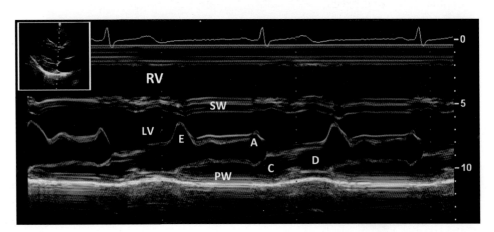

Figure 2.23 M-mode tracing of the mitral valve plane. The leaflets of mitral valve are two thin lines that widely separate in the beginning of the diastole in the point E. The leaflets move together near the middle line and then separate again after atrial systole in the point A. The small inbox shows how the 2D image was used to guide the position of the M-mode sampling line. LV, left ventricle; PW, posterior wall of the left ventricle; RV, right ventricle; SW, septal wall of the left ventricle septum.

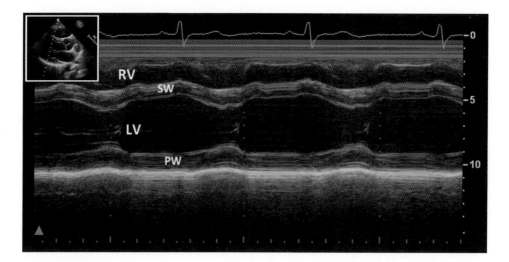

Figure 2.24 M-mode tracing of the left ventricle plane. The small inbox shows how the 2D image was used to guide the position of the M-mode sampling line. LV, left ventricle; PW, posterior wall of the left ventricle; RV, right ventricle; SW, septal wall of the left ventricle septum.

directly on the 2D plane. The M-mode tracing perpendicular to the LV long axis at papillary muscles is the reference imaging to measure the LV (➔ Fig. 2.24). However, more often than not, optimal long-axis view is not possible and LV is usually lining obliquely or present with an angulated septum: this makes M-mode measurements impossible and erroneous and, therefore, should be avoided. The accuracy of measurements in M-mode imaging is critically linked to the ability of achieving a perpendicular orientation of the echo beam relative to LV walls.

Measurements of the LV cavity dimension in diastole and systole and the thickness of the septum and the posterior wall are easily done in M-mode recordings and LV volumes and mass can be readily derived. Care should be taken to avoid confusion between LV walls and MV structures.

The classical M-mode orientation for LV measurements also allows measurement of the diastolic diameter of the RV. However, this approach yields a high measurement variability and is not widely used. M-mode recordings of the RV free wall are useful to study the pattern of motion when cardiac tamponade

is suspected. In A4C view, M-mode is also used to measure the tricuspid annular plane systolic excursion (TAPSE) that is useful in the evaluation of RV global function (➔ Fig. 2.25) (for details, see ➔ Chapter 11).

Pulmonary and tricuspid valves

The PV is usually easy to study with M-mode with the guide of the 2D PSAX view. The spatial orientation of the PV makes it impossible to study more than one leaflet movement at the same time in adults.

The basic normal pulmonary M-mode tracing (➔ Fig. 2.26) shows a posterior movement of the leaflet in systole and an anterior movement in diastole. A slight posterior movement of the leaflet related to atrial contraction called *a wave* is just after the ECG P wave (or just before QRS). The *point b* is the leaflet position at the beginning of systole and the *point c* the maximal posterior position in systole. The *point d* is the mark at the end of systole and the closure point of the valve is the *point e*. During diastole and just before the atrial contraction the leaflet moves

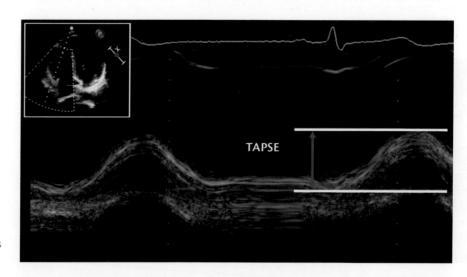

Figure 2.25 M-mode tracing of the tricuspid annular plane systolic excursion (TAPSE). The small inbox shows how the 2D image was used to guide the position of the M-mode over the tricuspid annulus in 2D echo image.

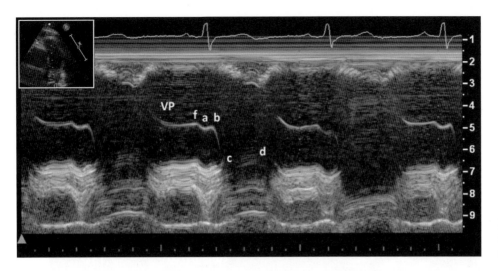

Figure 2.26 M-mode tracing of the pulmonic valve. See text for details.

slightly towards a more anterior position and the maximum excursion point is the *point f.*

The a wave is increased in pulmonary stenosis and decreased in pulmonary hypertension cases. A transient mid-systolic closure or notching of the PV is another marker of pulmonary hypertension.

The TV can be also studied with M-mode imaging. The tracings are similar to those obtained in the MV study but have little clinical utility.

Principles of echo measurements

Quantification of cardiac chamber size is one of the most important tasks of echocardiography. In fact, most of the diagnoses that are going to be included in the final report are mainly based on the measurements done during the study. Many of the basic echo measurements (e.g. LV mass) can have a deep impact on the perception of the referral physician regarding the prognosis and the management of the patient. This is the reason why care in the measurements and the accuracy of the results form part of the main basis of the quality of the echo study. There is an ASE-EAE joint document that offers clear guidelines and recommendations.[11]

Quantification of the left ventricle

LV wall thickness, dimensions, volumes, and mass are part of the basic measurement dataset of an echo study. Linear measurements based on M-mode or 2D imaging are most representative in ventricles of normal shape and function whereas volumetric measurements must be preferred in LVs with clear shape distortion or in patients with regional wall motion abnormalities. Parasternal views are the best option to do the measurements; PLAX view is the recommended option whereas PSAX view could be an alternative.

Left ventricular dimensions

The basic LV measurements are the IVS and PP thicknesses in diastole, the internal LV end-diastolic diameter (LVEDD), and LV end-systolic diameter (LVESD). Both 2D echo and M-mode can be used. M-mode, due to its high sample rate and high resolution, and due to the fact that there is a considerable amount of M-mode-based data and expertise on how to use it, is the perfect tool to work with. The measurements should be done over the LV minor axis at the level of MV leaflets tips (➲ Fig. 2.27). The specific point to measure IVS, PP, and LVEDD in the M-mode tracing is selected as the point at the onset of QRS or simply as the point in which there is the maximum separation between IVS and PP, whereas LVESD should be measured in the minimum separation point between LV walls. The major limitation of M-mode measurements is that there is a considerable amount of cases in which a correct perpendicular orientation of the echo beam in respect to LV walls is difficult to achieve even with 2D echocardiographic imaging guide. Non-parallel M-mode orientation is linked to obliquity and overestimation of measurements, and then with false diagnosis of LV dilation or hypertrophy.

Alternatively, measurements can be directly acquired from 2D echocardiographic imaging. When 2D echocardiographic imaging is used, it is recommended to do the measurements at MV chords level. IVS, PP thicknesses, and LVEDD must be assessed in the telediastolic frame, selected as the one corresponding to the QRS onset, the one following MV closure, or simply as the one in which the LV has its maximum size. LVESD measurement has to be done in the telesystolic frame, that means the one preceding MV opening or simply the one in which the LV is smallest.

Left ventricular mass

LV mass is usually estimated from linear LV dimensions using a mathematical model over LV shape. The most used method,

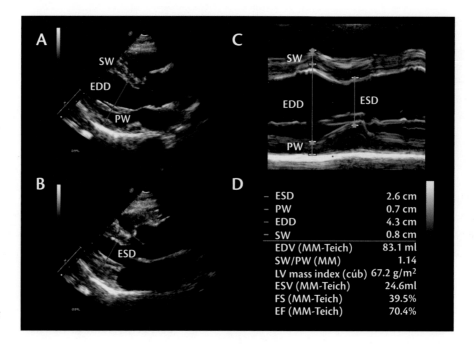

Figure 2.27 One-dimension-based left ventricle measurements. The basic four data can be achieved in 2D echo images (A and B) or in a M-mode tracing at left ventricle level (C). In any case, most echo machines can compute mass and ejection fraction when measurements are completed (D). EDD, end-diastolic diameter; EDV, end-diastolic volume; ESD, end-systolic diameter; ESV, end-systolic volume; EF, ejection fraction; FS, fractional shortening; PW, posterior wall; SW, septal wall.

validated in many studies by comparing with LV weight in autopsy and recommended by the EAE, is the formula:

$$\text{LV mass (g)} = 0.8 \times [1.04\,(\text{IVS} + \text{PP} + \text{LVEDD})^3 \\ - \text{LVEDD}^3] + 0.6 \tag{2.1}$$

This approach is useful only in patients without obvious distortions in LV shape. Most echo software makes the automatic calculation when measurements are done. However, care should be taken because measurements are cubed in the formula so that even the smallest error will be greatly magnified.

Relative wall thickness

Relative wall thickness (RWT) is calculated by the formula:

$$\text{RWT} = (2 \times \text{PP}) / \text{LVEDD} \tag{2.2}$$

It allows the evaluation of the pattern of the increase in LV mass as concentric or eccentric hypertrophy (➲ Fig. 2.28).

➲ Tables 2.1 and 2.2 show the reference limits for LV size and LV mass and geometry.

It is possible also to compute the mass of the LV with volumetric methods by computing the volume of the myocardium shell by the myocardium density. However, this approach is time consuming and is not used in clinical studies.

Left ventricular volumes

There are different approaches to calculate LV volumes. All of them are based on the fact that the LV has a regular shape that can be modelled in a mathematical formula.

There are linear methods such as those proposed by Teichholz or Quiñones that use the basic linear measurements to

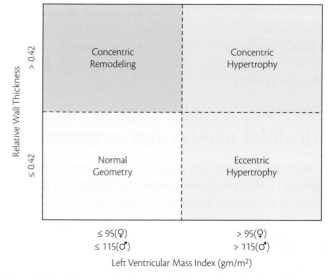

Figure 2.28 Evaluation of relative wall thickness (RWT). This calculation is useful to study the pattern of left ventricle hypertrophy. Reproduced with permission from Roberto M. Lang, Michelle Bierig, Richard B. Devereux et al (2006) Recommendations for chamber quantification Eur J Echocardiography 7, 79e108

compute volumes. These approaches are easy to use because calculations are again made automatically by the echo system software. However, they can result in inaccuracies due to the geometric assumptions needed to convert lineal dimensions in a 3D volume. Accordingly, the linear calculations of LV volume are not recommended for clinical practice.

The most commonly used 2D echocardiographic method to make a volumetric measurement of LV is the modified Simpson's rule. This approach is based on the calculation of the volume of a series of discs and in real practice requires drawing

Table 2.1 Reference limits and partition values of left ventricular size

	Women				Men			
	Reference range	Mildly abnormal	Moderately abnormal	Severely abnormal	Reference range	Mildly abnormal	Moderately abnormal	Severely abnormal
LV dimension								
LV diastolic diameter	3.9–5.3	5.4–5.7	5.8–6.1	≥6.2	4.2–5.9	6.0–6.3	6.4–6.8	≥6.9
LV diastolic diameter/BSA (cm/m²)	2.4–3.2	3.3–3.4	3.5–3.7	≥3.8	2.2–3.1	3.2–3.4	3.5–3.6	≥3.7
LV diastolic diameter/height (cm/m)	2.5–3.2	3.3–3.4	3.5–3.6	≥3.7	2.4–3.3	3.4–3.5	3.6–3.7	≥3.8
LV volume								
LV diastolic volume (ml)	56–104	105–117	118–130	≥131	67–155	156–178	179–201	≥201
LV diastolic volume/BSA (ml/m²)	**35–75**	**76–86**	**87–96**	**≥97**	**35–75**	**76–86**	**87–96**	**≥97**
LV systolic volume (ml)	19–49	50–59	60–69	≥70	22–58	59–70	71–82	≥83
LV systolic volume/BSA (ml/m²)	**12–30**	**31–36**	**37–42**	**≥43**	**12–30**	**31–36**	**37–42**	**≥43**

Values in bold are recommended and best validated.

Reproduced from Lang RM, Bierig M, Devereux RB, Flachskampf FA, Foster E, Pellikka PA, *et al.* on behalf of ASE, AHA, EAE and ESC. Recommendations for chamber quantification. *Eur J Echocardiogr* 2006; **7**(2):79–108.

Table 2.2 Reference limits and partition values of left ventricular mass and geometry

	Women				Men			
	Reference range	Mildly abnormal	Moderately abnormal	Severely abnormal	Reference range	Mildly abnormal	Moderately abnormal	Severely abnormal
Linear method								
LV mass (g)	67–162	163–186	187–210	≥211	88–224	225–258	259–292	≥293
LV mass/BSA (g/m²)	**43–95**	**96–108**	**109–121**	**≥122**	**49–115**	**116–131**	**132–148**	**≥149**
LV mass/height (g/m)	41–99	100–115	116–128	≥129	52–126	127–144	145–162	≥163
LV mass/height (g/m)²·⁷	18–44	45–51	52–58	≥59	20–48	49–55	56–63	≥64
Relative wall thickness (cm)	0.22–0.42	0.43–0.47	0.48–0.52	≥0.53	0.24–0.42	0.43–0.46	0.47–0.51	≥0.52
Septal thickness (cm)	**0.6–0.9**	**1.0–1.2**	**1.3–1.5**	**≥1.6**	**0.6–1.0**	**1.1–1.3**	**1.4–1.6**	**≥1.7**
Posterior wall thickness (cm)	**0.6–0.9**	**1.0–1.2**	**1.3–1.5**	**≥1.6**	**0.6–1.0**	**1.1–1.3**	**1.4–1.6**	**≥1.7**
2-D method								
LV mass (g)	66–150	151–171	172–182	≥183	96–200	201–227	228–254	≥255
LV mass/BSA (g/m²)	**44–88**	**89–100**	**101–112**	**≥113**	**50–102**	**103–116**	**117–130**	**≥131**

Values in bold are recommended and best validated.

Reproduced from Lang RM, Bierig M, Devereux RB, Flachskampf FA, Foster E, Pellikka PA, *et al.* on behalf of ASE, AHA, EAE and ESC. Recommendations for chamber quantification. *Eur J Echocardiogr* 2006; **7**(2):79–108.

the LV endocardium line from the MV ring in the end-diastolic and the end-systolic frames (◉ Fig. 2.29); the echo system software readily makes the calculations. Simpson's method can be used on a single plane in regular-shaped ventricles assuming that the orthogonal dimension should be equal; when there are shape distortions of wall motion abnormalities, measurements must be done over two orthogonal planes.

Quantification of the left atrium

The LA is measured at end-ventricular systole when the LA has the biggest dimension. The most used approach is to measure the anteroposterior linear dimension with 2D or M-mode

in PLAX view (◉ Fig. 2.30). As in the LV case, when M-mode sampling line is not perpendicular to LA, an inaccuracy of the measurement must be expected and 2D echocardiography-based measurement is the best option. Linear dimensions could be not representative of the complex shape of LA, which can be expanded in either of the other two non-studied axes. Therefore, they are not more recommended as the best assessment of LA size.

Measurement of the LA area in 2D imaging adds a second dimension and more accuracy to the measurement. To achieve this, the border of the atrium is drawn over the 2D image. By convention, the border should go directly from one side to the

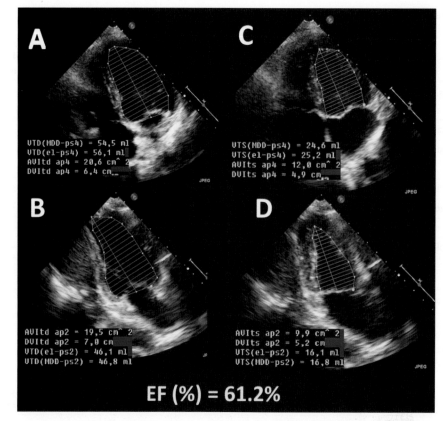

Figure 2.29 Volumetric measurements of the left ventricle. After drawing the endocardium line in end-diastolic frames in A4C (A) and A2C (B) views and the endocardium line in the end-systolic frames in A4C (C) and A2D (D) views, the system computes the volumes of the left ventricle and the ejection fraction (EF).

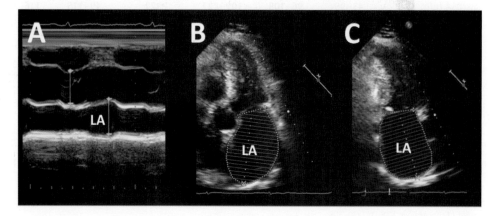

Figure 2.30 Measurements of left atrium. The classical measurement is the anteroposterior diameter in M-mode tracing (A). However, when left atrium size or morphology is abnormal is better to use the tracing of the area (B) or even better to use two orthogonal planes to compute volumes (B, C). LA, left atrium.

other of the MV ring, excluding the zone between mitral ring plane and mitral leaflets and must exclude pulmonary veins or the left appendage when seen.

The most precise measurement of the LA, but the least used in clinical practice, is volumetric, based on area-length or Simpson's methods. ➲ Table 2.3 shows the reference values for LA measurements.

Quantification of the right ventricle

The complex shape of the RV makes a quantitative approach an elusive question. RV size is usually assessed qualitatively by comparison with LV size.

RV free wall thickness could be measured using either 2D or M-mode in subcostal views (➲ Fig. 2.31). Normal RV thickness is less than 0.5cm. When facing the challenge to measure RV size, A4C view is usually the view selected. Care is needed to avoid a non-foreshortened RV apex. Measurements at end diastole of basal and mid-cavity RV diameters and longitudinal diameter are the most used methods (see ➲ Table 2.4 for normal values).

The RVOT can be measured in PSAX view at AoV size as the distance between the superior edge of the aortic annulus and the RV wall. PV annulus and main PA diameters can be measured in the RV outflow view.

Table 2.3 Reference limits and partition values for left atrial dimensions/volumes and for right atrial dimensions

	Women				Men			
	Reference Range	Mildly Abnormal	Moderately Abnormal	Severely Abnormal	Reference Range	Mildly Abnormal	Moderately Abnormal	Severely Abnormal
Atrial dimensions								
LA diameter (cm)	2.7–3.8	3.9–4.2	4.3–4.6	≥4.7	3.0–4.0	4.1–4.6	4.7–5.2	≥5.2
LA diameter/BSA (cm/m^2)	1.5–2.3	2.4–2.6	2.7–2.9	≥3.0	1.5–2.3	2.4–2.6	2.7–2.9	≥3.0
RA minor axis dimension (cm)	2.9–4.5	4.6–4.9	5.0–5.4	≥5.5	2.9–4.5	4.6–4.9	5.0–5.4	≥5.5
RA minor axis dimension/ BSA (cm/m^2)	1.7–2.5	2.6–2.8	2.9–3.1	≥3.2	1.7–2.5	2.6–2.8	2.9–3.1	≥3.2
Atrial area								
LA area (cm^2)	≤20	20–30	30–40	>40	≤20	20–30	30–40	>40
Atrial volumes								
LA volume (ml)	22–52	53–62	63–72	≥73	18–58	59–68	69–78	–79
LA volume/BSA (ml/m^2)	**22 ± 6**	**29–33**	**34–39**	**≥40**	**22 ± 6**	**29–33**	**34–39**	**≥40**

Values in bold are recommended and best validated.

Reproduced from Lang RM, Bierig M, Devereux RB, Flachskampf FA, Foster E, Pellikka PA, *et al.* on behalf of ASE, AHA, EAE and ESC. Recommendations for chamber quantification. *Eur J Echocardiogr* 2006; **7**(2):79–108.

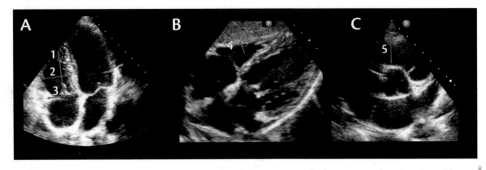

Figure 2.31 Useful measurements in the evaluation of the right ventricle. A) A4C view. 1 is the base to apex length; 2 the mid-ventricular level diameter; 3 the basal level diameter. B) Subcostal 4C view. 4 is the right ventricular wall thickness. C) SAX view at aortic valve level. 5 is the measurement of the right ventricular outflow tract.

Table 2.4 Reference limits and partition values of right ventricular and pulmonary artery size dimensions

	Reference range	Mildly abnormal	Moderately abnormal	Severely abnormal
RV dimensions				
Basal RV diameter (RVD#1) (cm)	2.0–2.8	2.9–3.3	3.4–3.8	≥3.9
Mid RV diameter (RVD#2) (cm)	2.7–3.3	3.4–3.7	3.8–4.1	≥4.2
Base-to-apex length (RVD#3) (cm)	7.1–7.9	8.0–8.5	8.6–9.1	≥9.2
RVOT diameters				
Above aortic valve (RVOT#1) (cm)	2.5–2.9	3.0–3.2	3.3–3.5	≥3.6
Above pulmonic valve (RVOT#2) (cm)	1.7–2.3	2.4–2.7	2.8–3.1	≥3.2
PA diameter				
Below pulmonic valve (PA#1) (cm)	1.5–2.1	2.2–2.5	2.6–2.9	≥3.0

Reproduced from Lang RM, Bierig M, Devereux RB, Flachskampf FA, Foster E, Pellikka PA, *et al.* on behalf of ASE, AHA, EAE and ESC. Recommendations for chamber quantification. *Eur J Echocardiogr* 2006; **7**(2):79–108.

Quantification of the right atrium

RA measurements should be done when needed in A4C view. The most used one is the minor axis dimension that extends from the lateral border of the RA to the interatrial septum.

Quantification of the aorta

Measurements should be done in PLAX view. The dataset should include measurements of the diameters of the aorta at AoV annulus, at the maximum diameter in the sinuses of Valsalva, in the sinotubular junction, and in the tubular portion of the ascending aorta.

Quantification of the inferior vena cava

The assessment of the IVC should be a part of every echo examination, due to its role in the estimation of pressures on the right side of the heart (see ➲ Chapter 11, 'Assessment of right ventricular haemodynamics'). The measurement should be done in the subcostal view, at 1–2 cm from the junction with the RA (➲ Fig. 2.32). Normal vena cava diameter is 1.5 cm. The change of size with respiration cycle should also be assessed (➲ Fig. 2.33).

The echocardiographic examination

The transthoracic echo evaluation is a standardized study that combines 2D echo and M-mode with colour, pulsed, continuous, and tissue Doppler imaging to make a comprehensive evaluation of chambers, valves, and flows of the heart. The minimal standard data digital acquisition protocol recommended by EAE guidelines[12] for a transthoracic echocardiography is summarized in ➲ Table 2.5.

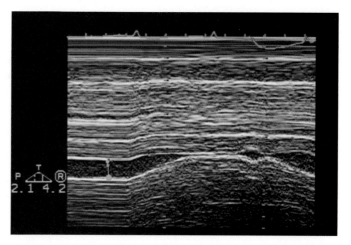

Figure 2.33 Inferior cava vein normal collapse. Image of subcostal view showing a normal collapse of inferior cava vein during patient inspiration.

Table 2.5 Minimal standard dataset acquisition protocol for transthoracic echocardiography

Parasternal	
Parasternal long-axis of LV	2D + Colour D + M-mode
Parasternal short-axis at aortic valve level	2D + Colour D + M-mode
Parasternal short-axis at mitral valve level	2D
Parasternal short-axis at mid-papillary level	2D
Parasternal RV inflow tract	2D + Colour D
Parasternal RV outflow tract	2D + Colour D
Transpulmonary velocities	PW Doppler
Apical	
Four-chamber view	2D + Colour D
Five-chamber view	2D + Colour D
Two-chamber view	2D + Colour D
Long-axis view	2D + Colour D
Transmitral velocities	PW Doppler
LV outflow tract velocities	PW Doppler
Transaortic outflow tract velocities	CW Doppler
Tissue Doppler at mitral annulus (septal, lateral)	TDI
Tricuspid regurgitant velocities	CW Doppler
Subcostal	
Four-chamber view	2D + Colour D
Vena cava view	M-mode
Suprastemal	
Long-axis view of aortic arch	2D + Colour D

LV, left ventricle; 2D, two dimensional echocardiography; Colour D, colour Doppler echocardiography; CW, continous wave-Doppler; PW, pulsed-wave Doppler; TDI, tissue Doppler.

Reproduced from Evangelista A, Flachskampf F, Lancellotti P, Badano L, Aguilar R, Monaghan M, *et al.* EAE recommendations for standardization of performance, digital storage and reporting of echocardiographic studies. *Eur J Echocardiogr* 2008; **9**(4):438–48.

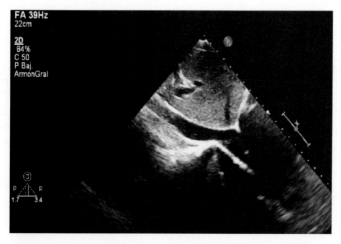

Figure 2.32 Measurements of the inferior cava vein. The figure shows an image of subcostal view at the level of inferior cava vein, measured at 1–2 cm from the junction with the RA.

Personal perspective

Transthoracic echocardiography has become the cardiac imaging tool of choice in many stable and emergency clinical conditions. The possibility of scanning the heart from multiple views only by manually rotating and angulating the transducer allows a complete cardiac evaluation in almost all patients. 2D echocardiography is the basis of morphological and functional assessment of the heart. Indeed, real-time visualization of cardiac structures not only makes the qualitative evaluation of cardiac structure and function extremely reliable, but also allows quantitative measurements of cardiac

dimensions, areas, and volumes. Thanks to availability of portable echo machines, transthoracic echocardiography can be easily performed and repeated at the bedside in the intensive care unit, as well as in the emergency room, catheterization laboratory, and operating room. Moreover, transthoracic echocardiography is largely spreading as a fundamental tool to guide invasive cardiac procedures. Although adequate confidence with technique and expertise in image acquisition and interpretation requires a learning curve, newer echo machines and softwares are improving their image resolution in order to facilitate diagnosis also in difficult clinical conditions.

References

1 Garcia Fernandez MA, Zamorano J. *Procedimientos en Ecocardiografía*. Madrid: McGraw Hill; 2004.

2 Henry WL, De Maria A, Gramiek R, King DL, Kisslo JA, Popp RL, *et al.* Report of the American Society of Echocardiography Committee on nomenclature and standards in two dimensional echocardiography. *Circulation* 1980; **62**:212–16.

3 Edwards WD, Tajik AJ, Seward JB. Standardized nomenclature and anatomic basis for regional tomographic analysis of the heart. *Mayo Clin Proc* 1981; **56**:479–97.

4 Weyman AE. *Principles and Practice of Echocardiography*, 3rd ed. Philadelphia, PA: Lea and Febiger; 1994, pp.99–123.

5 Lange LW, Sahn DJ, Allen HD, Golberg SJ. Subxiphoid crosssectional echocardiography in infants and children with congenital heart disease. *Circulation* 1979; **59**:513–18.

6 Goldberg BB. Supraesternal ultrasonography. *JAMA* 1971; **215**:245–9.

7 Feigenbaum H. *Echocardiography*, 7th ed. Philadelphia, PA: Lippincott Williams & Wilkins; 2009, pp.91–120.

8 Tei C, Tanaka H, Kashima T, Yoshimura H, Minagoe S, Kanehisa T. Real-time cross-sectional echocardiographic evaluation of the interatrial septum by right atrium–interatrial septum-left atrium direction of ultrasound beam. *Circulation* 1979; **60**:539–43.

9 American Society of Echocardiography Committee on Standards. Recommendations for quantification of the left ventricle by two dimensional echocardiography. *J Am Soc Echocardiogr* 1989; **2**:358–67.

10 Tajik AJ, Seward JB, Hagler DJ, Mair DD, Lie JT. Two–dimensional real-time ultrasonic imaging of the heart and great vessels: Technique, image orientation, structure identification, and validation. *Mayo Clin Proc* 1978; **53**:271–303.

11 Lang RM, Bierig M, Devereux RB, Flachskampf FA, Foster E, Pellikka PA, *et al.* on behalf of ASE, AHA, EAE and ESC. Recommendations for chamber quantification. *Eur J Echocardiogr* 2006; **7**(2):79–108.

12 Evangelista A, Flachskampf F, Lancellotti P, Badano L, Aguilar R, Monaghan M, *et al.* EAE recommendations for standardization of performance, digital storage and reporting of echocardiographic studies. *Eur J Echocardiogr* 2008; **9**(4):438–48.

Further reading

Evangelista A, Flachskampf F, Lancellotti P, Badano L, Aguilar R, Monaghan M, *et al.* EAE recommendations for standardization of performance, digital storage and reporting of echocardiographic studies. *Eur J Echocardiogr* 2008; **9**(4):438–48.

Lang RM, Bierig M, Devereux RB, Flachskampf FA, Foster E, Pellikka PA, *et al.*; on behalf ASE, AHA, EAE and ESC. Recommendations for chamber quantification. *Eur J Echocardiogr* 2006; **7**(2):79–108.

Additional online material

- 2.1 2D echo parasternal long-axis view.
- 2.2 2D echo right ventricle inflow view.
- 2.3 2D echo right ventricle outflow view.
- 2.4 2D echo parasternal short-axis view at aortic valve level.
- 2.5 2D echo parasternal short-axis view at mitral valve level.
- 2.6 2D echo parasternal short-axis view at papillary muscles level.
- 2.7 2D echo parasternal short-axis view at apical level.
- 2.8 2D echo apical four-chamber view.
- 2.9 2D echo apical five-chamber view.
- 2.10 2D echo apical two-chamber view.
- 2.11 2D echo apical three-chamber view.
- 2.12 2D echo subcostal four-chamber view.
- 2.13 2D echo subcostal short-axis view.
- 2.14 2D echo subcostal inferior vena cava view.
- 2.15 2D echo subcostal abdominal aorta view.
- 2.16 2D echo suprasternal long-axis view.

↪ For additional multimedia materials please visit the online version of the book (http://escecho.oxfordmedicine.com).

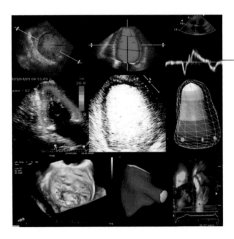

CHAPTER 3

Three dimensional echocardiography

M. Monaghan and S. Adhya

Contents

Summary

Three-dimensional (3D) echocardiography allows the real-time acquisition of volumes containing entire cardiac structures. The analysis of 3D volumes does not require any assumptions as to the shape of structures.

3D echocardiography is more accurate than two-dimensional (2D) in the assessment of left ventricular (LV) volumes, mass, and function, and is comparable to cardiac magnetic resonance imaging. This makes it an ideal modality for measuring LV function particularly when this will determine significant interventions such as implanting of cardioverter/defibrillators, biventricular pacing, and the commencement and continuation of cancer chemotherapy. 3D echocardiography makes it easy to visualize valves and define pathological mechanisms. 3D assessment of dyssynchrony, myocardial strain, and stress imaging are attractive.

However, 3D echocardiography is limited by the need for specialist software and lower spatial and temporal resolution when compared to 2D echocardiography.

Introduction

Three-dimensional (3D) echocardiography offers the possibility to visualize the heart in three dimensions without requiring mental reconstruction of multiple two-dimensional (2D) images. This offers advantages as the exact relation between different 2D cuts through the 3D volume is always known. Initial attempts required reconstruction of multiple 2D cuts into a 3D dataset, but recently full matrix arrays have allowed the acquisition of 3D volumes without manipulation of the probe.

In this chapter we will cover technical aspects of 3D acquisitions and the practical roles of 3D echocardiography in the assessment of cardiac function.

Technical aspects of full matrix 3D acquisition and analysis

Initial 3D images were created acquiring multiple 2D images that were digitally reconstructed and reformatted into rectangular voxels. However, 3D transducer technology has improved so that actually real-time 3D images are generated.

3D echocardiography transducers contain a matrix of piezo-electric elements, which allows a volume of the heart to be acquired simultaneously. Initial probes were unable to acquire a volume containing the whole heart in a single beat, and therefore the probe steered the volumes between heart cycles and stitched them together to build up a volume containing the entire heart. Currently there are commercially available systems that acquire a full volume in a single beat.

These advances have come at the cost of much lower volume rates than those seen in 2D echocardiography. Live 3D volumes often have volume rates of 20Hz or so, though parallel processing can allow up to 60 volumes per second. In patients who have a heart rate (HR) above 60 beats per minute, the number of volumes per heart cycle falls further. Acquiring multiple heart cycles with electrocardiogram (ECG) gating increases the temporal and spatial resolution, but at a cost of stitching artefacts that arise because of variability in HR as well as respiratory motion of the heart.

3D echocardiography is currently performed after 2D imaging, by using the same transducer, which also is able to scan two dimensionally: 2D images can be changed instantaneously into 3D images by selecting the 3D function. Multiple 2D images are displayed simultaneously with real-time 3D images. Cropping controls allow modification of 3D images, dissecting them from a full-volume pyramid in order to optimally visualize anatomical features of cardiac structures. Finally, 3D images can be rotated to any direction for viewing.

Software is necessary to display 3D volumes on 2D screens. 3D glasses have been used, but it is more common to use tools to crop into the 3D volume and then make measurements. The use of automated border tracking allows quick assessment of ventricular volumes and ejection fraction (EF), which would otherwise be overly laborious for routine use.

◗ Table 3.1 summarizes comparison between 2D and 3D echocardiography.

Left ventricular assessment

The most established use of 3D echo is in the assessment of LV volumes and function. 2D methods are limited due to geometrical assumptions that are incorrect in the presence of aneurysms or regional wall motion abnormalities (WMAs), as well as the problem of foreshortening. 3D echocardiography is not limited by these problems, and has been validated against cardiac magnetic resonance (CMR) imaging[1] and myocardial scintigraphy (see ◗ Chapter 8).[2] The enhanced accuracy results in less variability within and between different observers. This is clinically important as international guidelines suggest that decisions such as implantation of internal cardiovertor/defibrillators or monitoring of the cardiotoxic effects of chemotherapy are based on EF.

The rapid measurement of 3D volumes requires software for the analysis. A number of different software packages are available, but essentially they all require the user to define a number of points of the LV endocardial border and then extrapolate from these points the endocardial border for the whole ventricle throughout the cardiac cycle. The algorithms used for this extrapolation rely on border detection, or more recently speckle tracking (◗ Fig. 3.1; ◼ 3.1 and 3.2).

Several studies have suggested that 3D echo systematically underestimates volumes as compared to CMR measurements (see Chapter 8).[3]

3D echo has also been employed in the evaluation of LV mass. This is more challenging than volumes as it additionally requires determination of the epicardial border. Nevertheless, a number of studies have found it more accurate than M-mode and 2D echocardiography and comparable to CMR in normal subject[4,5] as well as in subjects with concentric LV hypertrophy[6] or WMAs[7].

Regional wall motion can also be assessed using 3D echocardiography. This has been shown to correlate well with 2D wall motion scoring and regional EF correlates with regional EF by CMR.[8] The true potential of this technique lies in rapid acquisition during stress imaging which will be discussed later in this chapter.

Dyssynchrony assessment is attractive, as the Prospect study has shown that traditional 2D markers of dyssynchrony have significant variability.[9] Our group developed the systolic dyssynchrony index (SDI) which is the standard deviation of times to minimum volumes of 16 different segments of the left ventricle.[10] This index has been shown to be elevated in impaired LV function and more so in left bundle branch block.[11] A number of groups have recently shown that this index is a useful predictor of benefit from biventricular pacing.[12,13] However, attention has been drawn to the fact that a single outlier segment significantly alters the SDI because it is a standard deviation measure, and that it may be difficult to define the time of minimum volume in segments that have small volume changes.[14]

Table 3.1 Comparison of 2D and 3D echocardiography

	Advantages	Limitations
2D echocardiography	Better temporal and spatial resolution Smaller probe which is easier to handle	Requires mental reconstruction of images
3D echocardiography	Does not require geometric assumptions when measuring areas or volumes	Limited temporal and spatial resolution Image drop out in part of the volumes Requires software to visualize 3D volumes on 2D screens

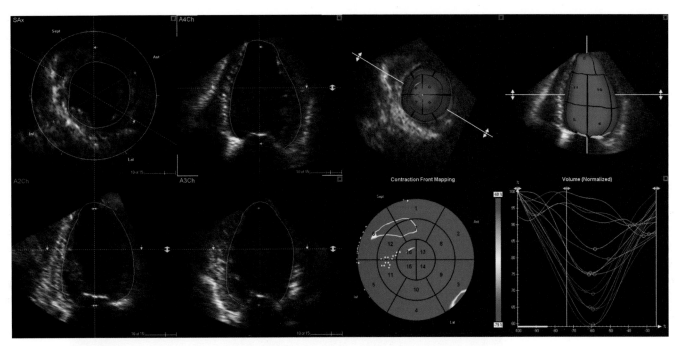

Figure 3.1 Left ventricular assessment. Measurement of left ventricular volumes is performed using specialized software. A few points are marked on the endocardial border, and the software generates a model of the left ventricle. In the four panels on the left the model is visualized in three standard long-axis and a short-axis view. The upper two right panels show the model in a short-axis and long-axis view. The lower 2 right panels displays a bull's-eye plot with a colour-coded volume representation, and the volume curves for the 16 segments. The volume curves show that the septal segments are out of phase with the rest of the ventricle so they are coloured blue on the bull's-eye plot. This patient had a high dyssynchrony index, met conventional criteria for biventricular pacing, and subsequently underwent this procedure.

Right ventricular assessment

The assessment of the right ventricle (RV) is particularly important in congenital heart disease and pulmonary hypertension. The complex crescentic shape of the RV has made this challenging using 2D echocardiography, and therefore another attractive use for 3D echocardiography. However, the position of the RV behind the sternum can cause echocardiographic drop-out particularly affecting the anterior wall and outflow tract of the RV. Endocardial definition is more difficult in the highly trabeculated RV than the LV. Initial studies found that 3D echo was not substantially better than 2D echo when compared to CMR reference.[15] This may be because it is difficult to determine the RV borders accurately on short axis CMR cuts that were optimized for the LV, as well as to visualize the tricuspid and pulmonary valves that define the basal segment. However, when specialized software designed to assess RV volumes is used for both 3D echo and CMR, the agreement between methods is good, though as with LV imaging the RV volumes are systematically lower than those found on CMR (➔ Fig. 3.2; ⬛ 3.3).[16–18]

Normal ranges have recently been published.[19] However, the variability between measurements appears to be of the order of ± 10%, which means that caution is required in the serial assessment of patients so subtle changes are not missed. Nevertheless, 3D echo promises to be a rapid, easily available modality to assess RV function, and is likely to lead to novel insights into the pathophysiology of cardiac diseases.

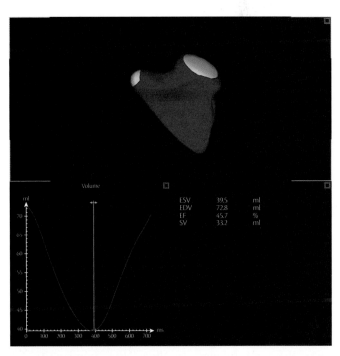

Figure 3.2 Right ventricular assessment. Specialized software exists for the analysis of right ventricular volumes. This tracks the endocardial border to generate a model and give systolic and diastolic volumes.

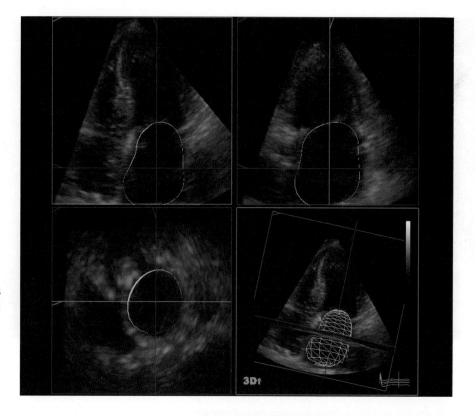

Figure 3.3 Atrial volumes and function assessment. Estimation of left atrial volumes can be performed on full volume acquisitions of the heart. After delineation of a few endocardial points, the software generates a 3D model. This figure demonstrates three orthogonal cut-planes (green, red, and blue boxes) through the volume and marks the other cut-planes, together with a projection of the 3D wire frame model showing the locations of the different cut-planes.

Atrial volumes and function

Left atrial (LA) enlargement is a marker of the severity and duration of elevated LA pressure. It predisposes to atrial fibrillation, stroke, and is a marker for worse cardiovascular outcomes. It is recommended that atrial volumes be measured from 2D cut planes, rather than linear measurements.[20] 3D echo is again attractive for this measurement, but it has not yet been validated against CMR imaging with specific acquisitions for the atria. Nonetheless, 3D atrial volumes are more sensitive to volume changes than 2D,[21] and 3D atrial volume predicts cardiac events in patients with significant LV dysfunction.[22] Transthoracic 3D has even been used to evaluate the LA appendage for thrombi[23] and shown to be superior to 2D echocardiography in measuring right atrial (RA) volume[24] (➲ Fig. 3.3).

Mitral valve disease

3D echocardiography makes it easy to get a surgeon's eye view of the mitral valve (MV). It allows easy identification of the section of mitral leaflet prolapse, planimetry of MV area both in mitral stenosis, and the measurement of the effective regurgitant orifice area (EROA) in mitral regurgitation. It is significantly easier for the non-echocardiographer, trainees, and surgeons to appreciate the mechanism of MV dysfunction. 3D transoesophageal echocardiography (TOE) offers better resolution than transthoracic echocardiography (TTE), and maintains these advantages. It allows the opportunity for intraoperative assessment for either surgical MV repair, or balloon valvuloplasty (➲ Fig. 3.4; ■ 3.4).

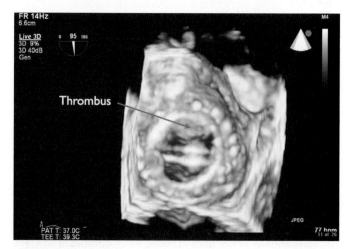

Figure 3.4 Mitral prosthesis assessment. 3D TOE is used here to image a prosthetic bileaflet mechanical mitral valve. The valve leaflets, valve ring, and sutures are clearly visible. The thrombus propagating from the valve ring is marked.

Research has focused on quantification and mechanism of mitral regurgitation, assessment of mitral stenosis, and assessment of the mitral annulus, particularly during surgical repair of the MV. Visualization of the anterior leaflet appears to be better than the posterior leaflet, probably because it is larger, and the posterior leaflet is best seen from the parasternal window, while the anterior leaflet is adequately visualized from both parasternal and apical windows[25] (➲ Fig. 3.5; ■ 3.5).

In mitral prolapse, determination of the segment of prolapse is more accurate with 3D TTE than 2D TTE[26] and has a similar

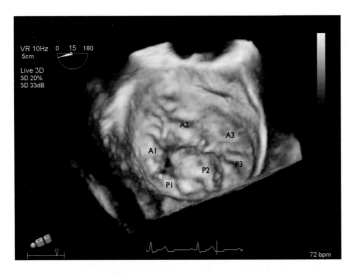

Figure 3.5 View of mitral valve leaflets and scallops. 3D TOE is used here to give a surgeon's eye view of the mitral valve looking from the left atrium. The middle scallop of the posterior leaflet (P2) is clearly seen to be prolapsing into the left atrium in systole. The other scallops—anterior 1 to 3 and posterior 1 and 3—are also marked.

accuracy to 2D TOE[27,28]. The functional anatomy of mitral regurgitation is also accurate compared to surgical findings.[29] A 3D regurgitant volume to LA volume ratio has been proposed as a marker of severity, though importantly the values were less than that derived from 2D measurements.[30] The regurgitant orifice area is usually elliptical rather than spherical. This results in an asymmetrical vena contracta and hemi-elliptical proximal flow convergence region. 3D colour flow imaging is therefore more accurate at measuring the vena contracta than single plane 2D imaging[31] and allows more accurate assessments of regurgitant volumes by PISA.[32]

Three studies have compared 2D, 3D, and cardiac catheterization assessments of mitral stenosis.[33–35] The mitral orifice area derived from 3D was closer to that derived invasively using the Gorlin formula than orifice areas derived from 2D echo including planimetry, pressure half-time, and flow convergence. It is therefore recommended that this should be the standard method for assessment of the orifice area.[36] Additionally these 3D measures have less interobserver variability than 2D measures. A 3D score of mitral stenosis has also been developed which may offer additional information than the Wilkins score.[37]

Mitral annulus size has been shown to be similar by 3D and CMR.[38] The addition of mitral annular assessment at the time of surgical repair can delineate if the normal saddle-shape of the annulus has been maintained.[39] This saddle-shape is important in reducing stress on the mitral leaflet and may lead to a more durable repair.

Aortic valve disease

2D echocardiography is very good in the assessment of aortic valve (AoV) disease. However, 3D echo offers additional benefits, particularly in the era of transcutaneous AoV implantation. Planimetry of the AoV with real-time 3D echo images showed good agreement with the standard 2D TOE technique, flow-derived methods, and cardiac catheterization data with the advantage of improved reproducibility.[40] It more accurately assesses the AoV annulus, which is often elliptical rather than the assumed spherical shape (➲ Fig. 3.6).

Figure 3.6 Aortic valve assessment. 3D TTE can be used to accurately planimeter valve areas. The green, red, and blue boxes show three different cut-planes through the volume containing the valve. Each box also demonstrates the other cut-planes. The lower right panel shows a 3D projection demonstrating the relationship between the cut-planes. The cut-planes are manipulated so that the red box contains the plane orthogonal to the valve axis at the level of the leaflet tips. The leaflets are manually delineated to give the valve area marked in yellow. 3D planimetry has the advantage that the plane in which planimetry is performed does not need to be co-axial with the ultrasound probe and can be precisely positioned in relation to the valve axis.

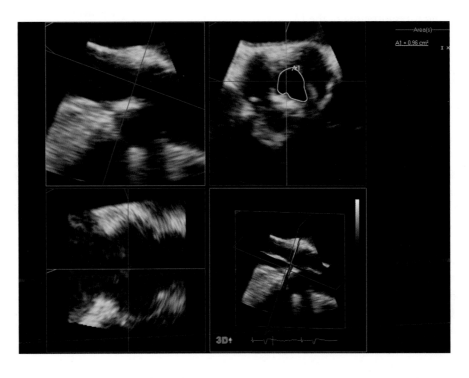

Tricuspid and pulmonary valve disease

Although less clinically important than left heart valvular function in adults, 3D echo allows the visualization of all three leaflets of the tricuspid valve (TV) simultaneously. However, the published data on 3D for tricuspid assessment outside congenital heart disease is limited. The fact that normal TVs are thin makes them challenging to image, but 3D echo has been shown to be useful in characterizing the valvular structure in rheumatic heart disease, as well as in pulmonary arterial (PA) hypertension.[41] 3D TOE may be useful for percutaneous procedures on the PV. For details regarding 3D assessment of TV, see ➲ Chapter 14c.

Basics in adult congenital heart disease: atrial septal defects

3D echocardiography is useful in the assessment of atrial septal defects (ASDs). It can accurately depict the whole defect and relations to the heart valves. 3D TTE has been compared to 2D TTE and 2D TOE. It more accurately depicts the anatomy of the defect,[42] and may obviate the need for contrast injection[43]. TOE is invaluable in pre-operative assessment to look for fenestrations and for accurate sizing of occluder devices.

Stress echocardiography, including 3D contrast echocardiography

2D echocardiography has limitations during stress echocardiography. Even with experienced echocardiographers, it may be difficult to avoid foreshortening of the LV and to ensure that concurrent images taken at different stages of stress are identical cuts to ensure imaging of the same segment throughout the stress protocol. Furthermore, taking several cuts requires time which is often a limiting factor in exercise stress echocardiography. 3D echo has the advantage of no foreshortening, and accurate registration of segments in serial stages of stress. Initial feasibility studies have been performed using ECG gated acquisitions in dobutamine stress echo and found a greater sensitivity and specificity than 2D echocardiography when compared with myocardial SPECT.[44] Furthermore, 3D echocardiography results in faster acquisition of images. The addition of contrast agents improves the accuracy of 2D echocardiography and has also been shown to be feasible in 3D echocardiography. The use of contrast also allows semiquantitative assessment of myocardial perfusion.[45] The limitations are a lower spatial and temporal resolution than 2D and therefore the number of volumes per cardiac cycle is fewer at the higher heart rates of peak stress. Single beat assessment is now available but it remains to be seen if this will offer significant advantages over gated acquisitions, though it may make treadmill exercise stress echocardiography achievable. Furthermore, software tools are commonly available to allow the side-by-side comparison of 2D cuts at different stages of stress. Not all 3D software packages have this capacity, but the ability of comparing multiple 2D short axis cuts from a 3D volume appears to be superior than tri-plane imaging.[46] The ability to obtain reproducible global and regional LV parameters during stress is another potential advantage of 3D in this context. An abnormal response to stress may include increasing LV volume, failure of LV EF to increase, and an increase in intraventricular dyssynchrony. Analysis of these parameters may decrease the subjectivity of current 2D stress echo.

Role of 3D transoesophageal echocardiography

3D TOE is useful for the assessment of valvular lesions and ASDs. It also lends itself to intraoperative imaging. In ASD and patent foramen ovale (PFO), 3D TOE can define the defect, its rim, and relation to the atrioventricular ring, which are important in planning closure. Furthermore, the intraoperative use of TOE can help accurate placement and decrease fluoroscopy times[47–49] (➲ Fig. 3.7; 🎬 3.6–3.8). 3D TOE has been used to perform trans-septal puncture, for mitral valvuloplasty[50] and atrial fibrillation ablation procedures.[51] TOE can guide catheters and ensure appropriate placement of balloon catheters in relation to the subvalvar apparatus[50]. In patients who are undergoing transcutaneous AoV implantation, the oval shape of the left ventricular outflow tract (LVOT) and AoV annulus means that care needs to be taken with sizing of the prosthetic valve. In our experience, 3D TOE is extremely helpful for sizing and for accurate placement prior to deployment[52] (➲ Fig. 3.8, 🎬 3.9).

Future advances

Improvements in technology will undoubtedly bring better spatial and temporal resolution. The integration of high quality 2D and 3D probes is likely to occur and make 3D imaging more convenient. Improvements to software should accelerate workflow and perhaps bring a greater degree of automation to many measurements with incremental benefits in interobserver variability. This may also assist the use of 3D echocardiography in stress imaging. In terms of techniques, 3D speckle tracking has recently become possible. This allows direct myocardial assessment in three dimensions, whereas movements of speckles outside of the imaged plane confound 2D speckle tracking. Regional myocardial strain can be calculated, and speckle tracking may improve endocardial tracking over border detection algorithms. However, clinical experience is currently limited. Regional myocardial strain using 3D and 2D speckle tracking have shown comparable

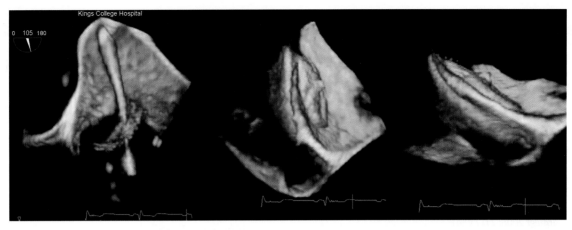

Figure 3.7 3D TOE view of patent foramen ovale. The left panel shows a 3D TOE volume of a catheter across a patent foramen ovale, with the left atrium at the top of the image, and the right atrium at the bottom. The middle and right panels demonstrate the deployed occluder device sandwiched across the defect with a small visible rim of atrial tissue.

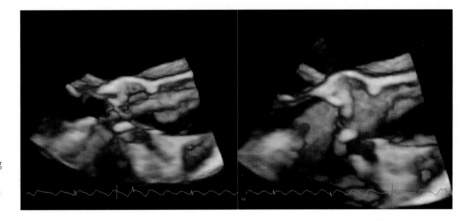

Figure 3.8 Positioning of the balloon catheter across the aortic valve. The left panel shows a balloon catheter across the aortic valve. The left ventricle is to the right, and the aortic root to the left of the image. The heart is paced rapidly to minimize motion of the valve. The right panel shows the inflated catheter. 3D is useful during the procedure for positioning of the balloon, particularly when valve implantation is being performed.

results, though 3D speckle had the advantage of being faster and able to assess more segments.[53] Another group have found that 2D and 3D measures were different, but 3D measures had a smaller range suggesting its superiority over 2D.[54]

Conclusion

3D echocardiography is at a similar stage to 2D echocardiography in the early 1980s. It is clearly easier for novices or trainees to appreciate cardiac structure, but requires post-processing and expertise with software to visualize structures. It is becoming an integral part of the routine echocardiographic examination, particularly for LV and valvular assessment. 3D TOE is a valuable adjunct to many invasive procedures. Future advances will make it easier to perform and analyse 3D volumes. Clinically the role of 3D echo in stress echocardiography, dyssynchrony assessment, and regional myocardial strain analysis is likely to expand.

Personal perspective

3D echocardiography has come a long way since it was first described in 1974. After initial laborious procedure that required careful manipulation of a probe, we now have highly advanced matrix array transducers that can acquire a full volume in real time. These advances have been mirrored in the computational power to manipulate the large datasets created, and in the user interface to display 3D images on 2D screens. The future is likely to bring 3D echocardiography into mainstream routine practice. Advances in technology and software will make it easier to acquire volumes, increase the automation of functional measurements, and store the data generated. Dedicated software packages will make it easier to apply 3D in stress echocardiography and perfusion imaging. Advances in 3D display hardware may have a significant impact on the human–computer interface. Clinical research will define the role of new 3D indices of cardiac function, particularly in dyssynchrony and strain imaging.

References

1 Kühl HP, Schreckenberg M, Rulands D, Katoh M, Schäfer W, Schummers G, et al. High-resolution transthoracic real-time three-dimensional echocardiography: quantitation of cardiac volumes and function using semi-automatic border detection and comparison with cardiac magnetic resonance imaging. J Am Coll Cardiol 2004; 43(11):2083–90.

2 Marsan NA, Henneman MM, Chen J, Ypenburg C, Dibbets P, Ghio S, et al. Real-time three-dimensional echocardiography as a novel approach to quantify left ventricular dyssynchrony: a comparison study with phase analysis of gated myocardial perfusion single photon emission computed tomography. J Am Soc Echocardiogr 2008; 21(7):801–7.

3 Mor-Avi V, Jenkins C, Kühl H, Nesser H-J, Marwick T, Franke A, et al. Real-time 3-dimensional echocardiographic quantification of left ventricular volumes: multicenter study for validation with magnetic resonance imaging and investigation of sources of error. J Am Coll Cardiol: Cardiovasc Imaging 2008; 1(4):413–23.

4 Jenkins C, Bricknell K, Hanekom L, Marwick TH. Reproducibility and accuracy of echocardiographic measurements of left ventricular parameters using real-time three-dimensional echocardiography. J Am Coll Cardiol 2004; 44(4):878–86.

5 Mor-Avi V, Sugeng L, Weinert L, MacEneaney P, Caiani EG, Koch R, et al. Fast measurement of left ventricular mass with real-time three-dimensional echocardiography: comparison with magnetic resonance imaging. Circulation 2004; 110(13):1814–8.

6 Yap S-C, van Geuns R-JM, Nemes A, Meijboom FJ, Mcghie JS, Geleijnse ML, et al. Rapid and accurate measurement of LV mass by biplane real-time 3D echocardiography in patients with concentric LV hypertrophy: comparison to CMR. Eur J Echocardiogr 2008; 9(2):255–60.

7 Pouleur A-C, le Polain de Waroux J-B, Pasquet A, Gerber BL, Gérard O, Allain P, et al. Assessment of left ventricular mass and volumes by three-dimensional echocardiography in patients with or without wall motion abnormalities: comparison against cine magnetic resonance imaging. Heart 2008; 94(8):1050–7.

8 Nesser H, Sugeng L, Corsi C, Weinert L, Niel J, Ebner C, et al. Volumetric analysis of regional left ventricular function with real-time three-dimensional echocardiography: validation by magnetic resonance and clinical utility testing. Heart 2007; 93(5):572–8.

9 Chung ES, Leon AR, Tavazzi L, Sun J-P, Nihoyannopoulos P, Merlino J, et al. Results of the Predictors of Response to CRT (PROSPECT) trial. Circulation 2008; 117(20):2608–16.

10 Kapetanakis S, Kearney MT, Siva A, Gall N, Cooklin M, Monaghan MJ. Real-time three-dimensional echocardiography: a novel technique to quantify global left ventricular mechanical dyssynchrony. Circulation 2005; 112(7):992–1000.

11 van Dijk J, Dijkmans PA, Götte MJW, Spreeuwenberg MD, Visser CA, Kamp O. Evaluation of global left ventricular function and mechanical dyssynchrony in patients with an asymptomatic left bundle branch block: a real-time 3D echocardiography study. Eur J Echocardiogr 2008; 9(1):40–6.

12 Marsan NA, Bleeker GB, Ypenburg C, Ghio S, Van De Veire NR, Holman ER, et al. Real-time three-dimensional echocardiography permits quantification of left ventricular mechanical dyssynchrony and predicts acute response to cardiac resynchronization therapy. J Cardiovasc Electrophysiol 2008; 19(4):392–9.

13 Soliman OII, Geleijnse ML, Theuns DAMJ, van Dalen BM, Vletter WB, Jordaens LJ, et al. Usefulness of left ventricular systolic dyssynchrony by real-time three-dimensional echocardiography to predict long-term response to cardiac resynchronization therapy. Am J Cardiol 2009; 103(11):1586–91.

14 Sonne C, Sugeng L, Takeuchi M, Weinert L, Childers R, Watanabe N, et al. Real-time 3-dimensional echocardiographic assessment of left ventricular dyssynchrony. J Am Coll Cardiol: Cardiovasc Imaging 2009; 2(7):802–12.

15 Kjaergaard J, Petersen CL, Kjaer A, Schaadt BK, Oh JK, Hassager C. Evaluation of right ventricular volume and function by 2D and 3D echocardiography compared to MRI. Eur J Echocardiogr 2006; 7(6):430–8.

16 Gopal AS, Chukwu EO, Iwuchukwu CJ, Katz AS, Toole RS, Schapiro W, et al. Normal values of right ventricular size and function by real-time 3-dimensional echocardiography: comparison with cardiac magnetic resonance imaging. J Am Soc Echocardiogr 2007; 20(5):445–55.

17 Jenkins C, Chan J, Bricknell K, Strudwick M, Marwick TH. Reproducibility of right ventricular volumes and ejection fraction using real-time three-dimensional echocardiography: comparison with cardiac MRI. Chest 2007; 131(6):1844–51.

18 Niemann PS, Pinho L, Balbach T, Galuschky C, Blankenhagen M, Silberbach M, et al. Anatomically oriented right ventricular volume measurements with dynamic three-dimensional echocardiography validated by 3-Tesla magnetic resonance imaging. J Am Coll Cardiol 2007; 50(17):1668–76.

19 Tamborini G, Marsan NA, Gripari P, Maffessanti F, Brusoni D, Muratori M, et al. Reference values for right ventricular volumes and ejection fraction with real-time three-dimensional echocardiography: evaluation in a large series of normal subjects. J Am Soc Echocardiogr 2010; 23(2):109–15.

20 Lang RM, Bierig M, Devereux RB, Flachskampf FA, Foster E, Pellikka PA, et al. Recommendations for chamber quantification. Eur J Echocardiogr 2006; 7(2):79–108.

21 Anwar AM, Soliman OII, Geleijnse ML, Nemes A, Vletter WB, Ten Cate FJ. Assessment of left atrial volume and function by real-time three-dimensional echocardiography. Int J Cardiol 2008; 123(2):155–61.

22 Suh I-W, Song J-M, Lee E-Y, Kang S-H, Kim M-J, Kim J-J, et al. Left atrial volume measured by real-time 3-dimensional echocardiography predicts clinical outcomes in patients with severe left ventricular dysfunction and in sinus rhythm. J Am Soc Echocardiogr 2008; 21(5):439–45.

23 Agoston I, Xie T, Tiller FL, Rahman AM, Ahmad M. Assessment of left atrial appendage by live three-dimensional echocardiography: early experience and comparison with transesophageal echocardiography. Echocardiography 2006; 23(2):127–32.

24 Müller H, Burri H, Lerch R. Evaluation of right atrial size in patients with atrial arrhythmias: comparison of 2D versus real time 3D echocardiography. Echocardiography 2008; 25(6):617–23.

25 Sugeng L, Coon P, Weinert L, Jolly N, Lammertin G, Bednarz JE, et al. Use of real-time 3-dimensional transthoracic echocardiography in the evaluation of mitral valve disease. J Am Soc Echocardiogr 2006; 19(4):413–21.

26 Beraud A-S, Schnittger I, Miller DC, Liang DH. Multiplanar reconstruction of three-dimensional transthoracic echocardiography improves the presurgical assessment of mitral prolapse. J Am Soc Echocardiogr 2009; 22(8):907–13.

27 Sharma R, Mann J, Drummond L, Livesey SA, Simpson IA. The evaluation of real-time 3-dimensional transthoracic echocardiography for the preoperative functional assessment

of patients with mitral valve prolapse: a comparison with 2-dimensional transesophageal echocardiography. *J Am Soc Echocardiogr* 2007; **20**(8):934–40.

28 Gutiérrez-Chico J, Zamorano Gómez J, Rodrigo-López J, Mataix L, Pérez de Isla L, Almería-Valera C, et al. Accuracy of real-time 3-dimensional echocardiography in the assessment of mitral prolapse. Is transesophageal echocardiography still mandatory? *Am Heart J* 2008; **155**(4):694–8.

29 Agricola E, Oppizzi M, Pisani M, Maisano F, Margonato A. Accuracy of real-time 3D echocardiography in the evaluation of functional anatomy of mitral regurgitation. *Int J Cardiol* 2008; **127**(3):342–9.

30 Sugeng L, Weinert L, Lang RM. Real-time 3-dimensional color Doppler flow of mitral and tricuspid regurgitation: feasibility and initial quantitative comparison with 2-dimensional methods. *J Am Soc Echocardiogr* 2007; **20**(9):1050–7.

31 Kahlert P, Plicht B, Schenk IM, Janosi R-A, Erbel R, Buck T. Direct assessment of size and shape of noncircular vena contracta area in functional versus organic mitral regurgitation using real-time three-dimensional echocardiography. *J Am Soc Echocardiogr* 2008; **21**(8):912–21.

32 Yosefy C, Levine RA, Solis J, Vaturi M, Handschumacher MD, Hung J. Proximal flow convergence region as assessed by real-time 3-dimensional echocardiography: challenging the hemispheric assumption. *J Am Soc Echocardiogr* 2007; **20**(4):389–96.

33 Sugeng L, Weinert L, Lammertin G, Thomas P, Spencer KT, Decara JM, et al. Accuracy of mitral valve area measurements using transthoracic rapid freehand 3-dimensional scanning: comparison with noninvasive and invasive methods. *J Am Soc Echocardiogr* 2003; **16**(12):1292–300.

34 Zamorano J, Perez de Isla L, Sugeng L, Cordeiro P, Rodrigo JL, Almeria C, et al. Non-invasive assessment of mitral valve area during percutaneous balloon mitral valvuloplasty: role of real-time 3D echocardiography. *Eur Heart J* 2004; **25**(23):2086–91.

35 Zamorano J, Cordeiro P, Sugeng L, Perez de Isla L, Weinert L, Macaya C, et al. Real-time three-dimensional echocardiography for rheumatic mitral valve stenosis evaluation: an accurate and novel approach. *J Am Coll Cardiol* 2004; **43**(11):2091–6.

36 Mannaerts HFJ, Kamp O, Visser CA. Should mitral valve area assessment in patients with mitral stenosis be based on anatomical or on functional evaluation? A plea for 3D echocardiography as the new clinical standard. *Eur Heart J* 2004; **25**(23):2073–4.

37 Anwar AM, Attia WM, Nosir YFM, Soliman OII, Mosad MA, Othman M, et al. Validation of a new score for the assessment of mitral stenosis using real-time three-dimensional echocardiography. *J Am Soc Echocardiogr* 2010; **23**:13–22.

38 Anwar AM, Soliman OII, Nemes A, Germans T, Krenning BJ, Geleijnse ML, et al. Assessment of mitral annulus size and function by real-time 3-dimensional echocardiography in cardiomyopathy: comparison with magnetic resonance imaging. *J Am Soc Echocardiogr* 2007; **20**(8):941–8.

39 Mahmood F, Subramaniam B, Gorman JH, Levine RM, Gorman RC, Maslow A, et al. Three-dimensional echocardiographic assessment of changes in mitral valve geometry after valve repair. *Ann Thorac Surg* 2009; **88**(6):1838–44.

40 Goland S, Trento A, Iida K, Czer LSC, De Robertis M, Naqvi TZ, et al. Assessment of aortic stenosis by three-dimensional echocardiography: an accurate and novel approach. *Heart* 2007; **93**(7):801–7.

41 Sukmawan R, Watanabe N, Ogasawara Y, Yamaura Y, Yamamoto K, Wada N, et al. Geometric changes of tricuspid valve tenting in tricuspid regurgitation secondary to pulmonary hypertension quantified by novel system with transthoracic real-time 3-dimensional echocardiography. *J Am Soc Echocardiogr* 2007; **20**(5):470–6.

42 Maffe S, Dellavesa P, Zenone F, Paino AM, Paffoni P, Perucca A, et al. Transthoracic second harmonic two- and three-dimensional echocardiography for detection of patent foramen ovale. *Eur J Echocardiogr* 2010; **11**(1):57–63.

43 Monte I, Grasso S, Licciardi S, Badano LP. Head-to-head comparison of real-time three-dimensional transthoracic echocardiography with transthoracic and transesophageal two-dimensional contrast echocardiography for the detection of patent foramen ovale. *Eur J Echocardiogr* 2010; **11**(3):245–9.

44 Matsumura Y, Hozumi T, Arai K, Sugioka K, Ujino K, Takemoto Y, et al. Non-invasive assessment of myocardial ischaemia using new real-time three-dimensional dobutamine stress echocardiography: comparison with conventional two-dimensional methods. *Eur Heart J* 2005; **26**(16):1625–32.

45 Bhan A, Kapetanakis S, Rana BS, Ho E, Wilson K, Pearson P, et al. Real-time three-dimensional myocardial contrast echocardiography: is it clinically feasible? *Eur J Echocardiogr* 2008; **9**(6):761–5.

46 Yoshitani H, Takeuchi M, Mor-Avi V, Otsuji Y, Hozumi T, Yoshiyama M. Comparative diagnostic accuracy of multiplane and multislice three-dimensional dobutamine stress echocardiography in the diagnosis of coronary artery disease. *J Am Soc Echocardiogr* 2009; **22**(5):437–42.

47 Bhan A, Kapetanakis S, Pearson P, Dworakowski R, Monaghan MJ. Percutaneous closure of an atrial septal defect guided by live three-dimensional transesophageal echocardiography. *J Am Soc Echocardiogr* 2009; **22**(6):753.e1–3.

48 Martin-Reyes R, López-Fernández T, Moreno-Yangüela M, Moreno R, Navas-Lobato MA, Refoyo E, et al. Role of real-time three-dimensional transoesophageal echocardiography for guiding transcatheter patent foramen ovale closure. *Eur J Echocardiogr* 2009; **10**(1):148–50.

49 Balzer J, van Hall S, Rassaf T, Boring Y-C, Franke A, Lang RM, et al. Feasibility, safety, and efficacy of real-time three-dimensional transoesophageal echocardiography for guiding device closure of interatrial communications: initial clinical experience and impact on radiation exposure. *Eur J Echocardiogr* 2010; **11**(1):1–8.

50 Eng MH, Salcedo EE, Quaife RA, Carroll JD. Implementation of real time three-dimensional transesophageal echocardiography in percutaneous mitral balloon valvuloplasty and structural heart disease interventions. *Echocardiography* 2009; **26**(8):958–66.

51 Chierchia GB, Capulzini L, de Asmundis C, Sarkozy A, Roos M, Paparella G, et al. First experience with real-time three-dimensional transoesophageal echocardiography-guided transseptal in patients undergoing atrial fibrillation ablation. *Europace* 2008; **10**(11):1325–8.

52 Bhan A, Dworakowski R, Smith LA, Maccarthy PA, Redwood S, El-Gamel A, et al. Does 3D transesophageal imaging add value to transcatheter aortic valve implantation? Experience in 150 cases. *J Am Coll Cardiol* 2010; **55**(10):A65.E610.

53 Pérez de Isla L, Balcones DV, Fernández-Golfín C, Marcos-Alberca P, Almería C, Rodrigo JL, et al. Three-dimensional-wall motion tracking: a new and faster tool for myocardial strain assessment: comparison with two-dimensional-wall motion tracking. *J Am Soc Echocardiogr* 2009; **22**(4):325–30.

54 Maffessanti F, Nesser H-J, Weinert L, Steringer-Mascherbauer R, Niel J, Gorissen W, et al. Quantitative evaluation of regional

left ventricular function using three-dimensional speckle tracking echocardiography in patients with and without heart disease. *Am J Cardiol* 2009; **104**(12):1755–62.

Further reading

Goland S, Trento A, Iida K, Czer LSC, De Robertis M, Naqvi TZ, *et al.* Assessment of aortic stenosis by three-dimensional echocardiography: an accurate and novel approach. *Heart* 2007; **93**(7):801–7.

Jenkins C, Chan J, Bricknell K, Strudwick M, Marwick TH. Reproducibility of right ventricular volumes and ejection fraction using real-time three-dimensional echocardiography: comparison with cardiac MRI. *Chest* 2007; **131**(6):1844–51.

Kapetanakis S, Kearney MT, Siva A, Gall N, Cooklin M, Monaghan MJ. Real-time three-dimensional echocardiography: a novel technique to quantify global left ventricular mechanical dyssynchrony. *Circulation* 2005; **112**(7):992–1000.

Kühl HP, Schreckenberg M, Rulands D, Katoh M, Schäfer W, Schummers G, *et al.* High-resolution transthoracic real-time three-dimensional echocardiography: quantitation of cardiac volumes and function using semi-automatic border detection and comparison with cardiac magnetic resonance imaging. *J Am Coll Cardiol* 2004; **43**(11):2083–90.

Mor-Avi V, Jenkins C, Kühl H, Nesser H-J, Marwick T, Franke A, *et al.* Real-time 3-dimensional echocardiographic quantification of left ventricular volumes: multicenter study for validation with magnetic resonance imaging and investigation of sources of error. *J Am Coll Cardiol: Cardiovas Imaging* 2008; **1**(4):413–23.

Perk G, Lang RM, Garcia-Fernandez MA, Lodato J, Sugeng L, Lopez J, *et al.* Use of real time three-dimensional transesophageal echocardiography in intracardiac catheter based interventions. *J Am Soc Echocardiogr* 2009; **22**(8):865–82.v

Soliman OII, Geleijnse ML, Theuns DAMJ, van Dalen BM, Vletter WB, Jordaens LJ, *et al.* Usefulness of left ventricular systolic dyssynchrony by real-time three-dimensional echocardiography to predict long-term response to cardiac resynchronization therapy. *Am J Cardiol* 2009; **103**(11):1586–91.

Sugeng L, Weinert L, Lang RM. Real-time 3-dimensional color Doppler flow of mitral and tricuspid regurgitation: feasibility and initial quantitative comparison with 2-dimensional methods. *J Am Soc Echocardiogr* 2007; **20**(9):1050–7.

Yang HS, Bansal RC, Mookadam F, Khandheria BK, Tajik AJ, Chandrasekaran K, *et al.* Practical guide for three-dimensional transthoracic echocardiography using a fully sampled matrix array transducer. *J Am Soc Echocardiogr* 2008; **21**(9):979–89; quiz 1081–2.

Zamorano J, Cordeiro P, Sugeng L, Perez de Isla L, Weinert L, Macaya C, *et al.* Real-time three-dimensional echocardiography for rheumatic mitral valve stenosis evaluation: an accurate and novel approach. *J Am Coll Cardiol* 2004; **43**(11):2091–6.

Online resource

European Society of Cardiology: 3D Echo Box. ✆ http://www.escardio.org/communities/EAE/3d-echo-box/Pages/welcome.aspx

Additional DVD and online material

▪ **3.1** Speckle tracking.

▪ **3.2** Assessment of LV volume and contractility.

▪ **3.3** Assessment of RV volume and contractility.

▪ **3.4** Assessment of mitral prosthesis.

▪ **3.5** View of MV leaflets and scallops.

▪ **3.6** 3D TOE view of patent foramen ovale.

▪ **3.7** 3D TOE view of patent foramen ovale.

▪ **3.8** 3D TOE view of patent foramen ovale.

▪ **3.9** Positioning of the balloon catheter across the aortic valve.

⊙ For additional multimedia materials please visit the online version of the book (✆ http://escecho.oxfordmedicine.com).

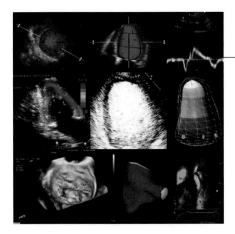

CHAPTER 4

Transoesophageal and intracardiac echocardiography

Christian Rost and Frank A. Flachskampf

Contents

Summary

Transoesophageal echocardiography (TOE), a minimal-risk, semi-invasive imaging procedure is nowadays an indispensable part of routine echocardiography. It is mainly necessary and indicated:

◆ To analyse some structures insufficiently seen transthoracically, such as the left atrial appendage or the thoracic aorta.

◆ In situations that prohibit the use of conventional transthoracic windows, such as the patient undergoing cardiac surgery.

As in transthoracic echocardiography (TTE), the TOE examination consists of a sequence of views defined by internal landmarks; unlike TTE, depending on the patient's tolerance and the clinical question, not all of these have to be obtained in every examination. Important typical indications for TOE are the search for signs of endocarditis, the search for cardiogenic emboli, diagnosis of left atrial (appendage) thrombi before cardioversion, diagnosis of aortic dissection, characterization of mitral and aortic valve pathology especially in the context of surgical repair, intraoperative monitoring of left ventricular function, and monitoring of interventional cardiac procedures monitored.

For some indications, intracardiac echocardiography has been found useful. This procedure involves insertion of a transducer-tipped catheter into the caval vein and advancement to the right heart, or intra-aortic placement. Applications are electrophysiological procedures, interventional closure of atrial septal defect, aortic stent placement, and others.

Introduction

Transoesophageal echocardiography (TOE) is a semi-invasive diagnostic procedure which uses the upper gastrointestinal tract to image cardiovascular structures, thus avoiding the problems for ultrasound imaging created by the thoracic ribcage and the lungs. It is therefore indicated when transthoracic echocardiography (TTE) is unable or unlikely to answer the clinical question, which may be related either to structures difficult to image transthoracically, e.g. the left atrial (LA) appendage, or to situations such as cardiac surgery or interventions which prohibit the use of classic echo windows. Being a semi-invasive procedure, a small risk of harm to the patient and some discomfort in the awake patient have to be considered.

TOE was introduced in the 1980s,[1] although early experiences with transoesophageal Doppler go back to the 1970s.[2] The probes first incorporated a transducer with a fixed horizontal (orthogonal to the shaft axis) two-dimensional (2D) cross-section and then evolved to biplane and nowadays multiplane transducers, in which the 2D cross-section can be rotated by 180 degrees by an electric motor. The marked improvement in the diagnosis of LA thrombi, of endocarditic vegetations and abscesses, and of aortic dissection afforded by TOE led to rapid dissemination and adoption,[3] and it has become a standard and indispensable technique which should be available in every echocardiographic laboratory as well as in every centre performing cardiac surgery.

In 2001, the Working Group on Echocardiography of the European Society of Cardiology (ESC) published the first TOE guidelines,[4] which were recently updated.[5] Cardiothoracic anaesthetists and cardiac surgeons became aware of the new possibility to monitor cardiac anatomy and function intraoperatively via the oesophagus, and to check operative results, especially in mitral valve (MV) repair, before closure of the chest.[6] The new technique was very quickly embraced and nowadays is considered standard, especially in cardiac valve surgery.

Equipment and training

Modern TOE transducers are multiplane (rotatable by 180 degrees inside their housing), operate at frequencies of 5–7MHz, and provide all echocardiographic modalities, especially Doppler modes (◗ Fig. 4.1A,B). The instrument tip that houses the transducer can be flexed mechanically in the lateral or anteroposterior direction. Most modern echo machines, including some portable devices, allow connection of a TOE transducer. The latest development is three-dimensional (3D) matrix transducers, which beside real-time 3D echo also provide all classic modalities. TOE transducers need to be properly maintained, by:

◆ Disinfection: this is necessary after each use and requires immersion of probe tip and shaft in a cleaning solution for 20–30min.

◆ Inspection for mechanical damage: it not only can affect the functions of the instrument, but also lead to a break of the electrical insulation, exposing the patient to the risk of electrical injury. Periodic checks for leakage current are therefore advised by the manufactures. In any case, visual inspection for damage, especially by the patient's teeth, is mandatory. A bite guard should be used with each examination (and properly disinfected thereafter), but physical damage to the probe can nevertheless occur.

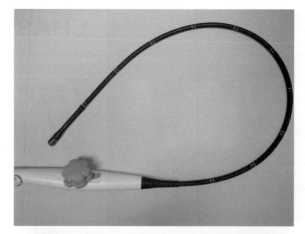

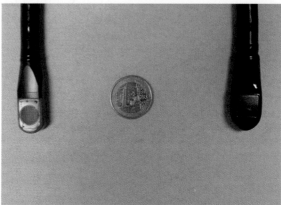

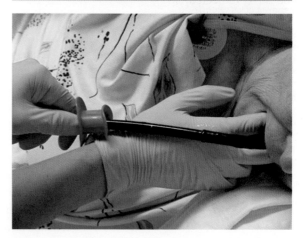

Figure 4.1 Equipment. A) Transoesophageal probe with handle (white) carrying knobs for tip flexion and rotation of plane, and transducer-tipped shaft (black). B) Transoesophageal probe tips encasing the transducer. Left, typical multiplane 2D probe, right, 3D matrix array probe. A €1 coin is shown for size comparison. C) Introduction of the probe guided by the examiners index and middle finger, with patient in a left lateral decubitus position. Note bite guard to be positioned after the probe has entered the upper oesophagus.

Correct maintenance should be documented in written notes. Standards for a TOE echo laboratory have been established by the European Association of Echocardiography (EAE),[7] specifying a minimum room size of 20m², cleaning and sterilizing equipment, suction, oxygen supply, resuscitation equipment and monitoring facilities for electrocardiogram (ECG), blood pressure, and oxygen saturation during TOE and subsequent recovery.

TOE competence requires acquisition of knowledge and practical skills by supervised training; for cardiologists, full competence in TTE is a prerequisite. Besides national regulations, the EAE and the European Association of Cardiac Anaesthesiologists have set up an accreditation procedure in TOE which requires individuals to train under a supervisor, to pass a multiple choice question exam, and to submit a log book of cases.[8]

Indications and risks

In general, TOE is indicated when important diagnostic information cannot be obtained by transthoracic examination. Cardiovascular structures better seen by TOE than transthoracically are the LA appendage, the pulmonary veins, the atrial septum, the superior vena cava, and the thoracic aorta. Mitral and aortic valvular abnormalities, in particular small vegetations and abscesses, and prosthetic valve abnormalities are generally better detected by TOE, and TOE affords superior imaging for valvular and other interventional procedures such as closure of patent foramen ovale (PFO) or atrial septal defects. On the other hand, in some patients and scenarios, transthoracic examination is very difficult or impossible (e.g. ventilated or intraoperative patients) and in this case TOE may be the only option for echocardiographic examination. In ➜ Table 4.1 a list of typical indications is summarized.

Serious complications of TOE are very rare and include:

◆ Laryngospasm.

◆ Arrhythmias (including cardiac arrest).

◆ Oesophageal perforation.

◆ Haemorrhage from oesophageal tumour.

Mortality is about 1 in 10 000.[9,10] If substantial resistance to introduction or advancement of the probe is encountered, upper endoscopy should be performed prior to a new attempt; the probe should never be forced. Oesophageal perforation may manifest with delay, causing fever, neck pain, and subcutaneous emphysema. Death during or immediately after TOE has been reported in patients with acute aortic dissection and ascribed to a sudden surge in blood pressure due to the examination. Therefore, blood pressure must be well controlled during an examination for suspected aortic dissection. Anticoagulation or thrombocytopenia raise the bleeding risk but are not strict contraindications to TOE. The most frequent problem during introduction of the probe is entrapment of the tip in the piriform recess, resulting in an elastic obstruction. Sedation may lead to hypoxia and apnoea. Methaemoglobinaemia due to the topical anaesthetic agents prilocaine and benzocaine has been observed in rare instances.[11] Endocarditis prophylaxis is not indicated for TOE.

The examination

Patient preparation

The patient should be asked about problems with swallowing or known upper gastrointestinal tract disease. Written informed consent should be obtained whenever possible and before sedation. The patient should fast for at least 4 hours before TOE. Most laboratories use topical oropharyngeal anaesthesia prior to probe insertion. Mild sedation, e.g. intravenous midazolam (2–4mg), is often beneficial, especially in younger patients, but use varies widely.

Introduction of the probe

The patient is positioned in a left lateral decubitus position to help drain saliva, with the head mildly flexed anteriorly (opposite to the position during tracheal intubation). An intravenous line should be in place both for sedation and in the event of complications, and a supply of oxygen as well as equipment for suction should be at hand, especially if sedation is used. During probe introduction and examination, ECG monitoring is mandatory, and oxygen saturation monitoring is useful. The probe is introduced into the mouth and the conscious patient asked to swallow. The probe can be guided by middle and index finger of the examiner to avoid deviation of the tip from the midline (➜ Fig. 4.1C). Some resistance is usually encountered at the upper oesophageal sphincter, which subsides if the patient actively swallows. If introduction fails, it may be helpful to attempt it again with the patient sitting up, or by increasing sedation; however, too much sedation renders the patient uncooperative. Once the probe has passed the upper oesophagus, the bite guard should be positioned and the probe advanced until at approximately 30–40 cm distance from the front teeth cardiac structures come into view.

General course of the examination

Unlike TTE, TOE is uncomfortable for the patient. Thus, depending on patient tolerance and circumstances, the examiner may restrict the examination to the main clinical indication, such as scanning the LA appendage and LA to rule out thrombi before the electrical cardioversion of atrial fibrillation. On the other hand, in the sedated or anaesthetized patient, a systematic and thorough approach yields maximal diagnostic benefit.

TOE views are defined by internal landmarks, not by specification of probe position and plane angulation. The manoeuvres available to the examiner to change the position of the view are:

◆ Plane rotation: to switch from transverse to longitudinal in biplane probes. 0 degrees denotes a transverse and 90 degrees a vertical position of the cross-sectional plane, with clockwise plane rotation when looking in the direction of the ultrasound beam.

Table 4.1 Principal TEE indications: essential views and structures in specific clinical situations*

1) Search for a potential cardiovascular source of embolism
Left ventricular apex or aneurysm (transgastric and low transoesophageal two-chamber views)
Aortic and mitral valve (look for vegetations, degenerative changes, or tumours, e.g. fibroelastoma)
Ascending and descending aorta, aortic arch
Left atrial appendage (including pulsed wave Doppler); note spontaneous contrast
Left atrial body including atrial septum; note spontaneous contrast
Fossa ovalis/foramen ovale/atrial septal defect/atrial septal aneurysm; contrast + Valsalva
2) Infective endocarditis
Mitral valve in multiple cross-sections
Aortic valve in long- and short-axis views; para-aortic tissue (in particular short-axis views of aortic valve and aortic root) to rule out abscess
Tricuspid valve in transgastric views, low oesophageal view, and right ventricular inflow–outflow view
Pacemaker, central intravenous lines, aortic grafts, Eustachian valve, pulmonary valve in high basal short-axis view of the right heart (inflow–outflow view of the right ventricle)
3) Aortic dissection, aortic aneurysm
Ascending aorta in long- and short-axis views; note maximal diameter, flap, intramural haematoma, para-aortic fluid
Descending aorta in long- and short-axis views, note maximal diameter, flap, intramural haematoma, para-aortic fluid
Aortic arch, note maximal diameter, flap, intramural haematoma, para-aortic fluid
Aortic valve (regurgitation—note mechanism, annular diameter, number of cusps)
Relation of dissection membrane to coronary ostia
Pericardial effusion, pleural effusion
Entry/reentry sites of dissection (use colour Doppler)
Spontaneous contrast or thrombus formation in false lumen (use colour Doppler to characterize flow/absence of flow in false lumen)
4) Mitral regurgitation
Mitral anatomy (transgastric basal short-axis view, multiple lower transoesophageal views). Emphasis on detection of mechanism and origin of regurgitation (detection and mapping of prolapse/flail to leaflets and scallops, papillary muscle and chordal integrity, vegetations, paraprosthetic leaks)
Colour Doppler mapping of regurgitant jet with emphasis on jet width and proximal convergence zone
Left upper pulmonary, and, if eccentric jet present, also right upper pulmonary venous pulsed Doppler
5) Prosthetic valve evaluation
Morphological and/or Doppler evidence of obstruction (reduced opening/mobility of cusps/discs/leaflets and elevated velocities by continuous wave Doppler)
Morphological and Doppler evidence of regurgitation, with mapping of the origin of regurgitation to specific sites (transprosthetic, paraprosthetic); presence of dehiscence/rocking of prosthesis
Presence of morphological changes in the prosthetic structure: calcification, immobilization, rupture, or perforation of bioprosthesis leaflets; absence of occluder in mechanical prostheses
Presence of additional paraprosthetic structures (vegetation/thrombus/pannus, suture material, strand, abscess, pseudoaneurysm, fistula)
6) Intraoperative TOE
Surgical valvular repair (mitral or aortic), with assessment of success before chest closure
Assessment of left and right global and regional ventricular function, as well as valve function, in patients during and after bypass surgery; monitoring of intracardiac air and venting
Assessment of left and right global and regional ventricular function, as well as valve function and aortic integrity, in patients with sudden intraoperative haemodynamic deterioration (including non-cardiac surgery)
Assessment of aortic pathology
7) TOE during interventional cardiac procedures
Mitral valvuloplasty (search for LA thrombi, guidance of trans-septal puncture, assessment of valvuloplasty result including post-valvuloplasty regurgitation
Interventional closure of atrial septal defects, patent foramen ovale, paraprosthetic leaks, or left atrial appendage
Percutaneous or transapical aortic valve implantation, including pre-interventional measurement of left ventricular outflow tract diameter
Percutaneous mitral valve repair

* Modified, with permission, from Flachskampf FA, Decoodt P, Fraser AG, Daniel WG, Roelandt JRTC; for the Subgroup on Transoesophageal Echocardiography and Valvular Heart Disease, on behalf of the Working Group on Echocardiography of the European Society of Cardiology. Recommendations for performing transoesophageal echocardiography. *Eur J Echocardiogr* 2001; **2**;8–21.

◆ Shaft rotation: clockwise or counterclockwise as seen from the examiner's viewpoint looking down the shaft of the probe.

◆ Anteflexion: to flex the tip mechanically upwards anteriorly, thereby usually improving contact with the anterior gastric or oesophageal wall.

◆ Retroflexion: to flex the tip upwards posteriorly, thereby often deteriorating transducer contact with the gastric or oesophageal wall.

◆ Sideward (lateral) flexion of the tip (to the right or left of the transducer face): it can be used instead of plane rotation to fine-tune views and improve contact with oesophageal or gastric wall, but is less important with the use of multiplane transducers.

◆ Probe advancement and withdrawal.

The complete examination comprises three major steps:

◆ The transoesophageal examination, with lower oesophageal views, mainly to image the ventricles (➲ Fig. 4.2), and upper transoesophageal views, mainly to image the valves, atria, and great vessels (➲ Figs. 4.3 and 4.4). However, sharply defined transducer positions or windows do not exist, since they vary individually and have to be adjusted for each view. Often, upper and lower transoesophageal views can be obtained from approximately the same transducer position

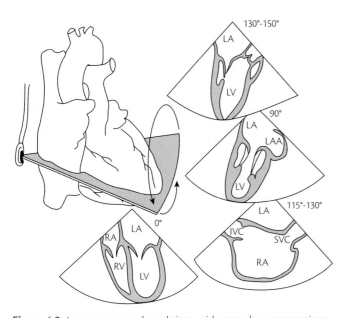

Figure 4.2 Lower transoesophageal views, with exemplary cross-sections corresponding to (counter-clockwise) the four-chamber view, two-chamber view, and long-axis view of the left ventricle (LV). A right atrial longitudinal (sagittal, bicaval) view is visualized at 90–120 degrees. IVC, inferior vena cava; LA, left atrium; LAA, left atrial appendage; RA, right atrium; RV, right ventricle; SVC, superior vena cava. Reproduced, with permission, from Flachskampf FA, Decoodt P, Fraser AG, Daniel WG, Roelandt JRTC; for the Subgroup on Transoesophageal Echocardiography and Valvular Heart Disease, on behalf of the Working Group on Echocardiography of the European Society of Cardiology. Recommendations for performing transoesophageal echocardiography. *Eur J Echocardiogr* 2001; **2**;8–21.

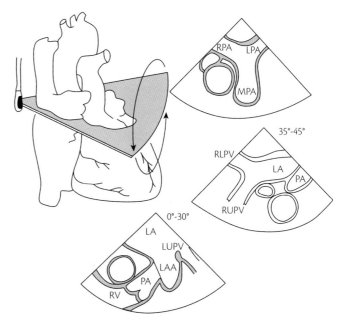

Figure 4.3 Upper transoesophageal views of the great vessels and atrial appendage (counterclockwise): the transverse view of the left atrial appendage (LAA) and the left upper pulmonary vein (LUPV) (0–30 degrees), the intermediate view of the ascending aorta (Ao), left atrium (LA), and right pulmonary veins, and with anterioflexion of the probe a transverse view of the ascending aorta, superior vena cava (SVC) and main pulmonary artery (MPA) with its bifurcation are obtained. LPA, left pulmonary artery; PA, pulmonary artery; RPA, right pulmonary artery; RUPV, right upper pulmonary vein; RV, right ventricle. Reproduced, with permission, from Flachskampf FA, Decoodt P, Fraser AG, Daniel WG, Roelandt JRTC; for the Subgroup on Transoesophageal Echocardiography and Valvular Heart Disease, on behalf of the Working Group on Echocardiography of the European Society of Cardiology. Recommendations for performing transoesophageal echocardiography. *Eur J Echocardiogr* 2001; **2**;8–21.

by flexing or extending the tip of the transducer, since the optimal oesophageal window often is small.

◆ The transgastric examination.

◆ The examination of the aorta.

The sequence of these elements may be chosen individually; many operators start with transoesophageal views, followed by transgastric views, and finally visualize the descending aorta and aortic arch pulling the instrument back from the position in the gastric fundus. Additional views are frequently necessary to better delineate pathological findings.

Lower transoesophageal views

With the instrument in the transverse position immediately above the diaphragm level, the orifice of the inferior vena cava (IVC), the right atrium (RA), the coronary sinus, and the tricuspid valve (TV) are visualized in a long-axis view. The anterior (or sometimes posterior) tricuspid leaflet is seen to the left, and the septal to the right on the screen. Retracting the probe, a (foreshortened) transoesophageal four-chamber view is obtained (➲ Fig. 4.5). The probe tip should be straightened to

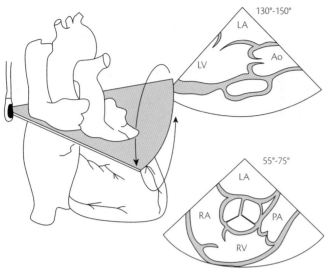

Figure 4.4 Transoesophageal views of the aortic valve. Transoesophageal views of the aortic valve in long-axis (130–150 degrees) and short-axis views (40–60 degrees). Ao, ascending aorta; LA, left atrium; LV, left ventricle; PA, pulmonary artery; RA, right atrium; RV, right ventricle. Reproduced, with permission, from Flachskampf FA, Decoodt P, Fraser AG, Daniel WG, Roelandt JRTC; for the Subgroup on Transoesophageal Echocardiography and Valvular Heart Disease, on behalf of the Working Group on Echocardiography of the European Society of Cardiology. Recommendations for performing transoesophageal echocardiography. *Eur J Echocardiogr* 2001; **2**;8–21.

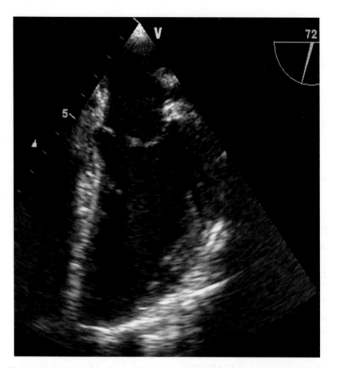

Figure 4.6 Transoesophageal two-chamber view.

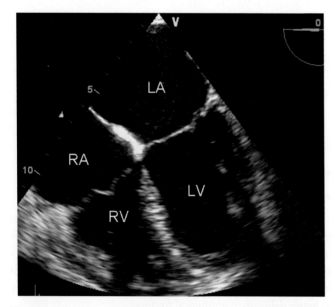

Figure 4.5 Transoesophageal four-chamber view. LA, left atrium; LV, left ventricle; PA, pulmonary artery; RA, right atrium; RV, right ventricle.

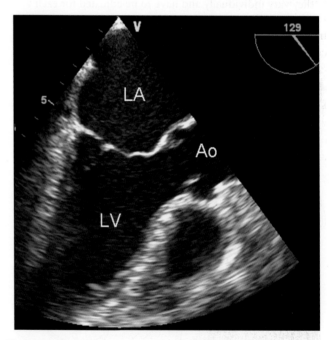

Figure 4.7 Transoesophageal long-axis view. Ao, ascending aorta; LA, left atrium; LV, left ventricle.

minimize foreshortening, as long as image quality is maintained. In the transoesophageal four-chamber view the left ventricle (LV) is on the right side of the sector and the right ventricle (RV) on the left; the LA is on top. The anterior mitral leaflet is seen on the left and the posterior on the right side; the septal tricuspid leaflet is on the right side and the anterior tricuspid leaflet on the left side. The transoesophageal two-chamber view

(● Fig. 4.6) is obtained at approximately 60–90 degrees, with the anterior wall to the right and the inferior wall to the left. Here, the posterior mitral leaflet is on the left side and the anterior leaflet on the right side. Frequently, the LA appendage is seen on the right side of the screen at the base of the LV. Plane rotation to 120–150 discloses the transoesophageal long-axis view of the LV (● Fig. 4.7), with the anterior mitral leaflet, the aortic valve (AoV) and ascending aorta, and the anteroseptal

LV segments on the right side, and the posterior mitral leaflet and posterior LV wall on the left side. The MV can be studied in detail (after appropriate depth reduction) in the same views enumerated for the LV. For further examination of the MV (see → Chapter 14b) 'Assessment of the mitral valve' section. Spontaneous echo contrast (*smoke*) in the LA and/or appendage should be noted; gain must be high enough to detect it.

Upper transoesophageal views

Anteflexion of the tip or withdrawal of the probe will display the AoV and both atria from an upper transoesophageal position. Pulmonary vein flow can be recorded by pulsed Doppler from both the left and the right upper pulmonary veins. Short- and long-axis views of the AoV (→ Figs. 4.8 and 4.9) should be obtained, generally the former at 40–70 degrees and the latter at 130–160 degrees. The long-axis view has the non-coronary aortic cusp on top and the right coronary cusp at the bottom (anteriorly); it also visualizes the ascending aorta coursing anteriorly of the right pulmonary artery (PA) (some retraction of the probe may be necessary to display this). The short-axis view shows the left coronary cusp in the upper right third, the non-coronary cusp in the upper left third, and the right coronary cusp in the lower third (anteriorly). Slightly withdrawing the transducer, the coronary ostia can be identified at approximately 2 o'clock (left coronary ostium) and 6 o'clock (right coronary ostium) of the circumference of the aortic root (→ Fig. 4.10A,B). The right coronary ostium is frequently visualized more easily in the long axis view of the AoV. Colour Doppler (CD) mapping should be performed in both AoV views. Spectral Doppler assessment of aortic flow velocities is better achieved in transgastric long-axis views due to more coaxial beam alignment. The short-axis view of the AoV

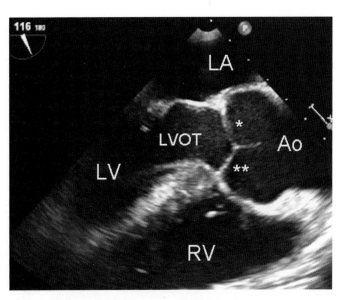

Figure 4.9 Long-axis view of the aortic valve. Long-axis view of the aortic valve with non-coronary (*) and right coronary leaflet (**), the left ventricular outflow tract (LVOT) and the ascending aorta (Ao). LA, left atrium; LV, left ventricle; RV, right ventricle.

(→ Fig. 4.11) also shows RA, TV, inflow and outflow tract of the RV, pulmonary valve (PV), and main pulmonary trunk in counterclockwise continuity. This view (sometimes called the RV inflow–outflow view) resembles an upside-down parasternal short-axis view of the same structures. CD evaluation of the TV and—less satisfactorily of—the PV can be performed. From an upper transoesophageal window, the atrial septum with the oval fossa should be visualized in at least two planes (transverse and longitudinal or sagittal view). The transverse view of the RA is usually a minor modification of the transoesophageal four-chamber view with reduced depth. It shows the LA on top, the atrial septum as an approximately horizontal structure, and the TV to the right. Neither caval vein is seen in this view. The longitudinal, sagittal, or bicaval view of the RA (at approximately 90 degrees, → Fig. 4.12) displays the orifices of the superior (right sector side) and inferior caval veins (left sector side) and the RA appendage; the TV is not seen. This view allows, in particular, the evaluation of the atrial septum for defects, aneurysms, and the foramen ovale; moreover, of pacemaker leads and intravenous lines including a small stretch of the superior vena cava. If patency of the foramen ovale is to be checked, echo contrast should be applied and monitored during spontaneous breathing and, importantly, on release of a Valsalva manoeuvre. Any kind of right heart echo contrast can be used, including agitated blood or air microbubbles, as long as they yield dense opacification of the RA (see → Chapter 7).

Views of cranial structures of the heart and great vessels are obtained by withdrawing and anteflecting the probe in the transverse (0 degree) plane from a position showing the MV in the centre of the sector. On the right side of the screen, the LA appendage is seen (→ Fig. 4.13); examination of this highly variable structure often requires additional plane rotation

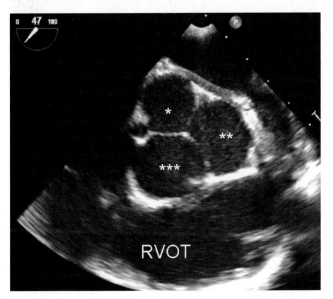

Figure 4.8 Short-axis view of the aortic valve. Short-axis view of the aortic valve with non-coronary (*), left coronary (**) and right coronary (***) leaflet and sinus. RVOT, right ventricular outflow tract.

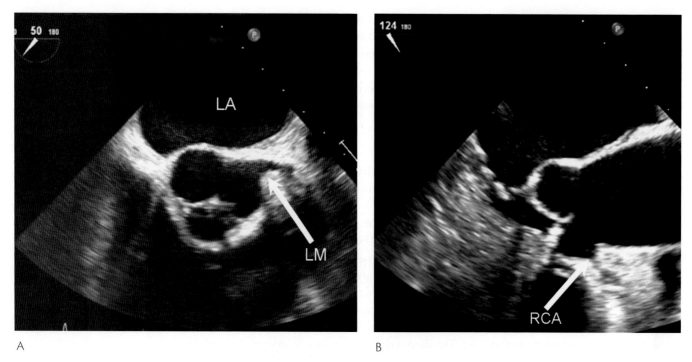

Figure 4.10 Take-off of the main coronary arteries. A) Modified short-axis view of aortic valve with take-off of the left main (LM) coronary artery (arrow). B) Modified long-axis view of aortic valve with take-off of the right coronary artery (RCA) (arrow). LA, left atrium.

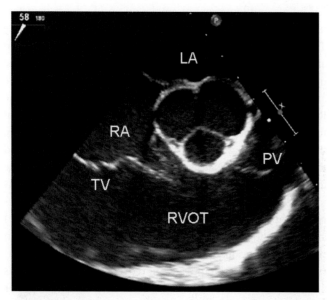

Figure 4.11 Short-axis view of aortic valve and right heart structures. LA, left atrium; PV, pulmonary valve; RA, right atrium; RVOT, right ventricular outflow tract; TV, tricuspid valve.

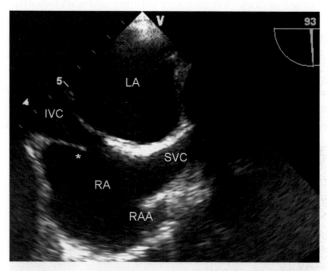

Figure 4.12 Bicaval view. Bicaval (sagittal, longitudinal) view of the right atrium (RA) with the orifices of the superior (SVC) and inferior caval veins (IVC). Next to the inferior caval vein, a Eustachian valve is displayed (*); next to the superior caval vein, the right atrial appendage (RAA) is visible; arrow, foramen ovale. LA, left atrium.

between 0 and 90 degrees. Pulsed wave (PW) Doppler recording of appendage flow is useful to assess the risk of thrombus formation. Further withdrawal and anteflexion displays the left upper pulmonary vein (➲ Fig. 4.14). Clockwise shaft rotation displays the short-axis view of the ascending aorta, accompanied on the left side by the superior vena cava (➲ Fig. 4.15), and on the right side by the main PA (➲ Fig. 4.16). The right PA courses to the

left side of the sector posteriorly of the ascending aorta. The left PA is poorly seen and courses to the right side of the sector.

The orifice of the right upper pulmonary vein is seen posterior to the superior vena cava, both in transverse and longitudinal views (➲ Fig. 4.15). This junction is the location of the transthoracically often poorly visualized sinus venosus atrial defects.

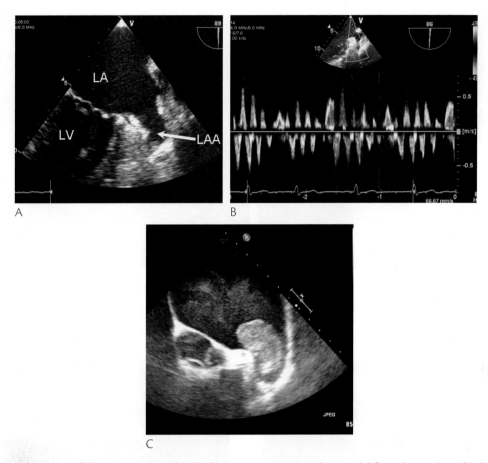

Figure 4.13 Transoesophageal view of left atrial appendage (LAA). A) Upper transoesophageal view with left atrial appendage. B) Pulsed Doppler recording of inflow and outflow velocities in the left atrial appendage in atrial fibrillation; the velocities are relatively high (mostly >25cm/s), indicating relatively low thrombotic risk. C) Large thrombus originating in the left atrial appendage of a patient in atrial fibrillation. Also note spontaneous echo contrast ('smoke') in the left atrium.

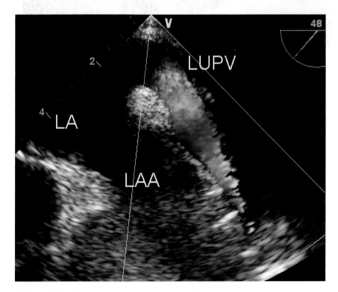

Figure 4.14 Transoesophageal view of left upper pulmonary vein (LUPV), next to the left atrial appendage (LAA), with colour Doppler image of blood flow directed into the left atrium (LA).

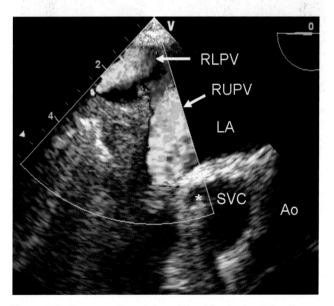

Figure 4.15 Transoesophageal view of blood flowing into left atrium (LA). Right pulmonary veins with blood flow directed into the left atrium (LA). Next to the pulmonary veins, the superior caval vein with a pacemaker wire (*) is seen. Ao, ascending aorta; RLPV, right lower pulmonary vein; RUPV, right upper pulmonary vein.

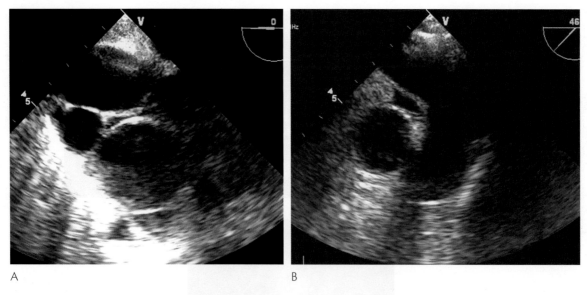

Figure 4.16 Transoesophageal view of great vessels. A) Upper transoesophageal view of ascending aorta, superior vena cava, and right pulmonary artery. B) Upper transoesophageal view of main pulmonary artery and pulmonary artery bifurcation.

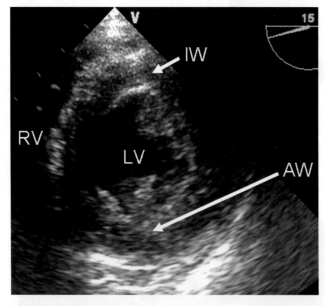

Figure 4.17 Transgastric short-axis view of the left ventricle (LV). AW, anterior wall; IW, inferior wall; RV, right ventricle.

Figure 4.18 Transgastric two-chamber view. Transgastric two-chamber view of left ventricle (LV) and left atrium, displaying also the mitral valve with papillary muscles and chordae tendineae. Note left atrial appendage (LAA).

Transgastric views

With the transducer in the gastric fundus, LV short-axis and two-chamber views are acquired (⊃ Figs. 4.17 and 4.18). In the LV short-axis view at the mid-papillary level (at 0 degrees), the anterolateral papillary muscle is seen at approximately 5 o'clock and the posteromedial approximately between 11 and 2 o'clock. The inferior wall is seen in the near field of the sector and the anterior wall at the bottom of the sector. In the LV two-chamber view (at 90 degrees), the apex, which often is not well visualized, is to the left and the MV to the right of the sector. The long-axis view of the LV, with assessment of left ventricular outflow tract (LVOT) and AoV, is obtained at approximately 100–120 degrees

and sometimes minor clockwise shaft rotation; this view is often difficult to obtain. Blood flow velocities in the LVOT or through the AoV can be documented. Additionally, or alternatively in case of difficulty in obtaining the long-axis view of the LV from the typical transgastric position, a deep transgastric long-axis view or five-chamber view, including the AoV, can be produced by advancing the probe further into the gastric fundus and using maximal anteflexion of the probe (*inverted* transducer position). Note that this view will display cardiac structures roughly like a transthoracic subcostal four-chamber view. The short-axis view of the MV (⊃ Fig. 4.19) is obtained by slightly withdrawing and anteflexing the instrument from the mid-papillary short-axis view position.

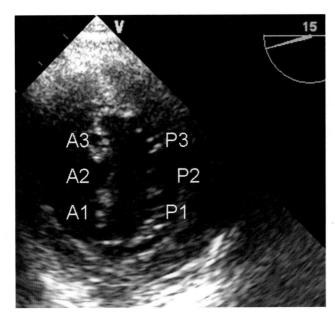

Figure 4.19 Transgastric short-axis view. Transgastric short-axis view of the mitral valve with visualization of the segments of the anterior (A1–3) and posterior leaflet (P1–3) (for detail, see text: ⊃ 'Assessment of the mitral valve').

Additional non-routine views of the right heart are generated by rotating the probe from the transgastric LV short-axis position to the right, positioning the RV in the centre of the sector, and steering the plane angulation first to approximately 30 degrees, producing a short-axis view of the TV, with the posterior leaflet to the upper left, the septal leaflet to the upper right, and the large anterior leaflet in the lower half of valve cross-section. A RV inflow view can be obtained by further rotation. At approximately 90 degrees a long axis of the RV inflow is seen. Further rotation discloses the right ventricular outflow tract (RVOT), with the PV located at the bottom of the sector.

Aortic views

Unless aortic pathology is the primary indication for a study, the thoracic aorta is usually examined at the end of the TOE examination. Between the abdomen and the aortic arch, the oesophagus and the descending aorta change their anterior–posterior relationships: at the diaphragm the oesophagus lies anterior to the aorta, at the aortic arch it is posterior. Therefore scanning the complete length of the thoracic descending aorta necessitates gentle rotation of the probe to maintain correct visualization of aortic walls (⊃ Fig. 4.20). Pathology should always be documented both in short- and long-axis views of the aorta. The take-off of the left subclavian artery can usually be seen, and often part of the distal arch and the supra-aortic branches can be visualized; probe shaft rotation may be useful to adjust the images.

Clockwise rotation and slight probe withdrawal at the junction of aortic arch and descending aorta displays the long axis of the aortic arch, with the anterior aortic arch wall in the far field of the sector, and partially the superior ascending aorta.

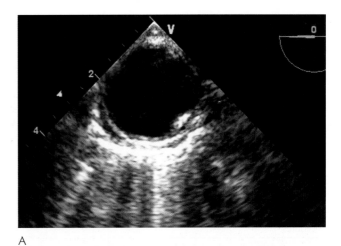

A

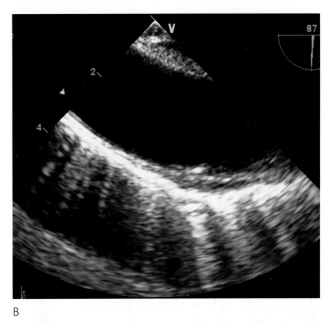

B

Figure 4.20 Short- and long-axis views of the descending thoracic aorta. Short- (A) and long-axis (B) views of the descending thoracic aorta. Note reverberation artefact in the long-axis view, creating false 'second lumen' in the far field. In the short-axis view an echodense atherosclerotic plaque is seen at 4 o'clock.

At 90 degrees, a short axis of the aortic arch is obtained. By rotating the transducer and advancing further into the oesophagus the distal portion of the ascending aorta may be recorded. However, due to the interposition of the trachea or left main bronchus, some portion of the arch or distal ascending aorta will usually not be visualized. The location of findings in the descending aorta can be described either by the distance of the probe tip to the frontal teeth, or by the cardiac structures at the same depth level.

3D TOE

3D TOE is a recent addition to the diagnostic armamentarium which is particularly suited for valvular heart disease and to accompany interventional procedures. 3D frame rates are

Table 4.2 Applications for 3D TOE

Mitral valve disease, especially mitral valve prolapse. The main advantage of 3D TEE is the accurate identification of location and extent of pathology (e.g., flail segments), particularly in en-face views ('surgeon's view') of the atrial side of the mitral valve

Aortic valve disease. 3D TEE helps to planimeter the valvular orifice area in aortic stenosis and the regurgitant orifice area in aortic regurgitation

Prosthetic valves, in particular to define location and extension of paraprosthetic leaks

Congenital heart disease, especially atrial septal defects

Guidance of percutaneous interventional procedures, especially closure of paraprosthetic leaks and atrial septal defects, and interventional valvular procedures

relatively low (25–28/s in *full volume*, higher for datasets recorded with a narrower sector angle). To obtain good quality, images and also CD should first be optimized in 2D mode, with special emphasis on gain and compression, and then re-adjusted in live 3D mode before final acquisition[12–14]. Typical applications where 3D TOE has been found to be useful are enumerated in Table 4.2.

Assessment of specific cardiac structures

Assessment of left ventricle

The six walls of the left ventricle and 17 segments (see Chapter 8) can be seen in the long axis using the standard mid-oesophageal views. These can be developed by placing the transducer at a mid-oesophageal depth of 30–40cm, and then rotating the multiplane transducer from the start position of 0–20 degrees, through to approximately 120 degrees. The depth of the transducer will not need to be altered although some retroflexion of the tip may be required to visualize the true apex and prevent a foreshortened image. The apical segments of the LV are often visualized, by gently advancing the probe, without rotation of the transducer, 2–4cm from the mid-cavity position. However, frequently the view is either poor or the deep transgastric view becomes apparent. The apical segments are therefore often best seen using the long-axis mid-oesophageal views.

The short axis of the LV may be assessed by developing the standard short-axis transgastric, mid cavity, and basal views. From the midcavity position (40–50cm, transducer angle 0–20 degrees, marked anteflexion) the probe is withdrawn gently and slowly until the basal view is developed and the mitral annulus becomes visible. The probe does not usually have to be rotated or turned.

Assessment of the mitral valve

TOE provides a multitude of possible cross-sections through the MV. The MV is seen in transgastric views either in the

transgastric two-chamber view (90 degrees), with the posterior leaflet at the top of the sector image and the anterior leaflet at the bottom, or in a short-axis view (0 degrees), which is somewhat more difficult to obtain with reasonable quality than by TTE.

From the transoesophageal window, the MV can be systematically scanned in three fundamental ways (Fig 4.21):

◆ By positioning it in the centre of the imaging sector and systematically steering the transducer through a 180 degree arc (Fig.4.17A).

◆ By systematically pulling back the probe from a *deep* to a *high* oesophageal position, with the cross-section fixed horizontally (0 degrees; Fig. 4.17B).

◆ By systematically rotating the probe shaft with the probe in a vertical (90 degrees) position (Fig.4.17C).

In practice, some combination of the three manoeuvres is used, depending on image quality, clinical question, and patient tolerance.

The transgastric long-axis view allows visualization of the papillary muscles and the chordae tendinae. Although the deep transgastric view will also allow visualization of the mitral leaflets, this view rarely adds to the evaluation of the MV.

Mitral regurgitation can be examined as to mechanism, location, and severity, as well as the likelihood of successful surgical repair assessed. Pathology such as prolapse and flail can be mapped to the segments of the mitral leaflets, to guide surgical repair techniques: the anterior and posterior leaflets meet at the medial and lateral commissures. Anterior and posterior leaflets typically are constituted by three distinct scallops: lateral (A1 and P1, respectively), central (A2 and P2, respectively), and medial (A3 and P3, respectively). The scallops are visualized by different views (Fig 4.21):

◆ A2 and P2 in transoesophageal four-chamber and long-axis view.

◆ A3 and P1, by rotating the image plane from 0 degree to 45 degrees.

◆ P3 and P1, by rotating the image plane of 60 degrees to 90 degrees to obtain the so-called *bicommissural view*

Moreover, by starting from a transoesophageal four-chamber view and tilting the image plane superiorly or slightly withdrawing the probe, A1 and P1 are visualized; whereas, by tilting posteriorly or advancing the probe, A3 and P3 are displayed. The entire anterior and posterior leaflets also are visualized by turning the probe rightward and leftward, respectively, from the two-chamber or bicommissural view.

TOE also offers easy access to pulmonary venous flow recording, especially of the left and right upper pulmonary vein. This is important in the assessment of severity of mitral regurgitation. Mitral prostheses are assessed in a similar way as the native MV. By systematic plane rotation, with the prosthesis centred in the imaging sector, the entire prosthesis and its full

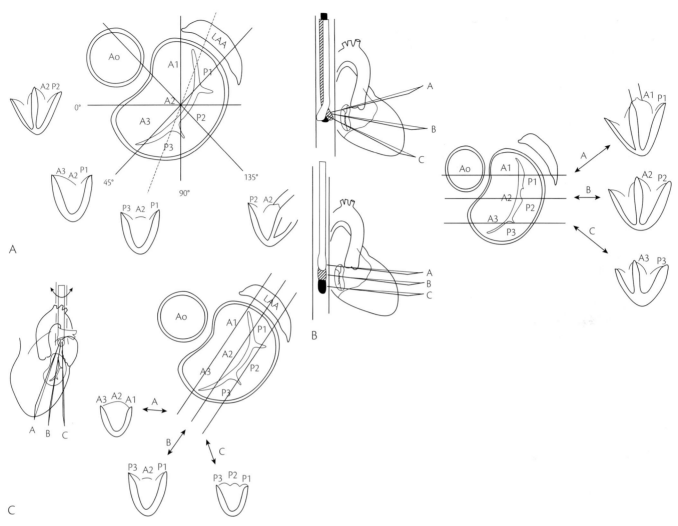

Figure 4.21 Examination of the mitral valve. Screen depiction of relative position of mitral leaflets and segments/scallops in typical transoesophageal cross-sections created by three different examination manoeuvres. Note that individual anatomy, especially scallop morphology, is variable. A1–3 anterior leaflet segments; P1–3 posterior leaflet segments; Ao, aortic valve; LAA, left atrial appendage. See text for details. Reproduced, with permission, from Foster GP, Isselbacher EM, Rose GA, Torchiana DF, Akins CW, Picard MH. Accurate localization of mitral regurgitant defects using multiplane transesophageal echocardiography. *Ann Thorac Surg* 1998; **65**:1025–31, with permission of Elsevier.

circumference can be scanned, particularly for endocarditic or thrombotic lesions or paraprosthetic leaks. Note that structures on the ventricular side of the prosthetic ring or occluder may be masked by prosthetic shadowing.

The new and old percutaneous interventions in MV disease (valvuloplasty or percutaneous repair) clearly benefit from TOE guidance, from the exclusion of thrombi to the guidance of trans-septal puncture to the deployment of devices, as in the EVEREST trial.[15] 3D TOE provides en face views of the MV as if seen by the surgeon after left atriotomy (➲ Fig. 4.22), which are felt to be advantageous for communication with the surgeon due to their intuitive appeal.[12,14] Paraprosthetic leaks are also well visualized in their spatial extent.

Assessment of the aortic valve

TOE frequently helps in assessing the AoV. Short- and long-axis views should be obtained with attention to optimal alignment. The AoV may be seen in the short axis using the mid-oesophageal short-axis view. This view may be acquired from the mid-oesophageal four-chamber view simply by withdrawing the probe 2–5cm and then rotating the transducer by up to 30 degrees to bring the cross-sectional image in full view. In the patient with a normal valve, the three leaflets of the aortic valve should be easily seen to open and close. This view may also be used to visualize the left coronary ostium and left main stem, and the right coronary ostium. Some modification may be necessary as the two coronary ostia are rarely visible in the same plane. The valve may be seen in the long axis by rotating the transducer by 80–100 degrees thereby developing the mid-oesophageal AoV long axis view. Changing the probe depth is not usually necessary. The mid-oesophageal long-axis view will also show the AoV leaflets, but this view is usually less useful than the mid-oesophageal AoV long-axis view.

The aortic valve may also be visualized using either the transgastric long-axis or deep transgastric views. The former view is

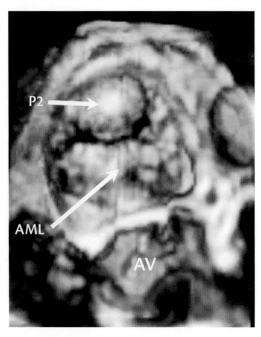

Figure 4.22 Mitral valve prolapse. 3D transoesophageal systolic image of a mitral valve with a prolapse of the P2 scallop of the posterior leaflet, seen from the left atrium ('surgeon's view'). The prolapsing segment balloons into the left atrium. AML, anterior mitral leaflet; AV, aortic valve.

acquired by obtaining the transgastric short-axis mid-chamber view and then rotating the transducer from zero to approximately 120 degrees; minor alterations in probe depth may be necessary. The latter view is acquired by advancing the probe to a depth of 45–55cm and the anteflexing the probe tip. This view may appear similar to the apical four-chamber view on TTE.

Mid-oesophageal views do not allow for an alignment of the Doppler beam parallel to the direction of blood flow through the AoV. The transgastric views are therefore necessary for a Doppler TOE assessment of the AoV. Either the transgastric long-axis or the deep transgastric view may be selected, but in practice it may be necessary to choose whichever gives the best signal and alignment.

Orifice area planimetry in aortic stenosis, though difficult in heavily calcified valves, may assist in the determination of severity. In aortic regurgitation, additional information about the mechanism (e.g. bicuspid valve, calcification/restriction, prolapse or flail, aortic dilation, and others) and the possibility of surgical repair can be expected from TOE.[16] Endocarditis vegetations, and in particular para-aortic abscesses (perivalvular aortic wall thickening with or without central echolucency) are much better visualized than transthoracically.

The aortic root is assessed in long-axis views, by withdrawing the probe slightly, showing the proximal part of the ascending aorta comprising the sinus of Valsalva located above the valve and the sinotubular junction (the narrowing above the sinus of Valsalva at the junction with the tubular part of the ascending aorta). Dilation of the aortic root, associated with hypertension, bicuspid valves or Marfan's disease,

frequently causes aortic regurgitation and is a risk factor for aortic dissection.

AoV prostheses are assessed in the same views as native AoVs to search for prosthesis-related complications such as obstruction, regurgitation, and endocarditis. However, it is not always possible to detect and quantify restricted occluder motion in aortic prostheses by TOE.[17] Short-axis views at the level of the sewing ring allow best to differentiate transprosthetic and periprosthetic leakage.

An emerging application of TOE is interventional or transcatheter (transapical or transfemoral) AoV implantation.[18,19] The aortic annulus diameter is of critical importance for selection of prosthetic size. Implantation of the prosthesis itself can be TOE-guided, although most laboratories use fluoroscopy. Immediately after deployment, TOE is important to evaluate aortic regurgitation. In severe paraprosthetic regurgitation, re-insufflation of the deployment balloon in the prosthesis may improve apposition of the prosthetic ring to the aortic wall and reduce regurgitation.

Assessment of the thoracic aorta

To start the examination of the thoracic aorta, at the level of the diaphragm (i.e. just as the mid-oesophageal four-chamber image is lost by advancing the probe) the probe is rotated through 180 degrees maintaining the angle of the transducer at 0 degrees. The descending aorta is seen in cross-section as the descending aorta short-axis view is acquired. It may be useful to alter the image focus and depth to more clearly examine the aortic wall. The probe may be withdrawn and re-advanced, thus examining the descending aorta in cross-section. The transducer may then be rotated through 90 degrees to acquire the long-axis view. Again, the probe may be withdrawn and advanced to examine the length of the descending aorta. The lack of anatomical landmarks in close proximity may make it difficult to accurately locate an abnormality. This may be facilitated either by noting the depth of the probe from the incisors, or by rotating the probe to orientate oneself to a cardiac landmark at a similar depth.

The ascending aorta may be viewed in the short and long axis. The mid-oesophageal ascending aorta short-axis view may be acquired from the mid-oesophageal short-axis aortic valve view by withdrawing the probe 3–5cm and rotating the transducer, usually reducing the angle of rotation by 20–30 degrees. Gently advancing and withdrawing the probe will bring the aortic root and ascending aorta into view in the centre of the display. Rotating the transducer tip through a further 90–100 degrees will develop the mid-oesophageal ascending aorta long-axis view.

If the probe is withdrawn to a depth of 20–25cm, with the transducer at 0 degrees of rotation, the upper oesophageal aortic arch long-axis view may be acquired. With the probe turned to the right, the distal arch is seen on the right of the display and the proximal arch to the left. Rotating the probe through 90 degrees allows the upper oesophageal short-axis view to be developed. Turning the probe to the right allows the proximal aortic arch to be viewed, and turning to the left views the distal arch. Turning the probe and retroflexing may bring the PA and PV into view to the left of the display.

Assessment of right heart chambers

Starting with the mid-oesophageal four-chamber view, the probe may be turned to the right to bring the TV into the centre of the display. The apical portion of the RV free wall is on the right of the display and the basal section on the left. The septal leaflet of the TV is seen on the right. The leaflet on the left is either the anterior or the posterior leaflet, depending on the image orientation. Gently advancing or withdrawing the probe a few centimetres may be necessary to visualize all the leaflets adequately.

The mid-oesophageal RV inflow/outflow view allows further examination of the TV, the PV, and the RV free wall. It is often easily acquired from the mid-oesophageal short-axis aortic view simply by further rotating the probe by 20–30 degrees; although it may be necessary to gently withdraw the probe by a few centimetres. The anterior leaflet of the TV is visible on the right of the display and the posterior leaflet on the left. Thus the mid-oesophageal four-chamber and mid-oesophageal RV inflow-outflow views should allow visualization of all three leaflets of the TV. The PV is also imaged using the mid-oesophageal RV inflow–outflow view, where the valve is visible on the right hand side of the display. The valve is seen in the long axis.

The RA may be visualized using the mid-oesophageal four-chamber view which may allow direct comparison of the size of the right and left atria. The RA may also be seen in part in the mid-oesophageal AV short axis and the mid-oesophageal RV inflow–outflow view. These may be useful views for checking the integrity of the atrial septum. Alternatively the mid-oesophageal bicaval view can be acquired from view mid-oesophageal long-axis view by turning the probe to the right (rotating the probe clockwise).

Finally, the transgastric RV inflow view may give useful information about the inferior RV free wall, the TV, and the tricuspid chordae tendinae. It is acquired by obtaining the transgastric short-axis mid-papillary view and turning the probe to the right to centre the right ventricle in the image display. The transducer is then rotated to between 100–120 degrees until the apex of the RV appears in the left hand side of the display. Non-standard transgastric views in the long and short axis may also be useful for further examining the TV leaflets, the PV, and the RVOT.

Perioperative TOE and TOE during cardiac interventions

Perioperative TOE was adopted early during the clinical dissemination of TOE and nowadays is firmly integrated in perioperative care especially of cardiac surgery patients, with particular emphasis on valve repair procedures, where it is considered indispensable (see also ⊕ Chapter 23). Specific guidelines for perioperative TOE have been published by cardiothoracic anesthesiologists.[20]

Perioperative TOE also is useful if acute cardiovascular derangements, e.g. hypotension and shock, occur in patients during or immediately after non-cardiac (e.g. abdominal or orthopaedic) surgery.

The increasing number of interventional or hybrid cardiac procedures has opened an additional field for TOE. If adequate sedation of the patient is obtained, TOE is ideally suited to accompany trans-septal puncture by directly showing the Brockenbrough needle indenting the atrial septum before puncture. A pericardial effusion is, of course, also immediately apparent. Similarly, positioning of occluding devices for PFO or atrial septal defects can be monitored, as well as occluders for ventricular septal defects or paravalvular leaks, with real-time information about impingement on other structures. TOE is standard before mitral valvuloplasty to exclude LA thrombi. The latest field for TOE deployment are the new interventional valve procedures: interventional AoV implantation, where TOE is important both to precisely define the LVOT diameter and the position of the prosthesis immediately before implantation, as well as procedural success immediately thereafter,[18,19] and interventional mitral repair, e.g. with the MitraClip® device.[15,21]

Intracardiac echocardiography

Equipment

Disposable catheters carrying miniaturized ultrasound transducers have been developed for intravascular and intracardiac use. While intravascular ultrasound has an established role in characterizing coronary artery lumen and wall morphology and complements coronary angiography, with special emphasis on atherosclerotic plaque burden, intracardiac echocardiography (ICE) is still not widely used. In principle, this technique uses catheter-mounted phased-array transducer which can be advanced via a wire into the heart chambers (mainly RA and RV) and through large vessels (mainly IVC or descending aorta). The catheter is introduced via a large sheath (8–10 French) and the transducer operates at frequencies of 5–10MHz, well above those in TTE (⊕ Fig. 4.23). Doppler modalities including CD are integrated. While these devices are able to furnish unobstructed, excellent high-resolution close-up views of cardiac and aortic structures (⊕ Fig. 4.24), their limitation are invasiveness with its attending risks and high cost, since the catheters are essentially for single-use, although some laboratories re-sterilize them. In many applications (see later), TOE is a less costly alternative. On the other hand, different from TOE, ICE causes only

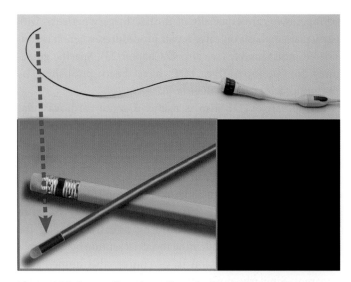

Figure 4.23 Intracardiac echocardiography. The 10F Acunav (Siemens Ultrasound) device is shown. The close-up shows the miniaturized 7mm long, 3.3mm thick, 64-element, 5–10MHz transducer incorporated into the catheter tip. Copyright by Siemens Ultrasound, Erlangen, Germany.

minimal patient discomfort during introduction of the sheath and thereafter is well tolerated without sedation.

Applications

The main clinical scenarios for which ICE has been found useful are:[22–24]

◆ Trans-septal puncture and closure of atrial septal defects or PFO, with the ICE catheter in the RA (➲ Fig. 4.24).

◆ Electrophysiological ablation procedures, including ablation of atrial fibrillation.

◆ Percutaneous AoV or PV implantation.

◆ Percutaneous LA appendage occlusion.

◆ Stent treatment of aortic dissection or other aortic disease of the descending aorta (including its abdominal portion), with the ICE catheter positioned in the IVC or in the aortic lumen.

Figure 4.24 Intracardiac echocardiography device. Left, atrial septum with patent foramen ovale (PFO), with colour Doppler. Right, Amplatzer septal occluder device after successful deployment. Note that, unlike transoesophageal images, these images show the right atrium (RA) on top, since the transducer is physically inside the right atrium. Ao, ascending aorta; LA, left atrium. Copyright by Siemens Ultrasound, Erlangen, Germany.

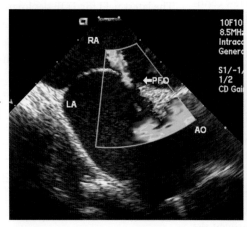
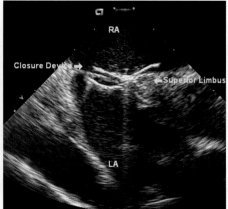

Personal perspective

TOE has substantially enriched the diagnostic armamentarium of the cardiologist, retaining the unique versatility and ubiquitous applicability that characterizes echo in general and distinguishes it from other imaging modalities. While 2D and Doppler capabilities of TOE are now mature, the image quality and time resolution of 3D TOE should—and will—further improve. Tissue Doppler so far has not been extensively used with TOE, but conceivably speckle-tracking based deformation imaging could be applied to TOE-imaged left and right ventricular segments. In recent years, the expanding array of interventional or hybrid procedures in

cardiology has created new fields for TOE. Many—but not all—operators regard TOE as a mandatory accompaniment to device closure of atrial septal defects, percutaneous AoV replacement, percutaneous MV repair, and other procedures. In some of these scenarios, ICE can replace TOE with the advantage of better patient tolerance, but at higher costs and higher invasiveness. ICE, on the other hand, seems almost ideally suited to monitor aortic procedures like stenting or dissection flap fenestration, but experience so far is very limited. Further miniaturization of probes very likely is technically possible, but may worsen contact of the probe with the oesophageal epithelium.

References

1 Schluter M, Langenstein BA, Polster J, *et al.* Transesophageal cross-sectional echocardiography with a phased array transducer system: Technique and initial clinical results. *Br Heart J* 1982; **48**:67–72.

2 Frazin L, Talano JV, Stephanides L, Loeb HS, Kopel L, Gunnar RM. Esophageal echocardiography. *Circulation* 1976; **54**:102–8.

3 Daniel WG, Mügge A: Transoesophageal echocardiography. *N Engl J Med* 1995: **332**:1268–1279.

4 Flachskampf FA, Decoodt P, Fraser AG, Daniel WG, Roelandt JRTC; for the Subgroup on Transoesophageal Echocardiography and Valvular Heart Disease, on behalf of the Working Group on Echocardiography of the European Society of Cardiology. Recommendations for performing transoesophageal echocardiography. *Eur J Echocardiography* 2001; **2**:8–21.

5 Flachskampf FA, Badano L, Daniel WG, Feneck RO, Fox KF, Fraser A, Pasquet A, Pepi M, Perez de Isla L, Zamorano J. Recommendations for transoesophageal echocardiography - 2010. *Eur J Echocardiogr* 2010; **11**:461–76.

6 Shanewise JS, Cheung AT, Aronson S, Stewart WJ, Weiss RL, Mark JB, *et al.* ASE/SCA guidelines for performing a comprehensive intraoperative multiplane transoesophageal echocardiography examination: recommendations of the American Society of Echocardiography Council for Intraoperative Echocardiography and the Society of Cardiovascular Anesthesiologists Task Force for Certification in Perioperative Transoesophageal Echocardiography. *J Am Soc Echocardiogr* 1999; **12**:884–900.

7 Nihoyannopoulos P, Fox K, Fraser A, Pinto F, on behalf of the Laboratory Accreditation Committee of the EAE. Laboratory standards and accreditation. *Eur J Echocardiogr* 2007; **8**:79–87.

8 Popescu BA, Andrade MJ, Badano LP, Fox KF, Flachskampf FA, Lancellotti P, *et al.* European Association of Echocardiography recommendations for training, competence, and quality improvement in echocardiography. *Eur J Echocardiogr* 2009; **10**: 893–905.

9 Côté G, Denault A. Transoesophageal echocardiography-related complications. *Can J Anaesth* 2008; **55**:622–47.

10 Jenssen C, Faiss S, Nürnberg D. Complications of endoscopic ultrasound and endoscopic ultrasound-guided interventions – results of a survey among German centers. *Z Gastroenterol* 2008; **46**: 1177–84.

11 Novaro GM, Aronow HD, Militello MA, Garcia MJ, Sabik EM. Benzocaine induced methemoglobinemia: Experience from a high-volume transoesophageal echocardiography laboratory. *J Am Soc Echocardiogr* 2003; **16**:170–5.

12 García-Orta R, Moreno E, Vidal M, Ruiz-López F, Oyonarte JM, Lara J, *et al.* Three-dimensional versus two-dimensional transoesophageal echocardiography in mitral valve repair. *J Am Soc Echocardiogr* 2007; **20**:4–12.

13 Sugeng L, Shernan SK, Weinert L, Shook D, Raman J, Jeevanandam V, *et al.* Real-time three-dimensional transoesophageal echocardiography in valve disease: comparison with surgical findings and evaluation of prosthetic valves. *J Am Soc Echocardiogr* 2008; **21**:1347–54.

14 Salcedo EE, Quaife RA, Seres T, Carroll JD. A framework for systematic characterization of the mitral valve by real-time three-dimensional transoesophageal echocardiography. *J Am Soc Echocardiogr* 2009; **22**:1087–99.

15 Silvestry FE, Rodriguez LL, Herrmann HC, Rohatgi S, Weiss SJ, Stewart WJ, *et al.* Echocardiographic guidance and assessment of percutaneous repair for mitral regurgitation with the Evalve MitraClip: lessons learned from EVEREST I. *J Am Soc Echocardiogr* 2007; **20**:1131–40.

16 de Waroux JB, Pouleur AC, Goffinet C, Vancraeynest D, Van Dyck M, Robert A, *et al.* Functional anatomy of aortic regurgitation: accuracy, prediction of surgical repairability, and outcome implications of transoesophageal echocardiography. *Circulation* 2007; **116**(11 Suppl):I264–9.

17 Montorsi P, De Bernardi F, Muratori M, Cavoretto D, Pepi M. Role of cine-fluoroscopy, transthoracic, and transoesophageal echocardiography in patients with suspected prosthetic heart valve thrombosis. *Am J Cardiol* 2000; **85**:58–64

18 Moss R, Ivens E, Pasupati S, Humphries K, Thompson CR, Munt B, *et al.* Role of echocardiography in percutaneous aortic valve implantation. *J Am Coll Cardiol* Imaging 2008; **1**:15–24.

19 Chin D. Echocardiography for transcatheter aortic valve implantation. *Eur J Echocardiogr* 2009; **10**:i21–9.

20 Practice guidelines for perioperative transoesophageal echocardiography: An updated report by the American Society of Anesthesiologists and the Society of Cardiovascular Anesthesiologists Task Force on Transesophageal Echocardiography. Anesthesiology 2010; 112 (Epub ahead of print)

21 Naqvi TZ. Echocardiography in percutaneous valve therapy. *J Am Coll Cardiol Cardiovasc Imaging* 2009; **2**:1226–37.

22 Vaina S, Ligthart J, Vijayakumar M, Ten Cate FJ, Witsenburg M, Jordaens LJ, *et al.* Intracardiac echocardiography during interventional procedures. *EuroIntervention* 2006; 1:454–64.

23 Kim SS, Hijazi ZM, Lang RM, Knight BP. The use of intracardiac echocardiography and other intracardiac imaging tools to guide noncoronary cardiac interventions. *J Am Coll Cardiol* 2009; **53**:2117–28.

24 Bartel T, Eggebrecht H, Müller S, Gutersohn A, Bonatti J, Pachinger O, Erbel R. Comparison of diagnostic and therapeutic value of transoesophageal echocardiography, intravascular ultrasonic imaging, and intraluminal phased-array imaging in aortic dissection with tear in the descending thoracic aorta (type B). *Am J Cardiol* 2007; **99**:270–4.

25 Foster GP, Isselbacher EM, Rose GA, Torchiana DF, Akins CW, Picard MH. Accurate localization of mitral regurgitant defects using multiplane transoesophageal echocardiography. *Ann Thorac Surg* 1998; **65**:1025–31.

Further reading

Flachskampf FA, Badano L, Daniel WG, Feneck RO, Fox KF, Fraser A, Pasquet A, Pepi M, Perez de Isla L, Zamorano J. Recommendations for transoesophageal echocardiography - 2010. *Eur J Echocardiogr* 2010; **11**:461–76.

Shanewise JS, Cheung AT, Aronson S, Stewart WJ, Weiss RL, Mark JB, *et al.* ASE/SCA guidelines for performing a comprehensive intraoperative multiplane transoesophageal echocardiography examination: recommendations of the American Society of Echocardiography Council for Intraoperative Echocardiography and the Society of Cardiovascular Anesthesiologists Task Force for Certification in Perioperative Transoesophageal Echocardiography. *J Am Soc Echocardiogr* 1999; **12**:884–900.

➲ For additional multimedia materials please visit the online version of the book (🕮 http://escecho.oxfordmedicine.com).

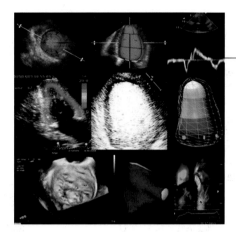

CHAPTER 5

Non-invasive haemodynamic assessment

Andrea Kallmeyer, José Luis Zamorano,
G. Locorotondo, Madalina Garbi,
José Juan Gómez de Diego and
Miguel Ángel García Fernández

Contents

Summary

The diagnostic power of two-dimensional (2D) echocardiography resides not only in its capability of providing anatomical information and of studying myocardial contractile function, but also in the possibility of performing a non-invasive haemodynamic assessment. Such non-invasive haemodynamic assessment is the subject of this chapter.

2D echocardiography, colour flow imaging, and Doppler modality make this haemodynamic assessment possible, by studying the following parameters:

◆ Blood flow velocities.

◆ Transvalvular pressure gradients.

◆ Valvular areas.

◆ Stroke volume, regurgitant volume, and regurgitant fraction.

◆ Cardiac function.

The application of these concepts in clinical practice will be explained through this chapter. They can be summarized in the following points:

◆ The study of valvular insufficiencies.

◆ The study of the valvular stenosis.

◆ The study of intracardiac shunts.

◆ The study of myocardial systolic and diastolic function.

◆ The estimation of intracardiac pressures.

Finally, non-invasive haemodynamic study represents an alternative to invasive procedures in some clinical circumstances and it is very important in the diagnostic and therapeutic decision making. Therefore, it is necessary for the cardiologist to understand how this echocardiographic study is performed, as well as its advantages and limitations.

Principles of Doppler echocardiography

The Doppler effect

The Doppler effect is based on the physical phenomenon of increase of sound frequency when an object moves towards the observer and of decrease of sound frequency when an object moves away from the observer. When applied to echocardiography, it measures blood flow velocities and directions in the vessels and heart chambers, because blood cells represent moving scatterers: they produce a *Doppler effect*. When the blood moves towards the echo transducer (which is the source of ultrasounds), sound wave frequency, reflected by red cells, increases. Frequency variance (named *frequency shift*) of the ultrasound waves which encounter them depends on the transmitted frequency, on the blood velocity, and on direction of the flow, as it follows the equation (⊃ Fig. 5.1):

$$f_r - f_0 = \Delta f = 2 \times f_0 \times (V \times \cos\theta /c) \tag{5.1}$$

where f_r is the reflected frequency, f_0 is the transmitted frequency, Δf is the frequency shift, v is the flow velocity, c is the speed of ultrasound in blood.

Frequency shift analysis generates a spectral display of blood flow direction (towards transducer above baseline and away below), velocity (distance from baseline), and amplitude (grey-scale brightness). Spectral analysis uses fast Fourier transformation, assuming constant flow (ignoring cardiac-cycle variations). Representative samples from the continuum of frequencies are given numeric values (digital transformation), displayed in grey-scale.

For every frequency shift, a band of frequencies reaches the transducer—*spectral broadening*—because of transit-time changes and non-constant flow sampling. The spectral trace is

thickened, blurring the peak, without influencing the mean. Turbulent flow favours spectral broadening. Doppler frequencies have audible range; higher velocities have higher pitch.

The moving scatterer velocity (V) is calculated with the *Doppler equation* from transmitted (f_0) and returning (f_r) frequency:

$$V = [c \times (f_r - f_0)] / [2f_0 \times (\cos\theta)] \tag{5.2}$$

where c is ultrasound speed in blood, that is 1540m/s. Then:

$$V = [1540m/s \times (f_r - f_0)] / [2f_0 \times (\cos\theta)]$$

Angle of incidence (θ) dependence gives accurate velocities for flow direction aligned incidence ($\cos\theta = 1$ for 0 or 180 degrees), no recordings for perpendicular incidence ($\cos\theta = 0$ for 90 degrees), and underestimated velocities for intermediate incidence.

Doppler imaging modalities

Continuous wave Doppler

This uses the frequency shift, transmitting and receiving continuously (with two separate piezoelectric elements) returning waves from the direction of interrogation, with no spatial resolution. It can measure high velocities.

Pulsed wave Doppler

This uses a different technique, transmitting intermittent short pulses with certain pulse repetition frequency (PRF) and sampling the returning waves' frequency with certain range gate (transmission–reception relation). Two samples within a wavelength quarter are needed to determine direction. Short wavelengths (high frequencies/high flow velocities) induce direction and even velocity value misinterpretation—*aliasing*. The highest appropriately interpreted frequency (*Nyquist limit*) is half the PRF. High PRF allows higher frequencies (velocities) assessment though predisposes to ambiguity artefact. Baseline shifting in the opposite direction may resolve aliasing, if the velocity peak can fit correctly in the display. Pulsed wave (PW) Doppler has spatial resolution within the sample volume. The maximum sampling depth is limited by ultrasound travelling time restricting PRF.

Colour Doppler

This is a PW Doppler-derived technique, using multiple (100–400) sample volumes along a multitude of scan lines to generate a real-time 2D superimposed colour-flow map. The number of pulses per sample volume is limited by a drop in frame rate. Frequency shift analysis with *autocorrelation* (comparison of a signal with itself in time to find a pattern) estimates mean velocity, variance (spread of velocities around the mean), and direction of flow. A pair of pulses determines a phase shift; two phase shifts (three pulses) enable velocity estimation. More pulses are

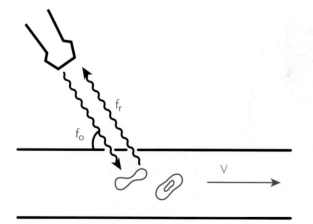

Figure 5.1 The Doppler effect. Schema indicating the Doppler effect in relation to blood flow: the transmitted ultrasounds with a frequency f_o detect blood flow and return to transducer with a frequency f_r higher or lower than the f_o, depending on direction of blood flow. Angle-dependence of Doppler analysis is also showed.

needed to increase accuracy or sensitivity to low velocities (slow flow). The depth is determined by arrival time (as for 2D).

Colour pattern depends on the orientation of the flow relative to the transducer and not on a specific flow. The direction is colour-coded blue away and red towards transducer (➲ Fig. 5.2A). This is the reason why the same flow can be seen with different colour Doppler (CD) patterns when studied from different windows. Colour hue and luminance (brightness) suggest mean velocity magnitude. There is a range of colour maps with different shades and readymade settings for optimal flow display. There is an option of variance display in added shades of green, to identify turbulent flow (mosaic of colours) (➲ Fig. 5.2B). CD suffers *aliasing* at high velocities (➲ Figs. 5.3 and 5.4). The instrument *scale* control changes PRF. By reducing PRF, an increase in examination depth increases aliasing throughout image depth. The Nyquist limit used in clinical imaging is below the maximum velocity of some normal cardiac flows (typically in the range of 60–80cm/s); that means that aliasing can be seen in physiological flows. This is especially true for the left ventricular (LV) inflow in parasternal long-axis (PLAX) and apical four-chamber (A4C) views and for LV outflow in PLAX and apical five-chamber (A5C) views. The detection of a small amount of regurgitation of mitral, tricuspid, and pulmonary valves is the rule even in healthy people when the study is done carefully. These small regurgitations should be considered as physiological and do not have clinical significance. In contrast, aortic regurgitation is an unusual finding in healthy people. *Sample size* increase gives better colour flow if we reduce the colour sector width (number of scan lines) to preserve frame rate. *Priority* selects a threshold for colour (or tissue) display and *persistence* uses signal averaging to give smooth appearance. Only one scan line is used for colour M-mode.

Normal Doppler flow patterns

CD flow is a tool widely used to assess patterns of intracardiac flows.[1,2] The appearance of unusual flows is the basis for the diagnosis of regurgitant valvular lesions, intracardiac shunts, and high-velocity flows that are linked to valvular stenosis.

Once the CD study has been performed, spectral Doppler must be performed to study the characteristics of blood flow across the valves, great vessels, and heart chambers.[3–5] PW Doppler is the preferred tool because it allows study of the flow at a specific point. Occasionally continuous wave (CW) Doppler should be used, especially when the goal is to avoid the underestimation of a potential high-velocity flow.

The challenge in spectral Doppler studies is to place the ultrasound beam parallel to the flow of interest. If there is a non-parallel alignment between the flow and the ultrasound beam, the Doppler tracing will be biased and the velocities underestimated. CD imaging is usually a useful reference map to place the Doppler sampling line in the right position.

Parasternal long-axis view

In PLAX view the ultrasound beam has a perpendicular orientation to the aortic valve (AoV) and mitral valve (MV) and, in consequence, a perpendicular orientation to LV inflow and LV outflow: the Doppler signal obtained is relatively weak. However, this is a useful plane to detect even small quantities of mitral and aortic regurgitation.

Ventricular inflow (➲ Fig. 5.5; ▣ 5.1) is seen as a broad red flow stream from the left atrium (LA) to the LV in diastole.

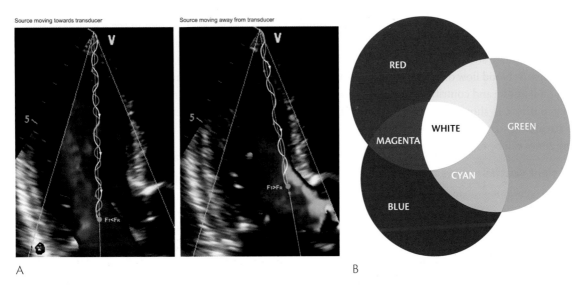

Figure 5.2 A) Colour Doppler mode. Through the mitral valve in diastole the scatterers move towards the transducer, which result in a higher received ultrasound frequency. Through the aortic valve in systole the blood moves away from the transducer (actually oblique in this case because of the anatomy of the left ventricular outflow tract), which results in a lower received ultrasound frequency. B) Colour Doppler mode. Colour flow maps used in colour Doppler images to code blood flow velocities. 5.2 B) Reproduced from Zamorano JL, Bax JJ, Rademakers FE, and Knuuti J (eds) (2010) The ESC Textbook of Cardiovascular Imaging, with kind permission from Springer Science + Business Media.

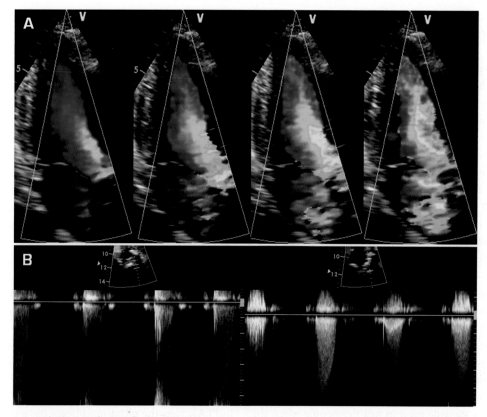

Figure 5.3 Doppler imaging. A) Aliasing of colour flow: Erroneous representation of flow direction with colour flow appears at too low Nyquist limit (too low scale). In the example, the scale was progressively reduced in purpose, to illustrate aliasing of flow in the left ventricular outflow tract in the absence of pathology. B) Spectral PW Doppler aliasing, High PRF ambiguity artefact, mirror image, and angle dependence: Spectral PW Doppler aliasing appears when the examined flow acceleration is too high for the Nyquist limit. Increasing the PRF may resolve the artefact, though in cases of very high accelerations may induce ambiguity artefact. Highly reflective spectral Doppler signal may give a mirror image on the other side of the baseline. Non-aligned Doppler interrogation cursor or loss of alignment because of respiratory translation of the heart results in subestimation of flow acceleration. In the example, the left-sided spectral recording is obtained for illustration purposes with PW Doppler in severe aortic stenosis, resulting in aliasing despite maximal PRF. There is ambiguity artefact—highly reflective signal displayed at the bottom of the image. In the right-sided spectral recording, CW Doppler was used resolving the aliasing and the ambiguity artefact. There is mirror image of the bright spectrum above the baseline.

In the early ventricular filling phase, blood flow velocity could be high enough to cause aliasing. The red colour pattern disappears in the diastasis phase and is seen again after the atrial contraction. A retrograde blood flow directed toward the LA can be found during mid-systole and contributes to valve closure.

Ventricular outflow is shown as a blue coded column of blood flow streaming from the LV towards the AoV. Again, some aliasing zones can be found.

Parasternal right ventricle views

These are specifically suited to study the right ventricular (RV) flows. The RV inflow view (➲ Fig. 5.6; ▪ 5.2) shows the flow from the RA to the RV as a wide red stream and the RV outflow view (➲ Fig. 5.7; ▪ 5.3) the flow from the RV to the main pulmonary artery (PA) as a blue column. Both views are perfectly oriented to study the regurgitation flows from right-side valves. The tricuspid regurgitation draws a blue column of flow directed back from the valve to the atrium in systole. The pulmonary valve (PV) regurgitation is seen as a red flame moving towards the RV in systole.

The spectral flow pattern in the RV outflow tract (RVOT) is a negative curve similar to that obtained in the LV outflow tract (LVOT) (➲ Fig. 5.8). However, due to the fact that RV usually works in a low pressure context, the right-side curve usually has a less steep acceleration slope, a rounded and lower mid-systolic peak and a less steeper deceleration slope. It is not uncommon to detect a holodiastolic flow due to a mild pulmonary regurgitation.

Parasternal short-axis view

The left PSAX view at AoV level (➲ Fig. 5.9; ▪ 5.4) is also useful to study the flow in the right cardiac chambers. The RA inflow appears in the image as a red coloured stream directed towards the tricuspid valve (TV), while the RV outflow can be seen as a blue column that fills the main PA.

Although aortic flow is fully perpendicular to image plane, the pattern of the flow in this plane can be also studied; this could be useful in some cases of aortic regurgitation to see the exact origin of the jet in the valve.

Other PSAX views are usually not studied with CD mode. However, CD mode can be useful at MV level to study eccentric

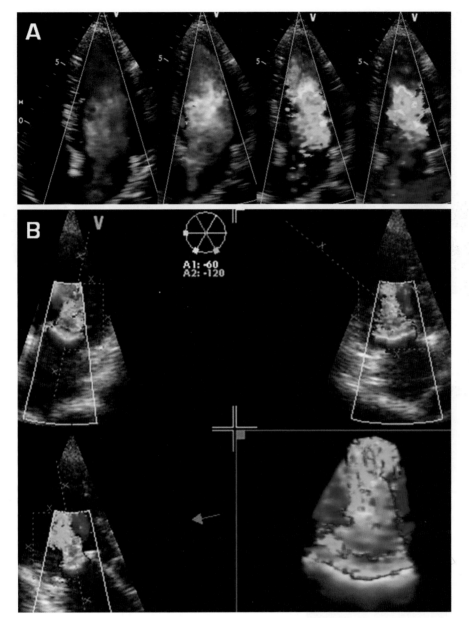

Figure 5.4 Aliasing of colour flow. A) Aliasing of colour flow: aliasing of flow during left ventricular filling was induced on purpose, by decreasing the scale. There is gradually more aliasing as the velocity decreases. There is no flow acceleration on the mitral valve area, suggesting that the aliasing is a technical and not a pathological phenomenon. B) Aliasing of colour flow at lesions: aliasing of colour flow may be useful to suggest existence of pathological flow acceleration. In the example, there is acceleration of flow in the mitral valve area during left ventricular filling, suggestive of existence of mitral stenosis. The phenomenon is present in colour flow 3D as well. In the example the 3D colour flow volume was post-processed by reducing tissue priority and increasing tissue threshold.

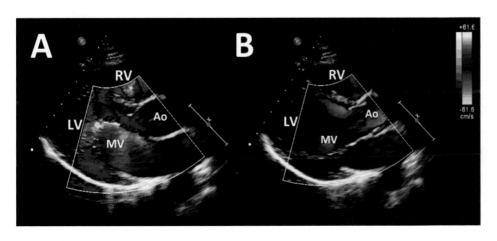

Figure 5.5 Colour flow Doppler in PLAX view. In diastole (A) main flow is a wide red column of flow streaming from the left atrium towards the left ventricle. In systole (B) the flow is a blue column from the left ventricle towards the aorta. Ao, aorta; LV, left ventricle; MV, mitral valve; RV, right ventricle.

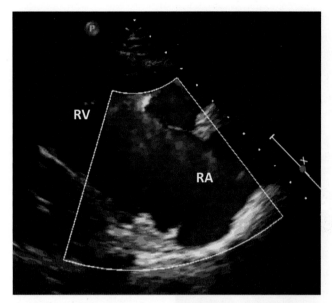

Figure 5.6 Colour flow Doppler in parasternal right ventricle inflow view. The main flow is a red column in diastole from the right atrium (RA) towards the right ventricle (RV).

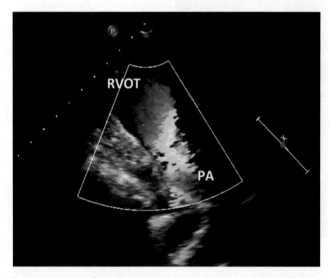

Figure 5.7 Colour flow Doppler in parasternal right ventricle outflow view. In this case, the main flow is a blue column in systole from right ventricle outflow tract (RVOT) towards the pulmonary artery (PA).

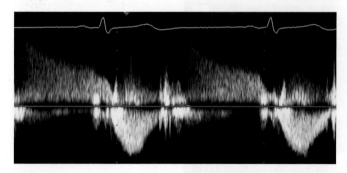

Figure 5.8 Continuous wave Doppler tracing of the right ventricle outflow.

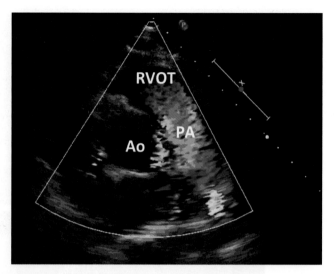

Figure 5.9 Colour flow Doppler in parasternal SAX view at aortic valve level. There is a blue column of flow in systole from right ventricle outflow tract (RVOT) towards the pulmonary artery (PA).

mitral regurgitation jets and at any level in cases of ventricular septal defect.

Apical views

Apical views are of a paramount importance in the CD analysis of intracardiac blood flows (➲ Fig. 5.10; ■ 5.5). The A4C view is the best one to study the LV inflow. The blood flow stream appears in diastole as a wide red column directed first towards the lateral ventricular wall and after towards the LV apex. The LV inflow across the mitral valve is obtained with PW Doppler, placing the sample volume at mitral leaflet tips guided by a 2D apical view (➲ Fig. 5.11). The flow velocity profile across the mitral valve has typically two peaks, which are in fact the Doppler translation of the M-mode tracing of the mitral valve (for transmitral diastolic flow pattern, see ➲ Chapter 9).

In systole the flow moves towards the outflow tract, away from the transducer, and the column becomes blue-coded. LV outflow is best studied in A5C view (➲ Fig. 5.12; ■ 5.6), because it offers the possibility to study the streaming of the flow column through the AoV and the aortic root. It is possible to see a small region of aliasing near the AoV in the outflow colour pattern especially in early systole.

PW Doppler is usually used to study the flow in the LVOT (see later). The spectral flow pattern of the LVOT (➲ Fig. 5.13) shows in systole a curve pointing down with very steep acceleration slope, a sharp peak in the very early systole, and a less steep deceleration slope. A thin vertical line after the flow profile due to the AoV closing click can be also seen. The flow pattern in the aortic side of the valve as seen with PW Doppler is very similar to the one obtained in the outflow tract when the AoV is normal, although velocity peak is slightly higher and a thin line before the flow due to the opening of the valve can be seen. In CW Doppler study both opening and closure marks

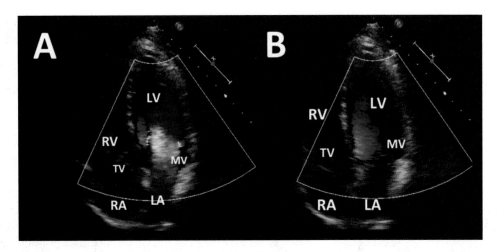

Figure 5.10 Colour flow Doppler in A4C view. In diastole (A) flow is a wide red column (better seen in left side of the heart) of flow streaming from the left atrium towards the left ventricle. In systole (B) the flow is a blue column from the left ventricle towards the aorta, that is best seen in A5C view. LA, left atrium. LV, left ventricle; MV, mitral valve; RA, right atrium; RV, right ventricle; TV, tricuspid valve.

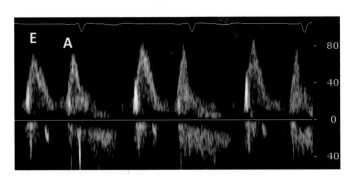

Figure 5.11 PW Doppler tracing of the left ventricle inflow. E is the first peak, placed in mid-diastole. A is the second peak and the easier to recognize because it is over the P wave in ECG or even easier immediately before the QRS complex.

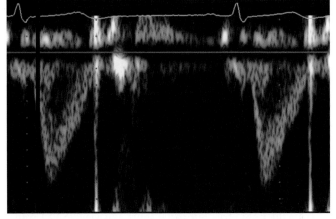

Figure 5.13 PW Doppler image showing the spectral analysis of blood flow in the LVOT.

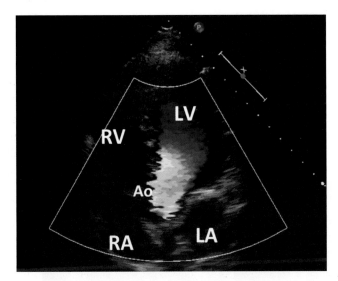

Figure 5.12 Colour flow Doppler in A5C view. This view allows study of the left ventricle outflow towards the aorta. This view is also very useful as a guide map to place the Doppler sampling line. Ao, aortic valve and aortic root; LA, left atrium; LV, left ventricle; RA, right atrium; RV, right ventricle.

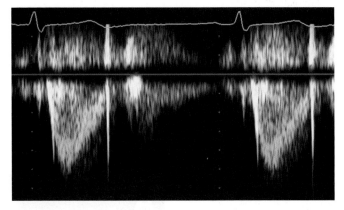

Fig 5.14 CW Doppler image showing the spectral analysis of blood flow in the LVOT.

can be recorded (◔ Fig. 5.14). ◔ Table 5.1 shows reference values.

LA filling by pulmonary veins can also be studied in A4C view. CD imaging shows the pulmonary vein flow as a red column joining the atrial roof. The LA filling flow can be studied placing a PW Doppler sampling volume in the pulmonary

Table 5.1 Left and right outflow tract velocities

	LVOT	RVOT
Maximal velocity (m/s)	0.88	0.72
	(0.47–1.29)	(0.36–1.08)
Ejection time (m/s)	286	281
	(240–332)	(212–350)
Acceleration time (m/s)	84	118
	(48–10)	(70–166)
Acceleration (m/s²)	11	6.1
	(5–17)	(3–9)
Flow velocity integral (cm)	20–25	

vein in apical A4C view (➲ Fig. 5.15). In difficult cases, transoesophageal echo is a good alternative to record a pulmonary vein flow.

The study of flow velocities across the TV is more accurate with PW Doppler from an apical view, although the parasternal right inflow view yields also good results. The morphological pattern of RV inflow is similar to the mitral flow pattern (➲ Fig. 5.16) (see ➲ Chapter 9).

Subcostal views

Subcostal views CD flow patterns are usually similar to those obtained from apical views. Subcostal four-chamber view is the best one to look for a patent foramen ovale that is shown, when present, as a red flame from the middle of the interatrial septum towards the right atria. Subcostal short-axis view (SAX) could be a good alternative to study the PV flow.

Suprasternal views

CD imaging in suprasternal views is largely focused on the study of the flow in the aorta. Ascending aorta flow is red-coloured (➲ Fig. 5.17; ☐ 5.7) and descending aorta flow is a blue column that can show some degree of aliasing.

The flow profile in the ascending aorta is seen as a positive curve with a steep acceleration slope, sharp peak, and less deceleration slope. The descending portion of the signal shows spectral widening caused by a broader range of blood flow velocities.

This pattern of flow is mirrored shaped compared to the flow in the aortic root obtained from the apical position (➲ Table 5.2).

A blood flow signal similar to those obtained in the ascending aorta except for direction (directed away from instead towards the transducer) is seen when a sample volume of PW Doppler is placed in the descending aorta in a suprasternal view. The average blood flow velocity in the ascending and the descending aorta is the same due to the fact that loss of volume directed to supra-aortic trunks is exactly compensated by lessening of the aorta calibre.

M-mode colour Doppler

CD imaging can be used over M-mode and this is simply the best tool to study the exact timing and the exact relationship to cardiac cycle of the flows. For example, this is the best way to measure the exact duration of a regurgitation jet over the entire systole (➲ Fig. 5.18).

Vena cava flow

The RA filling flow can be studied in the superior vena cava from the suprasternal or supraclavicular views or in a hepatic vein in subcostal window.

Coronary arterial blood flow

The coronary flow can be also studied in transthoracic echo. The sample volume of PW Doppler is usually placed over the central region of the left main trunk. The coronary flow is a double-peaked Doppler wave with higher velocity during diastole. This flow pattern is similar to those obtained with invasive methods.

Provocative manoeuvres

There are two specific manoeuvres that can be useful in very specific cases to achieve an improvement of some Doppler tracings:

1. *Carotid sinus massage,* which is a useful tool to better assess MV diastolic flow in patients with mitral stenosis. When carotid sinus massage is going to be performed, care should be taken to be sure to rule out a significant carotid artery

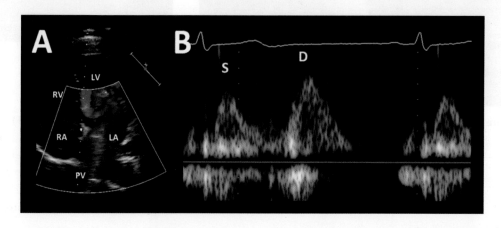

Fig 5.15 PW Doppler tracing of the flow of a pulmonary vein. In (A), an A4C view is used to find the pulmonary vein flow as a thin red stream towards the left atrium. In (B) the typical flow curve is seen, with systolic (S) and diastolic (D) main components.

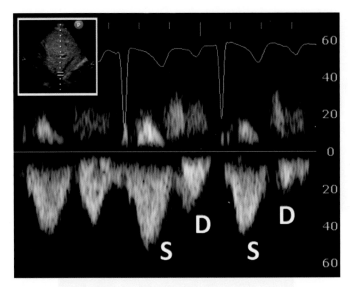

Fig 5.16 PW Doppler tracing of the flow of the inferior vena cava flow. In (A), the 2D echo imaging is used to guide to position the Doppler sampling line. In (B) the typical tracing is shown, again with systolic (S) and diastolic (D) main components.

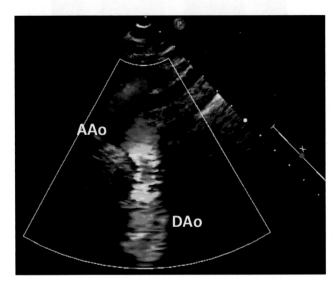

Fig 5.17 Colour flow Doppler in suprasternal long axis view. The flow is shown in red in the ascending aorta (AAo) and as a blue column in the descending aorta (DAo).

Table 5.2 Normal values for aortic and pulmonary flows

	Ascending Aorta Flow	Descending Aorta Flow	Pulmonary Artery
Maximal velocity (m/s)	1.17	1.07	0.84
	(0.59–1.75)	(0.50–1.79)	(0.56–1.33)
Ejection time (EX, ms)	263	261	300
	(216–310)	(202–302)	(197–403)
Acceleration time (AT, ms)	79	91	122
	(61–97)	(70–122)	(63–181)
Acceleration time (m/s²)	15	12	7.2
	(7–23)	(5–19)	(4–10)
Flow Integral (cm)	18-22		

disease; direct auscultation of the carotid to rule out a bruit that could be a marker is recommended.

2. *Valsalva manoeuvre*, which is performed by asking the patient for a forceful expiration (about 40mmHg) against a closed nose and mouth. It is helpful when there is a suspicion of a dynamic obstruction of the LVOT.

Haemodynamic parameters

Pressure gradients

The pressure gradients measure the differences of pressure between two cavities that are adjacent. In echocardiography, pressures can be estimated from the study of flow velocities, thanks to *Bernoulli's equation*. This is based on the principle of energy conservation, according to which when a fluid crosses a narrow orifice, an increase of pressure is produced due to an acceleration of the flow. The Bernoulli formula takes into consideration the convective acceleration, the acceleration of the flow, and the viscous friction. In its application in medicine, the acceleration of the flow is ignored (as the initial velocity of the flow is usually less than 1m/s and therefore is negligible), so the equation is reduced to:

$$(\text{Pressure 1} - \text{Pressure 2}) = \Delta P = 4 \times (\text{Velocity 1} - \text{Velocity 2})$$
$$\text{Pressure 2} < \text{Pressure 1} - \text{Velocity 2} < \text{Velocity 1}$$
$$\Delta P = 4 \times \text{Velocity}^2$$

(5.3)

➲ Figure 5.19 shows the simplification of Bernoulli's equation. The exceptions to this abbreviated formula are: injuries in tandem (which generate a higher initial velocity), long stenosis, and the phenomenon of recovery of pressures (which means that in the presence of a small ascending aorta, the pressure after an aortic valvular stenosis is higher due to the conversion of kinetic energy into potential energy. This phenomenon causes underestimation of transaortic pressure gradient in cases of aortic stenosis, AS, with small ascending aorta. For details, see ➲ Chapter 14a).

Time velocity integral

With echocardiography it is possible to measure the distance covered by the blood during each heart beat. In normal conditions the blood flow is laminar, so the elements of blood move parallel to the flow direction, with a higher velocity in the centre, in the shape of a parabola. The time velocity integral (TVI) is the result of adding all the individual velocities per unit of time and expresses the distance covered by the blood during one heart beat in centimetres.

In order to calculate the TVI, it is necessary to use the pulsed Doppler wave mode. The sample volume has to be positioned

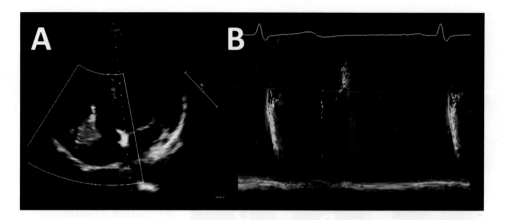

Fig 5.18 Colour flow Doppler over M-mode imaging. In (A) it is easy to see a tricuspid regurgitation jet as a blue blot form the right ventricle to the right atrium. Based on the size of the jet, it is tempting to consider the regurgitation as moderate. However, colour Doppler nicely shows in (B) that the blue jet is very brief, and in fact the tricuspid regurgitation is only mild.

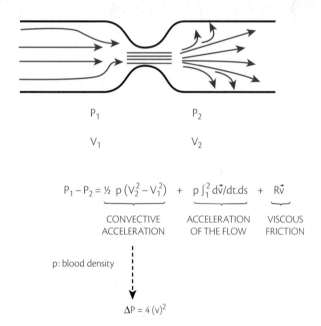

Figure 5.19 Simplification of Bernoulli's equation.

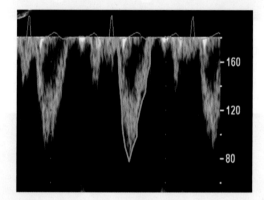

Figure 5.20 PW Doppler image of the LVOT flow.

in the point to study: for LVOT, mitral or tricuspid annulus, the apical views are most used, because they allow alignment with the flow. For the pulmonary one, the SAX is used instead. Once obtained the curve of Doppler, it is necessary to trace the external contour of curve. After that, the computer software gives directly the TVI value in centimetres (● Fig. 5.20).

The usefulness of TVI calculation is that it makes it possible to estimate volumes. These can be calculated using a mathematical formula according to which the volume of fluid that crosses an orifice (flow) is equal to the area of the orifice multiplied by the flow velocity through it.

$$\text{Flow (cc/s)} = \text{area (cm}^2) \times \text{velocity (cm/s)} \qquad (5.4)$$

By integrating flow velocity over the duration of flow, blood volume that crosses one valve is obtained by:

$$\text{Volume (cm}^3) = \text{area (cm}^2) \times \text{TVI (cm)} \qquad (5.5)$$

Assuming circular valvular orifices, the formula would be the following:

$$\text{Volume} = (\pi\, r^2) \times \text{TVI}$$

then

$$\begin{aligned}\text{Volume} &= [3.14 \times (D/2)^2] \times \text{TVI} \\ &= [0.785 \times D^2] \times \text{TVI}\end{aligned} \qquad (5.6)$$

where r is the valvular annulus radius and D is the valvular annulus diameter (● Fig. 5.21).

The ideal views to measure the diameters of the valvular annulus are the apical view for the mitral and the TV, and the long and short parasternal axis views for the AoV and the PV, respectively.

Thus, by calculating the blood volume that crosses one valve in every heart beat, the systolic volume or *stroke volume* (SV) is easily obtained. Then, the *cardiac output* (CO) can be determined multiplying SV by the heart rate (HR), as well as the *cardiac index* (CI), dividing the above mentioned result by the body surface area (BSA).

$$\text{CO} = \text{SV} \times \text{HR} \qquad (5.7)$$

$$\text{CI} = \text{CO/BSA} \qquad (5.8)$$

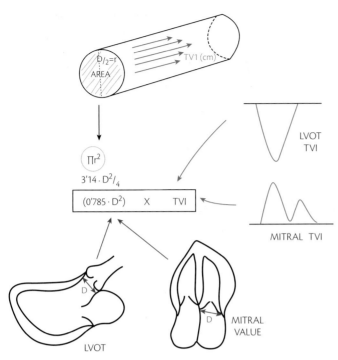

Figure 5.21 Schema indicating the method for calculating the LVOT flow volume and the mitral inflow volume. For this a measure of both the valvular annular diameters and the TVI is needed.

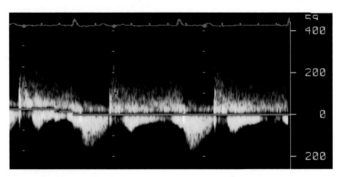

Figure 5.22 CW Doppler image of an aortic regurgitation.

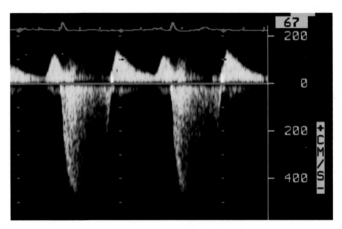

Figure 5.23 CW Doppler image of a mitral regurgitation.

However, this method has some limitations:

◆ With this method it is not possible to calculate the SV in cases of valvular insufficiencies or stenosis, in which the flow velocities are increased.

◆ Many mistakes can usually take place in measurement of the diameters of the valvular annulus.

◆ The valvular orifices are not always circular.

◆ In cases of irregular pacing it is necessary to calculate a mean value from the measurements of at least 10 heart beats.

Study of valvular insufficiencies

In case of valvular insufficiencies, the valvular orifice does not close hermetically in systole (for mitral and tricuspid pathologies), or in diastole (for aortic pathologies): these are the most common valvular insufficiencies. Due to such dysfunction, part of the blood flow returns to the previous heart chamber: to the LA or RA in the insufficiencies of the atrioventricular valves or to the ventricles when considering the insufficiencies of the great vessel valves (➲ Figs. 5.22 and 5.23).

This valvular dysfunction causes a progressive volume overload that results in expanding these cavities and impairing their contractile function.

For haemodynamic study of valvular insufficiencies the following methods can be used.

Volumetric method

The severity of valvular insufficiencies can be evaluated by determining the blood volume that returns backwards crossing the pathological valve. This blood volume is termed *regurgitant volume* (RVol).

For this purpose, it is important to remember the concept that in a normal heart the blood volume that crosses every valve is constant. In cases of valvular insufficiency (and in absence of dysfunction of other valves), the blood volume that crosses the pathological valve (total blood volume) is represented by forward blood volume (similar to that across a continent valve) plus RVol:

Volume across an insufficient valve = volume across a

normal valve + RVol

Then, RVol can be calculated by:

RVol = volume across an insufficient valve
− volume across a normal valve   (5.9)

The volumes will be calculated with the ➲ Equation 5.6 explained previously:

Volume = $(\pi\, r^2) \times$ TVI

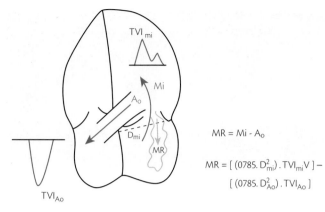

$$MR = Mi - A_o$$

$$MR = [\,(0785.\,D^2_{mi})\,.\,TVI_{mi}V\,] -$$
$$[\,(0785.\,D^2_{Ao})\,.\,TVI_{Ao}\,]$$

Figure 5.24 Schema indicating the volumetric method for calculating a regurgitant volume (RV). The example given is about the measure of the mitral regurgitant volume in case of a mitral insufficiency (also called mitral regurgitation). The RV in this case is the difference between the mitral inflow (represented as Mi in the image) and the LVOT flow volume (represented as Ao in the image).

Then, in order to calculate two different volumes, the valvular annulus diameters and the TVIs at two different cardiac sites have to be determined (→ Fig. 5.24).

For example:

◆ For the aortic insufficiency (in absence of mitral insufficiency):

$$\text{Aortic RVol} = \text{transaortic volume}$$
$$- \text{transmitral volume} \qquad (5.10)$$

◆ For the mitral insufficiency (in absence of aortic insufficiency):

$$\text{Mitral RVol} = \text{transmitral volume}$$
$$- \text{transaortic volume (LVOT)} \qquad (5.11)$$

Once the RVol is known, the *regurgitant fraction* (RF%) can be obtained as the proportion of the transvalvular volume which regurgitates referred to total transvalvular volume.

◆ For the aortic insufficiency:

$$\text{RF\%} = \text{aortic RVol/transaortic volume} \times 100 \qquad (5.12)$$

◆ For the mitral insufficiency:

$$\text{RF\%} = (\text{mitral RVol/transmitral volume}) \times 100 \qquad (5.13)$$

Another volumetric parameter also used to quantify the severity of an insufficiency is the cross-sectional area of the regurgitant flow, the so called *effective regurgitant orifice area* (EROA). This is obtained from the formula for calculation of volumes:

$$\text{RVol} = \text{Effective regurgitant orifice area (EROA)}$$
$$\times \text{TVI of the regurgitation} \qquad (5.14)$$
$$\text{EROA} = \text{RVol/TVI regurgitation}$$

The limitations of this method are:

◆ This method cannot be applied in cases of multiple valvular disease (in that case one might take the PV flow as a reference if it is not affected, but usually this valve is not visualized well enough).

◆ It is necessary to avoid accumulative mistakes, especially when measuring valve annular diameters.

◆ It is also necessary to optimize the Doppler signal and the image resolution parameters.

PISA method

Another way of studying the valvular insufficiencies (particularly mitral regurgitation) is the *proximal isovelocity surface area* (PISA) method or proximal isovelocity method. This procedure is based on the evidence that blood flow accelerates progressively as it approaches towards an orifice of regurgitation, where it creates a few concentric hemispheric shells. Each hemisphere displays the same velocity on its surface: at decreasing distance from the orifice, areas are smaller and velocities are higher. Because of the occurrence of aliasing phenomenon in the hemispheres, PISA velocity can be determined by CD flow aliasing: the velocity that produces the aliasing is named *velocity of aliasing*. It is necessary to adjust the colour scale by decreasing the velocity range and reducing the Nyquist limit to approximately 15–40cm/s, in order to obtain aliasing. The radius of the PISA is measured at mid-systole using the first aliasing, corresponding to a distinct red/blue interface. The image is optimized by lowering depth, narrowing the sector and using the zoom mode. In case of mitral insufficiency, in A4C view, the Doppler signal of the regurgitant jet shows a blue colour as it moves away from the transducer, but in proximity of regurgitant orifice the flow colour becomes red or yellow along isovelocity surface area (see → Chapter 14b) (→ Fig. 5.25).

In agreement with the principle of conservation of the mass, the flow in this surface of isovelocity (named Q1) is equal to the flow at the regurgitant orifice (named Q2). Again, the measure of the flow volumes will be obtained from the multiplication of areas by velocities:

◆ For Q1: the so-called PISA area multiplied for the velocity of aliasing.

◆ For Q2: the EROA multiplied for the peak mitral regurgitation velocity.

The PISA area represents area of hemisphere: its radius is the distance from the valvular orifice to the dome of the hemisphere (produced by the aliasing phenomenon). The most satisfactory hemispheric PISA image happens in mid systole. As it is a hemisphere, the area is calculated by the formula

$$\text{Hemisphere area} = 2\pi\,r^2$$

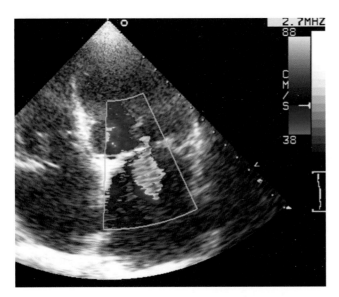

Figure 5.25 Example of PISA image of a mitral regurgitation. After diminishing the colour scale to approximately 38cm/s aliasing phenomenon occurs and the colour of the jet of regurgitation turns yellow, with the hemispheric image around the regurgitant orifice. The radius of this hemisphere is the so-called PISA radius.

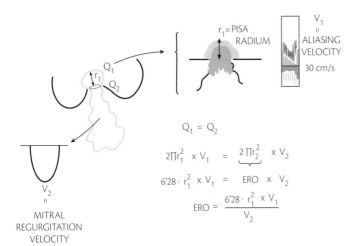

Figure 5.26 Schema indicating the PISA method for calculation of the ERO.

being *r* that radius (➲ Fig. 5.26). Therefore:

PISA area × velocity of aliasing
$\quad$ = EROA × peak velocity of the regurgitation $\qquad$ (5.15)

(6.28 × r^2) × velocity of aliasing
$\quad$ = EROA × peak velocity of the regurgitation flow

EROA = (6.28 × r^2) × velocity of aliasing/peak
$\quad$ × velocity of the regurgitation flow $\qquad$ (5.16)

This approach is based on the assumption that the maximal PISA radius occurs simultaneously with the peak regurgitant flow and the peak regurgitant velocity. In clinical practice, it is most common averaging PISA over the duration of flow, so that TVI of regurgitant flow replaces peak velocity, as follows:

EROA = (6.28 × r^2) × velocity of aliasing/TVI
$\quad$ of the regurgitant flow $\qquad$ (5.17)

The limitations of this method are:

◆ Sometimes it is difficult to obtain a good PISA image.

◆ It has to be considered that often a formula of the area of the hemisphere is used although perfect hemispheres cannot be obtained.

◆ It is necessary to use the zoom and because of this the resolution of the image may be worsened.

◆ The method is not useful for prosthetic valves and for very calcified valves.

◆ It is necessary to get a good alignment with the direction of the regurgitant flow.

Pressure half-time

The pressure half-time (PHT) represents the lapse of time in which the peak pressure gradient between two adjacent chambers decreases up to a half value.

PHT is commonly used to quantify severity of aortic insufficiency, as regurgitant jet is favoured by the high pressure difference existing between aortic vessel (systemic diastolic artery pressure) and LV at the beginning of diastole. With mild aortic insufficiency, the pressure drop in the aorta will occur slowly and PHT will have an elevated value. With increasing aortic insufficiency severity, the pressure drop in the aorta will occur more rapidly and LV diastolic pressure will significantly rise: thus, PHT tends to lessen, because the rapid decline in aortic pressure reflects a more rapid decline in Doppler velocity (see ➲ Chapter 14a).

PHT is measured by tracing the linear contour of continuous Doppler velocity signal of regurgitant jet and calculating the mean value between the highest and the lowest velocity values (➲ Fig. 5.27). In extreme cases, aortic and LV pressures may equalize and shows a triangular shape with a linear deceleration from the maximum velocity to baseline.

Study of valvular stenosis

Pressure gradients

The assessment of pressure gradients is fundamental in the study of valvular stenosis (as discussed previously).

Two different valvular pressure gradients have to be considered:

◆ Maximal gradient or instantaneous maximal gradient: it is possible to calculate the maximal pressure gradient, that exists when the flow crosses the stenosis, from the maximal

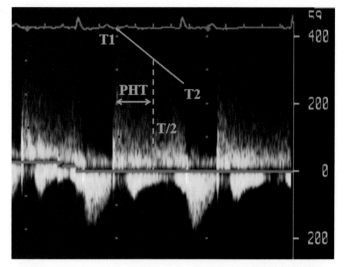

Figure 5.27 Schema indicating the PHT method for calculating severity of aortic regurgitant jet in a case of aortic insufficiency.

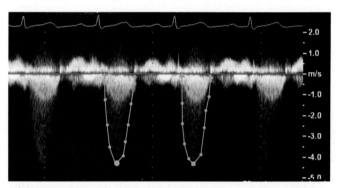

Figure 5.28 Aortic stenosis pressure gradients. CW Doppler image of the aortic pressure gradients in a patient with aortic valvular stenosis. The dome of the curve represents the maximal velocity, which correlates with the maximal gradient calculated with the Bernoulli's formula (explained previously: see ➲ Fig. 5.2). On the other hand, by tracing the curve we can obtain the mean gradient.

flow velocity measured at the peak of the curve by continuous Doppler

◆ Mean gradient: echocardiography allows determination of an average of all the different instantaneous pressure gradients, arising along passing flow. This gradient is obtained by tracing the external contour of the curve of CW Doppler (➲ Fig. 5.28).

The limitations of this approach are:

◆ A good alignment with the flow direction is required, as in other procedures.

◆ In cases of irregular paces an average of different measures (at least 10) needs to be determined.

◆ In some situations, flow velocity and therefore also gradients increase. Some examples are: hyperdynamic situations like hypovolaemia or anaemia, the volume overload secondary to valvular insufficiencies, etc. On the contrary, there are also

other circumstances, as, for example, systolic LV dysfunction, which causes a decrease of the gradients.

Details regarding pressure gradients of AS are explained in ➲ Chapter 14a.

Continuity equation

Calculation of valvular area needs to apply the same principle of conservation of the mass used in the cases of valvular insufficiencies: the flow before the stenosis has to be equal to that after stenosis. In agreement with the formula of calculation of volumes, the areas and the TVI before and at the level of stenosis have to be calculated (➲ Fig. 5.29).

$$\text{Area before stenosis (AREA1)} \times \text{TVI before stenosis (TVI 1)}$$
$$= \text{area of stenosis (AREA 2)} \times \text{TVI at stenosis (TVI 2)}$$

$$(5.18)$$

The limitations are the same as mentioned previously. Considering these, this method should be avoided:

◆ In cases of associated significant valvular insufficiencies.

◆ In cases of poor acoustic window.

◆ In absence of alignment with the flow direction.

◆ After a valvuloplasty (because in these cases correlation with invasive measurements is lower).

Pressure half-time

PHT is frequently used in cases of mitral stenosis, because it reflects the time lapse in which the transvalvular mitral diastolic gradient decreases up to half value: the smaller the orifice, the slower the rate of pressure decline. PHT is obtained by tracing the slope of the E-wave (see ➲ Chapter 9) by using CW Doppler. The tracing obtained is sometimes bimodal, the early part of the E-wave being more abrupt than the following part of the mitral flow. When this situation occurs, it is recommended to

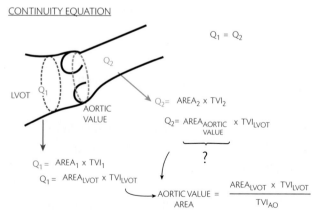

Figure 5.29 Schema indicating the continuity equation for the calculation of the aortic valve area in cases of aortic stenosis.

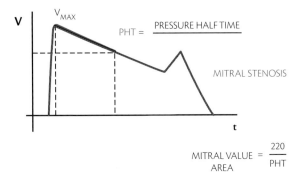

Figure 5.30 Schema indicating the PHT method for calculating mitral valvular area in cases of mitral stenosis.

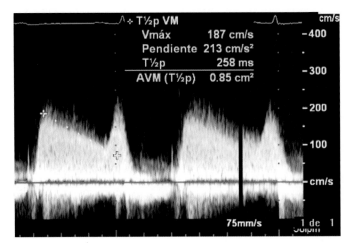

Figure 5.31 CW Doppler image of the mitral inflow in a patient with mitral stenosis.

measure the slope with the longer duration. In patients in atrial fibrillation, an average of five cycles should be measured.

Accordingly to measurements in the study by Halle, for an area of 1cm² the PHT value is 220 milliseconds ($\circleddash$ Figs. 5.30 and 5.31). Therefore, the following formula was obtained:

$$\text{Mitral valve area (MVA)} = 220/\text{PHT} \qquad (5.19)$$

An advantage of this method is that PHT is not affected by the angle between flow direction and ultrasound beam direction.

The limitations to this method are:

♦ In the presence of tachycardia, the measurement of the E-wave deceleration slope is difficult because the diastole is shortened.

♦ In cases of irregular paces, it would be necessary to measure at least 10 cycles.

♦ When the deceleration slope is not linear, it is recommended to omit the initial rapid slope and to measure the slope in the middle diastole.

♦ In cases of diastolic dysfunction, the mitral filling pattern is pathological.

♦ Immediately after a valvuloplasty (the first 3 days).

♦ In the presence of prosthetic valves, this method has not been validated and overestimates the areas.

♦ If there is a significant aortic regurgitation, the PHT becomes shorter because the increase in LV diastolic pressure (LVDP) promotes a more rapid mitral filling.

Another similar formula measures the time of deceleration of the E wave (DTE) (see $\circleddash$ Chapter 9) until the gradient of pressure becomes 0:

$$\text{MVA} = 750/\text{DTE} \qquad (5.20)$$

PISA method

The PISA method might also be used in cases of mitral stenosis. For this purpose, it is necessary to make a correction according to the angle if this is lower than 180 degrees (see $\circleddash$ Chapter 14b).

Study of the intracardiac pressures

Applying Bernoulli's formula ($\circleddash$ Equation 5.3), the pressures in different cardiac chambers can be assessed. For this purpose, the occurrence of some regurgitation flows is required, as indicated in the graph ($\circleddash$ Fig. 5.32):

♦ RV systolic pressure (RVSP): this is equal to the PA systolic pressure (PASP) and can be calculated by adding the tricuspid regurgitation (TR) gradient to the RA pressure (see $\circleddash$ Chapter 11, 'Assessment of right ventricular haemodynamics'). TR reflects the pressure difference between the systolic pressure of the RV and that of the RA. It is also important to measure RVOT and the PA velocities in order to know if there is an obstruction at that level that can account for an increase in the RVSP ($\circleddash$ Fig. 5.33).

♦ PA diastolic pressure (PADP): this can be assessed by adding the end-diastolic RV pressure (that is the same than the RA pressure) to the PA end-diastolic regurgitant gradient. Pulmonary regurgitation (PR) gradient is representative of the pressure difference between PA and RV in diastole ($\circleddash$ Fig. 5.32) (see $\circleddash$ Chapter 11, 'Assessment of right ventricular haemodynamics').

♦ LA systolic pressure: this is calculated by subtracting the mitral regurgitation maximal gradient from the LV systolic pressure (LVSP), that corresponds to the systolic blood pressure (SBP), in absence of an obstruction of the LVOT. Mitral regurgitation (MR) gradient reflects the pressure difference between LV and LA in systole ($\circleddash$ Fig. 5.32).

♦ LV diastolic pressure (LVDP): this can be obtained by subtracting the aortic end-diastolic regurgitant gradient from the diastolic blood pressure (DBP). Aortic regurgitation (AR) gradient reflects the pressure difference between the LV and the aorta in diastole ($\circleddash$ Fig. 5.32).

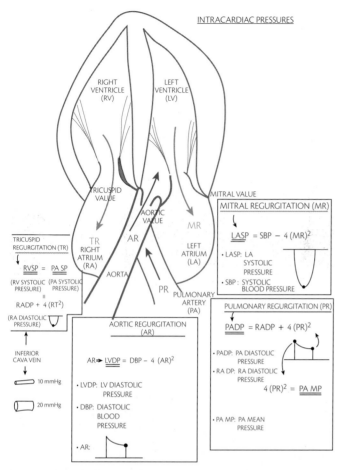

INTRACARDIAC PRESSURES

Figure 5.32 Estimation of intracardiac pressures. Schema indicating the formulae for calculating several intracardiac pressures. The main limitation is that the existence of a valvular regurgitation is required and that the right atrium pressure values are always estimated from the evaluation of the cava vein collapse.

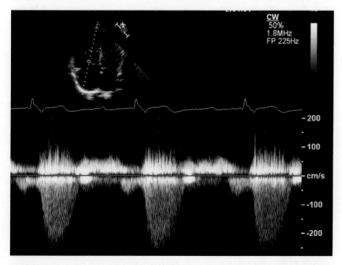

Figure 5.33 Tricuspid regurgitation. Example of the tricuspid regurgitation continuous Doppler wave image. The dome of the curve corresponds to the maximal tricuspid regurgitation pressure gradient.

♦ The LVDP can be also estimated from the diastolic mitral inflow pattern (see ➲ Chapter 9).

dP/dt

This parameter measures the variation of pressure depending on the time, during the isovolumetric contraction and allows the contractile function to be defined. During isovolumetric contraction there is no significant increase of atrial pressure (except in the acute mitral insufficiency). Therefore this value depends on the preload conditions, but not on the afterload.

A mitral or tricuspid insufficiency is required to calculate this parameter. Once the regurgitation curve is obtained by continuous Doppler, the time elapsed from the 1m/s to the 3m/s velocity steps or from a pressure of 4mmHg to 36mmHg has to be measured (➲ Fig. 5.34).

$$4 - 36mmHg = dP/dt = 32mmHg/time\ (s)$$
(Normal value: 1200mmHg/s)

Moreover, the measurement of the time constant of isovolumetric relaxation (Tau) can be performed. It corresponds to the negative dP/dt and the normal value is 30–40ms.

Resistances

Resistance is defined as the ratio of pressure gradient to flow. As Doppler echocardiography provides reliable measure of pressure gradients and flows, calculation of systemic and pulmonary vascular resistance is easily made.

Systemic vascular resistance

Data derived from cardiac catheterization shows that systemic vascular resistance (SVR), calculated as:

$$SVR = (mean\ aortic\ pressure\ -\ right\ atrial\ pressure)/CO$$

correlates with echocardiographic assessment of SVR as:

$$SVR = mitral\ regurgitation\ velocity/TVI_{LVOT}\qquad(5.21)$$

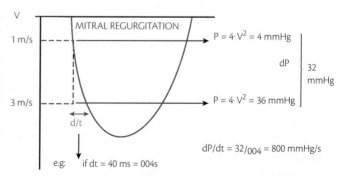

Figure 5.34 Example of the calculation of the dP/dt. In this example given, dP/dt is diminished which indicates the existence of systolic LV dysfunction.

In patients with aortic stenosis, mean aortic resistance appears to be less affected by transvalvular flow. So, mean aortic resistance can be assessed as:

Mean aortic resistance = mean pressure gradient/aortic flow

= (mean pressure gradient/√mean pressure gradient)/(flow/√mean pressure gradient)

= (28/√mean pressure gradient)/aortic valvular area

Pulmonary vascular resistance

Pulmonary vascular resistance (PVR) is considered as the pressure drop across the pulmonary bed (mean systolic pulmonary pressure minus mean left atrial pressure) divided by stroke volume. Because of difficulty in measuring left atrial pressure, there are two other way to calculate PVR. The first one is based on the estimation of pressure drop across the pulmonary vascular bed using the peak tricuspid regurgitant jet velocity and the stroke volume obtained from the TVI of the flow in the RVOT. The resulting ratio is multiplied by 10 to approximate PVR in Wood units:

$$PVR = 10 \text{ (peak tricuspid regurgitant jet velocity)}/TVI_{RVOT}$$
(5.22)

The second method to assess PVR is described in ➲ Chapter 11, 'Pulmonary vascular resistance'. Resistance values are expressed by Wood units

Study of communications between cardiac chambers

These parameters are very important to study intracardiac shunts (see ➲ Chapter 22) (➲ Figs. 5.35 and 5.36). The flow volume across the shunt correlates with its magnitude. It is calculated by dividing the pulmonary flow (named as Qp) by the systemic flow (named as Qs). For this purpose, the calculation of volumes using ➲ Equation 5.4 is required. The diameters of

ventricular outflow tracts should be measured in PLAX for LVOT and in SAX for RVOT.

$$Qp = Area_{RVOT} \times TVI_{RVOT}$$
(5.23)

$$Qs = Area_{LVOT} \times TVI_{LVOT}$$
(5.24)

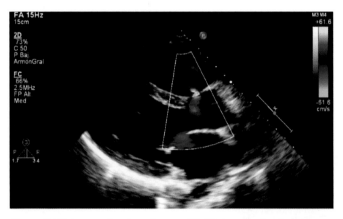

Figure 5.35 Intracardiac shunt. Image of PLAX view showing, by colour Doppler, a subaortic interventricular septal defect: note the blood flowing from left ventricle to right ventricle (red colour).

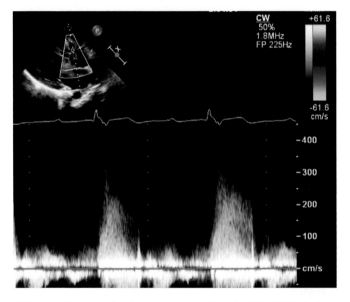

Figure 5.36 Intracardiac shunt assessment. Example of the CW Doppler assessment of intracardiac shunt at the level of subaortic interventricular septal defect.

Personal perspective

The haemodynamic assessment is one of the most important aims in the evaluation of cardiac function, not only for studying the myocardial dysfunction secondary to coronary artery disease, but also for studying cardiomyopathies and valvular diseases. Echocardiography is a very useful and important diagnostic technique because it provides anatomical information and evaluation of the myocardial contractile function, as well as the possibility of performing a non-invasive haemodynamic assessment. With this, we can measure the blood flow velocities, the transvalvular pressure gradients, the valvular areas, and other parameters of cardiac function. This non-invasive haemodynamic assessment is fundamental for decision making, not only due to the information that it provides, but also due to the fact that it can be an alternative to invasive procedures in some clinical circumstances. Thanks to the new image techniques in cardiology and the new image acquisition and processing tools, the importance of the echocardiographic haemodynamic assessment will increase and the actual methods may be improved. Thus, we consider that it is necessary for every cardiologist to understand how this echocardiographic study is performed, its advantages and limitations, and the future perspectives.

References

1 Omoto R, Kasai C. Physics and instrumentation of Doppler color flow zapping. *Echocardiography* 1987; **4**:467–83.

2 Kisslo J, Adams DB, Belkin RN. *Doppler color flow imaging.* New York: Churchill Livingstone; 1988.

3 Hatle L, Angelsen B. Doppler ultrasound in cardiology: physical principles and clinical applications, 2nd ed. Philadelphia, PA: Lea and Febiger; 1985.

4 García Fernández MA. *Principios y práctica del doppler cardíaco.* Madrid: McGraw Hill; 1995, pp.2–21.

5 Quiñones MA, Otto CM, Stoddard M, Waggoner A, Zoghbi WA. Recommendations for quantification of Doppler echocardiography: a report from the Doppler Quantification Task Force of the Nomenclature and Standards Committee of the American Society of Echocardiography. *J Am Soc Echocardiogr* 2002; **15**(2):167–84.

Further reading

Baumgartner H, Hung J, Bermejo J, Chambers JB, Evangelista A, Griffin BP, *et al.* Echocardiographic assessment of valve stenosis: EAE/ASE recommendations for clinical practice. *Eur J Echocardiogr* 2009; **10**:1–25.Evangelista A, Flachskampf F, Lancellotti P, Badano L, Aguilar R, Monaghan M, et al. EAE recommendations for standardization of performance, digital storage and reporting of echocardiographic studies. *Eur J Echocardiogr* (2008); 9(4):438–48.

García Fernández MA, Zamorano JL. *Procedimientos en ecocardiografía.* Madrdi: Mc Graw Hill; 2004: pp. 75–95.Garcia Fernández MA. *Principios del Doppler Cardíaco.* Madrid: Interamericana McGraw Hill; (2005).Oh JK, Seward JB, Tajik AS. *The Echo Manual,* 3rd ed. Philadelphia, PA: Lippincott Williams and Wilkins; (2007), pp.59–80.

Wittlich N, Erbel R, Drexler M. Color Doppler flow mapping of the heart in normal subjects. *Echocardiography* 1988; **5**:157.

Additional DVD and online material

- 5.1 Colour Doppler echo in PLAX.

- 5.2 Colour Doppler echo in parasternal right ventricle inflow view.

- 5.3 Colour Doppler echo in parasternal right ventricle outflow view.

- 5.4 Colour Doppler echo in PSAX at aortic valve level.

- 5.5 Colour Doppler echo in A4C view.

- 5.6 Colour Doppler echo in A5C view.

- 5.7 Colour Doppler echo in suprasternal long-axis view.

⊃ For additional multimedia materials please visit the online version of the book (⌕ http://escecho.oxfordmedicine.com).

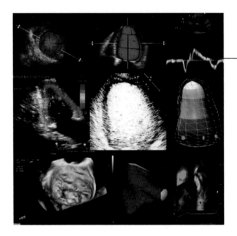

CHAPTER 6

Quantification of left ventricular function and synchrony using tissue Doppler, strain imaging, and speckle tracking

Jens-Uwe Voigt

Contents

Summary

Modern echocardiographic systems allow the quantitative and qualitative assessment of regional myocardial function by measuring velocity, motion, deformation, and other parameters of myocardial function.

Both colour Doppler (CD) and spectral Doppler modes provide one-dimensional estimates of velocity. From CD data only, further parameters can be derived. Tracking techniques have recently been introduced which provide all parameters two-dimensionally, but at the cost of lower temporal resolution.

Several clinical applications have been proposed, including regional and global systolic function assessment, evaluation of diastolic cardiac properties, and assessment of ventricular dyssynchrony.

This chapter provides an introduction to the method of Doppler- and tracking-based function assessment and provides a basis for understanding its different clinical applications.

Introduction

The evaluation of myocardial function by echocardiography is based on observing and interpreting the motion of tissue within the scan plane or volume. Currently, two techniques are available:

◆ Doppler-based velocity measurements.

◆ Tracking-based displacement measurements.

All other parameters (deformation, torsion, pressure gradients in the blood, etc.) are directly or indirectly derived from these two techniques.

Doppler-based velocity estimation

Principles

Doppler-based tissue velocity estimation, named tissue Doppler (TD), uses the known principles of spectral Doppler and colour Doppler (CD) echocardiography[1,2] (see ◐ Chapter 5).

A so-called *wall filter* which considers signal intensity and velocity is used to distinguish signals from tissue and blood motion. While the signal intensity of myocardium is higher than that of blood, velocity of the blood regularly exceeds velocities of the myocardium (◐ Fig. 6.1).

The options for influencing the colour or spectral tissue Doppler acquisition and display are then comparable to the

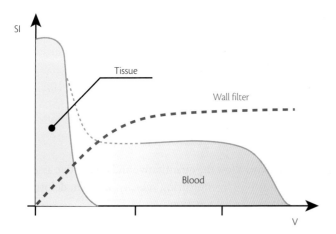

Figure 6.1 Wall filter curve. Velocity signals from tissue and blood can be distinguished by signal intensity (SI) and velocity (v). While blood usually moves fast and tissue slow, the tissue has higher signal intensities than blood.

known blood pool Doppler settings (◐ Fig. 6.2). Likewise, aliasing problems can occur in TD (◐ Fig. 6.3).

Furthermore, TD can be used over M-mode in selected cases: it paints in red movements of the myocardium towards the transducer and in blue movements of the myocardium away from the transducer. These colour patterns are useful for detailed studies of the movement of the myocardium (◐ Fig. 6.4).

Data acquisition

Spectral Doppler

Spectral Doppler acquisitions require a sample volume size and position to stay within the myocardial region of interest throughout the cardiac cycle. Scale, baseline, sweep speed, and gain adjustments need to be obtained. Care should be taken that the ultrasound beam is aligned with the direction of motion to be interrogated (◐ Fig. 6.5A). Depending on the view, only certain motion directions can be investigated with Doppler techniques (◐ Fig. 6.5B). In an apical view, velocity samples are usually taken at the basal end of the basal and mid, less frequent also in apical segments of each wall, i.e. an 18-segment model is used.

Colour Doppler

CD requires a high frame rate, preferably above 100, ideally around 140 or more frames per second (fps).[2] This can be achieved by reducing depth and sector width (of both grey-scale and Doppler sector), and by choosing a setting which favours frame rate over spatial resolution. Scale is set to a range which just avoids aliasing in any region of the myocardium. The image optimization should be done in the grey-scale display before switching to colour and acquiring. Care should be taken to

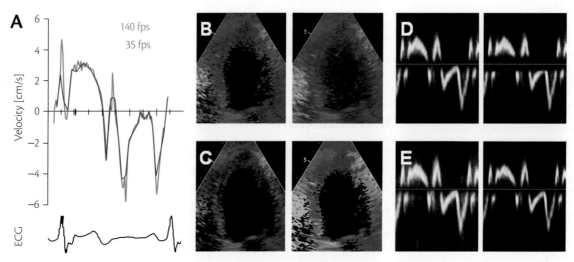

Figure 6.2 Settings for spectral and colour Doppler acquisition and display. A) High (green) and low (red) frame rate acquisition of the same velocity curve. Note the blunting of the sharper diastolic peaks. Isovolumic peaks are not valid any more. B) Tissue priority high (left) and low (right) as well as C) transparency high (left) and low (right) influence the display of colour data compared to the underlying grey-scale image. Data content of the acquisition is not affected. D) Low velocity reject low (left) and high (right) removes clutter signals around baseline. E) A threshold setting low (left) and high (right) suppresses weak signals in the background.

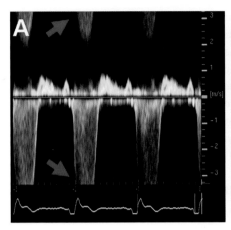
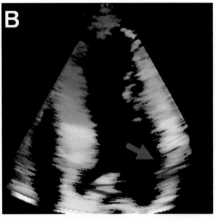

Figure 6.3 Aliasing (red arrows) in A) spectral Doppler; B) colour Doppler. (Modified from [31])

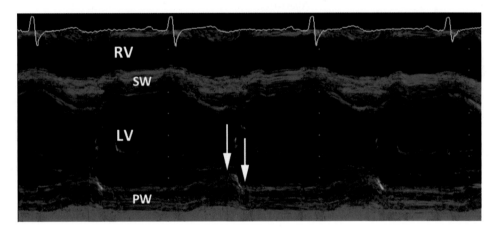

Figure 6.4 Tissue Doppler imaging over M-mode tracing of the LV. The myocardium is painted in red when moving towards the transducer and blue when moving away from the transducer. The changes of the direction of the movement of the myocardium (as, for example, the marked ones with white arrows) are easily tracked with the change of colour pattern. LV, left ventricle; PW, posterior wall; RV, right ventricle; SW, septal wall.

avoid reverberation artefacts. They will particularly disturb strain rate estimations over a wide area (➔ Fig. 6.6). As in CD, the motion direction to be interrogated should be aligned with the ultrasound beams. If needed, separate acquisitions per wall will facilitate this. Data should be acquired unsparingly over at least three beats (i.e. covering at least four QRS complexes) and stored in a raw data format.

For later classification of the different peaks, the additional acquisition of blood flow Doppler spectra of the in- and outlet valve of the interrogated ventricle is recommended. Opening and closing artefacts allow the exact definition of the cardiac time intervals (➔ Fig. 6.7).

Post-processing

Spectral Doppler

Spectral Doppler data cannot be further processed. Peak values or slopes are measured directly on the spectral display. Although it appears not completely consistent, most labs measure on the outer edge of the spectrum which results inevitably in slightly higher peak values compared to CD. ➔ Figure 6.8 shows normal curve patterns from the basal septum and lateral wall.

Colour Doppler

CD data can be displayed and post-processed in many ways. Two display concepts are used: colour coding with or without a straight or curved M-mode and reconstructed curves of regional function.

Colour-coded data develop their full potential in still frames and particularly in M-mode displays. In this way, they provide easy visual access to the regional and temporal distribution of a particular parameter within the entire wall (➔ Fig. 6.7).

Curve reconstructions are subsequently possible from any point within a stored data set (➔ Fig. 6.7). They allow the display of the exact time course of regional velocities or other parameters. An advantage of CD processing over pulsed wave (PW) Doppler is that the sample volume can track the motion of the myocardium and thus stay in the same region throughout the entire cardiac cycle (➔ Fig. 6.9). Curves can be generated and quantified with several commercial and non-commercial programs. The time course of a spectral Doppler velocity curve is similar to a colour-derived one. However, absolute values differ since the spectral curve is usually measured at the outer edge of the spectrum while CD data

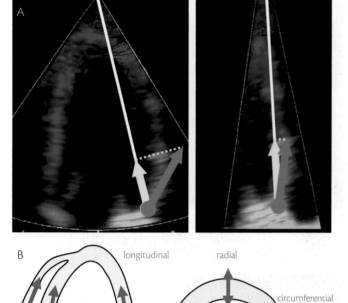

Figure 6.5 Data acquisition: spectral Doppler. A) Alignment of the Doppler beam with the wall. Left panel: measured velocities (yellow) are underestimated if the ultrasound beam is not well aligned with the motion to be interrogated (red). Right panel: narrow sector single wall acquisitions help to optimize data quality. B) Motion/deformation components which can be interrogated with Doppler techniques.

approximate the median velocity of a region. Therefore measurements from both methods cannot be used interchangeably.

CD data sets can be used to calculate derived parameters, such as motion (*displacement*), deformation and deformation rate (*strain and strain rate*), rotation, rotational deformation (*twist, torsion*) as well as to display the temporal course of events, such as the time of appearance of velocity peaks (*tissue synchronicity imaging*) or phase differences between myocardial regions (*VVI phase map*) (➲ Figs. 6.7 and 6.11).

Colour Doppler-derived parameters

Velocity

By default, CD imaging delivers velocity values, comparable to spectral Doppler. Data are given in cm/s.

Motion

Motion or displacement is the temporal integral of the tissue velocity, according to the following formula:

$$d = \int v dt \qquad (6.1)$$

where d is the displacement and v is the velocity. It describes the motion component of the tissue in the sample volume towards and away from the transducer during the cardiac cycle: the motion curve of the mitral ring derived from CD data should have the same shape and magnitude as the M-mode contour of the mitral ring at the same place.

Strain rate

Strain rate (SR) is the temporal derivative of myocardial deformation. It describes how fast the tissue changes its length. Strain rate is analytically identical to the spatial gradient of the tissue

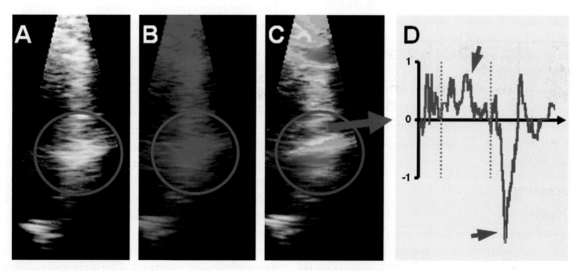

Figure 6.6 Data acquisition: colour Doppler. Reverberation artefacts are best recognized in the grey-scale image (A) and can be missed in the colour Doppler display (B). They become obvious again in the colour-coded strain rate display (B) as parallel yellow/blue lines of high intensity (C). If only the reconstructed curve from such a region is considered (D), artefacts may be mistaken as highly pathological curves mimicking 'systolic lengthening' or 'postsystolic shortening' (red arrows).

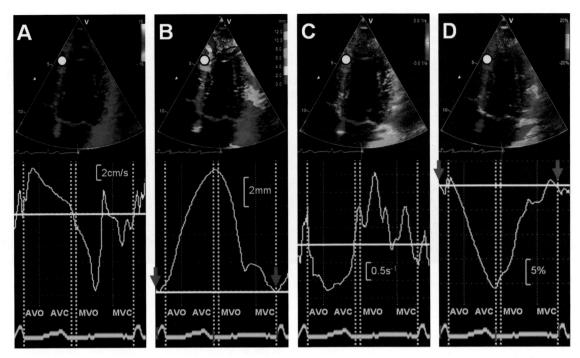

Figure 6.7 Function parameters. Different function parameters derived from one region of interest within the same colour Doppler data set. Top panels: colour-coded display, below curves, bottom: ECG. A) velocity, B) displacement, C) strain rate, D) strain. Note that in this case the baseline is—arbitrarily—set to the curve value (red arrows) at the automatically recognized begin of QRS (red opening bracket). (Modified from [31])

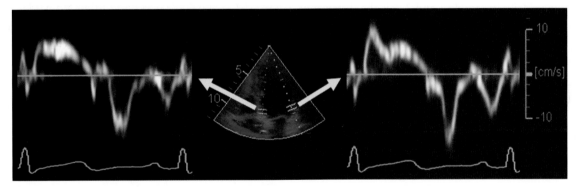

Figure 6.8 Post-processing: spectral Doppler. Normal tissue Doppler spectra from the basal septum (left) and the basal lateral wall (right). Note the different amplitude and shape of the curves.

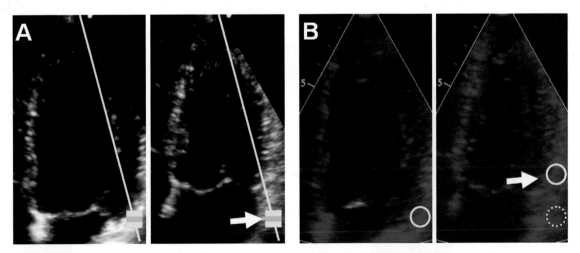

Figure 6.9 Post-processing: colour Doppler. A) The sample volume of a spectral Doppler remains in the same position throughout the cardiac cycle. Therefore, care has to be taken that the region to be interrogated is covered both in diastole and systole. B) In colour Doppler one can follow the myocardial motion during post-processing by manually adjusting the position of the region of interest (ROI) which allows it to stay in the same myocardial region throughout the cardiac cycle.

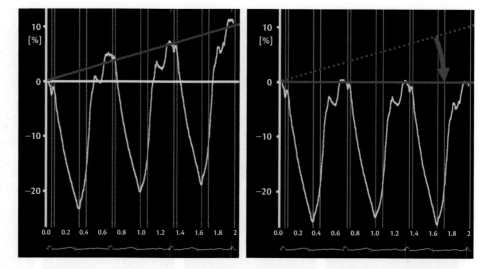

Figure 6.10 Strain and strain rate. Integration of velocity or strain rate data often results in considerable baseline shifts of the resulting motion or strain (left panel) curves. Most softwares allow a linear correction (right panel). Note that both systolic and diastolic values are influenced by this correction. (Modified from [31])

velocities and can be calculated from two velocity samples in a certain distance, which is done in echocardiography.[3,4] It is obtained by:

$$\text{A) } SR = \frac{dv}{dr} \qquad \text{B) } SR = \frac{v_2 - v_1}{r_2 - r_1} \qquad (6.2)$$

where v is the velocity in sample 1 and 2, r is the distance of sample 1 and 2 from the transducer. Strain rate is given in 1/s.

Strain

Strain or deformation describes the relative regional length or thickness change of myocardium. When interrogated with TD echocardiography, it is calculated as temporal integral of strain rate:

$$\varepsilon = \int SR \, dt \qquad (6.3)$$

where ε represents strain or deformation and SR is the strain rate as derived from colour TD. Strain is unitless and usually given in %.

Motion and deformation of the myocardium are cyclic processes with no defined beginning or end. Therefore, the position of the baseline (*zero line*) is arbitrary. Most analysis packages define *zero* automatically as the value at the begin of the QRS complex (red arrows in Fig. 6.7B,D) and report in measurements the actual position or length change relative to that. Although useful for a lot of applications, this approach may not work under certain circumstances, such as bundle branch blocks, wrong QRS detection in the ECG, etc. Care must be taken to use comparable references in all measurements within a lab (i.e. zero at beginning of QRS or mitral valve [MV] closure) and to consider the method used in publications.

Furthermore, the integration process (➲ Equations 6.1 and 6.3) often results in an erroneous baseline shift. Most softwares automatically apply a linear correction (➲ Fig. 6.10).

Tissue synchronicity imaging

Tissue synchronicity imaging (TSI) uses regular velocity data. Only the colour coding of the two-dimensional (2D) display is changed to a colour scale which codes the time of the first

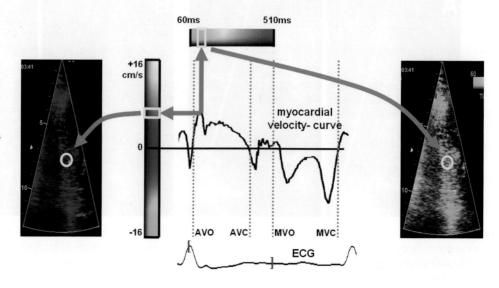

Figure 6.11 Principles of tissue synchronicity imaging. While regular colour Doppler displays encode the velocity of the myocardium (left panel), tissue synchronicity imaging (TSI) detects the first positive velocity peak in a certain time window (given by the red brackets on the ECG) and uses a green-red colour scale to encode the time to appearance of this peak, resulting in a motion delay display (right panel). Motion delays do not necessarily display contraction delays.

occurrence of a positive velocity peak after a certain point in time, such as beginning of QRS, aortic valve opening, etc (➔ Fig. 6.11). Measurement results are therefore given in ms.

Tracking-based motion estimation

Principles

Tissue tracking is based on analysing the image content of a given echo loop frame by frame and evaluating the recognized changes.[5] Analysis can be performed either at the level of radio-frequency data or at the level of the final grey-scale image. The latter is used in commercially available analysis software: certain patterns in the image (*speckles*) are recognized and their displacement is followed over time frame by frame. Since the frame rate of the echo loop is known, the velocity of single *points* within the tissue, but also the deformation and—theoretically—the deformation rate of a certain tissue region can be estimated (➔ Fig. 6.12).

In contrast to Doppler measurements, tissue tracking works in all directions within the image plane, i.e. it also identifies the direction of motion. With this, additional parameters become available.

Data acquisition

Tissue tracking requires regular grey-scale data of excellent quality. Reverberation artefacts, noise, and shadowing have to be avoided by all means. Within the image plane, no alignment between the motion direction to be interrogated and the ultrasound beam is necessary.

As in TD imaging, sector width and depth have to be adapted to allow frame rates as high as possible. Settings which increase frame rate on the cost of a reduced spatial resolution are less optimal, since lateral tracking within the image relies on beam density and would be directly negatively affected. Therefore, typical frame rates for tissue tracking rarely exceed 80fps which limits the technique mainly to the analysis of systolic events. Events during filling time may be assessed if frame rates are above 120–140fps, but any measurement during isovolumic intervals should be avoided as long as no higher frame rates can

be achieved (➔ Fig. 6.3A). For the same reason, tracking-based motion and deformation curves are more reliable than velocity and deformation rate.

A three-beat acquisition as for TD is recommended, although some softwares use single beats for analysis.

Post-processing

The single post-processing steps are vendor-specific but usually comprise a semi-automated selection of the region to be interrogated, a short waiting time for processing by the tracking algorithm, and a subsequent display of the tracking result.

The tracking result should be carefully checked on a subsegment scale, by visually comparing the motion of the tracking points to the motion of the underlying grey-scale data. Software which does not allow this control step should not be used. Estimates on tracking quality provided by the software may be considered, but cannot replace a careful visual inspection (➔ Fig 6.13; 🖥 6.1 and 6.2).

Tracking software post-processes the initially very noisy motion estimates further in order to produce clinically meaningful velocity, motion, and deformation results. This post-processing is vendor-specific and can hardly be controlled by the user. Knowledge on its principles, however, is useful for recognizing possible post-processing artefacts.

Due to the unfavourable signal-to-noise ratio of tracking estimates, smoothing over a wide myocardial region is needed. Particularly estimates across a wall and perpendicular to the ultrasound beam (e.g. radial strain in a four-chamber view) have to be handled with caution. Recognition of differences between myocardial layers appears difficult. Furthermore, several vendors use a priori knowledge on the overall motion pattern of a ventricle. The underlying algorithms influence the results for a certain myocardial region based on the behaviour of other regions within the same image which can lead to an underestimation of regional function differences in regional pathology.

On the other hand, the limited user interaction allows fast post-processing and a higher reproducibility of tracking results compared to Doppler and other *manual* echocardiographic measurements (🖥 6.3).

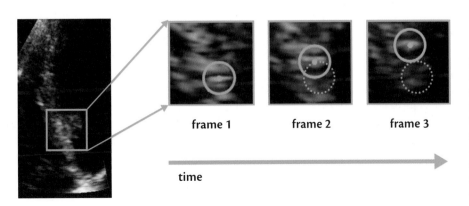

frame 1   **frame 2**   **frame 3**

time

Figure 6.12 Speckle tracking. Prominent speckles in the image are recognized and followed frame by frame. The measured displacement between frames allows calculation of velocity and direction of motion. Tracking several speckles allows the calculation of two-dimensional deformation. (Modified from [31])

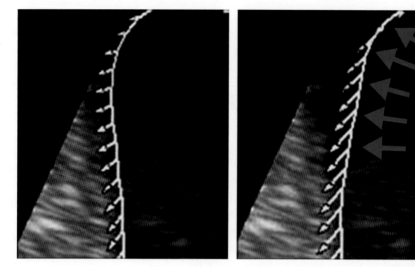

Figure 6.13 Tracking result. Careful visual inspection of the tracking result is mandatory. Detail of endocardial tracking in the apex. A) Good tracking. B) Bad tracking, since the line does not follow the myocardium. See also 🎞 6.1 and 6.2.

Tracking-derived parameters

Tissue tracking can provide all parameters known from TD, such as velocity, motion, deformation rate, and deformation (see earlier). Limitations due to frame rate and tracking quality have to be considered. Data are available in all directions within the image plane. By default, most tracking softwares provide options to select a display of results along or perpendicular to the endocardial border. In general, tracking results along the ultrasound beam are more reliable than those perpendicular to it. The temporal course of motion and deformation measured by tracking resembles Doppler data. Magnitude of parameters may differ due to the technique and due to the differing segmentation of the ventricle that includes the very apical region which is usually avoided in Doppler measurements.

Additional information can be derived by tracking (➲ Fig. 6.14). Vendor-specific differences are possible:

Rotation

Rotation is usually understood as an in-plane turning of the entire ventricle.[6] The axis of the rotational motion is automatically determined by the software. Values are given in degrees (°). Segmental rotation is difficult to define. The underlying tissue deformation is better described by circumferential strain.

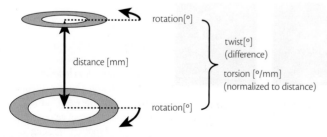

Figure 6.14 Parameters describing rotational deformation. Grey rings indicate apical and basal short-axis planes in which rotation is measured. Twist and torsion can be calculated as described in the text. (Modified from [31])

Rotation rate

This is the temporal derivative of rotation

$$RR = \frac{d\omega}{dt} \quad \text{with } RR = \text{rotation rate, } \omega = \text{rotation, } t = \text{time.} \quad (6.4)$$

where RR represents the rotation rate, ω the rotation and t the time. Rotation rate describes how fast the interrogated ventricular plane turns. Care should be taken that the underlying data set has a sufficient frame rate.

Twist and torsion

The words *twist* and *torsion* are not uniformly used. In principle, two entities have to be differentiated:

1 The difference in apical and basal rotation of a ventricle:

$$twist = \omega_{apex} - \omega_{base} \quad (6.5)$$

For this the term 'twist' will be used in the following. Twist is given in °. Image planes for measuring apical and basal rotation should be parallel and perpendicular to the left ventricular (LV) axis, which is rarely possible in the clinical setting. To what extend twist results are influenced by deviations from that rule is unknown.

2 The twist normalized to the distance between the two rotating planes:

$$torsion = \frac{\omega_{apex} - \omega_{base}}{d} \quad (6.6)$$

where d is the distance between planes. For this, the term 'torsion' will be used in the following. Torsion is given in °/mm. Although torsion has the theoretical advantage of being independent from LV length, the distance between the two image planes can not be exactly determined in 2D imaging.

Twist rate, torsion rate

Temporal derivatives are possible from both earlier mentioned parameters. Terms are not uniformly used in the literature.

Three-dimensional regional function estimation

Principles

With the evolution of three-dimensional (3D) imaging, *full volume* data set become available. Doppler-based function measurements are, in principle, possible in such data sets, but retain the limitation of one-dimensionality. Current 3D data sets have limited temporal and spatial resolution which makes tracking challenging. On the other hand, through-plane motion is no problem anymore, since motion can be detected in any direction in space. Further developments and study results have to be observed to give general recommendations on this topic.

Three-dimensional tracking derived parameters

In addition to the earlier mentioned, 3D tracking could provide principal strain, i.e. the regional direction and magnitude of the highest and lowest deformation of the myocardium. Furthermore, torsion estimates become more reliable because image planes can be set to be parallel while the exact distance is known.

Clinical assessment of myocardial function

Normal longitudinal velocity, displacement, strain rate, and strain curves are shown in ➲ Fig. 6.7. Depending on the pathology interrogated, changes occur in the amplitude of the systolic and/or diastolic peaks or in the time course pattern of the curve. In Doppler data, amplitude measurements are subject to higher variability while the time course of the curve is more robust. In tracking data, both rely on frame rate and tracking quality.

Interpretation of all functional parameters requires considering regional loading conditions, including pressures as well as size, shape, and conduction sequence of the ventricle. Specific changes in particular pathology are mentioned in the different chapters of the book.

Global systolic function

Doppler and tracking-based function measurements provide regional information. Velocity data in particular are subject to complex interactions between myocardial segments. Basal or mitral ring velocities can exemplify normal global function or homogeneous global dysfunction of a ventricle, but this is problematic in regional disease.

Ejection fraction

In combination with semi-automated contour detection, tracking algorithms can be used to automate and improve the assessment of ejection fraction (EF) in 2D (Simpson's method) or 3D (direct volume measurement) imaging.

Global strain

EF is an invaluable clinical parameter which can be provided by echocardiography in an accurate and reproducible manner. In clinical routine, uncertainties occur mostly in mildly reduced function. Global strain, usually defined as the average of longitudinal strain of the entire image plane or ventricle, is a new, mostly tracking-derived parameter which seems to offer comparable information to EF, but at lower inter- and intraobserver variability. Several larger studies have shown its superior predictive value for patient outcome.[7] Its normal ranges, assessment feasibility, and added value in the clinical routine remains to be determined. First experience indicates that values around −18% . . . −20% are normal and values around 12% are comparable to an EF of 35%.

Regional systolic function

Velocity and motion

These parameters are influenced by remote myocardial regions and overall heart motion. They have limited value for assessing regional function but may be used to prove normal function of an entire myocardial wall when basal peak systolic velocities are found to be normal. ➲ Table 6.1 shows normal values.[8,9] Averaged mitral ring velocities allow an estimation of the global longitudinal LV function.

Deformation

Deformation parameters (strain, strain rate) provide true regional information. The normal range of values[10] is shown in ➲ Table 6.2. Depending on the pathology, the general pattern of deformation can remain with just decreased peak values or, especially in regional disease (infarct scar, conduction delay, etc.), curve patterns will change regionally (➲ Fig. 6.15).

Longitudinal postsystolic shortening

Longitudinal postsystolic shortening (PSS) is the typical finding if ventricular function is inhomogeneous. It can be defined as shortening of the myocardium directly after aortic valve (AoV) closure. It occurs physiologically to a minor extent around the apical and basal septal region (➲ Fig. 6.16A). If PSS exceeds a fourth of the regional deformation, a pathological process is likely[11] (➲ Fig. 6.16B). Together with a reduced systolic function, PSS is a non-specific, but sensitive feature of regional ischaemia and scar. In the setting of stress echocardiography, a stress-induced PSS indicates regional ischaemia[12] (➲ Fig. 6.17B).

Table 6.1

A) Typical longitudinal velocities as measured with PW tissue Doppler from an apical window (adapted from [9], n=25, mean age 33 years (16-68)).

		Peak systolic	E wave	A wave
septal	apical	3.2 ± 0.9	4.3 ± 1.9	2.7 ± 1.1
	medial	5.4 ± 0.9	9.9 ± 2.9	6.2 ± 1.5
	basal	7.8 ± 1.1	11.2 ± 1.9	7.8 ± 2.0
lateral	apical	6.0 ± 2.3	5.5 ± 2.7	3.0 ± 2.4
	medial	9.8 ± 2.3	12.0 ± 3.3	5.7 ± 2.4
	basal	10.2 ± 2.1	14.9 ± 3.5	6.6 ± 2.4
inferior	apical	4.0 ± 1.7	5.2 ± 2.4	2.9 ± 1.8
	medial	6.6 ± 0.7	9.1 ± 2.7	6.4 ± 1.8
	basal	8.7 ± 1.3	12.4 ± 3.8	7.9 ± 2.5
anterior	apical	4.0 ± 1.5	3.9 ± 1.1	2.0 ± 1.5
	medial	7.7 ± 2.2	10.4 ± 3.0	5.5 ± 1.7
	basal	9.0 ± 1.6	12.8 ± 3.0	6.5 ± 1.6
RV free wall	apical	7.0±1.9	8.1±3.4	5.6±2.4
	medial	9.6±2.1	10.6±2.6	9.7±3.3
	basal	12.2±2.6	12.9±3.5	11.6±4.1

B) Typical systolic peak velocities as measured from a parasternal window (adapted from [9],n=30, mean age 31 years (21–56)).

	Radial				Circumferential	
	anterosept.	anterior	posterior	inferior	septal	lateral
medial	1.94±2.15	2.66±1.89	4.78±1.53	4.93±1.45	3.31±1.99	1.94±2.15
basal	−1.92±2.32	−2.64±1.85	4.65±1.51	4.85±1.37	−3.25±2.02	4.16±1.24

To what extent regional deformation measurements add to the diagnosis of viability and scar transmurality, remains to be determined.

Diastolic function/filling pressures

Mitral inflow patterns show a biphasic response with increasing filling pressures which complicates particularly the distinction of normal and severely disturbed diastolic function. Myocardial longitudinal velocities have been shown to reflect LV relaxation kinetics although being also dependent on LV function and preload. Therefore, the ratio of early mitral inflow (E) and early myocardial velocity (E′) was proposed as a clinically useful indicator of elevated filling pressures (see ➲ Chapter 9). Recent studies showed that in patients with reduced EF this parameter is less reliable and inflow velocities need to be considered in the first line. This is reflected in the differentiated recommendations of the EAE/ASE guidelines on evaluation of diastolic function[13] (➲ Fig. 6.17A,B and 6.18).

Clinical assessment of ventricular dyssynchrony

When included according to current guidelines,[14] 20–30% of patients do not respond to cardiac resynchronization therapy (CRT). Therefore, an echocardiographic assessment of intra- and interventricular mechanical dyssynchrony has been proposed to further improve patient selection and optimize pacing. At present, there is no robust evidence base for using advanced echocardiographic methods (motion/deformation imaging, 3D echo) in this clinical setting. Based on multiple studies, however, there is expert consensus that some of the techniques are useful to guide CRT.

Thus, evaluation for dyssynchrony comprises:

- LV volume and global function.

- Regional function assessment, focusing on scar regions and regional contraction sequence.

Table 6.2

A) Typical colour tissue Doppler derived longitudinal peak systolic strain rates and end systolic strains in volunteers (adapted from [10], n=146, mean age ca.33±19 years).

		Peak sys. strain rate [s-1] (mean±SD)	End sys. strain [%] (mean±SD)
septal	apical	−1,9 ± 0,7	−23 ± 6
	mid	−1,7 ± 0,5	−25 ± 5
	basal	−1,5 ± 0,6	−23 ± 7
anteroseptal	apical	−1,4 ± 0,5	−20 ± 4
	mid	−1,5 ± 0,5	−22 ± 5
	basal	−1,3 ± 0,5	−20 ± 6
anterior	apical	−1,6 ± 0,6	−21 ± 6
	mid	−1,5 ± 0,6	−21 ± 5
	basal	−1,5 ± 0,9	−16 ± 5
lateral	apical	−1,7 ± 0,8	−19 ± 5
	mid	−1,7 ± 0,8	−20 ± 6
	basal	−1,8 ± 1,1	−19 ± 6
posterior	apical	−1,6 ± 0,7	−22 ± 5
	mid	−1,6 ± 0,6	−22 ± 6
	basal	−1,6 ± 0,7	−21 ± 5
inferior	apical	−1,5 ± 0,5	−23 ± 5
	mid	−1,5 ± 0,6	−24 ± 6
	basal	−1,5 ± 0,4	−23 ± 6
mean	apical	−1,9 ± 0,7	−23 ± 6
	mid	−1,7 ± 0,5	−25 ± 5
	basal	−1,5 ± 0,6	−23 ± 7

B) Speckle tracking derived longitudinal peak systolic strain rates and end systolic strains in a population free of known heart disease (adapted from [29], n=1266, mean age 49±13 years). Note the rather low deformation values with this approach.

septal	apical	−1.08 ± −1.10	−17.80 ± −17.90
	mid	−1.10 ± −0.85	−17.90 ± −14.60
	basal	−0.85 ± −1.01	−14.60 ± −16.80
anteroseptal	apical	−0.95 ± −1.05	−16.10 ± −17.10
	mid	−1.05 ± −0.95	−17.10 ± -13.90
	basal	−0.95 ± −0.99	−13.90 ± −16.00
anterior	apical	−0.98 ± −1.01	−14.30 ± −17.40
	mid	−1.01 ± −1.07	−17.40 ± −17.70
	basal	−1.07 ± −1.02	−17.70 ± −16.80
lateral	apical	−1.03 ± −0.94	−14.60 ± −16.40
	mid	−0.94 ± −1.22	−16.40 ± −19.20
	basal	−1.22 ± −1.05	−19.20 ± −16.60
posterior	apical	−1.06 ± −1.05	−15.50 ± −17.00
	mid	−1.05 ± −1.10	−17.00 ± −17.00
	basal	−1.10 ± −1.07	−17.00 ± −16.50
inferior	apical	−1.08 ± −1.08	−17.60 ± −17.30
	mid	−1.08 ± −0.91	−17.30 ± −15.90
	basal	−0.91 ± −1.03	−15.90 ± −17.00
mean	apical	−1.04 ± −1.05	−16.40 ± −17.30
	mid	−1.05 ± −0.99	−17.30 ± −16.20
	basal	−0.99 ± −1.03	−16.20 ± −16.70

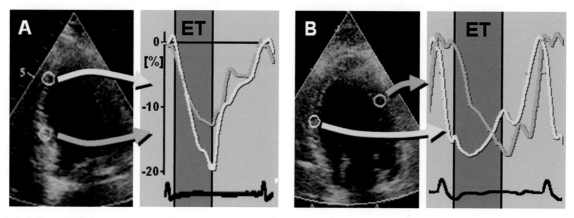

Figure 6.15 Pathological deformation patterns. A) Normal time course but reduced peak strain in the hypertrophic basal segment (green) compared to the normal apical segment (yellow). B) Disturbed strain pattern in LBBB. Shortening in septum (yellow) and lateral wall (green) is completely out-of-phase while the overall strain amplitude is comparable. ET, ejection time.

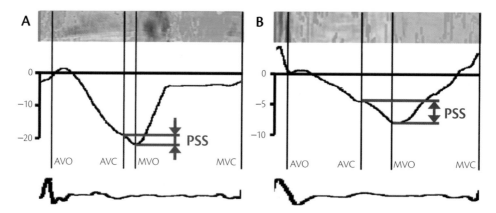

Figure 6.16 Longitudinal postsystolic shortening (PSS). PSS in strain rate curved M-mode (top panels), and strain curves (underneath). A) Physiological PSS usually occurs around the apical and basal septum and has a minor amplitude. B) Pathological PSS is often accompanied by reduced systolic function and exceeds 25–30% of the overall curve amplitude. (Modified from [31])

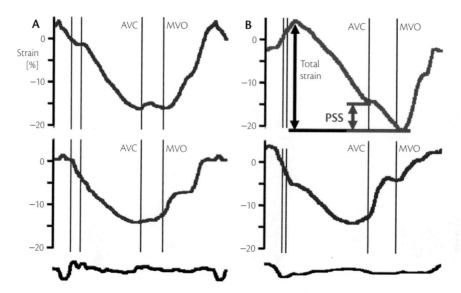

Fig 6.17 Longitudinal strain during sress echocardiography. Top panels: segment with ischaemic response. Bottom panels: segment with normal response. A) Baseline strain curves with normal patterns in both segments. B) Under peak dobutamine stress the normal segment shows still a normal curve pattern. The ischaemic response of the upper segment can be clearly seen by the newly developed marked postsystolic shortening (PSS). (Modified from [31])

♦ Interventricular dyssynchrony.

♦ Intraventricular dyssynchrony.

Echocardiography may be also applied for optimization of atrioventricular (AV) and interventricular (VV) delay pacemaker settings.

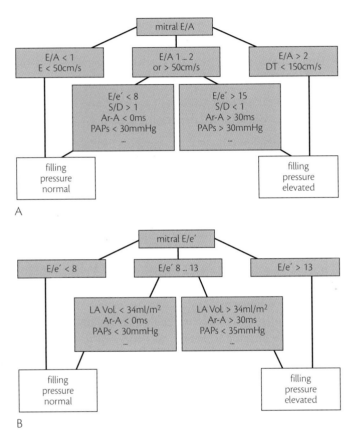

A

B

Figure 6.18 Filling pressures. A) Estimation of filling pressures of LV with reduced function (EF <50%). B) Estimation of filling pressures of LV with good function (EF >50%).

Assessment of left ventricular dyssynchrony for cardiac resynchronization therapy candidate selection

Left ventricular volume and global function

For determination of LV volume and EF see ➔ Chapter 8.

Regional function

In non-ischaemic cardiomyopathy, LV segments have reduced function of varying degree. In ischaemic disease, scar (thinner wall, hypo- or a/dyskinesia, brighter) may occur. Especially posterolateral scars reduce the chance of CRT response. Scar extent is inversely related to CRT outcome. A clear distinction between wall motion abnormality (reduced thickening) and dyssynchrony (delayed thickening) should be included in the echocardiographic report.

Typical features of a remodelled LV with left bundle branch block are (➔ Figs. 6.19 and 6.20; ▪ 6.4):

♦ Thin septum with minor, short contraction before or early during ejection.

♦ Normal or hypertrophied lateral wall with later contraction during ejection.

♦ *Rocking* motion of the LV apex as a result of the above.

♦ Short filling and ejection time intervals, long isovolumic time intervals.

Interventricular dyssynchrony

Conventional echocardiography assesses the difference between LV and RV pre-ejection time from PW Doppler traces of the RV outflow tract in parasternal short-axis view and LV outflow tract in apical five- and three-chamber views. A delay of more than 40ms is considered as marker of dyssynchrony.[15,16] Interventricular dyssynchrony has limited predictive value for a positive CRT response.

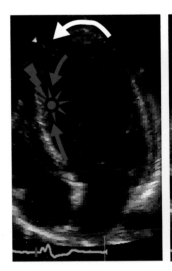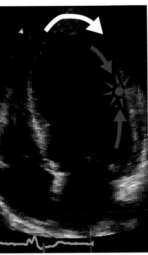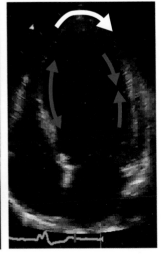

Figure 6.19 Typical contraction sequence in LBBB. A short initial (apical) septal contraction causes the apex to move septally. The lateral wall is activated with delay, pulling the apex laterally and stretching the septum. See also ▪ 6.4.

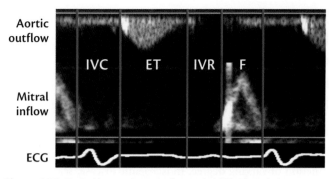

Figure 6.20 Typical haemodynamic changes in LBBB. The inferior vena cava (IVC) is long and the ejection delayed. The IVR is prolonged and the filling extremely short which reduces cardiac performace in addition to the myocardial dysfunction.

TD measures the onset of systolic motion in the basal RV free wall versus the most delayed basal LV segment. Asynchrony is assumed if the delay is greater than 56ms[17] (➲ Figs. 6.11 and 6.22).

Intraventricular dyssynchrony

This is the most important feature to evaluate. Already with conventional echo, visual inspection allows the recognition of the typical *apical rocking* which can predict CRT response[30] (➲ Fig. 6.19).

Conventional measurements which are considered suggestive for intraventricular dyssynchrony are an aortic pre-ejection time of greater than 140ms or a septal-to-posterior-wall motion delay (SPWMD) of more than 130–160ms. The latter can be obtained from parasternal M-mode by measuring the time delay of the maximum excursion of the two walls.[18] Predictive value and feasibility are disputed.[19] Colour TD or SR imaging may be used to improve reading LV time intervals.[20] The method is not applicable after septal or posterior infarction or in patients with aberrant septal motion due to high RV load.

TD allows measurement of the velocities of the mitral ring or basal and/or mid-myocardial segments from an apical window. Most parameters are based on the timing of the positive systolic velocity peak (➲ Fig. 6.21), few on the onset of systolic motion

or other features. With sufficient CD frame rate (>90/s), CD-derived and PW Doppler-derived timing data are interchangeable. Speckle tracking-derived data have worse temporal resolution. Global time events (AoV and MV opening and closure) should be considered when analysing Doppler traces. Automated algorithms for timing measurements need careful manual checking in each region of interest. The predictive value of these parameters is disputed:

- Time to peak systolic velocity in four basal segments (cut-off: dispersion >65ms).[21]

- Time to peak systolic velocity in six basal segments (cut-off: dispersion of >110ms).[22]

- Time to peak systolic velocity in six basal and six mid segments (cut-off: standard deviation > 33ms).[23]

- Onset of basal motion in three segments (septal, lateral, posterior) (cut-off: dispersion >60ms).[17]

It is often difficult to identify the timing of peak systolic velocity since there may be multiple systolic velocity peaks. Results of automated analyses (e.g. from TSI) have to be carefully checked. Evolving modalities such as 2D strain and 3D echocardiography may improve reproducibility and accuracy of predicting response to CRT in the future. LV dyssynchrony assessment is a challenging goal, since it cannot be considered an all-or-none phenomenon but a dynamic condition that may vary widely and can be dependent on loading conditions. Deformation imaging is theoretically superior to motion and velocity, however, only few studies on myocardial deformation parameters (strain, SR) are available. A higher noise and angle dependency of Doppler-derived measurements as well as the lower temporal resolution of tracking derived data limit the feasibility to use one of the following parameters (➲ Fig. 6.23):

- Time to peak radial strain in two basal segments (septal, posterior) (cut-off: dispersion >130ms).[20,24]

- Time to peak longitudinal strain in 12 basal and mid segments (cut-off: standard deviation >60ms).[20]

Figure 6.21 Difference in onset of systolic motion. The time difference between onset of motion in the basal right ventricular free wall and the most delayed basal segment of the left ventricle may be measured by pulsed wave or colour Doppler.

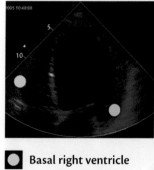

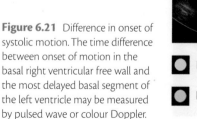
Basal right ventricle

Latest LV segment

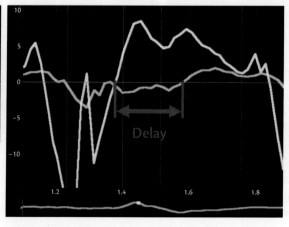

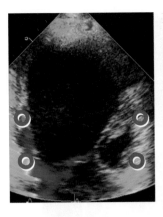
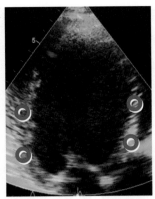
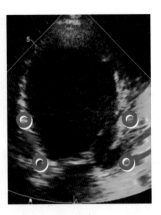

Figure 6.22 Most asynchrony parameters are based on the time to peak velocity measurements (Ts) in selected or all of the basal and mid segments of the LV. They can be conveniently measured using Tissue Synchronicity Imaging (see Fig. 6.11). Note that motion delays do not necessarily reflect contraction delays.

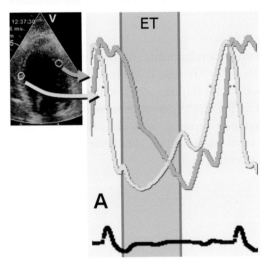
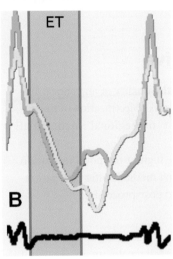

Figure 6.23 Deformation imaging. Longitudinal strain curves clearly show the asynchronous shortening of the different walls of the LV. A) CRT off: note the off-phase shortening in the septum and the lateral wall resembling a typical LBBB pattern. B) CRT on: mostly synchronous shortening in both walls during ejection time (ET) indicating a more effective LV function under CRT.

- Time of postsystolic contraction in 12 basal and mid segments (cut-off: sum of shortening time >760ms).[25]

3D echocardiography appears feasible for investigation of asynchrony, but temporal resolution limitations have to be considered. Currently, there is no sufficient evidence to recommend any approach or single parameter.

Determining the optimal site of pacing

The advantage of an echo-guided definition of the site of lead implantation has not yet been proven.

Optimization of cardiac resynchronization therapy settings

Optimization of AV and VV delays may improve the response rate to CRT.[26,27] Besides ECG parameters, echocardiographic data are used:

AV optimization

This seeks the best trade-off between the maximum number of paced beats and optimal LV filling. Its clinical value is disputed.

The optimal settings for varying physical activity or even body position are unknown. Optimization is usually attempted by changing the AV interval in 20-ms steps, allowing at least 10 beats of stabilization before haemodynamics data are acquired:

- LV filling time (attempt maximization).
- MV inflow VTI (attempt maximization).
- MV inflow A wave truncation (it is necessary to set a short AV interval to ensure LV stimulation. Then it is required to lengthen it again until A wave is just not truncated anymore).

AV optimization by LV outflow tract stroke volume or the Ritter formula is technically challenging and less reliable.

VV-optimization

The VV delay optimum is highly individual. Both left-first (majority) and right-first, as well as simultaneous pacing may prove optimal. For optimization, VV delay is changed stepwise in a range of ca. −80ms to +80ms and parameters are measured at each step (➲ Fig. 6.24). There is no consensus favouring a certain parameter for optimization. Both haemodynamic (LV stroke volume) and regional function data (interventricular

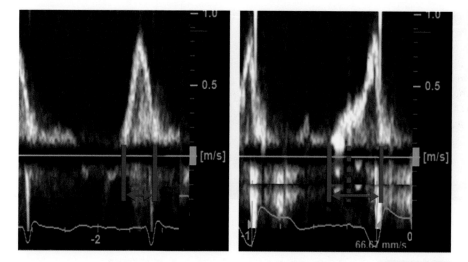

Figure 6.24 VV delay optimization. VV delay optimization should result in a longer filling time of the left ventricle. Note the gain in filling time in the right panel.

Personal perspective

Functional imaging improves the quality of an echocardiographic examination since it allows objectification of the traditionally visual assessment of regional myocardial function.

TD-based imaging offers the highest temporal resolution in cardiac imaging. New tracking methods offer new parameters and allow semi-automated post-processing.

Future developments will comprise the use of tracking methods in 3D echo datasets. Once the frame rate issue is solved, 3D tracking should allow more robust data without errors due to out-of-plane motion of speckles. Newly developed imaging methods could even allow a non-invasive assessment of parameters related to myocardial contractility.

dyssynchrony, time to peak systolic velocity in six basal segments, etc.) may be used.[28]

References

1 Doppler CJ. Über das farbige Licht der Doppelsterne. Abhandlung der Kgl. Böhmischen Gesellschaft der Wissenschaften 1842; **4**:465ff.

2 Sutherland GR, Hatle L (eds). *Doppler Myocardial Imaging – A Textbook*. Hasselt: BSWK bvba, 2006.

3 Heimdal A, Stoylen A, Torp H, Skjaerpe T. Real-time strain rate imaging of the left ventricle by ultrasound. *J Am Soc Echocardiogr* 1998; **11**:1013–9.

4 Edvardsen T, Gerber BL, Garot J, Bluemke DA, Lima JA, Smiseth OA. Quantitative assessment of intrinsic regional myocardial deformation by Doppler strain rate echocardiography in humans: validation against three-dimensional tagged magnetic resonance imaging. *Circulation* 2002; **106**:50–6.

5 Langeland S, Wouters PF, Claus P, Leather HA, Bijnens B, Sutherland GR, *et al*. Experimental assessment of a new research tool for the estimation of two-dimensional myocardial strain. *Ultrasound Med Biol* 2006; **32**:1509–13.

6 Helle-Valle T, Crosby J, Edvardsen T, Lyseggen E, Amundsen BH, Smith HJ, *et al*. New noninvasive method for assessment of left ventricular rotation: speckle tracking echocardiography. *Circulation* 2005; **112**:3149–56.

7 Stanton T, Ingul CB, Hare JL, Leano R, Marwick TH. Association of myocardial deformation with mortality independent of myocardial ischemia and left ventricular hypertrophy. *J Am Coll Cardiol: Cardiovasc Imaging* 2009; **2**:793–801.

8 Wilkenshoff UM, Sovany A, Wigström L, Olstad B, Lindstrom L, Engvall J, *et al*. Regional mean systolic myocardial velocity estimation by real time color Doppler myocardial imaging: a new technique for quantifying regional systolic function. *J Am Soc Echo* 1998; **11**:683–92.

9 Kukulski T, Hubbert L, Arnold M, Wranne B, Hatle L, Sutherland GR. Normal regional right ventricular function and its change with age: a Doppler myocardial imaging study. *J Am Soc Echocardiogr* 2000; **13**:194–204.

10 Herbots L. Quantification of regional myocardial deformation. Normal characteristics and clinical use in ischaemic heart disease. PhD Thesis. Acta Biomedica Lovaniensia. Leuven: Leuven University Press; 2006.

11 Voigt JU, Lindenmeier G, Exner B, Regenfus M, Werner D, Reulbach U, *et al*. Incidence and characteristics of segmental postsystolic longitudinal shortening in normal, acutely ischemic, and scarred myocardium. *J Am Soc Echocardiogr* 2003; **16**: 415–23.

12 Voigt JU, Exner B, Schmiedehausen K, Huchzermeyer C, Reulbach U, Nixdorff U, *et al*. Strain-rate imaging during dobutamine stress echocardiography provides objective evidence of inducible ischemia. *Circulation* 2003; **107**:2120–6.

13 Nagueh SF, Appleton CP, Gillebert TC, Marino PN, Oh JK, Smiseth OA, Waggoner AD, *et al*. Recommendations for the evaluation

of left ventricular diastolic function by echocardiography. *Eur J Echocardiogr* 2009; **10**:165–93.

14 Vardas PE, Auricchio A, Blanc JJ, Daubert JC, Drexler H, Ector H, *et al.* European Society of Cardiology; European Heart Rhythm Association. Guidelines for cardiac pacing and cardiac resynchronization therapy: the task force for cardiac pacing and cardiac resynchronization therapy of the European Society of Cardiology. Developed in collaboration with the European Heart Rhythm Association. *Eur Heart J* 2007; **28**:2256–95.

15 Cleland JG, Daubert JC, Erdmann E, Freemantle N, Gras D, Kappenberger L, *et al.*; CARE-HF study Steering Committee and Investigators. The CARE-HF study (CArdiac REsynchronisation in Heart Failure study): rationale, design and end-points. *Eur J Heart Fail* 2001; **3**:481–9.

16 St John Sutton MG, Plappert T, Abraham WT, Smith AL, DeLurgio DB, Leon AR, *et al.* Multicenter InSync Randomized Clinical Evaluation (MIRACLE) Study Group. Effect of cardiac resynchronization therapy on left ventricular size and function in chronic heart failure. *Circulation* 2003; **107**:1985–90.

17 Penicka M, Bartunek J, De Bruyne B, Vanderheyden M, Goethals M, De Zutter M, *et al.* Improvement of left ventricular function after cardiac resynchronization therapy is predicted by tissue Doppler imaging echocardiography. *Circulation* 2004; **109**: 978–83.

18 Pitzalis MV, Iacoviello M, Romito R, Guida P, De Tommasi E, Luzzi G, *et al.* Ventricular asynchrony predicts a better outcome in patients with chronic heart failure receiving cardiac resynchronization therapy. *J Am Coll Cardiol* 2005; **45**:65–9.

19 Marcus GM, Rose E, Viloria EM, Schafer J, De Marco T, Saxon LA, *et al.*; VENTAK CHF/CONTAK-CD Biventricular Pacing Study Investigators. Septal to posterior wall motion delay fails to predict reverse remodeling or clinical improvement in patients undergoing cardiac resynchronization therapy. *J Am Coll Cardiol* 2005; **46**:2208–14.

20 Mele D, Pasanisi G, Capasso F, De Simone A, Morales MA, Poggio D, *et al.* Left intraventricular myocardial deformation dyssynchrony identifies responders to cardiac resynchronization therapy in patients with heart failure. *Eur Heart J* 2006; **27**: 1070–8.

21 Bax JJ, Bleeker GB, Marwick TH, Molhoek SG, Boersma E, Steendijk P, *et al.* Left ventricular dyssynchrony predicts response and prognosis after cardiac resynchronization therapy. *J Am Coll Cardiol* 2004; **44**:1834–40.

22 Notabartolo D, Merlino JD, Smith AL, DeLurgio DB, Vera FV, Easley KA, *et al.* Usefulness of the peak velocity difference by tissue Doppler imaging technique as an effective predictor of response to cardiac resynchronization therapy. *Am J Cardiol* 2004; **94**: 817–20.

23 Yu CM, Fung WH, Lin H, Zhang Q, Sanderson JE, Lau CP. Predictors of left ventricular reverse remodeling after cardiac resynchronization therapy for heart failure secondary to idiopathic dilated or ischemic cardiomyopathy. *Am J Cardiol* 2003; **91**: 684–8.

24 Dohi K, Suffoletto MS, Schwartzman D, Ganz L, Pinsky MR, Gorcsan J 3rd. Utility of echocardiographic radial strain imaging to quantify left ventricular dyssynchrony and predict acute response to cardiac resynchronization therapy. *Am J Cardiol* 2005; **96**:112–6.

25 Porciani MC, Lilli A, Macioce R, Cappelli F, Demarchi G, Pappone A, *et al.* Utility of a new left ventricular asynchrony index as a predictor of reverse remodelling after cardiac resynchronization therapy. *Eur Heart J* 2006; **27**:1818–23.

26 Sogaard P, Egeblad H, Pedersen AK, Kim WY, Kristensen BO, Hansen PS, *et al.* Sequential versus simultaneous biventricular resynchronization for severe heart failure: evaluation by tissue Doppler imaging. *Circulation* 2002; **106**:2078–84.

27 van Gelder BM, Bracke FA, Meijer A, Lakerveld LJ, Pijls NH. Effect of optimizing the VV interval on left ventricular contractility in cardiac resynchronization therapy. *Am J Cardiol* 2004; **93**:1500–3.

28 Vanderheyden M, De Backer T, Rivero-Ayerza M, Geelen P, Bartunek J, Verstreken S, *et al.* Tailored echocardiographic interventricular delay programming further optimizes left ventricular performance after cardiac resynchronization therapy. *Heart Rhythm* 2005; **2**:1066–72.

29 Dalen H, Thorstensen A, Aase SA, Ingul CB, Torp H, Vatten LJ, *et al.* Segmental and global longitudinal strain and strain rate based on echocardiography of 1266 healthy individuals: the HUNT study in Norway. *Eur J Echocardiogr* 2010; **11**:176–83.

30 Szuli M, Tillekaerts M, Vangeel V, Ganame J, Willems R, Lenarczyk R, Rademakers F, Kalarus Z, Kukulski T, Voigt JU. Assessment of apical rocking: a new, integrative approach for selection of candidates for resynchronization therapy. *Eur J Echocardiogr* 2010; [Epub ahead of print] (PMID: 20615904).

31 Voigt Quantifizierung der Myokardfunktion in Flachskampf (Ed.): Praxis der Echokardiographie 3rd Edition, 2010, Thieme, Stuttgart.

Further reading

Sutherland GR, Hatle L (eds). *Doppler Myocardial Imaging – A Textbook.* Hasselt: BSWK bvba, 2006.

Additional DVD and online material

- 6.1 Detail of the tracking of the apical septum in a four-chamber view: good end-diastolic tracking, bad systolic tracking.

- 6.2 Detail of the tracking of the apical septum in a four-chamber view: good end-systolic tracking, bad diastolic tracking.

- 6.3 Speckle tracking in an apical three-chamber view of a patient after anterior infarction. Results can be displayed as colour overlay in the movie, segmental curves of function parameters (here: strain) or curved M-modes. Note the lower strain values in the anteroseptal region indicating myocardial dysfunction.

- 6.4 Typical motion pattern of a LV of a patient with left bundle branch block. See text and legend to ➲ Fig. 6.19 for description of features.

- ➲ For additional multimedia materials please visit the online version of the book (http://escecho.oxfordmedicine.com).

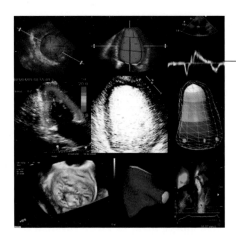

CHAPTER 7

Contrast echocardiography

L. Galiuto, R. Senior, and H. Becher

Summary

Contrast echocardiography is a non-invasive, well tolerated echocardiographic technique which employs ultrasound contrast agent in order to improve the quality of echocardiographic images, by enhancing blood flow signal.

Clinical usefulness of this echocardiographic imaging modality resides in the possibility of providing better acoustic signal in cases of poor quality images, with additional important information related to assessment of myocardial perfusion. Indeed, about one-third of echocardiographic images are affected by poor quality due to high acoustic impedance of the chest wall of the patients secondary to obesity or pulmonary diseases, not allowing detection of left ventricular endocardial border. Moreover, in patients with low ejection fraction and apical left ventricular aneurysm, intraventricular thrombus could be undetectable with standard echocardiography. Furthermore, coronary microcirculation cannot be assessed by standard echocardiography. Contrast echocardiography can be performed in all such conditions to improve diagnostic power of echocardiography.

The adjunctive role of contrast echocardiography is well defined in both rest and stress echocardiography in order to detect the endocardial border and intraventricular thrombi, to accurately measure ejection fraction, wall motion, and to assess myocardial perfusion.

The purpose of this chapter is to explain basic principles, feasibility, safety, major clinical applications, current indications, and further developments of contrast echocardiography.

Ultrasound contrast agents

Materials

On standard echocardiography, blood flow is usually not echogenic. Red blood cells are very weak backscatters due to the size and small difference in acoustic impedance between them and the surrounding serum. Only with slow-flowing blood or stasis does the blood becomes echogenic, because of the formation of aggregates of blood cells. With normal blood flow, the intensity of the backscattered signal from blood is usually too low, unless it is enhanced by an ultrasound contrast agent.[1]

Because air and other gases are much more potent than any liquids or solid particles in producing an useful echocardiographic signal, they constitute the basis of modern ultrasound contrast agents. In reality, the contrast effect is not caused by gas dissolved in a fluid, but is dependent on the presence of bubbles. Based on such evidence, two different types of gas bubbles have been developed as ultrasound contrast agents for use in clinical practice:

◆ Air microbubbles.

◆ Gas-encapsulated microbubbles.

Air microbubbles

Air microbubbles are produced by an agitation process of saline solutions with a small amount of air, resulting in formation of gas bubbles with a wide spectrum of size. These bubbles are unstable and tend to dissolve quickly in the blood, the smaller they are the faster they disappear. Such instability of the gas bubbles is exploited for some clinical indications: for example, they are commonly used for right-to-left intracardiac shunt detection. In fact, although the smaller bubbles are able to make their way through the capillary bed of the pulmonary circulation, they cannot be detected in the left heart chambers, due to a very quick disappearance. Only in the presence of an intracardiac or intrapulmonary shunt can bubbles reach the left heart.

Air microbubbles can be stabilized by adding a small amount of the patient's blood: the proteins in the plasma attach to the bubbles, but do not create a full shell. Similar effects can be obtained when using agitated gelatine solution instead of saline and blood. However, there is the small risk of an allergic reaction to gelatine and therefore agitated saline (air microbubbles) is recommended.

Gas-encapsulated microbubbles

These are manufactured contrast media, which are made by encapsulating a small amount of nitrogen or fluorocarbon gas (instead of air) in a shell. In this way, the instability is reduced, so that they can be used for left ventricular opacification (LVO) and arterial contrast, including tissue perfusion. In fact, when stabilized by a shell, microbubbles survive the journey from the venous injection side to the left ventricle and myocardial blood vessels.

The coated microbubbles size ranges from 1.1–8μm, similar to the size of red blood cells (◐ Fig. 7.1). The dimensions are made small enough to cross capillary beds (the pulmonary capillaries have the smallest calibre in the body, that is, 7μm). In this way they can survive during the passage through the pulmonary bed and provide useful cardiac enhancement. Their shells are not rigid, which allows them to travel through the capillary bed, without occluding it. The biological shell consists of albumin or phospholipids and is metabolized in the liver. The phospholipids are negatively charged in order to prevent aggregates of multiple microspheres which might block small arteries. All these agents contain a fluorocarbon gas, which is less soluble than air. High-molecular-weight gases are chosen for their slow diffusion, prolonging the bubbles' half-life in the circulation, where they are subject to mechanical trauma by heart valves and ultrasound beam. Usually, the perfluoro gases are preferred because they are biologically inert: in fact, the carbon chain has its hydrogen atoms completely replaced by elements such as fluorine or sulphur. The dissolved perfluorocarbon gas is exhaled through the lungs. The size and composition of the outer shell of the bubble and the encapsulated gas determine the microbubble's ultrasonic characteristics.

Worldwide there are three contrast agents approved for echocardiography (◐ Table 7.1).

Administration

One of the most advantageous features of ultrasound contrast agents is that they can be easily administered by a peripheral venous access. Because of the small volume injected, microbubbles

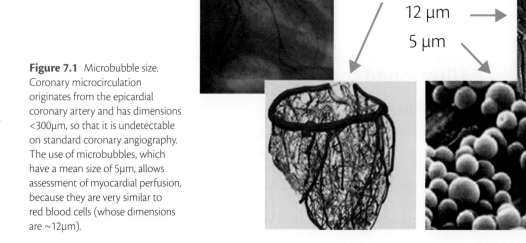

Figure 7.1 Microbubble size. Coronary microcirculation originates from the epicardial coronary artery and has dimensions <300μm, so that it is undetectable on standard coronary angiography. The use of microbubbles, which have a mean size of 5μm, allows assessment of myocardial perfusion, because they are very similar to red blood cells (whose dimensions are ~12μm).

< 300 μm

12 μm

5 μm

Table 7.1 Characteristics of currently available contrast agents for echocardiography

	Sonovue	**Optison***	**Luminity***
Gas	Sulfur hexafluoride	Perfluoropropane	Perfluoropropane
Bubble size	2–8 μm	3.0–4.5 μm	1.1–2.5 μm
Surface coating	Phospholipid	Human albumin	Phospholipid
Dosage**	Bolus: 0.3–0.5 ml	Bolus: 0.1–0.3 ml	Bolus: 1 ml
	Infusion: 0.5–1.5 ml/min		Infusion: 1–2 ml/min
Manufacturer	Bracco Diagnostic	GE Healthcare	Lantheus Medical Imaging

*EMEA approved but not marketed in Europe in 2009/2010 **for contrast specific imaging modalities

are also suitable for use as vascular tracers in patients with left ventricular (LV) contractile dysfunction, where volume overload should be avoided. Exam is better performed in fast conditions. The patient preparation requires insertion of an intravenous cannula usually into an antecubital vein. Ultrasound contrast agents can be injected through this line by:

◆ Bolus injection.

◆ Continuous infusion.

Slow bolus injections (0.2mL) of all agents is usually followed by slow 5mL saline flush over 20s. This modality allows both rapid flood and disappearance of bubbles from blood flow. It is not controllable or reproducible and is usually used to temporally enhance blood signal in order to detect an intracardiac shunt (by air microbubbles) or to improve endocardial border delineation (by gas-encapsulated microbubbles). Detection of intracardiac shunt by air microbubbles requires connection of the intravenous cannula to a three-way-tap or small-bore Y-connector (➲ Fig. 7.2).

Conversely, during continuous infusion, contrast agents are administered by an infusion pump at constant infusion rate (➲ Fig. 7.3). The pump can be prepared in a few minutes prior to the study or during baseline echo examination. Once infusion rate is planned, the pump can be kept in stand-by mode and then started up when necessary. Newer pumps also allow a bolus injection to be performed. Continuous infusion administration modality provides a constant bubble signal that is fundamental to assess myocardial perfusion. As air microbubbles rapidly dissolve, gas-encapsulated microbubbles are preferably employed.

However, microbubbles infusion requires attention, because:

◆ They are susceptible to the surrounding pressure: for instance, high pressure in a syringe or a thin line causes disruption of the shell and dissolution of the gas in the fluid. Therefore injection with high pressure and use of long and thin lines should be avoided.

◆ They tend to float in a fluid and to accumulate at the highest point of the syringe or vial. Therefore the vial or the syringe

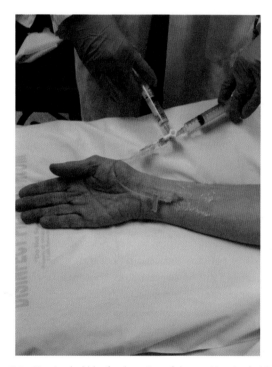

Figure 7.2 Air microbubbles for detection of shunts. Air microbubbles for detection of shunts: draw up a mixture of 8mL saline, 0.2mL air, and (ideally) 1mL of blood (from the patient!) into a syringe. Attach with a second syringe to a 3-way tap (use syringes with Luer locks to avoid the syringes bursting off). Force the mixture back and forth until frothy. Inject rapidly through a venous line inserted into an antecubital vein.

should be rolled between the hands or shaken before injection, in order to maintain solution heterogeneity. For SonoVue® a special pump is provided which constantly rotates (➲ Fig 7.3; 🎬 7.1).

Reology

Microbubbles do not seem to affect blood flow and behave in the same way as red blood cells. In fact, because their size and flexibility are similar to those of red blood cells, microbubbles constitute entirely intravascular agents. When administered intravenously, these agents flood the blood pool, mixing with red blood cells, and remain within the vascular compartment

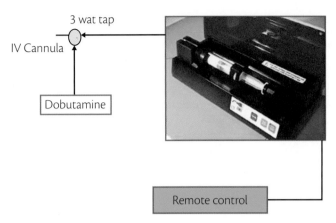

3 wat tap

IV Cannula

Dobutamine

Remote control

Figure 7.3 Infusion pump for constant infusion of microbubbles. Agitating the contrast prior to injection. The contrast agent should be injected within 30s after preparation.

unless there is active bleeding. In particular, they do not cross the endothelial layer and do not have as interstitial phase as do conventional contrast agents. Their contrast effect is closer to that of the labelled red blood cells used in nuclear medicine[2] than to that of agents used in X-ray and magnetic resonance studies.

Safety

Contrast echocardiography is safe. Several studies enrolling thousands of patients undergoing contrast echocardiography both at rest and during stress did not show a difference in mortality in patients who received contrast versus those who did not. Contrast agents can provoke side effects, which, however, are usually mild and transient.

Air microbubbles

A variety of transient side effects has been reported, including neurological and respiratory symptoms. The risk is low (<0.1%) and no residual side effects or complications were observed in a survey of the American Society of Echocardiography (ASE). However, during contrast echocardiography, precautions should be taken to prevent the injection of visible amounts of air, especially in patients with a right-to-left shunt.

Gas-encapsulated microbubbles

Side effects have been noted but they are usually mild and transient. Most frequent side effects of SonoVue® in clinical trials were:

- Headache (2.1%).
- Nausea (1.3%).
- Chest pain (1.3%).
- Taste perversion (0.9%).
- Hyperglycaemia (0.6%).

- Injection site reaction 0.6%).
- Paraesthesia (0.6%).
- Vasodilation (0.6%).
- Injection site pain (0.5%).

Serious adverse events are very rare (0.01%) and less frequent then for X-ray contrast agents. They may happen as acute sensitivity reactions (immunoglobulin E (IgE)-mediated type I), but **Complement Activation Related Pseudo Allergy** (CARPA) seems to be more typical for the contrast agents with a phospholipid membrane (➔ Table 7.2). In comparison to IgE-mediated reactions CARPA reactions need no prior exposure to the agent, the reaction is milder or absent upon repeated exposures, and spontaneous resolution is possible. Although serious adverse events are very rare, appropriate allergy and emergency equipment as well as a physician with knowledge in emergency medicine should be present or close by.

Only Optison® and Luminity® may be used in acute coronary syndromes, since the contraindication on their use in these conditions has been recently withdrawn by the US Food and Drug Administration (FDA), based on the evidence of their favourable risk–benefit profile and safety. Because SonoVue® has a similar safety profile, it is hoped that the European Medicines Agency (EMEA) will withdraw contraindication regarding use of this agent in acute coronary conditions. Actually, SonoVue® may be used 7 days after acute coronary syndrome. However, in all acute conditions, it is important to monitor vital signs and pulse oximetry for 30min after contrast administration. The only absolute contraindications for administration of contrast agents are in patients with:

- Known or suspected significant intracardiac shunts.
- Known hypersensitivity to the agent.

Intracoronary administration is also not approved and is considered contraindicated, although it has been performed without complications in thousands of patients with hypertrophic cardiomyopathy undergoing septal ablation.

Table 7.2 CARPA symptoms

Angioedema
Bronchospasm
Cyanosis
Hypotension
Low back pain
Pruritis
Urticaria
Tingling Sensation
Hypoxemia
Sneezing

Ultrasonic imaging of gas-encapsulated microbubbles

Bubbles–ultrasound interaction

Compared to red blood cells, the amplitude of the backscattered ultrasound signal is increased by microbubbles (➲ Fig. 7.4). Microbubbles' ultrasonic characteristics depend on their size, on the composition of the outer shell, and the encapsulated gas. Regarding size, microbubble ultrasound scatter is proportional to the sixth power of the radius, because they respond to the alternating compression and rarefaction cycles of the ultrasound wave by changing their diameter. This effect depends on the compressibility of gases. In addition, the more elastic the shell, the more easily it will be compressed in an ultrasonic field.

Moreover, the extent of the change depends on the acoustic power applied. In fact, as acoustic power of transmitted ultrasound increases, different types of microbubble responses occur, which provide various reflected signals (➲ Fig. 7.5).

Fundamental frequency

When the acoustic power is kept low, microbubble response to transmitted ultrasounds is *linear*, so the returning frequency is the same as transmitted frequency, the so-called *fundamental*

frequency. However, with the ultrasound system operating in fundamental frequency, microbubbles are barely visible with low signal to noise ratio.

Harmonic imaging

At higher acoustic pressures, the response of microbubbles to ultrasound(s) becomes *non-linear*. Indeed, while tissue is virtually incompressible, microbubbles expand and contract markedly, according to a natural oscillation frequency or *resonance* depending on their size. This behaviour results from the fact that the bubbles are able to expand more easily than they contract. Their diameter change is asymmetrical, since the gas tends to resist compression but expands more easily: this non-linear response alters the characteristics of the returned signals, so that the signal returning from the bubbles is a distorted version of the insonating wave. When the driving pressure changes of ultrasound are matched to this resonant frequency, bubbles become extremely efficient at translating the sound energy from the propagating sound wave into scattered signal. For a 3–7μm microbubble, the resonance frequency is around 3Mhz, which is the frequency of the standard echo transducers. This fortunate coincidence of the bubble size and the transducer frequency has allowed the development of contrast echocardiography (➲ Fig. 7.6). The harmonics emitted by the microbubbles, usually the second harmonic, can be used to image ultrasound contrast agents by tuning the receiver to the bubbles harmonic signal (➲ Fig. 7.7).

It is of note that when exposed to high-power ultrasound both the tissue and the microbubbles generate harmonic frequencies with a difference in amplitude (see ➲ Chapter 1, 'Ultrasound imaging principles'). As ultrasound propagates through tissue, a confounding signal occurs when harmonic imaging is used to detect bubbles. However, by decreasing the

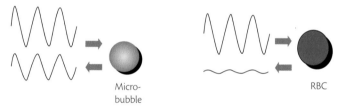

Figure 7.4 Microbubbles backscattered signal. Increase in amplitude of backscattered signal from microbubbles compared to red blood cell.

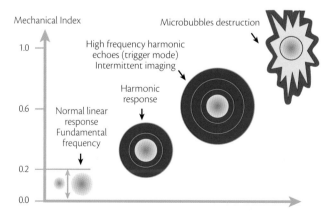

Figure 7.5 Different types of microbubbles response to ultrasounds. Schema indicating the interaction between transmitted ultrasound beam and microbubbles: microbubbles resonate at different increasing frequencies with increase of acoustic power, until they are destroyed by a high power ultrasound pulse (for details, see text).

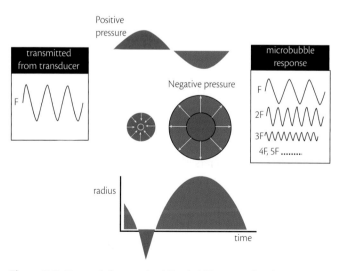

Figure 7.6 Harmonic frequencies. Microbubbles expand and contract in the acoustic field. They expand to a greater extent than compressing resulting in asymmetric oscillation. The resonating microbubbles emit harmonic frequencies to the frequency of the ultrasound transmitted by the ultrasound probe.

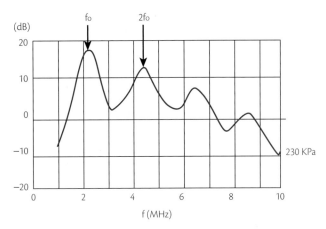

Figure 7.7 Frequency spectrum of an echo produced by microbubbles. Frequency spectrum of an echo produced by SonoVue® microbubbles when scanned with 2.25-MHz transducer. Ultrasound frequency is on the horizontal axis, with the relative amplitude on the vertical axis. A strong echo, at −13dB (2fo) with respect to the fundamental (fo) is seen at twice the transmitted frequency, that is known as the second harmonic. Peaks in the echo spectrum at third and forth harmonic frequency are also seen

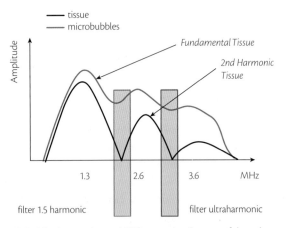

Figure 7.8 Ultraharmonics and 1.5 harmonics. Spectra of the echo received from tissue and contrast agents. Filters for ultraharmonic imaging and 1.5 harmonic imaging.

transmit power, the tissue harmonics are reduced, while the amplitude of the harmonic signals from microbubbles decreases to a lesser extent. Several signal processing sequences have been developed in order to cancel the signal from tissue and emphasize both *1.5 harmonic* and *ultraharmonic signal* from the microbubbles. By applying filters, the signals from tissue and contrast agent can be separated, thus improving the contrast-to-tissue signal ratio (➲ Fig. 7.8).

Power Doppler

At still higher ultrasound power, bubble oscillations become more complex, further increasing their non-linear response. By using the highest acoustic power, the bubbles will ultimately be disrupted, resulting in fragmentation into smaller bubbles or in release of free gas bubbles. A very strong signal originates from those multiple microparticles: this moving signal is easily and

efficiently detected by Doppler system. For several years, this *power Doppler modality*, which has the characteristic of imaging the total energy (*power*) of moving particles as detected by *Doppler* system, has been the most sensitive method for detection of microbubbles. However, movement of the heart muscle causes additional echoes, which can impair the contrast recordings. Furthermore, fragmentation of bubbles produces rapid dissolution of contrast agent volume, thus reducing the efficiency of contrast detecting. Different imaging modalities, recently developed, are able to distinguish microbubbles signal from tissue signal, by using a low-power acoustic pulse and avoiding bubbles destruction.

Ultrasound power

Mechanical index

The acoustic power generated by ultrasound beam in an acoustic field is measured as mechanical index (MI). As previously mentioned (see ➲ Chapter 1, 'Principles of ultrasound'), MI reflects the transmit power of the transducer, that is the normalized energy to which a target (such as a bubble) is exposed in an ultrasound field. It is an important parameter to optimize recordings in contrast echocardiography. It is defined by the following formula:

$$MI = P/\sqrt{f} \tag{7.1}$$

where P is the peak negative ultrasound pressure, f the ultrasound frequency. It is estimated at the focus of the ultrasound beam, lessens with increasing depth and towards the sector edges. Most ultrasound scanners have presets for contrast echocardiography with default MIs. However, it may be necessary to modify the transmit power in patient with particularly high or low attenuation.

The transmit power (measured by MI) is different from the gain which only amplifies or dampens the received ultrasound signals.

High-power contrast imaging

The most common high power contrast imaging modality is *harmonic power Doppler*. In this imaging modality, a high power ultrasound beam with MI greater than 1.0 produces bubbles fragmentation optimally visualized as Doppler signal.

This modality typically involves a dual-pulse technique where the difference in backscattered signal from two high MI pulses transmitted down each scan line is examined. It uses two consecutive identical pulses of sound and assesses the echoes of consecutive pulses. The first pulse hits the microbubbles and destroys it, and no echo is obtained on the following pulse. In addition, any tissue targets will also generate a signal. The second pulse will only generate a signal from tissue because all contrast will have been destroyed by the first pulse. The backscattered data from pulse 1 are subtracted from that derived from pulse 2, and the difference represents the contrast signal since the tissue signal cancels out. This is the maximal change in a Doppler modality. Newer high-power techniques also utilize ultraharmonic properties of the microbubble, which improves the detection of the 'signal' of the microbubble, from the 'noise' of the background tissue, since tissue produces very little ultraharmonic signal.

Low-power contrast specific imaging

Low-power imaging minimizes the signals from tissue and prolongs the persistence of the microbubbles. These modalities have been named according to the developing ultrasound system manufacturer: *Pulse Inversion, Power Modulation, Coherent (Cadence) Imaging.*

All these modalities rely on the fact that tissue only generates negligible harmonic frequencies at low ultrasound energy levels, whereas contrast microbubbles have a strong harmonic response. When alternate backscattered signals are received, which are perfectly out of phase or proportionally altered in amplitude, they are processed by the imaging software as being derived from tissue and therefore are filtered out and suppressed. All remaining 'non-linear' signals are considered to be derived from contrast microbubbles and are displayed. When using this kind of imaging modality, the image will normally be totally dark prior to contrast administration, confirming effective suppression of tissue data (➲ Fig. 7.9). Low-power contrast imaging modalities work by transmitting multiple pulses down each scan line. Alternate pulses are 180 degree out of phase with other or vary in magnitude of amplitude by a fixed ratio, or are a combination of both strategies (➲ Fig. 7.10).

➲ Table 7.3 lists the mechanical indices for different ultrasound techniques.

Imaging modalities

Intermittent

With all high-power contrast techniques, microbubbles are destroyed within the scan-plane and continuous imaging would result in rapid loss of contrast bubble signal. However, sending ultrasound signal intermittently and synchronized with cardiac cycle allows the creation of triggered imaging still frames.

Thus, although myocardial contractile function assessment is sacrificed, intermittent mode offers the best visualization of changes in microbubbles signal over time, with optimal signal-to-noise ratio (■ 7.2).

Real-time

In real-time mode, image acquisition is continuous along some cardiac cycles, so that microbubbles ultrasound signal intensity increases over time until it reaches the peak level in LV cavity and myocardial wall. In order to avoid bubbles destruction, MI should be kept low and low-power contrast specific imaging modality should be preferred. Continuous real-time imaging is very effective for LV endocardial border enhancement and myocardial perfusion assessment, since the contrast agent arrives at the region of interest and then washes out over 2–5min. Finally, this modality allows evaluation of myocardial perfusion combined with real-time assessment of contractile function (■ 7.3).

Pitfalls and artefacts

Several pitfalls and artefacts may occur during contrast echo examination. Recognition of such artefacts significantly improves image acquisition and interpretation:

- Attenuation: this is the reduction of the amplitude of ultrasound on its way through the human body. As a consequence, contrast intensity may be reduced at the bases of the heart, generating false basal contrast defect. This artefact is difficult to limit, since it is intrinsic in the nature of ultrasound imaging, but it is less frequent with continuous infusion of contrast and adjustment of the gain at greater depth. Attenuation has to be taken into account particularly in the assessment of contrast perfusion defect in the basal myocardial segments.

- Lateral shadowing is usually caused by a rib or lung tissue which blocks the penetration of ultrasound. It can be easily detected by a straight anechogenic area in the lateral field. Conversely, distal shadowing occurs when the volume of contrast media contained in heart chambers combined with ultrasound attenuation in the far field compromises the visualization of distal heart segments. This effect may be reduced

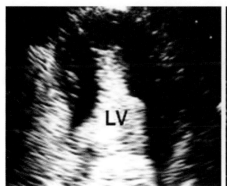
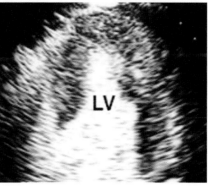

Figure 7.9 Low-power contrast-specific imaging. Example of low-power, contrast-specific imaging: clear demarcation can be seen between the contrast-enhanced cavity and the myocardium when the contrast bolus reaches the left ventricle and almost no signals in the myocardium (left), while myocardial opacification is displayed when the contrast reaches the myocardial vessels (right).

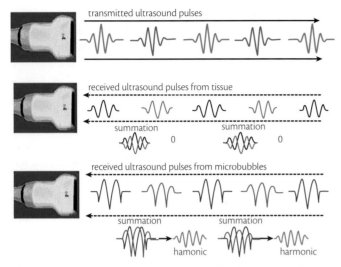

Figure 7.10 Power pulse inversion as an example of contrast specific imaging. A pulse of sound is transmitted into the body and echos are received from the contrast microbubbles and the tissue. A second pulse, which is an inverted copy of the first pulse, is then transmitted in the same direction and the two echos are summed. Echos from tissue are inverted copies of each other and are cancelled to zero. The microbubble echos are distorted echos of each other and the non-linear components of these echos will reinforce each other when summed, producing a strong harmonic signal.

Table 7.3. Mechanical Indices (MI) for different ultrasound techniques

	MI
Tissue harmonic imaging	>1.0
Contrast harmonic imaging	0.6
Low power contrast specific imaging	0.1-0.3
Power Doppler imaging	>1.0

optimizing the volume of contrast administered and preferring infusion to bolus (➲ Fig. 7.11).

◆ Apical drop out: the power of ultrasound is the strongest in the near field, thus destroying a larger amount of contrast and generating a swirling effect at the apical LV cavity and a false perfusion defect at the apex. It is crucial to recognize this artefact since the apex is the site of the majority of perfusion and contraction abnormalities. Positioning of ultrasound beam focus at the apex helps better and more reliable visualization of this segment.

◆ Lateral drop out: the power of ultrasound beam is reduced in the lateral field, thus even contrast images are ineffective in the lateral segments simulating perfusion defects. Thus artefact can be distinguished by true defect by the loss of the ultrasound signal in entire lateral sector, as opposed to contrast defect within the wall. When necessary, shifting lateral wall within the sector can be a useful method to optimize its visualization.

Left ventricular opacification

LVO is achieved by administration of microbubbles throughout:

◆ Continuous infusion, with the advantage that uniform LVO can be achieved without any significant attenuation artefacts.

◆ Slow bolus injection followed by 15–20mL saline flash, in order to avoid significant attenuation artefacts.

Because the microbubbles are destroyed during high power ultrasound imaging, it is preferable to perform lower-power

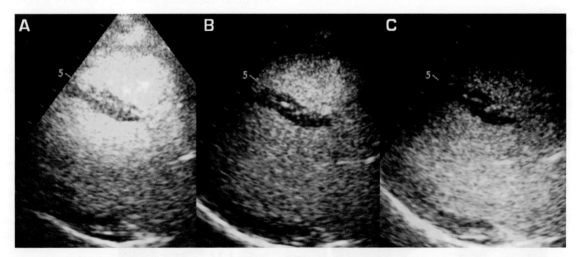

Figure 7.11 Pitfalls and artefacts. A) Blooming artefact and shadowing: fast administration or high dose of contrast can generate blooming artefact—bright appearance of contrast in the cavity which encompasses the myocardium as well. Shadowing reduces visualization of far-field structures. Starting contrast imaging with the parasternal instead of apical views puts the transducer near the highly reflective right heart and accentuates these artefacts. In the example, there is blooming in the right ventricle and above the interventricular septum and attenuation of image in the far field. B) Optimized appearance for comparison: A few cardiac cycles later, the image was optimized. C) Enhanced image in the far field in the late cardiac cycles in parasternal imaging (more rapid destruction of microbubbles in the near field).

imaging: this will allow uniform LVO and improved assessment of wall thickening. With improvement in transducer technology, frame rate greater than 30Hz may be obtained during low power imaging.

Two-dimensional (2D) echocardiography without contrast is known to significantly underestimate LV volumes by as much as 30–40% and LV ejection fraction (LVEF) by 3–6% in comparison to cardiac magnetic resonance (CMR) imaging. Contrast administration significantly improves border detection, LV volumes quantification, and EF measurement.[3] After myocardial infarction, contrast echocardiography correctly identifies patients with various degrees of LVEF: this is important both for accurate prognostication and for therapeutic intervention, such as implantation of an implantable cardioverter defibrillator. The improvement of contrast echocardiography accuracy in estimation of LV volume and EF is similar to that obtained by unenhanced three-dimensional (3D) echocardiography when compared to CMR.

Contrast echocardiography is actually the technique of choice for the evaluation of patients with:

◆ Suspected apical hypertrophic cardiomyopathy (➲ Fig. 7.12).

◆ LV non-compaction (➲ Fig. 7.13).

◆ Myocardial rupture and LV pseudoaneurysm.

◆ LV apical thrombus: it has to be excluded in patients with low LVEF (➲ Fig. 7.14), but unenhanced imaging of the LV apex is often confounded by near-field artefacts. With contrast administration, 90% of the scans provided a definitive diagnosis for establishing or excluding the presence of thrombus.

After contrast administration the proportion of uninterpretable images decreases significantly from 12% to 0.3% and that of technically difficult studies decreases from 87% to 10%. This leads to a significant avoidance of further diagnostic procedures in patients, primarily due to improved assessment of LV function. Medical therapy is sometimes inappropriate in some patients after interpretation of the contrast study, so that a significant impact on the clinical care is noted in most patients.

As recently stated by the ASE and European Association of Echocardiography (EAE), indications for LVO are:

◆ In difficult to image patients where two or more contiguous segments are not seen on non-contrast images.

◆ In patients requiring accurate assessment of LVEF regardless of image quality with the intention of increasing the confidence of the interpreting physician in assessing LV volumes and systolic function.

◆ In patients requiring confirmation or exclusion of LV structural abnormalities, intracardiac masses, and to enhance Doppler signals.

Myocardial perfusion

Physiological bases

Coronary microcirculation, which comprises myocardial vessels originating from large epicardial coronary arteries and having a diameter less than 300μm, contains about 90% of the total myocardial blood volume (MBV) and is mostly responsible for metabolic regulation of myocardial blood flow (MBF). MBF physiologically changes during cardiac cycle: at the end of systole most of the larger intramyocardial vessels have been emptied of blood and the majority of MBV resides within capillaries. Under normal conditions, the subendocardial flow is higher than the subepicardial flow (with a ratio of about 1.25:1), due to a greater subendocardial oxygen demand.

The capability of microbubbles to fill capillary vessels without diffusing in extravascular space has allowed use of contrast echocardiography to assess MBF. In fact, after opacifying LV cavity, microbubbles reach coronary microcirculation in a few minutes, providing an ultrasound signal that is a function of their concentration within myocardial wall.

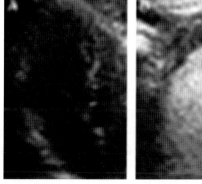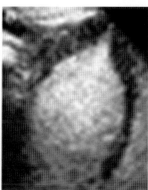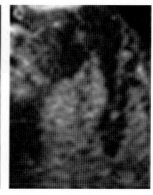

Figure 7.12 Apical hypertrophic cardiomyopathy. A) An unenhanced, three-chamber echocardiogram at rest in a 70-year-old lady referred for stress echocardiography to investigate breathlessness does not suggest any significant structural disease. B) Following administration of a contrast agent the characteristic spade-like LV cavity contour is fully appreciated and the diagnosis of apical hypertrophic cardiomyopathy is made. (Left image is taken at onset of diastole, right image at end-systole.)

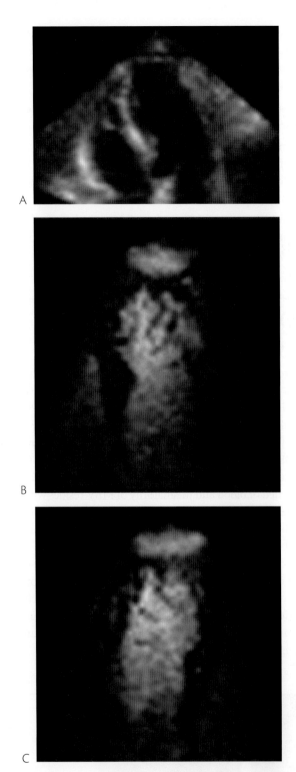

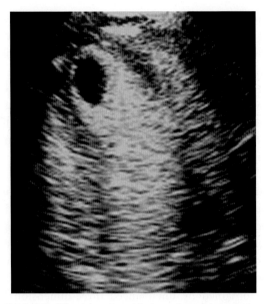

Figure 7.14 Apical thrombus. A mobile, large thrombus is clearly visualized on administration of ultrasound contrast agent in this patient who suffered an acute myocardial infarction in the anterior descending coronary artery territory.

Figure 7.13 LV non-compaction. A) The resting, unenhanced scan in a patient referred for stress echocardiography to investigate chest pain is of poor quality and non-diagnostic. B) After LV opacification, multiple deep trabeculations (arrows) of the LV myocardium are seen in the lateral (left image, four-chamber view) and posterior (right image, three-chamber view) walls involving the apex, typical of LV non-compaction.

Assessment of myocardial perfusion

Optimal myocardial perfusion assessment requires that contrast agent are administered by intravenous continuous infusion. Infusion rate can be adjusted depending on the degree of attenuation seen in LV cavity and should be kept constant. During microcirculation filling, signal intensity, proportional to bubble concentration, increases up to a peak value, beyond which it remains constant: once *steady-state* phase is achieved, bubble concentration represents capillary blood volume. Subsequently, if microbubbles are destroyed by a high MI pulse (*flash*), their signal temporarily disappears within the entire ultrasound field. After destruction, new microbubbles reach capillary vessels during the so-called *replenishment* phase: the rate of reappearance of microbubbles within myocardial wall provides a measure of microbubble velocity which ultimately reflects capillary blood velocity. After flash, at least a 15s cycle should be acquired for optimal replenishment analysis (◆ Fig. 7.15; ▣ 7.4).

Flash-replenishment method is useful to quantify myocardial perfusion. During replenishment, bubble ultrasound signal, displayed as *video-intensity*, is detected at different regular pulsing intervals. The signal intensity increases exponentially, according to the following function:

$$y = A\,(1 - e^{-\beta t}) \tag{7.2}$$

where *y* is the signal intensity, *A* is the plateau video-intensity, β reflects the rate of rise of video-intensity and, hence, microbubbles velocity and *t* represents the pulsing interval.[4] By computed analysis of myocardial perfusion, microbubble video-intensity is plotted against time, depicting a curve representative of exponential increase of ultrasound signal over time, as described by ◆ Equation 7.2. The plateau video-intensity (*A*) reflects the effective microbubble concentration, corresponding to

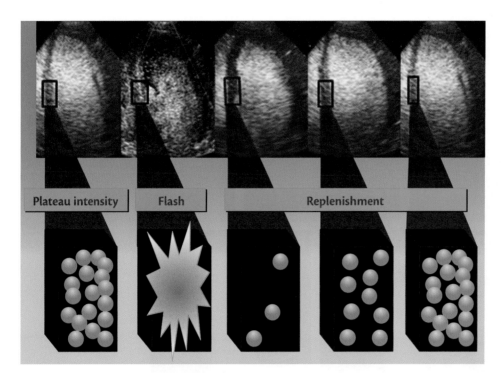

Figure 7.15 Flash-replenishment. Schema indicating the gradual refilling of coronary microcirculation by microbubbles following their destruction. The signal intensity increases up to a peak value, representative of achievement of the steady-state phase.

microvascular cross-sectional area and, hence, to MBV (➲ Fig. 7.16). The slope of the tangent to the curve, representing microbubbles velocity, is described by β parameter. Knowing both the MBV and microbubble velocity can then provide a measure of MBF:

$$MBF = A \times \beta \qquad (7.3)$$

Some automatic softwares provide LV perfusion maps, where video-intensity of each myocardial segment is encoded into different colours: such parametric imaging technique more rapidly enables assessment of MBF (➲ Fig. 7.16). Unfortunately, computed analysis is a more time-consuming method and does not recognize image artefacts.

A decreased microbubbles concentration and/or velocity within some myocardial segments denotes the presence of a coronary microvascular damage (MD).

At visual analysis of myocardial perfusion, the reduced, absent, and/or delayed opacification of any myocardial

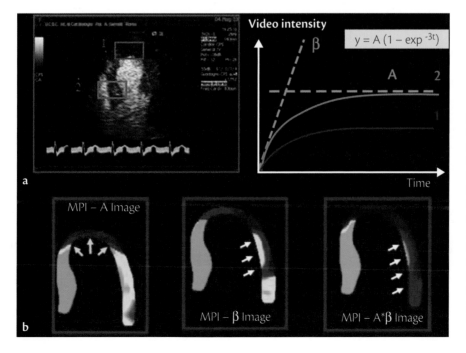

Figure 7.16 Computed analysis of myocardial perfusion. A) This panel displays the method for obtaining the replenishment curve: two regions of interest (ROIs) (red and blue boxes) are positioned along myocardial wall in different points, affecting by different degrees of myocardial perfusion. Computed analysis of video-intensity over time results in two distinct curves representative of blood volume and velocity in each ROI. B) In parametric images, blood volume, velocity, and flow are encoded into different colours.

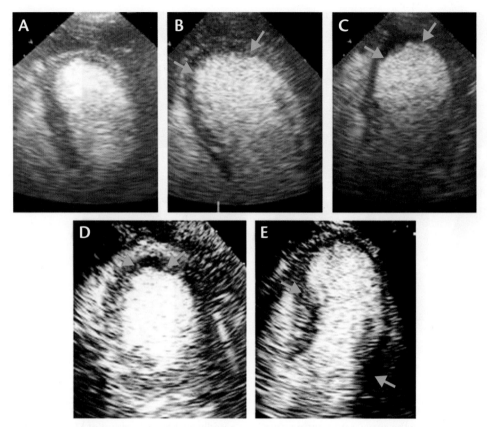

Figure 7.17 Visual assessment of myocardial perfusion. A) Example of a four-chamber apical view contrast echo study showing normal myocardial perfusion. B) Example of a four-chamber apical view contrast echo study showing a reduced/delayed perfusion of the LV apical wall (between arrows), corresponding to partial/functional microvascular damage. C) In this four-chamber apical view contrast echo study, the total absence of microbubbles signal within the LV apical wall identifies a large perfusion defect (between arrows), corresponding to a complete/structural microvascular damage. D) and E) While a parasternal short-axis view contrast echo study (D) shows a small transmural perfusion defect (between arrows), (E) displays a four-chamber apical view contrast echo study with a wide subendocardial perfusion defect that extent along septal, apical, and lateral LV walls (between arrows).

segments represent perfusion abnormalities. Such abnormal opacification appear as a black zone within myocardial wall and is named perfusion defect (PD) (➲ Fig. 7.17; ▣ 7.5).

PD can be easily visually assessed and measured by semi-quantitative or quantitative methods.

Semiquantitative analysis of perfusion defect

A single perfusion score is assigned to each myocardial segment, grading as:

1 = normal opacification

2 = reduced or delayed opacification

3 = absent opacification.

Finally, a Contrast Score Index (CSI) is achieved as:

Sum of all scores/Total number of segments   (7.4)

Quantitative analysis of perfusion defect

Zones without any opacification can also be visually quantitated by manually tracing the endocardial border length and the area of PD in four-, two-, and three-chamber views (➲ Fig. 7.18). The average of measurements obtained in all three views is expressed as contrast defect length (CDL) and contrast defect area (CDA), respectively. CDL and CDA are indexed as:

CDL% = (CDL/total endocardial border length) × 100   (7.5)

CDA% = (CDA/total LV wall area) × 100   (7.6)

Whereas CDL% is representative of transmural PD, the advantage of using CDA% to quantify perfusion abnormalities resides in the possibility of reliably measuring not only transmural, but also subendocardial PD (➲ Fig. 7.19).

Clinical applications

Usefulness of MCE has been widely recognized in several pathological conditions. This technique proves viability of hibernating or stunning myocardium with accuracy comparable to that of nuclear imaging tools.

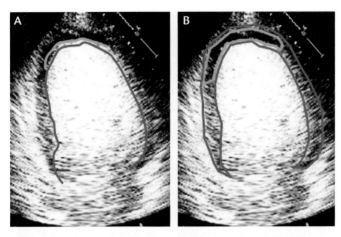

Figure 7.18 Assessment of transmural perfusion defect. A) The large transmural perfusion defect seen in four-chamber apical view can be measured by contrast defect length, representing the endocardial border length of contrast defect (green line) referred to total LV endocardial wall (blue line). B) The same perfusion defect can also be quantitated by contrast defect area (B), representing the area of contrast defect (green contour) referred to total LV wall area (blue contour).

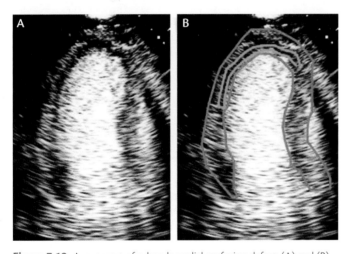

Figure 7.19 Assessment of subendocardial perfusion defect. (A) and (B) panels show a subendocardial perfusion defect in three-chamber apical view: it can be reliably quantified only by contrast defect area (B).

Myocardial infarction

In the setting of myocardial infarction, myocardial contrast echocardiography (MCE) can be performed to:

1) Establish extent of risk area as dark myocardial zone supplied by occluded artery, clearly distinguishable from normally opacified myocardium, in order to guide revascularization decision making.[5]

2) Evaluate no-reflow phenomenon, which is the lack of reperfusion of coronary microcirculation, despite optimal recanalization of infarct-related coronary artery by percutaneous coronary intervention. This phenomenon occurs in about half of patients with successfully treated acute myocardial infarction because of a MD, secondary to ischaemia/

reperfusion injury. Several structural and functional components affect such MD: atheroembolization, plugging of leucocytes and platelets, stasis of red blood cells, endothelial damage, tissue oedema, vasoconstriction.[6] When assessed at MCE, such MD appears as PD,[7] which can be sustained or spontaneously resolvable over time, with the former associated to worse prognosis.[8]

3) Measure infarct size in the subacute phase of myocardial infarction, because at that time PD extents within necrotic area.

4) Formulate post-infarct patient prognosis based on the presence and extent of no-reflow and infarct size.

Takotsubo syndrome

In takotsubo syndrome, reversible coronary MD, most reasonably responsible for transient mid-apical myocardial dysfunction, has been for the first time assessed and characterized by MCE. During acute phase, a large PD usually seen in the LV apical wall partially or completely resolves by means of adenosine vasodilator challenge. At follow-up, myocardial perfusion and associated contractile abnormalities appear totally restored.

Stable coronary artery disease

The ability of MCE to quantify MBF and coronary flow reserve in stable coronary artery diseases (CADs) has been widely demonstrated during stress echocardiography. Reduction of myocardial blood volume is proportional to disease entity: in the presence of critical epicardial stenosis, perfusion pressure of microcirculation is very low and capillary vessels collapse resulting in variable degrees of PD.

Hypertrophic cardiomyopathy

In patients with hypertrophic cardiomyopathy undergoing septal ablation, intracoronary administration of contrast agent has been done in order to depict the specific areas, perfused by selected branches, where ethanol has to be infused. The use of intracoronary contrast injection permits the dramatic reduction of the volume of ethanol required. However, although intracoronary injection of contrast agents has been performed in thousands of patients without complications, it is not approved and is considered contraindicated in the current guidelines on contrast echocardiography.

Stress contrast echo

Adjunctive role

Stress echocardiography is an excellent tool for the detection of myocardial ischaemia and for risk stratification. However, suboptimal images occur in approximately 30% of patients. Stress echocardiography relies on wall thickening abnormalities as a marker of myocardial ischaemia and for risk stratification, but it is known that perfusion defect precedes wall thickening abnormalities during demand ischaemia. With the advent of contrast echocardiography, not only improved image quality is obtained, but myocardial perfusion may also be assessed simultaneously when stress echo is performed using very low-power imaging.[9–13] For simultaneous assessment of perfusion and function, it is important to administer contrast agent by continuous infusion.

Left ventricular opacification

Contrast administration significantly improves not only the image quality but also endocardial border delineation, which leads to improved confidence and interpretation (➲ Fig. 7.20).

Contrast stress echo demonstrates improved diagnostic accuracy for the detection of CAD compared to the non-contrast echo. This is particularly so in patients in whom more than two contiguous segments are suboptimal before contrast administration.

Myocardial perfusion

In a normal myocardium subtended by a normal coronary artery, capillary flow is 1mm/s. This increases to 4–5mm/s during maximal hyperaemia which may be induced by vasodilator, inotropes, or exercise. When contrast echocardiography is performed at rest, microbubbles replenishment is complete in 5s in normal myocardium subtended by normal coronary artery. During stress, the replenishment takes 1s after microbubble clearance (➲ Fig. 7.21).

However, in the presence of a flow-limiting stenosis, during stress there is both reduction in capillary volume (signal intensity) and blood velocity. So, during the replenishment phase a subendocardial defect is seen which fills beyond 1–2s after the clearance of microbubbles.[14]

The protocols for performing stress myocardial perfusion imaging are shown in ➲ Figs. 7.22 and 7.23.

The mere observation of LVO improves wall motion assessment compared to non-contrast imaging; subtle subendocardial defects enhances appreciation of wall motion abnormalities. However, flash-replenishment imaging immediately during exercise can be challenging because of increased frequency of respiratory artefacts and the brief time window.

Coronary flow reserve

Coronary flow reserve (CFR) may be performed using both low and high MI imaging techniques. The MBF obtained in each of the myocardial segments in the apical views (preferably avoiding the basal segments) is assigned to the three vascular territories. The imaging process is repeated during stress myocardial imaging. The ratio of the peak and that of resting flow indicates CFR:

$$CFR = peak\ MBF/resting\ MBF \tag{7.7}$$

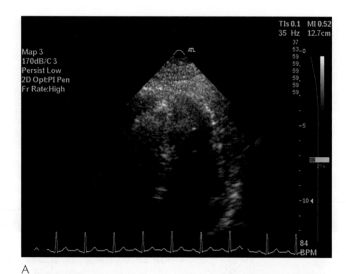

A

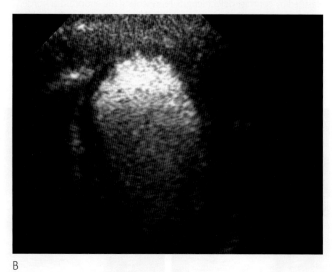

B

Figure 7.20 Contrast for left ventricular opacification during stress echo. A) Example of four-chamber apical view during a stress echo study: note the poor quality of image that affect assessment of regional wall motion. B) Contrast administration significantly improves the image quality and endocardial border delineation during stress echo as well as during rest echocardiography.

Many studies in various cardiovascular pathological conditions showed that CFR assessed by MCE can accurately evaluate not only the presence but also severity of CAD.[15–17]

Three-dimensional contrast echocardiography

Intracardiac shunts

Transthoracic and transoesophageal 3D echocardiography can be used to localize the orifice in the interatrial septum. With 2D techniques it is sometimes not possible to decide whether contrast appearing in the left atrium is coming through the pulmonary veins or through a patent foramen ovale. The preparation

Ms IL

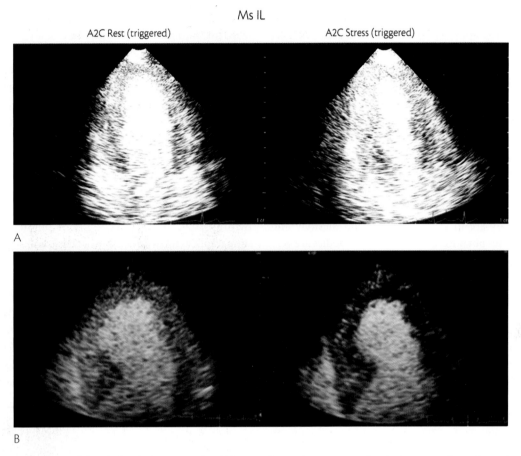

Figure 7.21 Contrast for myocardial perfusion during stress echo. A) In case of normal coronary arteries, during stress echocardiography, the replenishment of coronary microcirculation by microbubbles is complete and lasts only a few seconds (left panel = rest; right panel = stress). B) In the presence of a flow-limiting stenosis, during stress echocardiography, a subendocardial perfusion defect is seen in a few seconds after microbubbles destruction (left panel = rest; right panel = stress).

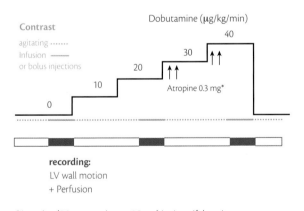

Figure 7.22 Dobutamine stress protocol. Schema indicating the dobutamine contrast stress protocol with different timing of infusion of inotropic agent and ultrasound contrast agent. Reproduced with permission from Senior R, Becher H, Monaghan M et al (2009) Contrast echocardiography: evidence-based recommendations by European Association of Echocardiography European Journal of Echocardiography; 10: 194–212.

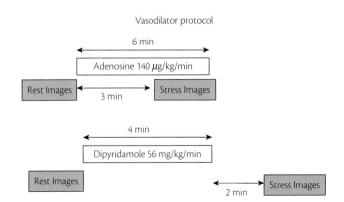

Figure 7.23 Adenosine and dipyridamole stress protocol. Schema indicating the adenosine (at the top) and dipyridamole (at the bottom) stress protocol with timing of infusion of vasodilator agents. Reproduced with permission from Senior R, Becher H, Monaghan M et al (2009) Contrast echocardiography: evidence-based recommendations by European Association of Echocardiography European Journal of Echocardiography; 10: 194–212.

of the contrast agent and injection are not different from 2D contrast echocardiography. 3D recordings are obtained over several cycles with using real-time imaging.

Left ventricular opacification

Contrast 3D echo is the most accurate echocardiographic method for assessing LV volumes and EF. For accurate measurements of LV volumes and EF, contrast should be used not only in datasets with poor native image quality.

Poor endocardial definition is more frequent in 3D echocardiography than in 2D echocardiography. Intravenous contrast agents enhance endocardial border definition and are as useful in 3D echo as they are in 2D studies. LV end-diastolic and end-systolic volumes obtained from contrast 3D studies are very close to the volumes measured in CMR studies, whereas end-diastolic volumes obtained from native 2D echo and native 3D echo are up to 40% or 15% lower than those measured with CMR.

All contrast agents used for 2D echocardiography can be used. Up to 50% higher dosages of the contrast agents are needed for 3D contrast echocardiography compared to 2D contrast echocardiography. The higher contrast dose is required since the matrix probe used for real-time 3D echocardiography transmits more ultrasound energy and destroys the contrast microbubbles more easily. As for 2D contrast echocardiography,

an infusion of contrast is preferable over bolus injections (start with1mL/min SonoVue® and increase by 0.2-mL steps if LV opacification is incomplete or contrast swirling is seen).

Presets which are available on echo scanners provide real-time 3D echocardiography with contrast. In order to achieve a high frame rate, lowest line density should be used. This reduces spatial resolution, but is necessary to avoid near-field microbubble destruction and to achieve a wider sector angle.

Training and accreditation

Before using contrast agents, both physicians and cardiac sonographers must have acquired basic and stress echocardiography training. The use of contrast agents requires a level of experience and performance initially under guidance or supervision. Physicians, sonographers, and nurses should be competent in the administration of contrast agents, aware of the indications and contraindications, and able to manage adverse events. Personnel involved in contrast use should attend courses, etc. to learn the use of contrast, performance, and interpretation of contrast-enhanced images, particularly assessment of perfusion. In fact, experience with contrast agent for LVO is a prerequisite for moving on to assess perfusion and function with contrast agents.

Personal perspective

Contrast echocardiography has gained a crucial role in everyday clinical practice since it significantly improves the image quality during both rest and stress echocardiography. Furthermore, it provides additional important information on myocardial perfusion. In fact, contrast echocardiography can be safely performed at bedside in order not only to assess cardiac structures and function, but also to obtain a comprehensive evaluation of myocardial perfusion and a reliable measure of coronary flow reserve. Although a specifically devoted learning curve is necessary to achieve adequate confidence with technique and expertise in image acquisition and interpretation, contrast echocardiography reduces the need for additional, costly, and more hazardous tests and spares the patients further invasive investigations. Furthermore, the possibility of live visualization of coronary microvascular flow and function, allows myocardial contrast echocardiography to define novel pathogenetic mechanisms of diseases specifically affecting coronary microcirculation.

References

1 Becher H, Burns PN, Handbook of Contrast Echocardiography, Springer 2000.

2 Jayaweera AR, Edwards N, Glasheen WP, Villanueva FS, Abbott RD, Kaul S. In vivo myocardial kinetics of air-filled albumin microbubbles during myocardial contrast echocardiography. Comparison with radiolabeled red blood cells, *Circ. Res* 1994; **74**:1157–65.

3 Senior R, Andersson O, Caidahl K, Carlens P, Herregods, Jenni R, Kenny A, Melcher A, Svedenhag J, Vanoverschelde JL, Wandt BW, Widgren BR, Williams G, Guerret P, la Rosee K, Agati L, Bezante G. Enhanced Left Ventricular Endocardial Border Delineation with an Intravenous Injection of SonoVue, a New Echocardiographic Contrast Agent: A European Multicenter Study, Echocardiography, 2000; **17**:705–11.

4 Wei K, Jayaweera AR, Firoozan S, Linka A, Skyba DM, Kaul S. Quantification of myocardial blood flow with ultrasound-induced destruction of microbubbles administered as a constant venous infusion. *Circulation* 1998; **97**:473–83.

5 Villanueva FS, Myocardial Contrast Echocardiography in Acute Myocardial Infarction, *Am J Cardiol* 2002; **90**(suppl):38J–47J.

6 Kloner RA, Ganote CE, Jennings RB, The "No-Reflow" Phenomenon after Temporary Coronary Occlusion in the Dog, *The Journal of Clinical Investigation*, 1974; **54**:1496–1508.

7 Galiuto L, Garramone B, Scarà A, *et al.* on behalf of the AMICI Investigators. The Extent of Microvascular Damage During

Myocardial Contrast Echocardiography Is Superior to Other Known Indexes of Post-Infarct Reperfusion in Predicting Left Ventricular Remodeling. Results of the Multicenter AMICI Study. *J Am Coll Cardiol* 2008; **51**:552–9.

8 Galiuto L, Lombardo A, Maseri A, Santoro L, Porto I, Cianflone D, Rebuzzi AG, Crea F. Temporal evolution and functional outcome of no reflow: sustained and spontaneously reversible patterns following successful coronary recanalisation, *Heart* 2003; **89**: 731–37.

9 Senior R, Monaghan M, Main ML, Zamorano JL, Tiemann K, Agali L *et al*. Detection of coronary artery disease with perfusion stress echocardiography using a novel ultrasound imaging agent: two phase 3 international trials in comparison with radionuclide perfusion imaging. *Eur J Echocardiogr* 2009; **10**:26–35.

10 Dolan MS, Riad K, El-Shafei A, Puri S, Tamirsa K, Blerig M *et al*. Effect of intravenous contrast for left ventricular opacification and border definition on sensitivity and specificity of dobutamine stress echocardiography compared with coronary angiography in technically difficult patients. *Am Heart J* 2001; **142**:908–15.

11 Shimoni S, Zoghbi WA, Xie F, Kricsfeld D, Iskander S, Gobar L *et al*. Real-time assessment of myocardial perfusion and wall motion during bicycle and treadmill exercise echocardiography; comparison with single photon emission computed tomography. *J Am Coll Cardiol* 2001; **37**:741–7.

12 Rainbird AJ, Mulvagh S, Oh JK, McCully RB, Klarich KW, Shub C *et al*. Contrast dobutamine stress echocardiography clinical practice assessment in 300 consecutive patients. *J Am Soc Echocardiogr* 2001; **14**:375–8.

13 Plana JC, Mikati IA, Dokainish H, Lakkis N, Abukhalti J, Davis R *et al*. A randomized cross-over study for evaluation of the effect of image optimization with contrast on the diagnostic accuracy of dobutamine echocardiography in coronary artery disease. *J Am Coll Cardiol Cardiac Imaging* 2008; **1**:145–2.

14 Wei K, Mulvagh SL, Carson L, Davidoff R, Gabriel R, Grim RA *et al*. The safety of Definity and Optison for ultrasound image enhancement: a retrospective analysis of 78,383 administered contrast doses. *J Am Soc Echocardiogr* 2008; **21**:1202–6.

15 Senior R, Janardhanan R, Jeetley P, Burden L. Myocardial contrast echocardiography for distinguishing ischemic from nonischemic first-onset acute heart failure: insights into the mechanism of acute heart failure. *Circulation* 2005; **112**:1587–93.

16 Hayat SA, Dwivedi G, Jacobsen A, Kinsey C, Senior R. Effects of left bundle branch block on cardiac structure, function perfusion and perfusion reserve: implications for myocardial contrast echocardiography versus radionuclide perfusion imaging for the detection of coronary artery disease. *Circulation* 2008; **117**: 1832–41.

17 Moir S, Haluska BA, Jenkins C, McNab D, Marwick TH. Myocardial blood volume and perfusion reserve responses to combined dipyridamole and exercise stress: a quantitative approach to contrast stress echocardiography. *J Am Soc Echocardiogr* 2005; **18**:1187–93.

Further reading

Jenkins C, Moir S, Chan J, Rakhit D, Haluska B, Marwick TH, *et al*. Left ventricular volume measurement with echocardiography: a comparison of left ventricular opacification, three-dimensional echocardiography, or both with magnetic resonance imaging. *Eur Heart J* 2009; **30**(1):98–106.

Kurt M, Shaikh KA, Peterson L, Kurrelmeyer KM, Shah G, Nagueh SF, *et al*. Impact of contrast echocardiography on evaluation of ventricular function and clinical management in a large prospective cohort. *J Am Coll Cardiol* 2009; **53**:802–10.

Lim TK, Burden L, Janardhanan R, Ping C, Moon J, Pennell D, *et al*. Improved accuracy of low-power contrast echocardiography for the assessment of left ventricular remodeling compared with unenhanced harmonic echocardiography after acute myocardial infarction: comparison with cardiovascular magnetic resonance imaging. *J Am Soc Echocardiogr* 2005; **18**:1203–7.

Malm S, Frigstad S, Sagberg E, Larsson H, Skjaerpe T. Accurate and reproducible measurement of left ventricular volume and ejection fraction by contrast echocardiography: a comparison with magnetic resonance imaging. *J Am Coll Cardiol* 2004; **44**:1030–5.

Mor-Avi V, Jenkins C, Kuhl HP, Nesser HJ, Marwick TH, Franke A, *et al*. Real-time 3-dimensional echocardiographic quantification of left ventricular volumes: multicenter study for validation with magnetic resonance imaging and investigation of sources of error. *J Am Coll Cardiol: Cardiovasc Imaging* 2008; **1**(4):413–23.

Olszewski R, Timperley J, Cezary S, Monaghan M, Nihoyannopoulos P, Senior R, *et al*. The clinical applications of contrast echocardiography. *Eur J Echocardiogr* 2007; **8**:S13–S23.

Reilly JP, Tunick PA, Timmermans RJ, Stein B, Rosenzweig BP, Kronzon I, *et al*. Contrast echocardiography clarifies uninterpretable wall motion in intensive care unit patients. *J Am Coll Cardiol* 2000; **35**:485–90.

Senior R, Becher H, Monaghan M, Agati L, Zamorano J, Vanoverschelde JL, Nihoyannopoulos P. EAE Recommendations. Contrast echocardiography: evidence-based recommendations by European Association of Echocardiography. *Eur J Echocardiogr* 2009; **10**:194–212.

Thanigaraj S, Schechtman KB, Perez JE. Improved echocardiographyic delineation of left ventricular thrombus with the use of intravenous second-generation contrast image enhancement. *J Am Soc Echcocardiogr* 1999; **12**:1022–6.

Additional DVD and online material

▥ 7.1 Functioning of pump for continuous infusion of contrast agents.

▥ 7.2 Intermittent imaging modality.

▥ 7.3 Real time imaging modality.

▥ 7.4 Flash-replenishment.

▥ 7.5 Transmural perfusion defect.

▥ 7.6 Subendocardial perfusion defect.

↻ For additional multimedia materials please visit the online version of the book (🔊 http://escecho.oxfordmedicine.com).

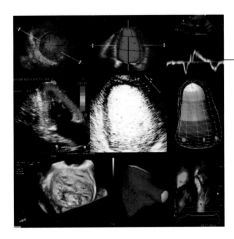

CHAPTER 8

Assessment of systolic function

Alexandra Gonçalves, Pedro Marcos-Alberca, Peter Sogaard, and José Luis Zamorano

Contents

Summary

This chapter describes the different modalities for assessment of systolic function by transthoracic echocardiography. Firstly, the basic principles of physiology and the determinants of left ventricular (LV) performance are considered, followed by a systematic appraisal of the methodologies for global LV systolic function assessment. Starting with M-mode echocardiography, passing through the traditional two-dimensional echocardiography evaluation to three-dimensional echocardiography approaches, main strengths and limitations are described. Power Doppler usefulness, regarding stroke volume calculations and dP/dt measurement are summarily explained, taking into consideration the usual pitfalls found in daily practice. There is a section dedicated to regional systolic function evaluation, with the recommendations for standardized LV division and differential characteristics of wall motion abnormalities. Additionally, more recent approaches with tissue Doppler imaging and strain analyses for global and regional LV function assessment are described. Finally, a section is dedicated to right ventricle systolic function which describes all modalities of evaluation.

Introduction

The assessment of left ventricular (LV) systolic function is one of the mainstays for echocardiography use. It has a huge impact on medical decisions, device implantation, and heart surgery recommendations, in addition to providing important prognostic information.[1,2] It is a part of routine echocardiography examination, but since the first attempts with the M-mode approach, several improvements regarding reproducibility and accuracy were made with two-dimensional (2D) and recently with three-dimensional (3D) echocardiography. More sophisticated methods such as strain imaging, based on Doppler or speckle tracking techniques, provide a quantitative measurement of the contractility of the myocardium and gradually are gaining a place in common daily practice.

Determinants of left ventricle performance

The ventricle works as a pump generating pressure and ejecting a volume of blood. The normal relationship between LV pressure and ejection is usually presented as LV pressure variation versus LV volume, as shown in ➲ Fig. 8.1. Ventricular performance is the result of cardiac inotropic state (*contractility*) plus two independent loading variables, the *preload* and the *afterload*.

♦ *Contractility* is the force generated at any given end-diastolic volume and may be defined as the quality of cardiac muscle that determines performance, independently of loading conditions.[3] Each myocardial cell is capable of varying the amount of tension generated during contraction, which mainly results from the calcium bound to the troponin complex of the myofilaments. The myocardial fibres are orientated in the subendocardium of the LV following a right-handed helix, whereas the ones from the subepicardium present a left-handed spiral (➲ Fig. 8.2).[4] Contraction of these fibres leads to a counterclockwise twisting of the apex, relative to the basis on its long axis.[4] During systole, the extent of torsion is linearly related to the ejection of blood,[5] therefore, the stroke volume is also a function of contractility. However, its part in the haemodynamic process is difficult to study because it is affected by the loading conditions, and no load independent index of basal contractile state has been described.

♦ *Preload* is the force which stretches the myofibrils at rest. Fibre extension depends on the myocardial compliance, or *muscle stiffness*, and the degree of filling.[6] Preload is generally estimated as the LV end-diastolic pressure, diameter, or volume. The Frank–Starling mechanism describes the relationship between ventricular end-diastolic volume and ventricular performance, which might be calculated by stroke volume, cardiac output, and/or stroke work. As preload affects the initial fibre length, it influences LV systolic performance,[3] and within physiological limits, an increase in LV preload improves myocardial contraction on the basis of the Frank–Starling mechanism.

♦ *Afterload* is the force exerted by the myocardium after the onset of contraction, or the force per unit area acting in the direction in which the fibres lie in the ventricular wall. It can be estimated using the Laplace law, which describes the systolic wall stress (afterload) as directly related to pressure and radius and inversely related to wall thickness.[7] Consequently, changes in ventricular volume, wall thickness, as well as systemic vascular resistance or aortic impedance affect the afterload. The classical example is the acute increase in systolic pressure, causing an increase in the afterload, which results in stroke volume reduction in an inadapted LV. In contrast, an acute increase in systolic pressure can result in increased afterload.[8] In the normal heart, stroke volume is minimally affected by changes in afterload, whereas in the failing heart small changes in afterload can generate important changes in stroke volume.[9]

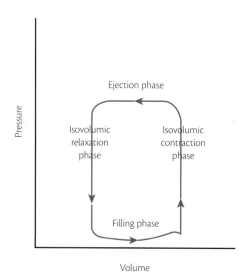

Figure 8.1 Pressure–volume relationship. Classic loop of pressure-volume relationship of a normally contracting left ventricle with the four phases of the cardiac cycle. Adapted from Zipes D, Libby P, Bonow R, Braunwald E (eds) *Braunwald's Heart Disease*, 7th edn. Philadelphia, PA: Elsevier Saunders; 2005, p.1572. Copyright Elsevier (2005).

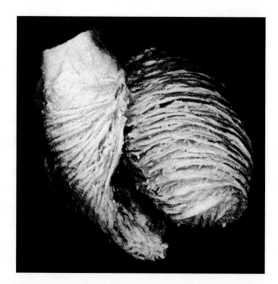

Figure 8.2 Myocardial fibers orientation. Dissection of a normal heart illustrating myocardial fibers orientation. In this model the left handed spiral orientation of the subepicardium fibers is demonstrated. Adapted with permission from Sanchez-Quintana D, Garcia Martinez V, Hurle JM. Myocardial fiber architecture in the human heart. Anatomical demonstration of modifications in the normal pattern of ventricular fiber architecture in a malformed adult specimen. *Acta Anat* (S. Karger AG, Basel) 1990; 138(4):352–8.

Table 8.1 Formulas for measurements of left ventricular systolic function

	Formula	Units	Possible methods
Stroke volume (SV)	LVEDV − LVESV	mL	M-mode; 2DE; 3DE
Stroke volume	TVI (LVOT) × 2∏(LVOTd/2)^2	mL	M-mode; 2DE
Ejection fraction	SV/LVVd	%	M-mode; 2DE; 3DE
Fractional shortening (FS)	(LVDd − LVDs)/LVDd	%	M-mode; 2DE
Velocity of circumferential shortening (Vcf)	FS/ET	circumference/s	M-mode; 2DE
Fractional area change	(ASxd − ASxs)/ASxd	%	2DE; 3DE
Cardiac output (CO)	SV × HR	L/min	M-mode; 2DE; 3DE
Cardiac index (CI)	CO/BSA	L/min/m^2	M-mode; 2DE; 3DE

2DE, two-dimensional echocardiography; 3DE, three dimensional echocardiography; ASxd, short axis left ventricle diastolic area; ASxs, short axis left ventricle systolic area; BSA, body surface area; ET, ejection time; HR, heart rate; LVDd, left ventricle diastolic diameter; LVEDV, left ventricle end-diastolic volume; LVESV, left ventricle end systolic volume; LVOT, left ventricle outflow tract; LVSd, left ventricle systolic diameter; TVI, time velocity integral;

Global left ventricle systolic function

The most common quantitative approach of LV systolic function is the ejection fraction (EF), defined by the fraction of volume ejected during each ventricle contraction (➲ Table 8.1). It is a global index which expresses myocardial fibre shortening, requires the estimation of LV volumes, and it is affected by preload and afterload.[10]

M-mode

The initial attempts at LV function quantification were based on one-dimensional, M-mode linear measurements of the LV internal dimension in diastole and systole, using *Teichholz or Quinones* methods (➲ Fig. 8.3). Parameters such as *fractional shortening* and *velocity of circumferential shortening* are assessed with low intraobserver and interobserver variability and provide an adequate measurement of ventricular function, in the presence of normal geometry and symmetric function.[11–14] When these conditions are assembled, the diastolic measurement is a reasonable assessment of the size of the LV and the resultant fractional shortening is a reliable index of systolic function (➲ Table 8.1). Its normal value is ≥30%. However, fractional shortening is a specific marker of LV basal contractility and does not necessarily reflects global LV function in patients with regional wall motion abnormalities (WMAs).

In the calculation of velocity of circumferential shortening, the minor axis represents a circle of known diameter from which the circumference can be calculated and the rate of change of circumference determined. This index has the advantage of providing the amplitude of the ejection and its velocity; however, this method is rarely used at present time.[15]

Another linear measurement providing indirect quantitative evaluation of LV systolic function is the quantification of the *distance between the E point of the anterior mitral leaflet and the basal portion of the interventricular septum (IVS).*[16] The ratio of mitral excursion to LV size reflects the EF. Typically, there is a

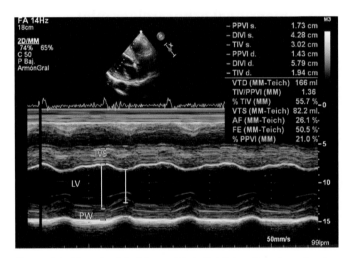

Figure 8.3 M-mode of the left ventricle in PLAX view. Two-dimensional anatomically-guided M-mode of the left ventricle, keeping a perpendicular orientation in relation to the cardiac long axis and interventricular septum. Left ventricle internal dimension in diastole and systole are acquired for estimation of left ventricle systolic function, according to the Teichholz method. IVS, interventricular septum; LV, left ventricle; PW, posterior wall.

relative linear correlation between the degree of annular and mitral excursion during systole and the global systolic function. Thus, in the presence of a normal mitral valve (MV) and in the absence of other factors that interfere with MV opening, as severe aortic regurgitation (AR), a distance less than or equal to 5mm from the E point (maximal early opening) represents a normal EF.[17] Moreover, the magnitude of motion from the base of the heart towards the apex during ventricular contraction is directly proportional to systolic function, interestingly, this is the same principle used in tissue Doppler (TD) imaging of the mitral annulus velocities, for determination of diastolic and systolic function.[18]

Spatial resolution of the M-mode beam is superior to that of 2D echocardiography. However, pitfalls on 3D geometric assumptions of Teichholz or Quinones methods must be regarded. The linear line has to be perpendicular to the septum, but, even if using 2D-guided M-mode measurements, it may not be possible to align the beam in a truly perpendicular fashion to the long axis of the ventricle, which is an essential condition to reflect the true minor-axis dimension. The M-mode measurements typically overestimates the true minor-axis of the LV by 6–12mm, in comparison with 2D minor-axis dimensions.[16] These mathematical assumptions are not valid in the presence of regional myocardial disease, since they may underestimate the severity of dysfunction, when only a normal region is interrogated, or conversely overestimate the abnormality, if it transits through the WMA exclusively. For those reasons 2D echocardiography methods have supplanted these measurements and M-mode LV systolic function estimation is no longer recommended for clinical practice.

Two-dimensional echocardiography

2D echocardiography provides superior spatial resolution for determining LV size, and the estimation of the LV ejection fraction (LVEF) can be made either qualitatively, by visual inspection of global and regional function, with the so-called *eyeball method* or quantitatively, by means of geometric assumptions of the LV cavity shape.

Qualitative assessment

Global function is usually described as *normal, hyperdynamic,* or *depressed*. Hyperdynamic is usually associated with high-output syndromes or with a response to exercise or pharmacological stress. In the presence of depressed systolic function, its severity may be characterized as *mild, moderate,* or *severe*, according to the cut-off values presented in ➲ Table 8.2. The qualitative global function evaluation is no longer recommended as the reference methodology in clinical practice. However, it presents a good correlation with Simpson's method, as long as all projections are regarded and interpreted by an experienced operator,[19] and it is still recommended for cross-checking the quantitative data obtained.[20]

Quantitative assessment

Regarding quantitative methods, the *fractional area change* (FAC) estimates LV function in the parasternal short-axis (PSAX) view. It calculates the fraction of area change along the cardiac cycle of a symmetrically contracting ventricle (➲ Table 8.1). FAC is considered a reasonable global estimate of LV function and correlates well with EF, because approximately two-thirds of the LV stroke volume is generated by the contraction of the mid-papillary region of the LV. The normal value is ≥45%. Conversely, it is not accurate if WMAs are present as it does not take into account abnormal areas of myocardium that are not imaged through this view.[21]

Another useful method is the *midwall fraction and shortening*, since the contraction of muscle fibres in the LV mid-wall may better reflect intrinsic contractility than the contraction of fibres at the endocardium. Its benefit is based on the fact that the circumferential fibres, which predominate in the mid-wall of the left ventricle, are orientated in the same direction of the stress vector. It is particularly useful in LV systolic function evaluation of patients with concentric hypertrophy[22] and it can be estimated from linear measures of wall thicknesses, along with diastolic and systolic cavity sizes.[22,23]

The *area–length method* is an alternative process to calculate LV volumes and EF, assuming a bullet-shaped LV. The LV cross-sectional area is traced in PSAX view and the LV length is taken from the midpoint of the MV annulus to the apex in apical four-chamber (A4C) view. All measurements are repeated in end-systole and in end-diastole and the volume is mathematically computed, according to the following formula:

$$\text{LV volume} = (5 \times \text{area} \times \text{length}) / 6 \qquad (8.1)$$

There are few variations on area–length formulas based on different assumptions regarding the LV geometric shape[24] (e.g. truncated ellipse, cylinder, and cone). This method may be used when poor apical definition prevents accurate tracing of LV endocardial border.

Table 8.2 Reference limits of different parameters of left ventricle systolic function

| | Male | | | | Female | | | |
	Reference range	Abnormal Mild	Moderate	Severe	Reference range	Abnormal Mild	Moderate	Severe
M mode								
Endocardial fractional shortening, %	25–43	20–24	15–19	≤14	27–45	22–26	17–21	≤16
Mid-wall fractional shortening, %	14–22	12–13	10–11	≤10	15–23	13–14	11–12	≤10
2D mode								
Ejection fraction, %	≥55	45–54	30–44	<30	≥55	45–54	30–44	<30

Adapted from Lang RM, Bierig M, Devereux RB, Flachskampf FA, *et al.* Recommendations for chamber quantification. *European Journal of Echocardiography* 2006; **7**(2): 79–108.

The first attempts to simplify and automatize LV volumes determination were done using the *acoustic quantification*. This technique for automatic border detection, is based on conventional 2D ultrasound imaging, modified to detect and track blood-tissue interfaces in real time, according to their quantitative acoustic properties.[25] This allows on-line demonstration of the LV cavity area, fractional area change, volumes and EF.[26] This method is not commonly used nowadays, but its concept underlies modern approaches such as 3D echocardiography.

The most frequently used technique for LV volume measurement is the *biplane method of discs (modified Simpson's rule)*, which is the method currently recommended by the American Society of Echocardiography and the European Association of Echocardiography for ejection fraction estimation (➲ Fig. 8.4).[20] This methodology is based on the principle of calculation of total LV volume as the summation of a series of elliptical discs of equal height, equally spaced along the long axis of the LV.[16] The cross-sectional area in ideal conditions is based on both diameters, obtained from the A2C and A4C views. LV end-diastolic and end-systolic volumes (LVEDV and LVESV, respectively) are measured in A4C and A2C view. LVEF is calculated as:

$$EF_{A4C} = (LVEDV_{A4C} - LVESV_{A4C}/VESV_{A4C})/LVEDV_{A4C} \times 100 \quad (8.2)$$

$$EF_{A2C} = (LVEDV_{A2C} - LVESV_{A2C})/LVEDV_{A2C} \times 100 \quad (8.3)$$

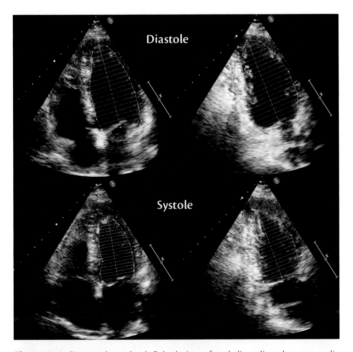

Figure 8.4 Simpson's method. Calculation of end-diastolic volume, systolic volume, stroke volume, and ejection fraction by the Simpson's method adapted for two-dimensional echocardiography. The operator outlines the left ventricle area in apical four- and two- chambers, both in diastole and in systole. The software divides the areas of the mutual projections into discs of equal height and automatically calculates the diastolic and systolic volumes and the resultant ejection fraction.

Mean EF is obtained as an average of A4C and A2C EF values. However, if there are not two appropriate orthogonal views, one plane is used and the area is assumed to be circular. Trabeculations and papillary muscles should be included as part of the LV cavity, and, if the definition of the endocardial border is not clear, the intravenous administration of contrast agents might be used for better delineation of the border (see ➲ Chapter 7). When less than 80% of the endocardial border is adequately visualized, the use of contrast agents is highly recommended.[27]

As well as the EF, Simpson's method also indicates the stroke volume, which corresponds to the amount of blood volume ejected in each cardiac cycle, measured as the difference between the LV end-diastolic volume and LV end-systolic volume. The stroke volume can also be obtained with 3D full volume echocardiography, or with the use of Doppler measurements as explained later.

The main limitations of this method are the foreshortening of the ventricular apex and the possible tangentially A2C view acquisition. The former results in inaccurate assessment of the LVEF, and most frequently on its overestimation. Conversely, the tangentially A2C view acquisition causes underestimation of the true LV volume. Moreover, in cases of asymmetries in ventricular geometry or WMAs, a single-plane view seems less accurate.

It is of note that this method presents additional limitations, such as the myocardial dropout: it is minimized with the use of tissue harmonic imaging and contrast echocardiography. Care should be taken to keep the transducer at the true apex and the ultrasonic cross-sectional beam at the centre of the LV. Correct image acquisition is obtained when the apex is visualized as the thinnest area of the LV and it does not move towards the base during diastolic filling.[16] Although LV volumes might be indexed for body surface area (BSA), and data suggest that LVEF is to some extent higher in healthy women than in men,[28,29] the same cut-off in men and woman is used for LV systolic function classification (➲ Table 8.2).

Several studies have evaluated the accuracy of 2D echocardiography for measurement of LVEF in comparison to radionuclide or contrast ventriculography.[30,31] It was noted that those three techniques show a high correlation and a moderate agreement.[30] However, the current gold standard method for LV volumes and function evaluation is cardiac magnetic resonance (CMR)[32] and LV evaluation by 3D echocardiography appears to be the closest method regarding accuracy and reproducibility.[33,34]

Three-dimensional echocardiography

3D echocardiography imaging clearly has improved the accuracy in the evaluation of LV volumes, EF, and WMAs.[35] Multiple studies have demonstrated higher levels of agreement and

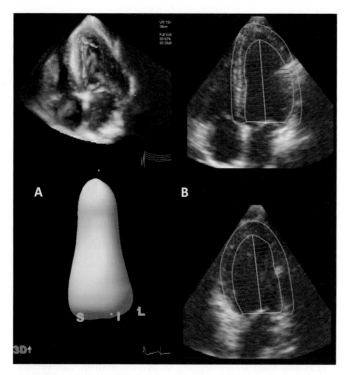

Figure 8.5 3D calculation of ejection fraction. A) Left ventricle ejection fraction calculation using 3D with direct volumetric analysis. B) Left ventricle ejection fraction calculation using 3D with biplane approximation.

reproducibility between the 3D echocardiography approach and gold-standard techniques, such as radionuclide ventriculography and CMR, as compared to conventional 2D echocardiography methodology.[33,34] Moreover, 3D echocardiography evaluation of the LV has shown the ability to detect slight changes in LV volumes over time, that were not detectable by 2D echocardiography.[36]

Despite the high reproducibility and high correlation with CMR values, several studies have reported a significant underestimation of 3D echocardiography LV volumes, when compared with CMR.[36,37] Different explanations have been presented, regarding acquisition and different analysis between the techniques, but no study has conclusively identified the main sources of error. One possible explanation is the different methodology of analysis performed when using 3D echocardiography. The direct volumetric analysis is the most accurate approach by a semiautomated detection of the LV endocardial surface. It measures many hundreds of points over the LV surface and does not rely on geometric modelling.[38,39] However, an alternative evaluation is based on the selection of two anatomically correct non-foreshortened 2D views and LV volume is calculated using a biplane approximation. Thus it still presents the limitation of reliance on geometric modelling (⊃ Fig. 8.5). However, even if using 3D direct volumetric analysis, a significantly underestimation of LV volumes quantification has been described.[38,39] Some studies revealed bias related to image quality[35,40] and to the individual ability in the clear differentiation between the myocardium and the trabeculae,

at time of endocardial visualization. This limitation might be overcome with systematic methodology of assessment.

Doppler evaluation

Using the Doppler system, dP/dt and stroke volume can be estimated (see ⊃ Chapter 5). If restricted to the early phases of systole, during isovolumic contraction, dP/dt is a relatively load-independent measure of ventricular contractility.[41] Originally, this was a determination resultant from the intraventricular pressure curves, achieved in invasive haemodynamic studies, with a high-fidelity micrometer catheter in the catheterization laboratory. Using echocardiography, it can be calculated with a good correlation with invasive haemodynamic data, as long as the patient presents with mitral regurgitation (⊃ Fig. 8.6).[42] In the presence of significant mechanical dyssynchrony dP/dt may be reduced, as a consequence of contractile dyssynchrony in spite of global preserved systolic function.

Stroke volume can be estimated not only by the biplane Simpson method and 3D full volume echocardiography, but also as the product of the left ventricular outflow tract (LVOT) area and LVOT time velocity integral (TVI) (⊃ Table 8.1) (see ⊃ Chapter 5). The normal value is 50–80mL. The Doppler method presents several potential sources of error. It presumes a flat velocity profile across the cross-sectional area of the LVOT, but Doppler flow spectrum usually is parabolic. Moreover, the cross-sectional area of the LVOT is usually calculated assuming a circular geometry, but really it is often elliptical, as recently shown with 3D echocardiography.[43] The efforts to apply a formula for elliptical geometry resulted in minimal improvements in accuracy and had no widespread clinical recognition. Any inaccuracy in measuring the LVOT may create a substantial error in flow calculation, taking into account the

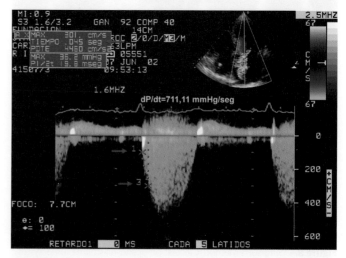

Figure 8.6 Calculation of dP/dt using the spectrogram of mitral regurgitant flow obtained by continuous Doppler. The dP/dt was calculated by measuring the time spent in the acceleration flow from 1m/s (4mmHg) at 3m/s (36mmHg). The difference (32mmHg) divided by the acceleration time in seconds results in the dP/dt, in mmHg/s. The normal value is above 1000mmHg/s. The patient in the example has an abnormal dP/dt.

square of the radius introduced in the recommended formula (see ➲ Equation 5.6) (➲ Table 8.1).

Furthermore, stroke volume as well as EF are afterload-dependent parameters, thus they are dependent on the pressure developed and on impedance against which the LV has to contract. Therefore, the preload decrease (e.g. severe anaemia) or afterload increase (e.g. aortic stenosis, severe hypertension) negatively affects LV systolic function and might cause a false underestimation of it. Conversely, the pathological decrease in afterload (e.g. mitral regurgitation, or interventricular septal defect) can cause a false impression of preserved LV function even in the presence of a serious myocardial compromise.[8] Moreover, in cases of significant intravascular volume changes, as occurs in haemodialysis, patients can present significant variations in EF, accordingly to the volume status.[44] As a result, stroke volume results from the interaction of multiple factors and it can be a false indicator of systolic function.

The systolic acceleration time (LVOTacc) is another index of LV systolic function, independent from loading conditions.[45] It is calculated as peak LVOT velocity divided by the time needed to achieve this velocity. It was found to relate linearly to LV maximal elastance and to be correlated with dP/dt.[45]

Tissue Doppler imaging

Tissue Doppler (TD) imaging measures myocardial motion velocity (see ➲ Chapter 6). In addition to diastolic function evaluation, it also allows estimation of global and regional LV systolic performance.[46]

Annular velocity in systole has shown a good correlation with the LVEF, over a wide range of ventricular function. Usually, the systolic velocity of the mitral annulus is superior to 6cm/s (➲ Fig. 8.7)[47] and has a strong correlation with normal EF.

Even though TD imaging of the mitral annulus reproduces the global LV systolic and diastolic function, regional function can also be assessed with myocardial velocity measurement in each segment.[47] This is a sensitive marker of ischaemia, as patients with a first myocardial infarction and normal systolic and diastolic LV function, determined by conventional Doppler methods, showed decreased mitral annular systolic and diastolic velocities as determined by TD, compared to healthy subjects.[48] Moreover, a decreased peak systolic velocity is a sensitive marker of mildly impaired LV systolic function, even in patients with a normal LVEF,[49] or in the early subclinical phase of hypertrophic cardiomyopathy, when mutations occur without the presence of cardiac hypertrophy.[50]

However, TD is not independent from preload. Studies in patients who underwent haemodialysis, showed that both systolic and diastolic TD velocities of the left and right ventricles were preload-dependent, even though the lateral mitral annulus was more resistant to preload changes than the septal mitral annulus or the lateral tricuspid annulus.[44.]

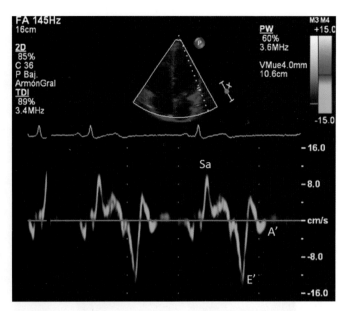

Figure 8.7 Tissue Doppler imaging of mitral annular velocities. Spectral mitral annular velocities obtained by tissue Doppler imaging from the lateral mitral annulus, recorded from an apical four-chamber view. E′, early diastolic wave; A′, late diastolic wave; Sa, systolic wave.

Index of global myocardial performance

The index of global myocardial performance (IMP) or Tei index reflects global systolic and diastolic LV performance and is expressed by the formula:

$$IMP = ICT + IRT/ET \qquad (8.4)$$

where *ICT* is the isovolumic contraction time, *IRT* is the isovolumic relaxation time, and *ET* the ejection time. Such time intervals can all be obtained using TD imaging. The normal value of the index is 0.4. Systolic dysfunction causes a prolonged ICT and a reduction of ET, while diastolic impairment prolongs the IRT. In patients with heart failure the Tei index is greater than 0.5.

Myocardial strain

After TD imaging derived strain and strain rate[51,52], improvements in strain analysis with evaluation by speckle tracking have occurred (see ➲ Chapter 6). Recently 3D speckle tracking analysis has been reported as a faster and more complete method to assess LV longitudinal and radial strain (➲ Fig. 8.8).[53]

While LVEF describes myocardial pump function, strain calculates the true contractility of the myocardium: it is less load-dependent, since it is not influenced by compensatory mechanisms such as ventricular dilation, which might result in a normal stroke volume even if the contractility is reduced. Accordingly, the main factors that influence regional myocardial deformation are the intrinsic contractility, which is affected by tissue perfusion and electrical activation,[54] the cavity pressure, whose influence is associated to the local ventricular geometry, the different segments interaction,[55] and the tissue

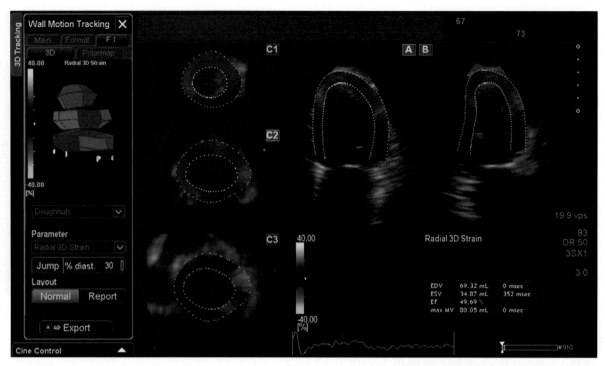

Figure 8.8 Speckle tracking analysis. Left ventricle systolic function and radial strain assessed with 3D speckle tracking analysis. Complex computation allows the calculation of the segmental, meridian, and global strain of the left ventricle. Rotational and torsional derivatives are calculated quickly. (Requires clinical validation.)

intrinsic elasticity. Consequently, LV strain evaluation is highly appropriate for assessment of systolic function in patients with apparently normal EF or with regional WMAs.[56] Moreover, it has the ability to discriminate different ischaemic substrates, ranging from acute ischaemia, over-stunning, to chronic ischaemia with subendocardial fibrosis.[57] Peak systolic strain-rate and end-systolic strain regional velocities reduce linearly with regional myocardial perfusion; in the presence of subendocardial fibrosis, simultaneous postsystolic deformation develops (➲ Fig. 8.9).[58] These changes increase with dobutamine infusion, while in normal tissue an increasing strain and strain rate is observed. In contrast, when stimulated with dobutamine, chronic infarction segments show a modest deformation increase, especially in the presence of transmurality infarction. Stunned myocardium shows reduced deformation at rest, associated with postsystolic deformation, however, when stimulated with dobutamine, systolic deformation approximately returns to normal and postsystolic deformation almost disappears.[57] In order to improve patient selection for cardiac resynchronization therapy (CRT), a novel combined index by radial strain echocardiography has been developed, which might be a predictor of response to CRT[59] (see later).

Regional systolic function

Myocardial walls are divided according to the distribution of the coronary arteries (➲ Fig. 8.10). In order to study contractile function within each perfused territory, LV myocardial wall is usually distinguished into different segments. Evaluation of regional systolic function results from contractility assessment of these segments. Although there is some degree of variability, there is a direct correlation between the LV segments and the coronary arteries that allows diagnosis of which coronary artery is affected when a segmental contraction anomaly is seen.

There are two main models widely used to guide LV segmentation. In 1989 the American Society of Echocardiography recommended a 16-segment model. In this model, the LV is divided in walls first, and in a second step, walls are divided in segments (➲ Fig. 8.11). The RV attachment defines the septum that is divided in anterior septum and inferior septum. Continuing counterclockwise the remaining walls are labelled as inferior, inferolateral, anterolateral, and anterior. There could be some confusion with the nomenclature due to the fact that the inferolateral wall has also previously been called *posterior* and the anterolateral simply *lateral*. Each wall is sectioned in basal segments, defined by the MV and papillary chords, and mid-ventricular segments defined by papillary muscles. So, at basal and mid-ventricular levels six segments are defined. In the most apical third of the ventricle, the segmentation system changes slightly and there are only four segments (anterior, septal, inferior, and lateral).[60] In 2002, the American Heart Association described a 17-segment model in an attempt to establish segmentation standards applicable to all types of imaging (➲ Fig. 8.11). The main difference from the previous 16-segment model is the addition of the *apical cap* as segment

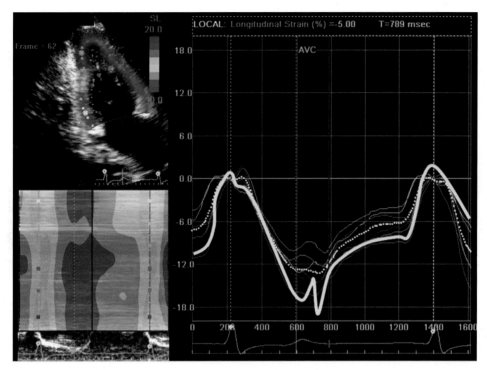

Figure 8.9 Speckle tracking in hypertrophic cardiomyopathy. Left ventricle longitudinal strain assessed with 2D speckle tracking in a patient with hypertrophic cardiomyopathy. In the highlighted yellow curve, post-systolic deformation is illustrated.

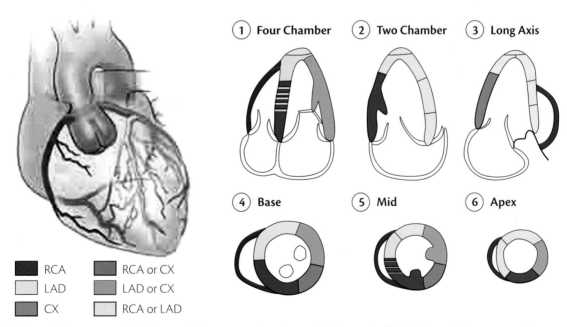

Figure 8.10 Left ventricular segmentation. Left ventricular segments from three apical views and mid-PLAX view with the corresponding coronary artery distribution. Cx, circumflex artery; LAD, left anterior descending artery; RCA, right coronary artery. Reproduced from Roberto M. Lang, Michelle Bierig, Richard B. Devereux *et al.* (2006) Recommendations for chamber quantification. *Eur J Echocardiography* **7**, 79 e108.

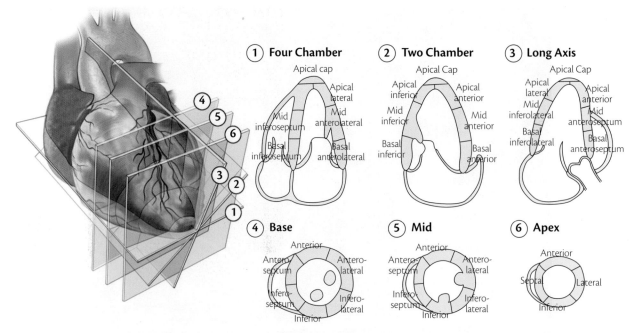

Figure 8.11 Seventeen-segment model. Segmental analysis of LV walls based on schematic views following the 17 segment model. Reproduced with permission from Roberto M. Lang, Michelle Bierig, Richard B. Devereux et al (2006) Recommendations for chamber quantification *Eur J Echocardiography* 7, 79e108.

number 17, defined as the myocardium beyond the end of LV cavity.[61] Either 16- or 17-segment systems are used for echocardiographic studies, although the 17-segment model should be predominantly used for studies comparing between myocardial perfusion imaging modalities and the 16-segment model is still appropriate for studies assessing WMAs, because the seventeenth segment (tip of the apex) does not move.[20]

It is recommended that each segment is analysed individually (and, even better, twice using overlapping information from different planes) and scored on the basis of its systolic motion and thickening. The segments are scored as:

1 = normal motion.

2 = hypokinesis.

3 = akinesis (no thickening).

4 = dyskinesis (paradoxical outwards systolic motion).

5 = aneurismal (diastolic and systolic deformation).

The wall motion score index (WMSI) is derived from the sum of all scores divided by the number of segments visualized. The total score obtained is related to the necrosis or ischaemia extension and allows a semiquantitative assessment of LV systolic function. This score has presented a better reproducibility then EF in global function evaluation even though it is not so frequently used.[62] Moreover, WMSI has been shown to be an important prognostic indicator in patients with coronary artery disease. An inherent limitation is the interobserver and intraobserver variability, although interpretation by experienced readers is reproducible.[15]

Results of the regional LV evaluation can be reported in a bull's-eye graph similar to nuclear imaging (➲ Fig. 8.12), where each myocardial segment is represented as a part of a whole circle. In this circle the septum is represented to the left, the anterior wall in the upper part, the lateral wall to the right, and the inferior wall in the lower part. Basal segments are represented in the outer part of the circle and the apex in the centre. The scoring in such a representation can be represented as a number or with a colour-coded system and makes it easier to understand where the abnormal segments are.

In the presence of important lesions, causing a significant decrease in myocardial perfusion, changes in the function of the affected segment occur. These changes might be temporary and disappear once coronary flow returns to normal, or persist if myocardial necrosis takes place. The regional assessment of LV systolic function is assessed with the analysis of endocardial excursion toward the centre of the ventricle and systolic thickening of each segment in multiple views. Usually the proximal inferoposterior and lateral walls contract rather later than the septum and inferior wall causing some expected segmental heterogeneity. Additionally, a greater absolute and percentage change of endocardial excursion and myocardial thickening from diastole to systole at the base when compared with the apex is typically found.

Using 3D echocardiography, along with the LVEF, a mathematical model showing the regional function of the 16 or 17 segments can be assessed (➲ Fig. 8.13). This LV volume model comes with a graph (➲ Fig. 8.14) showing each segment volume variation according to time throughout the cycle.

Left Ventricular Segmentation

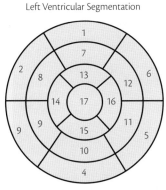

1. basal anterior	7. mid anterior	13. apical anterior
2. basal anteroseptal	8. mid anteroseptal	14. apical septal
3. basal inferoseptal	9. mid inferoseptal	15. apical inferior
4. basal inferior	10. mid inferior	16. apical lateral
5. basal inferolateral	11. mid inferolateral	17. apex
6. basal anterolateral	12. mid anterolateral	

A

Coronary Artery Territories

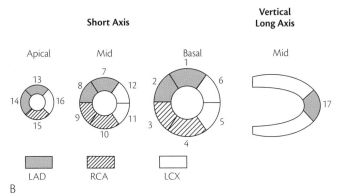

B

Figure 8.12 Bull's-eye graph in regional left ventricle evaluation.
A) Representation of each left ventricle segment in the bull's-eye graph.
B) Corresponding coronary artery territories. Modified from Steven C. Port
(1999) Imaging guidelines for nuclear cardiology procedures, Part 2. J Nucl
Cardiol. 6: G47–G84, with permission from Elsevier.

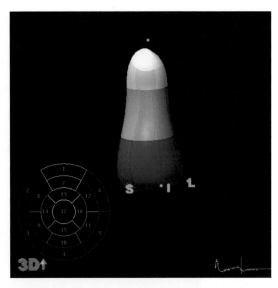

Figure 8.13 3D left ventricular systolic volume. Left ventricular systolic
volume with the 17-segment segmentation identified by different colours,
assessed with 3D echocardiography.

Assumptions regarding regional function and asynchrony can be made, since in the presence of a dyssynchronous ventricle there is dispersion in the timing of the point of minimum volume for each of the 16 or 17 segments. The degree of dispersion can be calculated through the measurement of the time standard deviation to achieve minimum volume and then correcting that for the R–R interval. This permitted the development of a systolic dyssynchrony index that can be used to quantify the degree of LV dyssynchrony resulting from the comparison of all segments.[64] This index has shown a good sensitivity and specificity in predicting short- and long-term response to CRT (see also ➔ Chapter 6); however, the most accurate cut-off in the systolic dyssynchrony index, in order to improve patient selection for CRT, is still a matter of debate.[65]

Several conditions distinct from coronary artery disease may result in WMAs. Occasionally, atypical WMAs such as tardokinesis (delayed systolic contraction) or early relaxation can be found. This occurrence might be difficult to appreciate in real-time 2D echocardiography, but TD or strain quantification tools may help in its evaluation. Those findings are generally considered a normal variant, most noted during stress echocardiography at high heart rates. The most frequent non-ischaemic WMAs are as a consequence of *conduction system abnormalities* such as RV paced rhythm, premature ventricular contractions, or left bundle branch block. Usually left bundle activation precedes right bundle in 10–20ms; however, in the presence of left bundle branch, the initial septal activation sequence is reversed and the RV and right side of the ventricular septum are firstly activated, resulting in the characteristic WMA with initial downward motion of the ventricular septum, followed by paradoxical septal motion and then consequent full thickening of the ventricular septum. The differential diagnosis of WMAs caused by conduction system abnormalities or ischaemia might be challenging. Probably the most valuable sign is the myocardial thickening, which is observed after the early ventricular contraction in patients with bundle branch block.[66] Another common form of non-ischaemic wall WMA is abnormal septal motion, observed after any form of cardiac surgery with pericardium opening. It results from the amplified anterior motion of the heart within the thorax due to loss of pericardial constraint and the concrete aetiology of the WMA is still a matter of debate. When it occurs, septal thickening is preserved although its motion is abnormal. Finally, conditions involving pericardial constriction, or abnormal ventricular interaction caused by RV volume or pressure overload may be the origin of WMA of the IVS. It is a consequence of exaggerated ventricular differential filling, often with respiratory variation, mainly as a consequence of volume overload or pericardial constriction.[67] Using PSAX view, the degree of septal flattening during systole and diastole is useful to differentiate volume

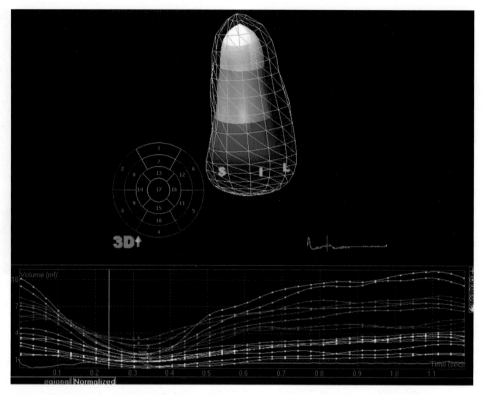

Figure 8.14 Volume variation curves. Left ventricular segments volume variation curves presented in the graph, according to time, throughout the cardiac cycle, assessed with 3D echocardiography.

from pressure overload. The *eccentricity index* allows qualitative assessment, with the calculation of the ratio of two orthogonal minor axes at the level of LV chordae, measured from the PSAX view. A normal expected LV shape would have a ratio of 1.0, whereas cases of septal flattening result in an eccentricity index greater than 1.0.[67]

Global right ventricular systolic function

RV presents a complex shape (➲ Fig. 8.15); consequently, the assessment of its morphology and function requires integration of multiple echocardiographic views and it is difficult to model geometrically, especially in pathological conditions.[20] Even though echocardiography is the most common form of evaluation of RV structure and function, its complex geometry, irregular endocardial surface, and the retrosternal position, make CMR the most accurate method for assessing RV volume and function.[68]

RV mass is approximately one-sixth that of the LV, which is a consequence of a low-impedance, highly distensible pulmonary vascular system with significantly lower pressures comparable to left-sided pressures. Similar to LV, RV systolic function

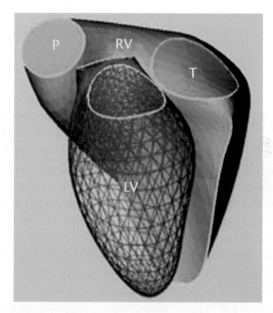

Figure 8.15 Three dimensional reconstructions of the right ventricle illustrating its complex shape in a normal subject. Reproduced from Sheehan F, Redington A. The right ventricle: anatomy, physiology and clinical imaging. *Heart* 2008; 94(11):1510–5 with permission from BMJ Publishing Group Ltd.

is a reflection of contractility, preload, afterload, rhythm, AV synchrony, and ventricular interdependence. However, its contraction is more complex. It presents a sequential pattern, starting with the contraction of the inlet and trabeculated myocardium and ending with the contraction of the infundibulum (approximately 25–50ms apart), having the latter a longer duration of contraction.

In contrast to the LV contraction mechanism, twisting and rotational movements do not contribute significantly to RV contraction, whose shortening is greater longitudinally than radially. Moreover, because of the higher surface-to-volume ratio of the RV, a smaller inward motion is required to eject the same stroke volume. RV function evaluation remains mostly qualitative in clinical practice; however, several studies have recently emphasized the importance of RV function in the prognosis of a variety of cardiopulmonary diseases, as a result a routine quantification of RV function is needed.[69,70] Evaluation of size and function of right heart chambers is extensively described in ➲ Chapter 11.

One of the most common used methods is the measurement of the tricuspid annulus systolic excursion (TAPSE) (➲ Fig. 8.16): its systolic excursion presents a moderate correlation with RV ejection fraction measured by radionuclide.[71] TD imaging measurements of myocardial velocities at lateral level within tricuspid annulus, also allows quantitative assessment of RV systolic function (➲ Fig. 8.17). Longitudinal TD-derived RV strain and strain rate were found significantly higher in the RV compared with the LV, and with maximal values in the mid-RV free wall. However, strain and strain rate analysis are still a matter of investigation in RV systolic function evaluation. The previously described methods are summarized in ➲ Table 8.3.

It is also possible to study the regional function of the RV. The main segments are anterior, lateral, inferior, and RV outflow tract (RVOT) walls. Again, the combination of views gives the most accurate evaluation (➲ Fig. 8.18).

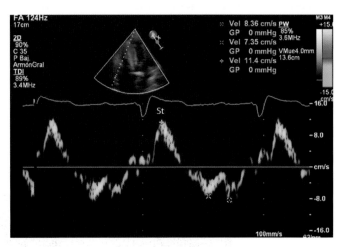

Figure 8.17 Tissue doppler imaging myocardial velocities. Measurement of myocardial velocities at lateral level within the tricuspid annulus using tissue Doppler imaging. St, velocity of the systolic tissue Doppler signal in the tricuspid annulus.

The introduction of 3D echocardiography in clinical practice, with the ability of volumes calculations without geometric assumptions was immediately regarded as having the potential to overcome the geometric limitations of 2D techniques (➲ Fig. 8.19). However, new dedicated RV quantification software has only recently been developed and validated in contrast CMR and radionuclide ventriculography as gold standards.[72] Despite optimal correlation, it was observed, that like LV volumes, RV volumes calculated by 3D echocardiography were slightly underestimated, when compared with CMR RV volumes calculation. The accuracy of this method has been analysed in patients with different pathologies,[73] and normal reference range values for RV volumes and function have been already published (➲ Table 8.4).[74] However, there are some concerns about reproducibility and this dedicated software is not yet widespread.[75]

Conclusion

The estimation of LV systolic function is one of the most frequent practices in echocardiography, but its accurate report is fundamental for the assurance of correct therapeutic strategies. In general, it is assessed with computation of EF using M-mode, 2D, or 3D echocardiography. However, its result is load-dependent and all methods of assumption have inherent limitations, which must be known and taken into consideration while performing the evaluation. Supplementary quantitative methods for analysis of myocardial function, such as TD and strain, are gaining a place, and in spite of the technical limitations, at this time they present an effective contribution for the determination of systolic function of either the left or right ventricle.

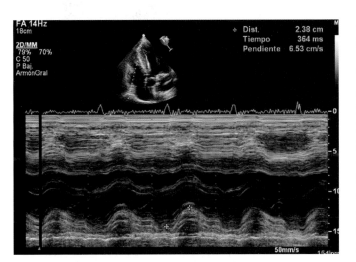

Figure 8.16 Tricuspid annulus systolic excursion (TAPSE), measurement using M-mode echocardiography.

Table 8.3 Indices of RV contractility

Functional parameters	Normal value	Load dependence*	Clinical utility
RVEF, %	61 ± 7% (47%–76%)	+++	Clinical validation, wide acceptance
RVFAC, %	>32%	+++	Good correlation with RVEF
TAPSE, mm	>15	+++	Simple measure not limited by endocardial border recognition. Good correlation with RVEF
Sm annular, cm/s	>12	+++	Good sensitivity and specificity for RVEF <50%
Strain	Basal: 19 ± 6 Mid: 27 ± 6 Apical: 32 ± 6	+++	Correlates with stroke volume
Strain rate, s⁻¹	Basal: 1.50 ± 0.41 Mid: 1.72 ± 0.27 Apical: 2.04 ± 0.41	++	Correlates with contractility
RVMPI	0.28 ± 0.04	++	Global non-geometric index of systolic and diastolic function, prognostic value PH, CHD

CHD, congenital heart disease; PH, pulmonary hypertension; RVEF, right ventricle ejection fraction; RVFAC, right ventricle fractional area change; RVMPI, right ventricle myocardial performance index; Sm, tissue Doppler maximal systolic velocity at the tricuspid annulus; TAPSE, tricuspid annular plane systolic excursion.

Adapted from Haddad F, Hunt SA, Rosenthal DN, Murphy DJ. Right ventricular function in cardiovascular disease, part I: Anatomy, physiology, aging, and functional assessment of the right ventricle. *Circulation* 2008; **117**(11):1436–48.

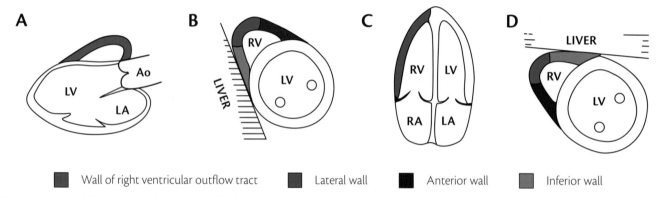

Wall of right ventricular outflow tract   Lateral wall   Anterior wall   Inferior wall

Figure 8.18 Regional analysis of right ventricle walls. A) Parasternal long-axis view. B) Apical four-chamber view. C) Parasternal short-axis view. D) Subcostal short-axis view. Ao, aorta; LA, left atrium; LV, left ventricle; RA, right atrium. RV, right ventricle.

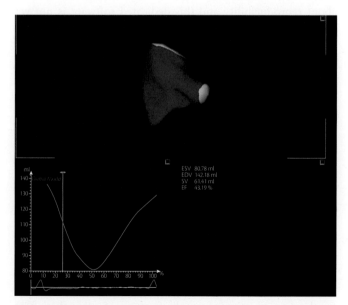

Figure 8.19 Calculation of right ventricle systolic function, using 3D echocardiography dedicated software. (Clinical validation in progress.)

Table 8.4 Reference ranges for 3D echocardiographic RV ejection fractions by age decile

Age decile (years)	Men	Women	All
<30	62 ± 6	69 ± 9	66 ± 8
30–39	64 ± 8	69 ± 7	66 ± 8
40–49	64 ± 8	71 ± 7	66 ± 8
50–59	65 ± 6	67 ± 8	66 ± 7
60–69	68 ± 9	67 ± 10	67 ± 9
>70	65 ± 6	71 ± 7	68 ± 7
All	64 ± 8	69 ± 8	67 ± 8

Adapted from Tamborini G, Marsan NA, Gripari P, *et al.* Reference values for right ventricular volumes and ejection fraction with real-time three-dimensional echocardiography: evaluation in a large series of normal subjects. *J Am Soc Echocardiogr* 2010; **23**(2):109–15.

Personal perspective

During the last two decades an impressive evolution in echocardiography occurred. Since the first methodology of quantification with M-mode, simpler and more accurate measurements of LV systolic function, using 2D or more recently 3D echocardiography with automated edge-detection algorithms have been developed.

Interestingly, more than two decades ago, Feigenbaum predicted the future of echocardiography with the development of new clinical techniques, the ability to identify tissue types, 3D echocardiography, and new techniques for quantitating echocardiographic data.[76] These predictions have become reality. However, the most common approach of LV systolic function evaluation at present time is still the measurement of EF by 2D echocardiography. Despite its reproducibility and reliability, even if performed with 3D echocardiography,

EF is affected by preload and afterload. New methods of myocardium contractile quantification as TD and strain imaging have been developed, but no independent index of basal contractile state has been described so far. Upcoming advances in understanding the molecular cardiac physiology may help echocardiography to find even better indexes. Continuous advances in feasibility and accuracy on the interpretation of LV systolic function are expected, taking into consideration the vast clinical and economical impact of the therapeutic decisions based on this data. On the other hand, the increase in computing power has allowed the miniaturization of devices. In the near future there are prospects for a new model of cardiology, which incorporates an ultrasound stethoscope in daily practice. However, we should keep in mind that technology will always have its limitations and the operator view must remain critical without overlooking potential pitfalls.

References

1 Vahanian A, Baumgartner H, Bax J, Butchart E, Dion R, Filippatos G, et al. Guidelines on the management of valvular heart disease: the Task Force on the Management of Valvular Heart Disease of the European Society of Cardiology. Eur Heart J 2007; 28:230–68.

2 Task Force for Diagnosis and Treatment of Acute and Chronic Heart Failure (2008) of European Society of Cardiology, Dickstein K, Cohen-Solal A, Filippatos G, McMurray JJ, Ponikowski P, et al. ESC Guidelines for the diagnosis and treatment of acute and chronic heart failure (2008): the Task Force for the Diagnosis and Treatment of Acute and Chronic Heart Failure (2008) of the European Society of Cardiology. Developed in collaboration with the Heart Failure Association of the ESC (HFA) and endorsed by the European Society of Intensive Care Medicine (ESICM). Eur Heart J 2008; 29(19):2388–442.

3 Sheehan F. Ventricular shape and function. In: Otto C (ed) Practice of Clinical Echocardiography, 3rd edn, Philadelphia, PA: Saunders Elsevier; 2007, p.212–36.

4 Streeter DD, Jr: Gross morphology and fiber geometry of the heart. In: Berne RM, Sperelakis N, Geiser S (eds) Handbook of Physiology. Baltimore, MD: Williams & Wilkins 1979, pp. 61–112.

5 Beyar R, Yin F, Hausknecht, Weisfeldt M, Kass D. Dependence of left ventricular twist –radial shortening relations on cardiac cycle phase. Am J Physiol 1989; 257: H1119–H1126.

6 Gaasch WH, Battle WE, Oboler AA, Banas JS Jr, Levine HJ. Left ventricular stress and compliance in man. With special reference to normalized ventricular function curves. Circulation 1972; 45(4):746–62.

7 Badeer, HS. Contractile tension in the myocardium. Am Heart J 1963; 66:432.

8 Goldfine H, Aurigemma GP, Zile MR, Gaasch WH. Left ventricular length-force-shortening relations before and after surgical correction of chronic mitral regurgitation. J Am Coll Cardiol 1998; 31(1):180–5.

9 Cohn JN. Vasodilator therapy for heart failure. The influence of impedance on left ventricular performance. Circulation 1973; 48(1):5–8.

10 Oh JK, Seward JB, Tajik J. Assessment of Systolic Function and Quantification of Cardiac Chambers. In: Oh JK, Steward JB, Tajik AJ (eds) The Echo Manual, 3rd ed. Philadelphia, PA: Lippincott Williams & Wilkins 2006; p.109–20.

11 Ilercil A, O'Grady MJ, Roman MJ, Paranicas M, Lee ET, Welty TK, et al. Reference values for echocardiographic measurements in urban and rural populations of differing ethnicity: the strong heart study. J Am Soc Echocardiogr 2001; 14:601–11.

12 Nidorf SM, Picard MH, Triulzi MO, Thomas JD, Newell J, King ME, et al. New perspectives in the assessment of cardiac chamber dimensions during development and adulthood. J Am Coll Cardiol 1992; 19:983–8.

13 Pearlman JD, Triulzi MO, King ME, Newell J, Weyman AE. Limits of normal left ventricular dimensions in growth and development: analysis of dimensions and variance in the two-dimensional echocardiograms of 268 normal healthy subjects. J Am Coll Cardiol 1988; 12:1432–41.

14 Devereux RB, de Simone G, Pickering TG, Schwartz JE, Roman MJ. Relation of left ventricular midwall function to cardiovascular risk factors and arterial structure and function. Hypertension 1998; 31:929–36.

15 Marcos-Alberca P, Zamorano JL, Garcia Fernandez MA. Valoración de la función cardíaca. In: Zamorano JL, Garcia Fernandez MA (Eds) Procedimientos en ecocardiografia. McGrawHill; 2004, pp.57–74.

16 Feigenbaum H, Armstrong WF, Ryan T. Evaluation of systolic and diastolic function of the left ventricle. In: Feigenbaum's Echocardiography, 6th ed. Philadelphia, PA: Lippincott Williams & Wilkins; 2005, pp.138–69.

17 Ahmadpour H, Shah AA, Allen JW, Edmiston WA, Kim SJ, Haywood LJ. Mitral E point septal separation: a reliable index of left ventricular performance in coronary artery disease. Am Heart J 1983; 106:21–8.

18 Pai RG, Bodenheimer MM, Pai SM, Koss JH, Adamick RD. Usefulness of systolic excursion of the mitral anulus as an index of left ventricular systolic function. *Am J Cardiol* 1991; **67**(2):222–4.

19 Stamm RB, Carabello BA, Mayers DL, Martin RP. Two-dimensional echocardiographic measurement of left ventricular ejection fraction: prospective analysis of what constitutes an adequate determination. *Am Heart J* 1982; **104**:136–44.

20 Lang RM, Bierig M, Devereux RB, Flachskampf FA, Foster E, Pellikka PA, *et al.*; Chamber Quantification Writing Group; American Society of Echocardiography's Guidelines and Standards Committee; European Association of Echocardiography. Recommendations for chamber quantification: a report from the American Society of Echocardiography's Guidelines and Standards Committee and the Chamber Quantification Writing Group, developed in conjunction with the European Association of Echocardiography, a branch of the European Society of Cardiology. *J Am Soc Echocardiogr* 2005; **18**(12):1440–63.

21 Folland ED, Parisi AF, Moynihan PF, Jones DR, Feldman CL, Tow DE. Assessment of left ventricular ejection fraction and volumes by real-time, two-dimensional echocardiography. A comparison of cineangiographic and radionuclide techniques. *Circulation* 1979; **60**(4):760–6.

22 de Simone G, Devereux RB, Roman MJ, Ganau A, Saba PS, Alderman MH, *et al.* Assessment of left ventricular function by the midwall fractional shortening/end-systolic stress relation in human hypertension. *J Am Coll Cardiol* 1994; **23**:1444–51.

23 Shimizu G, Zile MR, Blaustein AS, Gaasch WH. Left ventricular chamber filling and midwall fiber lengthening in patients with left ventricular hypertrophy: overestimation of fiber velocities by conventional midwall measurements. *Circulation* 1985; **71**: 266–72.

24 Folland ED, Parisi AF, Moynihan PF, Jones DR, Feldman CL, Tow DE. Assessment of left ventricular ejection fraction and volumes by real-time, two-dimensional echocardiography. A comparison of cineangiographic and radionuclide techniques. *Circulation* 1979; **60**(4):760–6.

25 Perez JE, Waggoner AD, Barzilai B, Melton HE, Miller JG, Sobel BE. On-line assessment of ventricular function by automatic boundary detection and ultrasonic backscatter imaging. *J Am Coll Cardiol* 1992; **19**:313–20.

26 Spencer KT, Bednarz J, Mor-Avi V, DeCara J, Lang RM. Automated endocardial border detection and evaluation of left ventricular function from contrast-enhanced images using modified acoustic quantification. *J Am Soc Echocardiogr* 2002; **15**(8):777–81.

27 Nahar T, Croft L, Shapiro R, Fruchtman S, Diamond J, Henzlova M, *et al.* Comparison of four echocardiographic techniques for measuring left ventricular ejection fraction. *Am J Cardiol* 2000; **86**:1358–62.

28 Celentano A, Palmieri V, Arezzi E, Mureddu GF, Sabatella M, Di MG, *et al.* Gender differences in left ventricular chamber and midwall systolic function in normotensive and hypertensive adults. *J Hypertens* 2003; **21**:1415–23.

29 Gerdts E, Zabalgoitia M, Bjornstad H, Svendsen TL, Devereux RB. Gender differences in systolic left ventricular function in hypertensive patients with electrocardiographic left ventricular hypertrophy (the LIFE study). *Am J Cardiol* 2001; **87**:980–3.

30 Naik MM, Diamond GA, Pai T; Soffer A, Siegel RJ. Correspondence of left ventricular ejection fraction determinations from two-dimensional echocardiography, radionuclide angiography and contrast cineangiography. *J Am Coll Cardiol* 1995; **25**(4):937–42.

31 Starling, MR, Crawford, MH, Sorenson, SG, *et al.* Comparative accuracy of apical biplane cross-sectional echocardiography and gated equilibrium radionuclide angiography for estimating left ventricular size and performance. *Circulation* 1981; **63**:1075.

32 Bellenger NG, Burgess MI, Ray SG, Lahiri A, Coats AJ, Cleland JG, *et al.* Comparison of left ventricular ejection fraction and volumes in heart failure by echocardiography, radionuclide ventriculography and cardiovascular magnetic resonance; are they interchangeable? *Eur Heart J* 2000; **21**(16):1387–96.

33 Jenkins C, Bricknell K, Hanekom L, Marwick TH. Reproducibility and accuracy of echocardiographic measurements of left ventricular parameters using real-time three-dimensional echocardiography. *J Am Coll Cardiol* 2004; **44**:878–86.

34 Nikitin NP, Constantin C, Loh PH, Ghosh J, Lukaschuk EI, Bennett A, *et al.* generation 3-dimensional echocardiography for left ventricular volumetric and functional measurements: comparison with cardiac magnetic resonance. *Eur J Echocardiogr* 2006; **7**:365–372.

35 Mor-Avi V, Sugeng L, Lang RM. Real-time 3-dimensional echocardiography: an integral component of the routine echocardiographic examination in adult patients? *Circulation* 2009; **119**(2):314–29.

36 Jenkins C, Bricknell K, Chan J, Hanekom L, Marwick TH. Comparison of two- and three-dimensional echocardiography with sequential magnetic resonance imaging for evaluating left ventricular volume and ejection fraction over time in patients with healed myocardial infarction. *Am J Cardiol* 2007; **99**:300–6.

37 Pouleur AC, le Polain de Waroux JB, Pasquet A, Gerber BL, Gerard O, *et al.* Assessment of left ventricular mass and volumes by three-dimensional echocardiography in patients with or without wall motion abnormalities: comparison against cine magnetic resonance imaging. *Heart* 2008; **94**:1050 –7.

38 Jacobs LD, Salgo IS, Goonewardena S, Weinert L, Coon P, Bardo D, *et al.* Rapid online quantification of left ventricular volume from real-time three-dimensional echocardiographic data. *Eur Heart J* 2006; **27**:460–8.

39 Soliman OI, Krenning BJ, Geleijnse ML, Nemes A, Bosch JG, van Geuns RJ, *et al.* Quantification of left ventricular volumes and function in patients with cardiomyopathies by real-time three-dimensional echocardiography: a head-to-head comparison between two different semiautomated endocardial border detection algorithms. *J Am Soc Echocardiogr* 2007; **20**:1042–1049.

40 Tighe DA, Rosetti M, Vinch CS, Chandok D, Muldoon D, Wiggin B, *et al.* Influence of image quality on the accuracy of real time three-dimensional echocardiography to measure left ventricular volumes in unselected patients: a comparison with gated-SPECT imaging. *Echocardiography* 2007; **24**:1073–80.

41 Tei C, Nishimura RA, Seward JB, Tajik AJ. Noninvasive Doppler-derived myocardial performance index: correlation with simultaneous measurements of cardiac catheterization measurements. *J Am Soc Echocardiogr* 1997; **10**(2):169–78.

42 Bargiggia GS, Bertucci C, Recusani F, Raisaro A, de Servi S, Valdes-Cruz LM, *et al.* A new method for estimating left ventricular dP/dt by continuous wave Doppler-echocardiography. Validation studies at cardiac catheterization. *Circulation* 1989; **80**:1287–923.

43 Khaw AV, von Bardeleben RS, Strasser C, Mohr-Kahaly S, Blankenberg S, Espinola-Klein C, *et al.* Direct measurement of left ventricular outflow tract by transthoracic real-time 3D-echocardiography increases accuracy in assessment of aortic valve stenosis. *Int J Cardiol* 2009; **136**(1):64–71.

44 Drighil A, Madias JE, Mathewson JW, El Mosalami H, El Badaoui N, Ramdani B, et al. Haemodialysis: effects of acute decrease in preload on tissue Doppler imaging indices of systolic and diastolic function of the left and right ventricles. Eur J Echocardiogr 2008; 9(4):530–5.

45 Bauer F, Jones M, Shiota T, Firstenberg MS, Qin JX, Tsujino H, et al. Left ventricular outflow tract mean systolic acceleration as a surrogate for the slope of the left ventricular end-systolic pressure-volume relationship. J Am Coll Cardiol 2002; 40(7):1320–7.

46 Greenberg NL, Firstenberg MS, Castro PL, Main M, Travaglini A, Odabashian JA, et al. Doppler-derived myocardial systolic strain rate is a strong index of left ventricular contractility. Circulation 2002; 105(1):99–105.

47 Gulati VK, Katz WE, Follansbee WP, Gorcsan J 3rd. Mitral annular descent velocity by tissue Doppler echocardiography as an index of global left ventricular function. Am J Cardiol 1996; 77(11): 979–84.

48 Alam M, Witt N, Nordlander R, Samad BA. Detection of abnormal left ventricular function by Doppler tissue imaging in patients with a first myocardial infarction and showing normal function assessed by conventional echocardiography. Eur J Echocardiogr 2007; 8(1):37–41.

49 Sanderson JE. Heart failure with a normal ejection fraction. Heart 2007; 93(2):155–8.

50 Nagueh SF, Bachinski LL, Meyer D, Hill R, Zoghbi WA, Tam JW, et al. Tissue Doppler imaging consistently detects myocardial abnormalities in patients with hypertrophic cardiomyopathy and provides a novel means for an early diagnosis before and independently of hypertrophy. Circulation 2001; 104(2):128–30.

51 Marwick TH. Measurement of strain and strain rate by echocardiography: ready for prime time? J Am Coll Cardiol 2006; 47(7):1313–27.

52 Blessberger H, Binder T. Non-invasive imaging: Two dimensional speckle tracking echocardiography: basic principles. Heart 2010; 96(9):716–22.

53 Pérez de Isla L, Balcones DV, Fernández-Golfín C, Marcos-Alberca P, Almería C, Rodrigo JL, et al. Three-dimensional-wall motion tracking: a new and faster tool for myocardial strain assessment: comparison with two-dimensional-wall motion tracking. J Am Soc Echocardiogr 2009; 22(4):325–30.

54 Guccione JM, Le Prell GS, de Tombe PP, Hunter WC. Measurements of active myocardial tension under a wide range of physiological loading conditions. J Biomech 1997; 30:189–92.

55 Claus P, Weidemann F, Dommke C, Bito V, Heinzel FR, D'hooge J, et al. Mechanisms of postsystolic thickening in ischemic myocardium: mathematical modelling and comparison with experimental ischemic substrates. Ultrasound Med Biol 2007; 33:1963–70.

56 Edvardsen T, Helle-Valle T, Smiseth OA. Systolic dysfunction in heart failure with normal ejection fraction: speckle-tracking echocardiography. Prog Cardiovasc Dis 2006; 49:207e14.

57 Bijnens B, Claus P, Weidemann F, Strotmann J, Sutherland GR. Investigating cardiac function using motion and deformation analysis in the setting of coronary artery disease. Circulation 2007; 116:2453–64.

58 Bijnens BH, Cikes M, Claus P, et al. Velocity and deformation imaging for the assessment of myocardial dysfunction. Eur J Echocardiogr 2009; 10:216e26.

59 Inden Y, Ito R, Yoshida N, Kamiya H, Kitamura K, Kitamura T, et al. Combined assessment of left ventricular dyssynchrony and contractility by speckled tracking strain imaging: a novel index for predicting responders to cardiac resynchronization therapy. Heart Rhythm 2010; 7(5):655–61.

60 Schiller NB, Shah PM, Crawford M, DeMaria A, Devereux R, Feigenbaum H, et al. Recommendations for quantitation of the left ventricle by two-dimensional echocardiography: American Society of Echocardiography committee on standards, subcommittee on quantitation of two-dimensional echocardiograms. J Am Soc Echocardiogr 1989; 2:358–67.

61 Cerqueira MD, Weissman NJ, Dilsizian V, Jacobs AK, Kaul S, Laskey WK, et al. Standardized myocardial segmentation and nomenclature for tomographic imaging of the heart: a statement for healthcare professionals from the cardiac imaging committee of the council on clinical cardiology of the American Heart Association. Circulation 2002; 105:539–42.

62 Kan G, Visser CA, Koolen JJ, Dunning AJ. Short and long term predictive value of admission wall motion score in acute myocardial infarction. A cross sectional echocardiographic study of 345 patients. Br Heart J 1986; 56:422–7.

63 Monaghan M. Role of real time 3D echocardiography in evaluating the left ventricle. Heart 2006; 92:131–6.

64 Kapetanakis S, Siva A, Corrigan N, Cooklin M, Kearney MT, Monaghan MJ. Real-time three-dimensional echocardiography. A novel technique to quantify global left ventricular mechanical dyssynchrony. Circulation 2005; 112:992–1000.

65 Soliman OI, Geleijnse ML, Theuns DA, van Dalen BM, Vletter WB, Jordaens LJ, et al. Usefulness of left ventricular systolic dyssynchrony by real-time three-dimensional echocardiography to predict long-term response to cardiac resynchronization therapy. Am J Cardiol 2009; 103(11):1586–91.

66 Geleijnse ML, Vigna C, Kasprzak JD, Rambaldi R, Salvatori MP, Elhendy A, et al. Usefulness and limitations of dobutamine-atropine stress echocardiography for the diagnosis of coronary artery disease in patients with left bundle branch block. A multicentre study. Eur Heart J 2000; 21(20):1666–73.

67 Kingma I, Tyberg JV, Smith ER. Effects of diastolic transseptal pressure gradient on ventricular septal position and motion. Circulation 1983; 68(6):1304–14.

68 Lorenz CH, Walker ES, Morgan VL, Klein SS, Graham TP Jr. Normal human right and left ventricular mass, systolic function, and gender differences by cine magnetic resonance imaging. J Cardiovasc Magn Reson. 1999; 1:7–21.

69 Sun JP, James KB, Yang XS, Solankhi N, Shah MS, Arheart KL, et al. Comparison of mortality rates and progression of left ventricular dysfunction in patients with idiopathic dilated cardiomyopathy and dilated versus non dilated right ventricular cavities. Am J Cardiol 1997; 80:1583–7.

70 Spinarova L, Meluzin J, Toman J, Hude P, Krejci J, Vitovec J. Right ventricular dysfunction in chronic heart failure. Eur J Heart Fail 2005; 7:485–9.

71 Ueti OM, Camargo EE, Ueti AA, de Lima-Filho EC, Nogueira EA. Assessment of right ventricular function with Doppler echocardiographic indices derived from tricuspid annular motion: comparison with radionuclide angiography. Heart 2002; 88: 244–8.

72 Niemann PS, Pinho L, Balbach T, Galuschky C, Blankenhagen M, Silberbach M, et al. Anatomically oriented right ventricular volume measurements with dynamic 3-dimensional echocardiography validated by 3-Tesla magnetic resonance imaging. J Am Coll Cardiol 2007; 50:1668–76.

73 Accuracy and reproducibility of real-time 3-dimensional echocardiography for assessment of right ventricular volumes and ejection fraction in children. *J Am Soc Echocardiogr* 2008; 21: 84–9.

74 Tamborini G, Marsan NA, Gripari P, Maffessanti F, Brusoni D, Muratori M, *et al.* Reference values for right ventricular volumes and ejection fraction with real-time three-dimensional echocardiography: evaluation in a large series of normal subjects. *J Am Soc Echocardiogr* 2010; **23**(2):109–15.

75 Mor-Avi V, Sugeng L, Lindner JR. Imaging the forgotten chamber: is the devil in the boundary? *J Am Soc Echocardiogr* 2010; **23**(2):141–3.

76 Feigenbaum H. Future applications for the evaluation of ventricular function using echocardiography. *Am J Cardiol* 1982; **49**:1330–6.

Further reading

Blessberger H, Binder T. Non-invasive imaging: Two dimensional speckle tracking echocardiography: basic principles. *Heart* 2010; **96**(9):716–22.

Feigenbaum H, Armstrong WF, Ryan T. Evaluation of systolic and diastolic function of the left ventricle. In: *Feigenbaum's Echocardiography*, 6th ed. Philadelphia, PA: Lippincott Williams & Wilkins; 2005, pp.138–69.

Haddad F, Hunt SA, Rosenthal DN, Murphy DJ. Right ventricular function in cardiovascular disease, part I: Anatomy, physiology, aging, and functional assessment of the right ventricle. *Circulation* 2008; **117**(11):1436–48.

Kapetenakis S, Siva A, Corrigan N, Cooklin M, Kearney MT, Monaghan MJ. Real-time three-dimensional echocardiography.

A novel technique to quantify global left ventricular mechanical dyssynchrony. *Circulation* 2005; **112**:992–1000.

Lang RM, Bierig M, Devereux RB, Flachskampf FA, Foster E, Pellikka PA, *et al.*; Chamber Quantification Writing Group; American Society of Echocardiography's Guidelines and Standards Committee; European Association of Echocardiography. Recommendations for chamber quantification: a report from the American Society of Echocardiography's Guidelines and Standards Committee and the Chamber Quantification Writing Group, developed in conjunction with the European Association of Echocardiography, a branch of the European Society of Cardiology. *J Am Soc Echocardiogr* 2005; **18**(12):1440–63.

Marwick TH. Measurement of strain and strain rate by echocardiography: ready for prime time? *J Am Coll Cardiol* 2006; **47**(7):1313–27.

Monaghan M. Role of real time 3D echocardiography in evaluating the left ventricle. *Heart* 2006; **92**:131–6.

Mor-Avi V, Sugeng L, Lang RM. Real-time 3-dimensional echocardiography: an integral component of the routine echocardiographic examination in adult patients? *Circulation* 2009; **119**(2):314–29.

Oh JK, Seward JB, Tajik J. Assessment of Systolic Function and Quantification of Cardiac Chambers. In: Oh JK, Steward JB, Tajik AJ (eds) *The Echo Manual*, 3rd ed. Philadelphia, PA: Lippincott Williams & Wilkins 2006; p.109–20.

Tamborini G, Marsan NA, Gripari P, Maffessanti F, Brusoni D, Muratori M, *et al.* Reference values for right ventricular volumes and ejection fraction with real-time three-dimensional echocardiography: evaluation in a large series of normal subjects. *J Am Soc Echocardiogr* 2010; **23**(2):109–15.

↪ For additional multimedia materials please visit the online version of the book (⌘ http://escecho.oxfordmedicine.com).

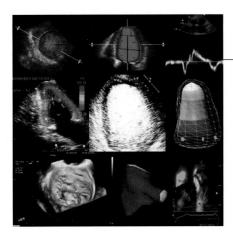

CHAPTER 9

Assessment of diastolic function

Maurizio Galderisi and Sergio Mondillo

Contents

Summary

Modern assessment of left ventricular (LV) diastolic function should be based on the estimation of degree of LV filling pressure (LVFP), which is the true determinant of symptoms/signs and prognosis in heart failure.

In order to achieve this goal, standard Doppler assessment of mitral inflow pattern (E/A ratio, deceleration time, isovolumic relaxation time) should be combined with additional manoeuvres and/or ultrasound tools such as:

◆ Valsalva manoeuvre applied to mitral inflow pattern.

◆ Pulmonary venous flow pattern.

◆ Velocity flow propagation by colour M-mode.

◆ Pulsed wave tissue Doppler of mitral annuls (average of septal and lateral E' velocity).

In intermediate doubtful situations, the two-dimensional determination of left atrial (LA) volume can be diagnostic, since LA enlargement is associated with a chronic increase of LVFP in the absence of mitral valve disease and atrial fibrillation.

Some new echocardiographic technologies, such as the speckle tracking-derived LV longitudinal strain and LV torsion, LA strain, and even the three-dimensional determination of LA volumes can be potentially useful to add further information. In particular, the reduction of LV longitudinal strain in patients with LV diastolic dysfunction and normal ejection fraction demonstrates that a subclinical impairment of LV systolic function already exists under these circumstances.

Introduction

The assessment of left ventricular (LV) diastolic function and of LV filling pressure (LVFP) is an important part of the standard Doppler echocardiographic examination, particularly in patients who refer for symptoms (mainly dyspnoea) and signs of heart failure (HF). It allows integration of the evaluation of LV systolic functional parameters in systolic HF and to differentiate this entity from HF with normal ejection fraction (EF), in which the alteration of LV diastolic properties represents the main determinant of either onset or progression of the disease.

However, although in clinical practice it may be convenient to distinguish LV dysfunction as either systolic or diastolic, it has to be taken into account that each component of the cardiac cycle is functionally dependent on the other. In this view, the assessment of LV diastolic function now appears more complex than it seemed in the past two decades and a comprehensive approach including quantitative analysis of multiple (also systolic) measurements should be encouraged.

Physiology of diastole

LV has two alternating functions: systolic contraction and diastolic filling. Although in normal hearts transition from contraction to relaxation begins much earlier than LV end-systole, i.e. at 16–20% of the ejection period and even prior to aortic valve (AoV) opening when LV contractility is severely impaired, the traditional definition of diastole (in ancient Greek language the term διαστολε means *expansion*), includes the part of the cardiac cycle starting at the AoV closure—when LV pressure falls below aortic pressure—and finishing at the mitral valve (MV) closure.

A normal LV diastolic function may be clinically defined as the capacity of the LV to receive a LV filling volume able in its turn to guarantee an adequate stroke volume, operating at a low pressure regimen. In merely descriptive terms, diastole can be divided into four phases:

1) *Isovolumetric relaxation*: this is the period occurring between the end of LV systolic ejection (AoV closure) and the opening of the MV, when LV pressure continues its rapid fall while LV volume remains constant. This period is mainly attributed to the active LV relaxation, with a lower, variable contribution of elastic recoil of the contracted fibres. Relaxation shares with contraction the same molecular processes of transient activation of the myocyte and is subjected to the control of load, inactivation, and asynchrony.

2) *LV rapid filling*: this begins when LV pressure falls below left atrial (LA) pressure and the MV opens. During this period the blood has an acceleration which achieves a maximal velocity, directly related to the magnitude of atrioventricular pressure, and stops when this gradient ends. This period represents a complex interaction between LV suction (*active relaxation*) and viscoelastic properties of the myocardium (*compliance*).

3) *Diastasis*: this occurs when LA and LV pressures are almost equal and LV filling is essentially maintained by the flow coming from pulmonary veins—with LA representing a passive conduit—with an amount depending of LV pressure, function of LV *compliance*.

4) *Atrial systole*: this corresponds to LA contraction and ends at the MV closure. This period is mainly influenced by LV compliance, but depends also on the pericardial resistance, the atrial force, and the atrioventricular synchrony (*electrocardiogram-derived PR interval*).

Globally, LV filling is determined by the interaction between LVFP and filling properties, which are, in their turn, regulated by extrinsic determinants—mainly pericardial restraint and ventricular interaction—and by intrinsic factors such as chamber stiffness (cardiomyocytes and extracellular matrix), myocardial tone, chamber geometry, and LV wall thickness.

Increased LVFP is the main pathophysiological consequence of diastolic dysfunction. It is mainly determined by filling and passive properties of LV walls but may be additionally controlled by incomplete LV relaxation and alterations of myocardial diastolic tone.

Main morphological and functional correlates of diastolic dysfunction include LV concentric geometry (hypertrophy and remodelling), LA enlargement and function, and pulmonary arterial (PA) hypertension.

Invasive and non-invasive approach to left ventricular diastolic function

Cardiac catheterization allows assessment of the pressure–volume relationship along the overall cardiac cycle (➲ Fig. 9.1).

LVFP are considered abnormally elevated when the mean pulmonary capillary wedge pressure (PCWP) is higher than 12mmHg or when LV end-diastolic pressure (LVEDP) is higher than 16mmHg.

Other main haemodynamic measurements of LV diastolic function include:

◆ τ(*Tau*), which is time constant of the isovolumic-pressure decline and represents a reliable measure of the rate of LV relaxation (normal values <48ms).

◆ The $\Delta P/\Delta V$ ratio, an expression of LV end-diastolic myocardial stiffness.

Non-invasive Doppler recording of transmitral and pulmonary venous flow, as well as of tissue Doppler (TD), measure

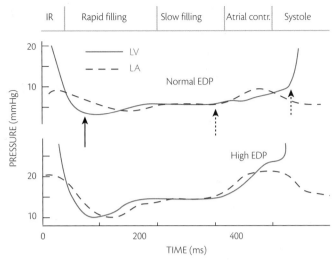

Figure 9.1 Invasive and non-invasive assessment of LV diastolic function. The four phases of diastole marked in relation to invasive pressure recordings from the LV and the LA in anesthetized dogs. The upper panel is recorded at a normal EDP (= 8mmHg). After the first cross-over corresponding to the end of IR and mitral valve opening, rapid filling (transmitral Doppler-derived peak E velocity) occurs and, when LV pressure exceeds LA pressure, mitral flow decelerates until the second pressure cross-over. This is followed by slow filling (diastasis) with almost no pressure gradient between LV and LA. During atrial contraction (transmitral Doppler-derived A velocity) LA pressure again exceeds LV pressure. The lower panel is recorded at end-diastolic pressure of 24mmHg (volume loading). The pressure differences appear larger: atrial contraction induces a sharp rise in LV pressure and LA pressure strongly exceeds this elevate LV pressure. EDP, end-diastolic pressure; IR, isovolumic relaxation; LA, left atrial pressure; LV, left ventricular pressure. Solid arrow, LV minimal pressure, dotted arrow, LV pre-A pressure, dashed arrow, LV EDP. Reproduced with permission from Nagueh SF *et al* (2009) Recommendations for the Evaluation of Left Ventricular Diastolic Function by Echocardiography *Eur J Echocardiogr* **10**(2): 165–193.

velocities and *time intervals*, whose variations occur in relation to analogous variations of LA and LV pressures (see also ➲ Chapter 6). The majority of these measurements and parameters have been validated against invasive measurements provided by cardiac catheterization. Thus, Doppler parameters provide important information about dynamics of LV filling and LV diastolic properties during disease evolution or improvement and are currently used in clinical practice.

The integrated approach to left ventricular diastolic function

The modern approach of Doppler echocardiography to LV diastolic function aims to quantify the degree of LVFP more than simply classifying Doppler-derived diastolic patterns. The increase of LVFP initially represents a compensatory mechanism, able to maintain LV stroke volume in the normal range but, over time, it also becomes the main determinant of dyspnoea and a prognostic indicator.

The mitral inflow velocity profile can be used to initially characterize LV filling dynamics, but the combination of different techniques and/or manoeuvres is needed in order to allow for an effective clinical staging of LV diastolic dysfunction.

Mitral inflow

Mitral inflow velocities are recorded by pulsed wave (PW) Doppler in the apical four-chamber (A4C) view. Using colour flow imaging as a guide, a 1–3-mm sample volume is placed at the level of mitral leaflet tips (➲ Fig. 9.2).

Spectral mitral velocity pattern should be obtained at end-expiration and at sweep speed of 50–100mm/s, in order to improve Doppler temporal resolution and, thus, reproducibility of time interval measurements. All the measurements should be averaged over three consecutive cardiac cycles in patients in sinus rhythm and over over cardiac cycles in patients with atrial fibrillation.

Mitral inflow measurements include:

◆ Peak of early filling (*E velocity*).

◆ Peak of late atrial filling (*A velocity*).

◆ The E/A ratio.

◆ Deceleration time (DT) of E velocity.

◆ Isovolumic relaxation time (IVRT), which can be obtained by placing the PW Doppler sample volume in between LV inflow and outflow to simultaneously display the end of aortic ejection and the onset of mitral E velocity.

Velocities are expressed in m/s and time intervals in ms (➲ Fig. 9.3).

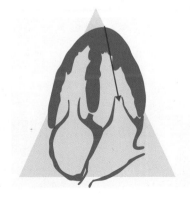

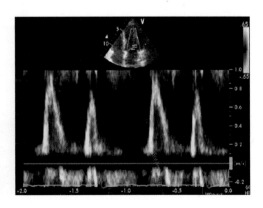

Figure 9.2 Mitral inflow pattern recording. Schema for appropriate placement of PW Doppler-derived sample volume of mitral inflow at the tips of the mitral leaflets (left panel) and Doppler-derived mitral inflow pattern (right panel).

With the sample volume at the level of the mitral annulus, where the Doppler signal is more stable, additional measurements can be obtained:

* *Mitral A velocity duration* (ms).

* *Atrial filling fraction* (AFF%), which is calculated by:

$$AFF\% = (VTI_{A\ velocity} / VTI_{total\ mitral\ inflow}) \times 100 \qquad (9.1)$$

Caution should be used when measuring E velocity DT in patients with sinus tachycardia (overlapping of E and A velocity), by prolonging the slope of E velocity into the A waveform until the baseline. Atrial fibrillation is obviously associated with the absence of A velocity.

E velocity mainly reflects the LA–LV pressure gradient during early diastole, being subjected to preload changes and alterations of LV relaxation, while A velocity is influenced by LA–LV pressure gradient during late diastole, mainly affected by LV compliance and LA function. Determinants of DT include LV relaxation, LV diastolic pressures after MV opening, and LV compliance.

Diastolic filling patterns

Diastolic filling patterns can be classified by the combined quantitative analysis of E/A ratio and DT. They traditionally include:

* Normal pattern, characterized by E/A ratio = 1–2, DT = 150–200ms, and IVRT = 50–100ms.

* Pattern of delayed relaxation (*grade I* of diastolic dysfunction), characterized by E/A ratio <1, DT ≥240ms, and IVRT ≥100ms.

* Pseudonormal pattern (*grade II* of diastolic dysfunction), characterized by E/A ratio of 0.8–1.5.

* Reversible restrictive pattern (*grade III* of diastolic dysfunction), characterized by E/A ratio ≥2, DT <160ms, and IVRT ≤80, which reverse after manoeuvres inducing preload reduction, such as the Valsalva manoeuvre (see later).

* Irreversible restrictive pattern (*grade IV* of diastolic dysfunction), characterized by E/A ratio ≥2, DT <160ms, and IVRT ≤80, in the absence of reversal after manoeuvres inducing preload reduction.

◐ Figure 9.4 shows progression of LV diastolic dysfunction into different grades.

Delayed relaxation occurs in uncomplicated arterial hypertension and/or diabetes mellitus, when LVFP should be considered still normal by definition (except for patients with severely delayed relaxation). However, an E/A ratio less than 0.8 and a DT greater than 200ms can already suggest a mild diastolic dysfunction.

Because of the load dependence of its measurements, pseudonormal filling pattern cannot be unmasked by the simple evaluation of mitral inflow pattern, unless it is evaluated during a Valsalva manoeuvre (see later).

The main clinical application of Doppler-derived LV filling concerns patients with advanced HF and dilated cardiomyopathy where mitral inflow measurements correlate better than EF with LVFP, functional classes, and prognosis. In fact, during the progression of HF, transmitral E/A ratio exhibit a 'U-shape' behaviour which has also prognostic reflexes: subjects with E/A ratio less than 1 (delayed relaxation) and higher than 1.5 (likely restrictive pattern) are both associated with increased mortality.

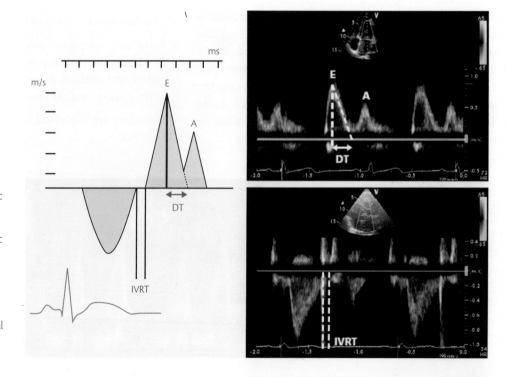

Figure 9.3 Measurement of mitral inflow indices of LV diastolic function. Methodology of measurement of Doppler-derived mitral inflow indices of LV diastolic function. Left panel: diagram of measurements. Right upper panel: mitral inflow pattern. Right lower panel: measurement of IVRT. A, mitral inflow A velocity; DT, E velocity deceleration time; E, mitral inflow E velocity; IVRT, isovolumic relaxation time.

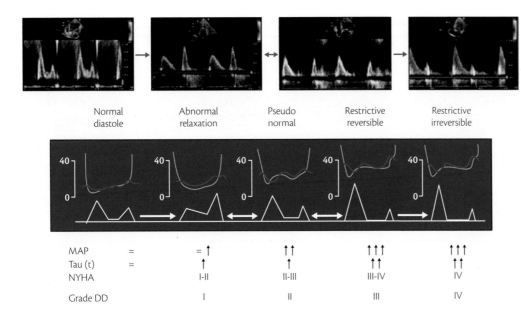

	Normal diastole	Abnormal relaxation	Pseudo normal	Restrictive reversible	Restrictive irreversible
MAP	=	= ↑	↑↑	↑↑↑	↑↑↑
Tau (t)	=	↑	↑	↑↑	↑↑
NYHA		I-II	II-III	III-IV	IV
Grade DD		I	II	III	IV

Figure 9.4 Stages of LV diastolic dysfunction. The progressive stages of LV diastolic dysfunction according to PW Doppler-derived mitral inflow patterns. MAP, mean atrial pressure; NYHA, New York Heart Association. Modified from Nishimura RA, Tajik J. Evaluation of diastolic filling of left ventricle in health and disease: Doppler echocardiography is the clinician's Rosetta Stone. *J Am Coll Cardiol* 1997; **30**: 8-18, with permission from Elsevier.

In particular, the restrictive filling pattern is associated with unfavourable prognosis if it is irreversible (grade IV). A DT less than 130ms predicts worse prognosis after acute myocardial infarction and in patients with dilated cardiomyopathy. Conversely, the intermediate range (E/A ratio = 0.8–1.5), has no significant prognostic impact because it encompasses patients with normal or unidentified pseudonormal patterns.

Additional factors such as variations of LV end-diastolic and end-systolic volumes, and elastic recoil also affect mitral inflow measurements. When defining normal values of mitral inflow velocities and time intervals the influence of age and heart rate (HR) should be taken into account because both aging (slowing of myocardial relaxation) and tachycardia (restriction of diastolic filling time) induce a reversal of E/A ratio, with increase of atrial contribution to LV filling. With increasing age, DT increases, while, with increasing HR, DT shortens. Also P–R interval, cardiac output (CO), mitral annulus size, and LA function can influence LV filling pattern. ➲ Table 9.1 summarizes the normal values of American Society of Echocardiography/European Association of Echocardiography recommendations for mitral inflow diastolic measurements according to age groups.

The non-invasive estimation of left ventricular filling pressure

In order to provide a non-invasive estimation of the degree of LVFP, an accurate evaluation of diastolic function can be performed by additional analyses such as Valsalva manoeuvre, pulmonary venous flow, and/or LA volume determination. Alternatively, the combination of PW TD or velocity flow propagation with transmitral inflow may be extremely useful to

characterize LVFP. The combination of mitral inflow pattern and PW TD of mitral annular velocity has gained relevance in clinical practice.

Valsalva manoeuvre

The Valsalva manoeuvre (see also ➲ Chapter 5, 'Principles of Doppler echocardiography') is applied during the recording of the mitral inflow. During the strain phase of the manoeuvre, LV preload is reduced and changes in LV filling features allows normal and pseudonormal patterns to be distinguished: in normal pattern both E and A velocity are reduced proportionately, without changes of E/A ratio, whereas in pseudonormal pattern—characterized by mild to moderate increase of LA pressure in a patient with LV delayed relaxation—mitral inflow changes to a pattern of delayed relaxation, i.e. E velocity decreases, DT prolongs, and A velocity increases or remains unchanged, with a consequent reversal of E/A ratio (➲ Fig. 9.5).

A decrease of 50% or more in E/A ratio during Valsalva manoeuvre strongly suggests an increase of LVFP but smaller changes are not always associated with a normal diastolic function. For a successful Valsalva manoeuvre, the operator needs to maintain a correct sampling at the mitral leaflet tips during all of the manoeuvre duration and the patient must produce a sufficient increase in intrathoracic pressure. This represents the main limitation since not everyone is able to correctly perform the manoeuvre (about 60% of patients in the clinical setting).

Pulmonary venous flow

PW Doppler assessment of pulmonary venous flow can be performed in A4C view by sampling the right upper pulmonary vein (PV) under the guidance of colour flow imaging (➲ Fig. 9.6).

Table 9.1 Normal values for Doppler-derived diastolic measurements

Parameter	Age 16–20 years	Age 21–40 years	Age 41–60 years	Age >60 years
E/A ratio	1.88 ± 0.45	1.53 ±0.40	1.28 ± 0.25	0.96 ± 0.18
	(0.98–2.72)	(0.73–2.33)	(0.78–1.78)	(0.60–1.32)
E velocity DT (ms)	142 ± 18	166 ± 14	181 ± 19	200 ± 29
	(104–180)	(138–194)	(143–219)	(142–258)
IVRT (ms)	50 ± 9	67 ± 8	74 ± 7	87 ± 7
	(32–68)	(51–83)	(60–88)	(73–101)
A duration (ms)	113 ± 17	127 ± 13	133 ± 13	138 ± 19
	(79–147)	(101–153)	(107–159)	(100–176)
S/D ratio	0.82 ± 0.18	0.98 ± 0.32	1.21 ± 0.2	1.39 ± 0.47
	(0.46–1.18)	(0.34–1.62)	(0.81–1.62)	(0.45–2.33)
AR (m/s)	16 ± 10	21 ± 8	23 ± 3	25 ± 9
	(1–36)	(5–37)	(17–29)	(11–39)
AR duration (ms)	66 ± 39	96 ± 33	112 ± 15	113 ± 30
	(1–144)	(30–162)	(82–142)	(53–173)
Septal e′	14.9 ± 2.4	15.5 ± 2.7	12.2 ± 2.3	10.4 ± 2.1
	(10.1–19.7)	(10.1–20.9)	(7.6–16.8)	(6.2–14.6)
Lateral e′	20.6 ± 3.8	19.8 ± 2.9	16.1 ± 2.3	12.9 ± 3.5
	(13–28.2)	(14–25.6)	(11.5–20.7)	(5.9–19.9)

Data are expressed as mean ± SD (95% confidence interval).

A, A velocity; AR, atrial reverse velocity; D, diastolic velocity; DT, deceleration time; E, E velocity, e′, annular e′ velocity; IVRT, isovolumic relaxation time; S, systolic velocity.

Modified from Nagueh SF, *et al. Eur J Echocardiogr* 2009.

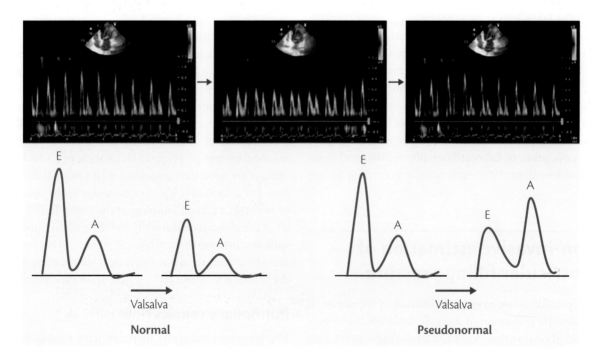

Figure 9.5 Valsalva manoeuvre applied to LV mitral inflow pattern. In healthy subjects the preload reduction induced by the manoeuvre induces an amplitude reduction of both E and A peak velocities (lower left panel). In patients with pseudonormal/restrictive pattern the manoeuvre unmasks a pattern of LV delayed relaxation, i.e. reduction of E peak velocity and increase of A peak velocity (lower right panel).

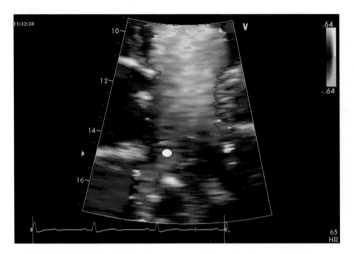

Figure 9.6 PW Doppler sample volume in the right upper pulmonary vein. Methodology for appropriate colour-guided sampling of PW Doppler sample volume in the right upper pulmonary vein (see white circle), in apical four-chamber view.

For optimal recording, the transducer should be angulated superiorly such that the AoV is seen, the sample volume (2–3-mm) should be placed 0.5cm into the PV and the wall filter settings be low enough in order to distinguish the onset and the end of atrial reversal velocity.

Measurements of pulmonary venous flow pattern include:

- Peak systolic (S) velocity.
- Peak diastolic (D) velocity, which corresponds temporarily to the mitral inflow E velocity.
- The S/D ratio.
- Peak atrial reversal (AR) velocity, which corresponds temporarily to the mitral inflow A velocity.

The time duration of AR velocity is also measured. Velocities are expressed in m/s and time intervals in ms (⮕ Fig. 9.7)

In the presence of prolonged P–R interval, two systolic velocities (S1 and S2) are visualizable and, because S1 is related to atrial relaxation, S2 should be used to compute the S/D ratio. Atrial fibrillation is associated with a blunted S velocity and absence of AR velocity. In general, pulmonary venous inflow pattern is influenced by age: values of its components according to age groups are reported in ⮕ Table 9.1.

AR velocity is influenced by atrial preload, LA contractility and, in particular, by LVEDP. For this reason, when LVEDP increases, both the amplitude and the duration of AR velocity increase, whereas the duration of mitral inflow A velocity decreases: of consequence, the time difference between AR duration and mitral inflow A velocity duration increases by more than 30ms (⮕ Fig. 9.8)

This cut-off point value is highly predictive of increased LVFP. The AR–A duration is particularly useful in clinical practice since it is relatively age-independent (AR velocity can increase with age but usually does not exceed 35cm/s) and is able to identify even patients with elevated LVEDP but normal mean LA pressure, that is, an initial stage of LVFP increase. It also is accurate in patients with normal EF, MV disease, and hypertrophic cardiomyopathy. The prognostic role of AR–A difference has been demonstrated after acute myocardial infarction, in ischaemic, and idiopathic dilated cardiomyopathy,

The main limitation of pulmonary venous flow recording is that its feasibility that does not exceed 80%. This is related to the difficulty of obtaining high-quality recording suitable for measurements. A primary factor limiting the reliability of pulmonary venous flow is the disturbance of atrial contraction, particularly in patients with sinus tachycardia and atrioventricular block (long P–R interval).

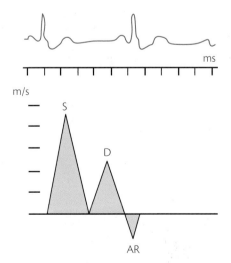
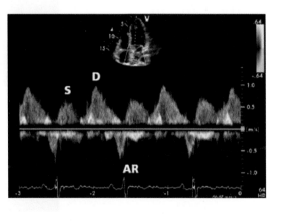

Figure 9.7 Measurement of pulmonary venous flow velocities. Methodology of measurement of pulmonary venous flow velocities. Diagram of measurements (left panel) and Doppler–derived pulmonary venous flow pattern (right panel). AR, atrial reverse velocity; D, early diastolic velocity; S, systolic peak velocity.

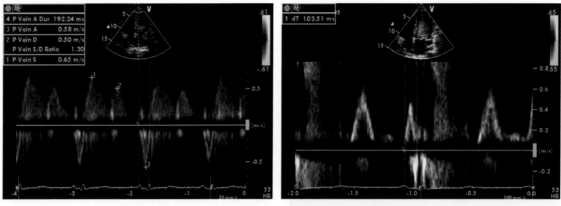

AR velocity duration – A velocity duration = 192.24 – 103.51 = 88.73 msec

Figure 9.8 Diagnosis of increased LVFP. Example of combined use of pulmonary venous flow derived AR velocity (left panel) and mitral inflow A velocity (right panel) to diagnose an increase of LVFP. In this patient the difference AR–A duration (= 88.73ms) is indicative of LVFP increase.

Colour M-mode flow propagation velocity

Regional differences in myocardial relaxation exist during diastole. In normal subjects there is a wave of relaxation originating at the apex and moving toward the base, which results in a LV base-to-apex pressure gradient and allows blood flow to be sucked into the LV. With the development of LV diastolic dysfunction, the regional relaxation differences are less evident and the intraventricular pressure gradient determining LV filling is reduced or even absent. Colour M-mode of the mitral inflow, recorded by placing M-mode cursor in the direction of the mitral inflow jet seen on the colour Doppler (CD) map, may be utilized to assess LV relaxation: it provides temporal, spatial, and velocity information. Among different methods described for calculating the *velocity flow propagation* (Vp, cm/s) from LV base to apex, the slope method is the most widely used due to its least variability (⊃ Fig. 9.9).

The slope method measures the slope of the line of the first aliasing velocity during early filling, measured from the MV plane to approximately 4cm distal into LV cavity, in A4C view, using a narrow colour flow sector and adjusting the gain to reduce noise. Colour flow baseline is shifted below the Nyquist limit so that the central highest velocity is blue.

In normal LV, values of Vp are greater than 30cm/s. During HF and myocardial ischaemia a slowing of Vp occurs, it being consistent with a reduction of apical suction. Since Vp characterizes LV relaxation, the ratio between E velocity and Vp (*E/Vp ratio*) is directly proportional to LA pressure and can be used to estimated LVFP: a E/Vp ratio of 2.5 or more predicts PCWP higher than 15mmHg with reasonable accuracy in most patients with depressed EF.

Caution in the interpretation of E/Vp ratio is recommended in the presence of LV concentric hypertrophy or remodelling,

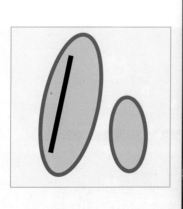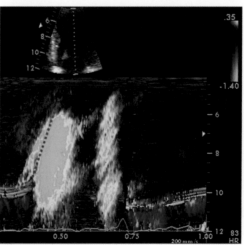

Figure 9.9 Colour M-mode flow propagation velocity. Methodology of velocity flow propagation by colour M-mode. Left panel: diagram of measurements. Right panel: colour M-mode derived flow propagation velocity. Flow propagation velocity (Vp) is measured as the slope of the first aliasing velocity in the early filling, measured from the mitral valve to 4cm distally into LV cavity. Alternatively, the slope of the transition between from no colour to colour is measured.

which themselves can induce an increase of Vp, and in patients with normal LV volumes and EF, who may present misleadingly normal Vp despite increased LVFP.

Pulsed wave tissue Doppler annular diastolic velocities

PW TD of the mitral valve ring represents an integral part of study of diastolic function. A PW Doppler sample volume is placed at 1cm within the septal or lateral MV insertions of MV leaflets over an A4C view. Gain and velocity scale should be set adequately, and minimal angulation should be maintained between the ultrasound beam and the plane of cardiac motion. TD recording should be obtained at end-expiration, at a sweep speed of 50–100mm/s. All the measurements should be averaged over three consecutive cardiac cycles in patients in sinus rhythm and over five cardiac cycles in patients with atrial fibrillation.

The TD tracing pattern shows a rounded wave facing upwards (SM) in systole and two sharper waves facing downwards in diastole, which are similar, but inverted and with lower velocity peaks, to mitral inflow waves.

PW TD measurements include (⊖ Fig. 9.10):

- Early diastolic velocity (E′).
- Late (atrial) diastolic velocity (A′).
- The E′/A′.
- Systolic velocity (S′).

Annular velocities are expressed in cm/s. PW TD can unmask subtle changes in LV relaxation by identifying low *e′* (<10cm/s).

The measurement of diastolic time intervals (E′ deceleration time and relaxation time, both in ms) does not appear to provide incremental information. However, the difference between the time occurring from QRS onset to mitral inflow E velocity and the time occurring from QRS onset and e′ onset (T_{E-e}′) can be useful in certain situations (⊖ Fig. 9.11). When calculating T_{E-e}′ ratio, the matching of RR intervals for measuring both time intervals (time to E and time to e′) is needed. This measurement is strongly influenced by the *Tau* and LV minimal pressure and provides incremental information when e′ velocity has its limitations (e.g. MV disease including annular calcification, surgical rings, mitral stenosis, mitral prosthesis, moderate to severe primary mitral regurgitation). Under these circumstances also the *IVRT/T_{E-e}′ ratio* can be applied: a value lower than 2 has good accuracy in predicting elevated LVFP). For the evaluation of LV global diastolic function it is recommended to record and measure TD signals at both septal and lateral mitral annulus and their average

Some operators prefer TD sampling of the septal annulus because it moves parallel to the ultrasound beam and is less influenced by the translation movement of the heart; others encourage the sampling at the junction between LV lateral wall and mitral annulus since septal velocities are conditioned by the right ventricular interaction. Recent studies have shown that E/lateral E′ ratio has the best correlation with LVFP in patients with normal EF. The rationale of averaging septal and lateral values is derived from the observation that E′ velocities are significantly greater at the lateral location than at the septal placement of the annulus. Thus, single-site measurements can be used in the presence of globally normal or abnormal LV systolic function whereas the average of the two site measurements is absolutely needed in patients with LV regional dysfunction.

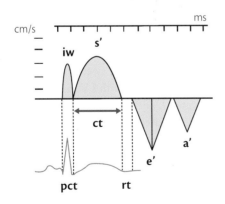

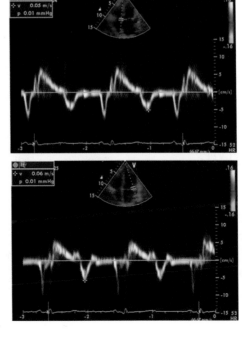

Figure 9.10 Measurement of PW tissue Doppler of the mitral annulus. Methodology of measurement of PW tissue Doppler of the mitral annulus. Diagram of measurements (left panel) and PW tissue Doppler pattern of septal annulus (right upper panel) and of lateral annulus (right lower panel). By PW tissue Doppler both annular velocities and time intervals can be measured but, in the clinical practice, the measurement of velocities is preferred. a′, atrial velocity; ct, contraction time; e′, early diastolic; ivv, isovolumic velocity; pct, pre-contraction time; rt, relaxation time; s′, systolic velocity.

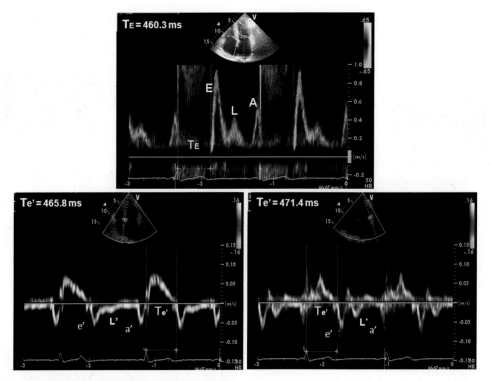

Figure 9.11 Comparison between mitral inflow PW Doppler and mitral annulus PW tissue Doppler. Doppler standard mitral inflow pattern (upper panel) and pulsed tissue Doppler of septal and lateral mitral annulus (lower left and right panels respectively) in a patient referring for acute heart failure. At the same heart rate, $T_{e'}$ at both septal and lateral side of the mitral annulus (465.8ms and 471.4ms respectively) are longer than T_E (= 460.3ms). In addition, both standard Doppler and tissue Doppler show triphasic diastolic patterns because of the presence of a mid-diastolic velocity. $T_{E\text{-}e'}$ and triphasic diastolic pattern (in presence of sinus bradycardia) are useful markers of increased LVFP. A, transmitral atrial velocity, a', myocardial atrial velocity, E, transmitral early diastolic peak velocity, e', myocardial early diastolic velocity, L, transmitral mid-diastolic velocity, l', myocardial mid-diastolic velocity, T_E, time from ECG R wave peak to E onset, $T_{e'}$, time from ECG R wave peak to e' onset.

a' velocity is influenced by LA function (the higher the function, the higher the a') and LVEDP (the higher the LVEDP, the lower the a'), while E' velocity is determined by LV relaxation. The reduction of E' velocity is minimally influenced by preload changes in patients with delayed relaxation while it increases with preload increase in normal or increased relaxation (➲ Fig. 9.12).

PW TD is highly reliable: E/e' ratio predicts invasively estimated LVFP with good accuracy and has been demonstrated to be an independent prognosticator in the clinical setting. TD-derived velocities are influenced by age and their values according to age groups are reported in ➲ Table 9.1.

Different cut-off point values of normality for E/e' ratio exist in relation with the choice of the site measurement:

◆ In the case of septal site, E/e' ratio <8 indicates normal LVFP and values >15 predict elevated LVFP.

◆ In the case of lateral site, E/e' ratio >12 is associated with high LVFP.

◆ When averaging septal and lateral values, E/e' ratio >13 should be used to define a undoubtedly LVFP increase.

The role of left atrial volume

Left atrial (LA) cavity exerts three important physiological roles: contractile pump, reservoir function, and conduit

(see ➲ Chapter 10). LA dilation occurs as a consequence of mitral disease and/or atrial fibrillation but also in response to impaired LV filling. In this view, LA volume is a cornerstone to provide information into the chronicity of LVFP. For details regarding LA size and volume assessment, see ➲ Chapter 10.

The meaning of pulmonary arterial systolic pressure

Since increased pulmonary arterial systolic pressure (PASP) is evident in symptomatic patients with LV diastolic dysfunction, correlates with elevated LVFP, and is potently associated with mortality, it can also be used to identify an increase of LVFP when no lung disease is diagnosed. Accordingly, in the absence of pulmonary outflow obstruction, the estimation of PASP can be obtained by utilizing the measurement of the peak velocity of tricuspid regurgitation (➲ Fig. 9.14) (for details, see ➲ Chapters 5 and 11)

Clinical recommendations for echo laboratories

The assessment of LV diastolic function should always consider LVFP and LV volumes. At normal LVFP, the normal LV shows end-diastolic volumes necessary to guarantee an adequate

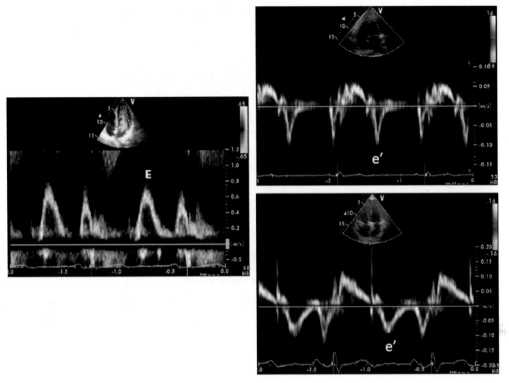

Figure 9.12 E/E′ calculation. Methodology for calculating the ratio between mitral inflow E peak velocity (left panel) and tissue Doppler derived ε′ of the mitral annulus: average of septal (right lower panel) and lateral ε′ (right upper panel).

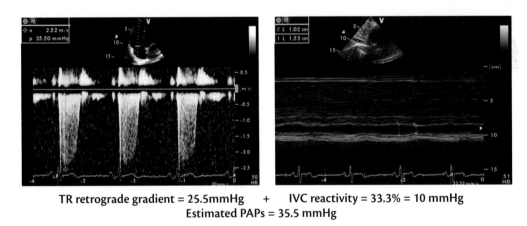

TR retrograde gradient = 25.5mmHg   +   IVC reactivity = 33.3% = 10 mmHg
Estimated PAPs = 35.5 mmHg

Figure 9.13 Methodology for non-invasive estimation of RA pressure. The value of tricuspid regurgitation retrograde pressure gradient derived by CW Doppler is summed to an estimation of right pressure given by the respiratory reactivity of IVC to obtain PAS. In the present case a patient referring for dyspnoea, with E/e′ ratio = 10 has an estimated PAS = 35.5mmHg which is indicative of increased LVFP. IVC, inferior vena cava; PAS, pulmonary arterial systolic pressure.

stroke volume. The stiff heart has similar volumes at higher pressures or, alternatively, normal pressures and smaller volumes (➲ Fig 9.15).

Non-invasive assessment of LVFP can present the same differences in patients with depressed or normal LV chamber systolic function:

◆ In patients with depressed LV systolic function (EF ≤55%) the mitral inflow pattern, in particular DT, can be used per se to estimate LVFP degree with reasonable accuracy when the E/A

ratio is ≥2. For E/A ratio ranging between <2 and ≥1, the use of additional Doppler parameters is required (➲ Fig. 9.16). A change ≥0.5 of E/A ratio with the Valsalva manoeuvre, a pulmonary venous flow S/D ratio <1 and a AR–A duration ≥30ms, an E/Vp ≥2.5, and an E/e′ ratio (using E′ average) ≳15 strongly suggests the presence of increased LVFP.

◆ In patients with normal EF the estimation of LVFP should be based on the determination of E/E′ ratio (using e′ average): values ≤8 indicates normal LVFP and values ≥13 identify

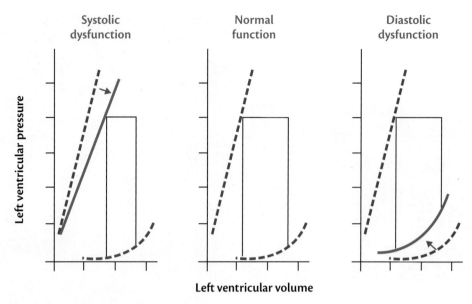

Figure 9.14 Pressure–volume relationship. Diagram of LV pressure–volume loops in systolic dysfunction (left panel), normal heart (central panel), and diastolic dysfunction (right panel). Systolic dysfunction is characterized by decreased performance, function, and contractility with LV end-diastolic pressure-volume line displaced downward and to the right, and normal diastolic properties. Diastolic dysfunction is characterized by increased chamber stiffness, with the diastolic pressure-volume displaced upward and to the left, while systolic properties are normal.

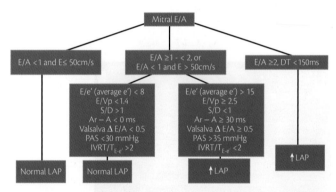

Figure 9.15 Diagnostic algorithm for the estimation of LVFP in patients with depressed EF.

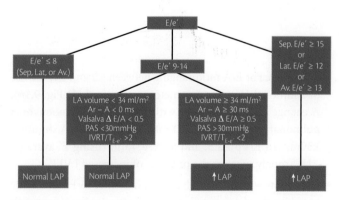

Figure 9.16 Diagnostic algorithm for the estimation of LVFP in patients with normal EF.

increased LVFP; for E/e′ ratio ranging from 9–13, one of the following additional measurements are required for diagnosing an increase of LVFP: LA volume index ≥34mL/m^2 (see ➲ Chapter 10), AR–A duration difference ≥30ms, a reduction ≥0.5 of E/A ratio with Valsalva manoeuvre or a PASP ≥35mmHg (➲ Fig 9.17). The accuracy of E/Vp ratio is not very good and should be avoided in this clinical setting.

In general, it has to be taken into account that Doppler echocardiographic measurements of LV diastolic function show individual biological (day-to-day) variability in relation with changes of afterload, preload, and sympathetic tone. In this view, an integrated approach combining multiple parameters has always to be preferred. In addition, cut-off points for identifying abnormal patients should consider age and, possibly, HR. Aging naturally deteriorates LV relaxation and in subjects older than 60 years without a history of cardiovascular disease, an E/A ratio of less than 1 with DT greater than 200ms should be judged normal for age.

New methods for the evaluation of left ventricular diastolic function

Diastolic stress echocardiography

Any stress on the heart, including simple sinus tachycardia, is also a powerful diastolic stress, since the positive lusitropic (enhanced LV relaxation) effects of adrenergic stress (or exercise)

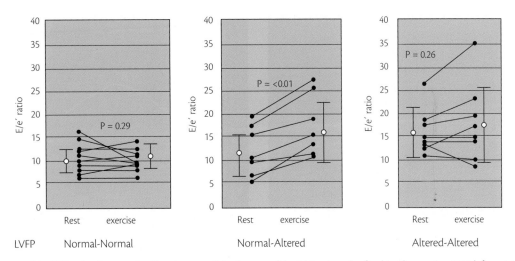

Figure 9.17 Changes of the E/E' ratio after exercise. The three possible changes of the E/e' ratio early after bicycle exercise. LVFP, left ventricular filling pressure. Modified from Ha JW, Oh JK, Pellikka PA, Ommen SR, Stussy VL, Bailey KR, Seward JB, Tajik AJ. Diastolic stress echocardiography: a novel noninvasive diagnostic test for diastolic dysfunction using supine bicycle exercise Doppler echocardiography. *J Am Soc Echocardiogr* 2005;**18**:63–68, with permission from Elsevier.

induce better LV filling in a shorter time. In fact, the normal diastolic response to stress includes an initial stage corresponding to LV end-systolic volume reduction (due to increased contractility) and LV end-diastolic volume increase, a plateau at intermediate to high stress level, up to a point when LV diastolic reserve is exhausted and LV filling declines. This decline occurs at lower HR in the presence of LV diastolic dysfunction: the lower the diastolic LV filling, the lower the stroke volume and, for any given level of LV systolic dysfunction, the worse the prognosis.

The diastolic stress echo can be particularly useful in patients reporting unexplained dyspnoea but presenting normal LV systolic function and LVFP at rest. The E/e' ratio can be successfully applied for that objective since it is an accurate representation of LA pressure (as shown by simultaneous acquisition with cardiac catheterization) and can be measured at the end of an aerobic stress such as supine bicycle exercise. Changes in mitral and PW TD septal velocities with exercise in healthy subjects correspond to an increase of both E and e' velocities, without significant variation of E/e' ratio (➲ Table 9.2). In patients

with LV delayed relaxation, the exercise-induced e' increase is much less than that of transmitral E velocity such that the E/e' ratio increases.

Summarizing, subjects can present three possible response to the exercise:

◆ Normal (at rest)–normal (post-exercise): no significant change of E/e' ratio.

◆ Normal (at rest)–altered (post-exercise): E/e' ratio is normal at rest but increases abnormally after exercise.

◆ Altered (at rest)–altered (post-exercise): E/e' ratio is abnormally high at rest and remains high after exercise.

The second response to stress is an important option to unmask mechanisms of diastolic dysfunction and HF (➲ Fig. 9.18).

The rationale of performing this assessment after the exercise completion is based on the observation that in cardiac patients E velocity increase remains stable for a few minutes after the exercise cessation and the delayed recording of transmitral pattern avoids the problems in measuring appropriately E peak velocity deriving from the fusion of E and A velocities at faster HR, i.e. at the maximal exercise. CW Doppler signal of tricuspid regurgitation can be additionally evaluated in order to provide quantitative information on PASP increase induced by exercise.

Diastolic stress echo can also be performed with dobutamine infusion: it has shown to provide prognostic information.

Potential limitations of diastolic stress test include:

◆ Patients with LV regional dysfunction.

◆ Mitral valve disease.

◆ Atrial fibrillation.

Table 9.2 Changes in mitral and tissue Doppler septal velocities in healthy subjects

Variable	Baseline	Exercise
E peak velocity (cm/s)	73 ± 19	90 ± 25
A peak velocity (cm/s)	69 ± 17	87 ± 22
DT (ms)	192 ± 40	176 ± 42
e' (cm/s)	12 ± 4	15 ± 5
E/ e' ratio	6.7 ± 2.2	6.6 ± 2.5

Modified from Nagueh SF *et al. J Am Soc Echocardiogr* 2009.

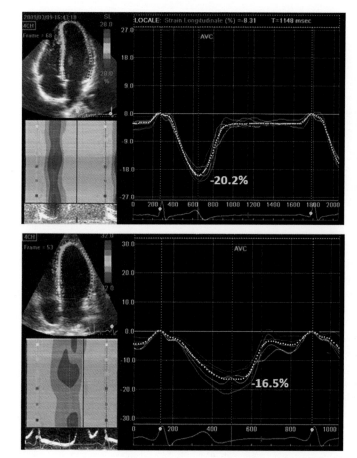

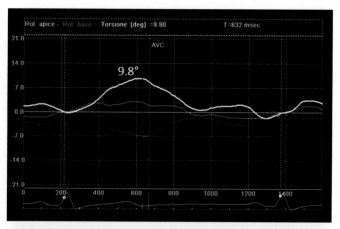

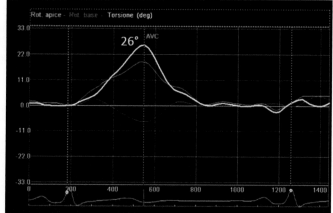

Figure 9.18 Speckle tracking-derived longitudinal strain. Comparison of STE-derived longitudinal strain in a healthy subject (upper panel) and in a hypertensive patient with LV diastolic dysfunction and normal EF (lower panel). Longitudinal strain is reduced in the hypertensive patient.

Figure 9.19 Speckle tracking-derived LV torsion. Comparison of STE-derived LV torsion in a healthy subject (upper panel) and in a hypertensive patient with LV diastolic dysfunction and normal EF (lower panel). LV torsion is higher in the hypertensive patient, it contributes to the maintenance of EF in the normal range. AVC, aortic valve closure.

Deformation measurements and torsion

Two-dimensional-derived speckle tracking echocardiography (STE) provides semiautomated elaboration of at least partially load-independent indices of LV contractility and allows quantification of LV longitudinal, radial, and circumferential deformation and deformation rate of myocardium (see ➲ Chapter 6).

Myocardial strain and strain rate can provide very important information regarding diastolic dysfunction. In particular, LV longitudinal strain appears to be reduced in patients with isolated diastolic HF when EF is still preserved and parameters of Doppler-derived diastolic function are altered (➲ Fig. 9.19)

This kind of information can also be obtained alternatively by a simple PW TD quantitative analysis of systolic velocities (s′) of the mitral annulus which have been demonstrated to have values ranging in between those found in healthy controls and patients with LV systolic HF.

Also speckle tracking-derived diastolic measurements have shown important aspects in this clinical setting: early diastolic strain rate correlates with the degree of myocardial interstitial fibrosis and the invasive time constant of LV relaxation. In addition, the ratio between transmitral E velocity and global strain rate (SR) measured during isovolumic relaxation (E/SR IVR) predict LVFP degree in patients with ratio of E/E′ ratio ranging from 8–15 and normal EF.

Furthermore, when *LV torsion* is viewed from the apex, the apex rotates counterclockwise and the base rotates clockwise in systole (*twisting*), with the opposite motion in diastole (*untwisting*). LV torsion is maintained or even accentuated in order to keep a normal EF in patients with *isolated* diastolic failure who present a preserved LV systolic function (➲ Fig. 9.20). The reduction in LV untwisting with attenuation or loss of diastolic suction contributes to LV diastolic dysfunction.

Personal perspective

The assessment of LV diastolic function should be approximated to a non-invasive haemodynamic evaluation, in order to obtain an estimation of LVFP degree—a true determinant of symptoms/sign and prognosis in patients with either systolic or diastolic heart failure—and of PASP, whose increase is recognized in the presence of LV diastolic dysfunction.

A comprehensive assessment of LV diastolic function should also take into account LV geometry (concentric in the case of isolated diastolic heart failure), LV end-diastolic volume (increased in LV systolic failure, reduced or normal in diastolic failure), and LA volume (increased in the presence of a chronic increase of LVFP). Efforts should be aimed at unmasking subclinical deterioration of LV systolic function by using advanced technologies (STE-derived longitudinal strain) or even the simple PW TD quantitation of s' velocity of the mitral annulus.

Further reading

Galderisi M. Diastolic dysfunction and diastolic heart failure: diagnostic, prognostic and therapeutic aspects. *Cardiovasc Ultrasound* 2005; **3**:18.

Ha JW, Oh JK, Pellikka PA, Ommen SR, Stussy VL, Bailey KR, *et al.* Diastolic stress echocardiography: a novel noninvasive diagnostic test for diastolic dysfunction using supine bicycle exercise Doppler echocardiography. *J Am Soc Echocardiogr* 2005; **18**:63–8.

Lang RM, Bierig M, Devereux RB, Flachskampf FA, Foster E, Pellikka PA, *et al.*; Chamber Quantification Writing Group; American Society of Echocardiography's Guidelines and Standards Committee; European Association of Echocardiography. Recommendations for chamber quantification: a report from the American Society of Echocardiography's Guidelines and Standards Committee and the Chamber Quantification Writing Group, developed in conjunction with the European Association of Echocardiography, a branch of the European Society of Cardiology. *Eur J Echocardiogr* 2006; **7**:79–108.

Nagueh SF, Appleton CP, Gillebert TC, Marino PN, Oh JK, Smiseth OA, *et al.* Recommendations for the evaluation of left ventricular diastolic function by echocardiography. *Eur J Echocardiogr* 2009; **10**:165–93.

Nishimura RA, Tajik J. Evaluation of diastolic filling of left ventricle in health and disease: Doppler echocardiography is the clinician's Rosetta Stone. *J Am Coll Cardiol* 1997; **30**:8–18.

Paulus WJ, Tschöpe C, Sanderson JE, Rusconi C, Flachskampf FA, Rademakers FE, *et al.* How to diagnose diastolic heart failure: a consensus statement on the diagnosis of heart failure with normal left ventricular ejection fraction by the Heart Failure and Echocardiography Associations of the European Society of Cardiology. *Eur Heart J* 2007; **28**:2539–50.

Quinones MA, Otto CM, Stoddard M, Waggoner A, Zoghbi WA. Recommendations for quantification of Doppler echocardiography: a report from the Doppler Quantification Task Force of the Nomenclature and Standard Committee of the American Society of Echocardiography. *J Am Soc Echocardiogr* 2002; **15**(2):167–84.

Tsang TS, Barnes ME, Gersh BJ, Bailey KR, Seward JB. Left atrial volume as a morphophysiologic expression of left ventricular diastolic dysfunction and relation to cardiovascular risk burden. *Am J Cardiol* 2002; **90**:1284–99.

Wang J, Khoury DS, Thohan V, Torre-Amione G, Nagueh SF. Global diastolic strain rate for the assessment of left ventricular relaxation and filling pressures. *Circulation* 2007; **115**:1376–83.

Yu CM, Sanderson JE, Marwick TH, Oh JK. Tissue Doppler imaging a new prognosticator for cardiovascular diseases. *J Am Col Cardiol* 2007; **49**:1903–14.

Zile MR, Brutsaert DL. New concepts in diastolic dysfunction and diastolic heart failure: Part I: diagnosis, prognosis, and measurements of diastolic function. *Circulation* 2002; **105**: 1387–93.

Zile MR, Brutsaert DL. New concepts in diastolic dysfunction and diastolic heart failure: Part II: causal mechanisms and treatment. *Circulation* 2002; **105**:1503–8.

➲ For additional multimedia materials please visit the online version of the book (🔖 http://escecho.oxfordmedicine.com).

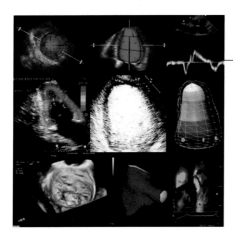

CHAPTER 10

Assessment of left atrial function

Río Aguilar-Torres

Summary

The left atrium (LA) plays an important role in cardiovascular performance, not only as a mechanical contributor, elastic reservoir, and a primer for left ventricular filling, but also as a participant in the regulation of intravascular volume through the production of atrial natriuretic peptide.

Although LA diameter in the parasternal long-axis view has been routinely employed, LA volume is a more robust marker for predicting events than LA areas or diameters. The assessment of LA performance based on two-dimensional volumetrics, Doppler evaluation of mitral, pulmonary vein flow, and annular tissue Doppler, as well as deformation imaging techniques, may provide incremental information for prognostic purposes and for the evaluation of severity and duration of conditions associated with LA overload.

The aims of this chapter are to explain the basics of LA function, and to describe the role of Doppler echocardiography techniques, and how to implement them, for the non-invasive evaluation of LA in clinical practice.

Introduction

The main mechanical function of the left atrium (LA) is to facilitate and modulate the filling of the left ventricle (LV) with blood returning from the lungs. This is accomplished during LV systole as a reservoir for the inflow volume from pulmonary veins, as a conduit during early LV diastole transferring blood stored in the atrium, and from the pulmonary veins, to the LV, and finally, as a booster pump that enhances LV end-diastolic filling.

The LA was the first cardiac chamber to be analysed employing echocardiography. Although LA assessment has been proven to be very useful in many cardiovascular diseases, the assessment of LA function is complex due to a variety of reasons:

◆ For geometrical assumptions, LA shape is not as simple as LV due to the presence of the LA appendage, confluence of pulmonary veins, and the interatrial septum.

◆ As the size of the LA varies during the cardiac cycle, the temporal sampling should be adequate when precise estimations of dimensional changes are required.

◆ No other imaging technique, except echocardiography, can be used as a gold-standard for the evaluation of LA dynamic changes. Although cardiac magnetic resonance (CMR) provides adequate spatial resolution, temporal sampling is insufficient for the assessment of fast changes in dimensions, especially when irregular and fast rhythms are present.

◆ Assessment of LA pressure (LAP), fundamental for the evaluation of important functional parameters (i.e. compliance, elastance), is invasive and technically difficult. In addition, LAP is only partially determined by intrinsic LA function due to the fact that LV function and volume status have important influences on it.

Doppler echocardiography, including recent developments, like tissue Doppler imaging (TDI), three-dimensional (3D) echocardiography, and myocardial deformation techniques, constitutes the more extensive set of tools for dimensional and functional evaluation of LA providing important parameters for the assessment of therapeutic interventions and for monitoring prognosis in a wide variety of cardiovascular diseases.

Left atrial function

During LV systole and isovolumic relaxation, when the mitral valve (MV) is closed, LA works as a distensible *reservoir* accommodating blood flow from the pulmonary veins and storing elastic energy generated by systolic descent of the mitral annular plane, in the form of pressure. During early LV diastole, the elastic energy is returned facilitating early LV filling. Then the LA behaves as a *conduit* that starts with MV opening and terminates before LA contraction allowing passive emptying during early ventricular diastole and diastasis (see ➲ Chapter 9). Finally, at end-diastole LA is also a muscular pump (*booster*), which operates depending on its own pre-load according to the Frank–Starling mechanism, which contributes to maintaining adequate LV end-diastolic volume by actively emptying (➲ Table 10.1).

The understanding of each of these functions is crucial to correctly interpret phasic changes in dimensions and the patterns of flow into and out of the LA during the cardiac cycle both in normal hearts and in pathological conditions (➲ Fig. 10.1).

Table 10.1 LA function: phases

	PHASE I *RESERVOIR*	**PHASE II** *CONDUIT*	**PHASE III** *PUMP BOOSTER*
PERIOD	Mechanical systole, including isovolumic periods (IVC and IVR).	- Early diastole and diastasis.	- Late diastole (atrial contraction) in Sinus Rhythm (SR).
BEGGINING	Mitral Valve Closure (MVC)	- Mitral Valve Opening (MVO)	
	- ~ End of A Doppler wave	- ~ Beggining of E	- ~ Beggining of A-wave
	- ~ Beggining of QRS (ECG)	- ~ End of T-wave (ECG)	- ~ Beggining of P-wave. (ECG)
END	MVO.		- MVC
	- ~ Beggining of E	- ~ Beggining of Doppler A-wave.	- ~ End of A-wave.
	- ~ End of T-wave (ECG)	- ~ Beggining of P-wave. (ECG)	- ~ Beggining of QRS (ECG)
VOLUME CHANGE	- INCREASES (Filling)	- DECREASES (Passive emptying)	- DECREASES (Late emptying)
	- LA starts at its minimum volume and reaches its Maximal volume at the end of phase I	- Early rapid relatively short descent	- Minimum LA volume at the end of atrial contraction.
		- Minimal volume changes in LA during diastasis.	
		- Volume at the end of Phase II corresponds to preload for LA contraction	
PRESSURE CHANGE	INCREASES	- DECREASES	- INCREASES (in SR)
	From low pressure, "x" descent, peaking at "v" wave	- Early rapid descent ("y" descent)	- Peaks at "a" wave
	QRS	T	P

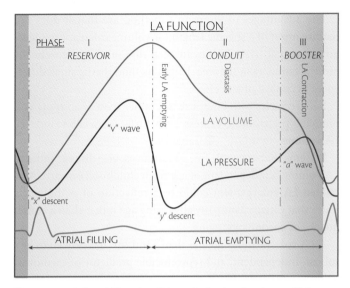

Figure 10.1 Left atrial function. Schema indicating the phases of LA function, volume, and pressure changes over the cardiac cycle.

Assessment of left atrial dimensions

Echocardiographic examining views for left atrial evaluation

Due to its ovoid shape and the variable angulations that the major axis of LA usually presents in respect to the LV major axis, the longest dimension of the LA may not lie in the longitudinal plane. The recommended planes for better assessment of LA anatomy, shape, and dimensions are:

♦ Parasternal long-axis (PLAX) view.

♦ Parasternal short-axis (PSAX) view.

♦ Apical four-chamber (A4C) view.

♦ Apical two-chamber (A2C) view.

♦ Apical three-chamber (A3C) view.

As the interatrial septum is orthogonal to ultrasound scan lines in the subcostal long-axis view, this projection is preferred for an adequate assessment of this structure.

Left atrial dimensions

Use of a standardized approach for LA size assessment is recommended. The use of a single diameter to assess LA dimension assumes that the chamber expands and contracts symmetrically, maintaining a constant shape and not taking into account that the LA often enlarges asymmetrically.

During the cardiac cycle, the LA expands primarily by elongating in the superoinferior and anteroposterior directions, mainly due to the systolic descent of the mitral annular plane (that suctions like a syringe) but also due to the elevation of the aortic roof during the ejective period (▣ 10.1).

In fact, the LA is more spherical at ventricular end-systole than at end-diastole because the medial–lateral contribution to dimensional changes is usually of lower magnitude. LA dimensions are usually measured just before MV opening, during LV end-systole, because volume is greatest at this point, the chamber has a more spherical shape, and, thus, a single dimension is more representative of LA cavity volume.

Such measurements can be done with either M-mode or two-dimensional (2D) mode from the PLAX view. For each view the transducer should be angled to maximize LA size.

Measurement of LA linear dimension

In PLAX view, the M-mode scan line should be directed orthogonal to aortic root and LA walls. According to European Association of Echocardiography/ American Society of Echocardiography (EAE/ASE) guidelines the convention for M-mode assessment is to measure from the leading edge of the posterior aortic wall to the leading edge of the posterior LA wall. However, to avoid the variable extent of space between the LA and aortic root, the trailing edge of the posterior aortic is recommended.

Normal LA anteroposterior dimension ranges from 19–40mm and the LA/aortic root ratio should be equal or less than 1.1/1. This method is the simpler; however, it is neither reproducible nor accurate, and insensitive to changes in LA size (➲ Fig 10.2).

Measurement of LA volume

The measurement of LA volume enables accurate assessment of the asymmetric remodelling of the LA. In addition, LA volume is a more robust marker for predicting events than LA areas or diameters. LA volume reflects the cumulative effects of increased filling pressures over time: due to this reason LA volume has been called the 'glycosylated haemoglobin of diastolic dysfunction'.

Volume is the recommended dimension for the evaluation of LA size and should be determined in all clinical studies in which

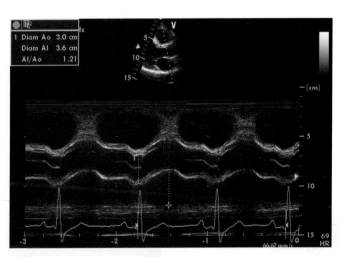

Figure 10.2 Left atrial size measurement. M-mode left atrial linear size.

atrial distortion would make the information provided by the anteroposterior dimension misleading, and in follow-up studies where quantitative accuracy is important.

2D biplane method

In clinical practice, for LA volume measurement 2D biplane methods are recommended because the majority of prior research and clinical studies have used these options. Either the Simpson's rule (method of discs) or the area–length method is valid (➲ Table 10.2).

After tracing the LA cavity areas, the measurement software package automatically calculates the LA volume in millilitres according to the modified summation of discs method or using the area–length formula (➲ Fig. 10.3):

$$\text{LA volume (mL)} = (0.85 \times \text{A4C area} \times \text{A2C area}) / \text{Length}$$

(10.1)

Table 10.2 Modified biplane methods

LA measurement:

Modified biplane Simpson's rule or area–length method

How to calculate it:

Step 1. Use 2 orthogonal planes of the LA (usually A4C and A2C views)

Step 2. Obtain the best image quality, optimizing sector width and place focal zones distally for better lateral resolution in the far-field and increasing gain just to the point on which image drop-outs in the atrial walls have disappeared

Step 3. Avoid LA foreshortening to obtain maximal LA size (discrepancies in length measured from the two orthogonal planes should be ≤5mm)

Step 4. Select adequate frames for measurement. For maximal LA volume select end-systolic frame (just before mitral valve opening, end of T wave on ECG)

Step 5. LA area border planimetry, the inferior border should be the mitral annular plane and endocardial tracing should exclude atrial appendage and pulmonary veins

Step 6. Long axis LA: orthogonal to mitral annulus plane from its midpoint to superior margin of LA*.

* As small discrepancies are acceptable, the most common option is to average the two lengths from the 4-chamber and 2-chamber views.

The advantages of Simpson's method are that it does not require input of a specific length for volume calculation, incorporates small irregularities in each disc, and is theoretically more accurate than the area–length method (being small differences in clinical practice).

LA size varies with body size: so, rather than as absolute volumes it is preferable to express 'body surface area (BSA) indexed LA volume', in mL/m^2 (➲ Table 10.3)

It seems that in people free of cardiovascular disease, indexed LA volume is independent of age from childhood onward. Age-related LA enlargement could be a reflection of pathological states that often accompany advancing age rather than a consequence of chronologic aging.

A LA volume index greater than 34mL/m^2 has proven to be a robust, independent, and reproducible predictor of cardiovascular events (atrial fibrillation, heart failure, ischaemic stroke, and death) in large follow-up studies.

Real-time 3D echocardiography

As real-time 3D echocardiography does not rely on any geometrical assumption, and is not subject to plane positioning errors (which can lead to chamber foreshortening), these

Table 10.3 2D-echocardiographic reference LA volume indexed values in adults

Normal LA indexed (BSA) maximum volume:	22 ± 6mL/m^2
Normal LA indexed (BSA) minimum volume:	9 ± 4mL/m^2
Normal mean total emptying volume:	13.5 ± 4.3mL/m^2
Mild LA enlargement (>1 SD from mean normal):	28–33mL/m^2
Moderate LA enlargement (>2 SD from mean):	34–40mL/m^2
Severe LA enlargement (> 3 SD from mean):	>40mL/m^2

*Established using 2D biplane methods.

As a continuous variable, LA volume is best used as such instead of using cut-off values.

After correction by BSA, gender has little influence, and reference values and cut-off values are the same for either male or female irrespective of age.

SD, standard deviation

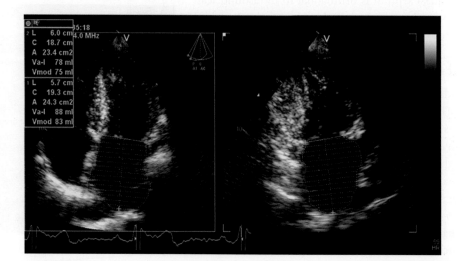

Figure 10.3 Calculation of left atrial 2D volume. Biplanar LA volume using A4C and A2C views. Calculations according to A-L formula.

methods are appealing alternatives for measuring LA volumes. However, a relatively low frame rate might preclude an accurate and reproducible assessment of LA volume change throughout the cardiac cycle and may prove to be the preferred method of LA volume assessment in large studies in the future (➲ Figs. 10.4 and 10.5; ◨10.2 and 10.3).

➲ Tables 10.4 and 10.5 summarize causes of LA enlargement and conditions of LA smaller than expected, respectively

LA volume measurements should be considered in conjunction with a patient's age, clinical status, other chambers' volumes, and Doppler parameters.

Assessment of left atrial function

Volumetric assessment of left atrial function

In addition to LA size, the assessment of LA performance based on the 2D volumetric method may provide incremental information for the evaluation of severity and duration, of conditions associated with LA, of volume or pressure overload, and for predicting events.

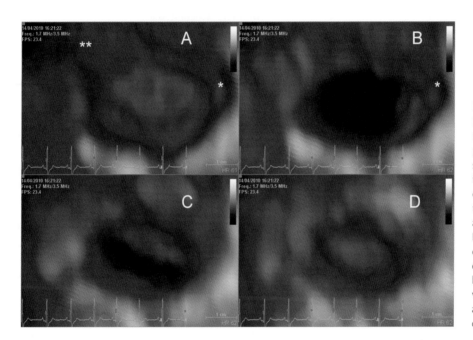

Figure 10.4 Real-time 3D imaging of left atrium. Views from the LA roof at the right superior pulmonary vein level. Mitral valve is seen at the bottom of the images in four different phases of the cardiac cycle. Interatrial septum appears at the right-side. * fosa valis; ** left atrial appendage. A) End-systolic, LA maximal expansion. B) Early-diastole, beginning of passive emptying. C) Diastasis, immediate before LA contraction (pre-A volume). D) Minimal atrial volume after LA contraction (end of LV diastole).

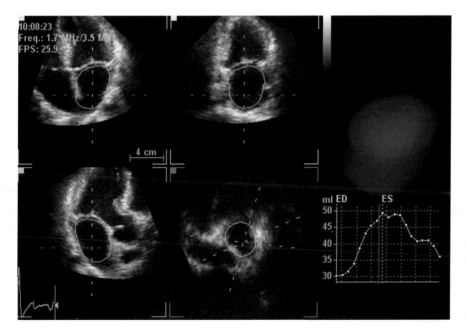

Figure 10.5 3D echocardiography assessment of left atrial volume. LA volume calculation using 3D echo and automatic tracking of wall. The curve represents changes in volume throughout the cardiac cycle.

Table 10.4 Causes of LA enlargement

Atrial pressure overload:

Diastolic dysfunction

Mitral valve stenosis

Cor triatriatum

Stiff LA syndrome: marked decrease in compliance due to wall fibrosis or calcification

Atrial volume overload:

Atrial fibrillation or flutter

Mitral valve regurgitation

Left-to-right shunts:

Atrial septal defect

Ventricular septal defect

Patent ductus arteriosus

High-output states (usually with generalized four-chamber enlargement):

Anaemia

Arteriovenous fistulas

Athletes in the absence of cardiovascular disease

Other causes:

Congenital aneurysms of the LA: more frequently confined to the atrial appendage

Left juxtaposition of atrial appendages

Unroofed coronary sinus

Post-surgical abnormalities:

Atrial baffles

Atrial anastomosis (heart transplant)

Table 10.5 Causes of smaller than expected LA

Foreshortened views: are the commonest cause of an apparently small LA

Left-to-right shunts with bypass of LA: total or partial anomalous pulmonary venous connection with or without ASD

External compression:

Enlarged aorta (root aneurysm as in Marfan's syndrome, chronic aortic dissection)

Extracardiac masses or structures (elevation and change in angulation of LA): hiatal hernia

LA rotation due to extreme RA dilation

Other: hypoplasia of the left heart

The basic LA volumes are:

- **Maximal LA volume (LAV$_{max}$):** is the volume at end-systole (timed to the moment immediately before MV opening or end of T-wave on electrocardiogram [ECG]).

- **Minimal LA volume (LAV$_{min}$):** occurs at MV closure (timed to QRS onset on ECG).

- **Volume pre-A (LAV$_{pre-a}$):** is the volume immediately before atrial contraction (timed to the onset of the P-wave). This volume represents LA preload before atrial contraction. It has been shown that, according to the Frank–Starling's

mechanism, active LA pumping function improves with greater LA pre-A volumes, only to a certain point, beyond which LA starts to deteriorate.

It is recommended to always employ all of these volumes indexed by BSA.

LA volumes representing changes throughout the cardiac cycle can be calculated (➲ Fig 10.6):

1) **Reservoir volume,** that is considered as filling or expansion volume, is calculated as:

$$LAV_{max} - LAV_{min} \qquad (10.2)$$

2) **Active pumping volume**, that is considered as LA stroke volume, is calculated as:

$$LAV_{pre-A} - LAV_{min} \qquad (10.3)$$

Atrial systole also causes contraction at the inner circular muscle layer of the pulmonary vein's entry into the LA. This sphincter-like effect seems to prevent important flow back during atrial active emptying, if pressure gradients are adequate. In pathological conditions, with elevated LV end-diastolic pressure (LVEDP), as pulmonary veins compliance is greater than LV compliance, the total amount of the retrograde flow into the pulmonary veins will increase.

3) **Conduit volume** is not easily measured, because, while the MV is open, some blood flows directly from the pulmonary veins. Thus it is estimated as LA passive emptying plus direct blood flow from pulmonary veins to LV and calculated as:

$$LV \text{ stroke volume } - LA \text{ stroke volume} \qquad (10.4)$$

As it can be easily inferred, a reciprocal relation exists between conduit and reservoir and pump booster functions of the LA (➲ Fig. 10.7)

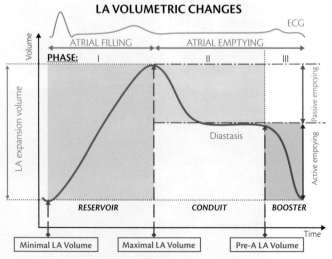

Figure 10.6 Assessment of left atrial function. Schema showing volumetric assessment of LA function.

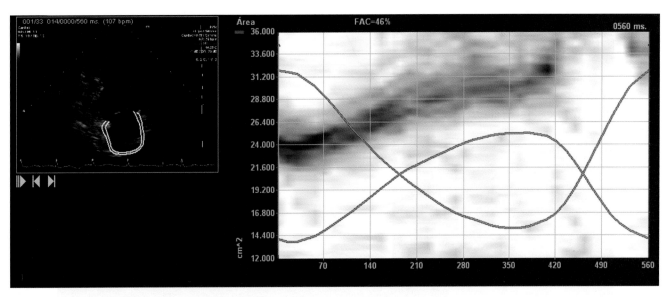

Figure 10.7 Left atrial volume change during cardiac cycle. Curves, representing simultaneous reciprocal changes in LV (top) and LA areas (bottom) in one cardiac cycle.

The change in total LA volume is not equivalent to the volume entering the LV during ventricular diastole, even in the absence of mitral regurgitation or shunt at the atrial level, because some flow enters the LV directly from pulmonary veins during passive LV filling and also a variable amount of blood flows back to pulmonary veins during atrial contraction phase.

When sinus rhythm is present, it has been estimated that, in subjects with normal diastolic function, reservoir, conduit and booster pump functions, relative contributions of the LA to the LV filling is approximately 40%, 35%, and 25%, respectively. As LV diastolic dysfunction progresses, the booster pump and the reservoir functions increase, decreasing conduit function. However, when LV filling pressure is high and diastolic dysfunction is very advanced, LA serves predominantly as a conduit.

Both conduit and pump function varies with age. With advanced age, active pumping accounts for less of total emptying.

Although many other indices have been described for specific purposes, the main functional parameters that can be derived from volumetric assessment are described in ➲ Table 10.6.

Echocardiographic equipment from different vendors allow the use of automatic motion tracking of endocardial border based on diverse algorithms (acoustic quantification, speckle tracking, boundary detectors based on optical flows). The main advantages of these techniques are that they are fast and simple and may provide several indices for LA function assessment derived from LA volume curves. However, when employing automatic tracking, an exquisite verifying is needed, in order to avoid mistakes in traces and timing (selection of end-systolic or end-diastolic frames). As a rule of thumb for automatic tracking systems, the greater the image quality is, the greater the accuracy of automatic tracking (➲ Fig. 10.8).

Doppler assessment of mitral inflow

Doppler analysis of transmitral flow velocities and time intervals may provide fundamental information for the assessment of LA–LV diastolic interaction and function, being considered a mandatory part of each echocardiographic study.

In fact, mitral inflow Doppler pattern enables the classification of diastolic dysfunction, according to E/A ratio and DT (see ➲ Chapter 9). These parameters, however, are influenced by many simultaneous haemodynamic variables that make it very difficult to obtain pure information about the functional status and performance of LA (➲ Table 10.7).

Table 10.6 Basic indices of LA function based in volumes

Reservoir function: ($+\Delta$, positive volume change)

Filling or expansion volume :
$$LAV_{max} - LAV_{min}$$
Expansion index:
$$([LAV_{max} - LAV_{min}]/LAV_{min}) \times 100$$
Diastolic emptying index:
$$([LAV_{max} - LAV_{min}]/LAV_{max}) \times 100$$

Conduit function: ($-\Delta$, negative volume change)

Passive emptying index :
$$([LAV_{max} - LAV_{pre-a}]/LAVmax) \times 100$$
Passive emptying percent of total emptying:
$$([LAVmax - LAV_{pre-a}]/[LAVmax - LAVmin]) \times 100$$

Booster pump function: ($-\Delta$, negative volume change)

Active emptying index :
$$([LAV_{pre-a} - LAV_{min}]/LAV_{pre-a}) \times 100$$
Active emptying percent of total emptying:
$$([LAV_{pre-a} - LAV_{min}]/[LAV_{max} - LAV_{min}]) \times 100$$

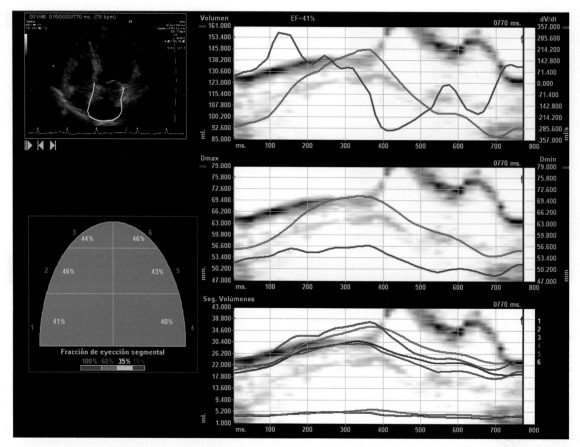

Figure 10.8 Automatic endocardial border tracking based on boundary detectors. Upper panel: curves representing changes in LA volume (orange line), volume/time (blue line). Mid panel: changes in diameter. Lower panel: regional contribution of different LA segments to volumetric changes.

Table 10.7 Mitral inflow Doppler analysis determinants for the assessment of LA–LV diastolic interaction

E-wave peak velocity and deceleration time (DT)	A-wave*
LA–LV pressure gradient during early diastole	LA–LV pressure gradient during late diastole
Determinants:	Determinants:
LV preload	LV compliance (LVEDP)
LV relaxation	LA contractile function
LV elastic recoil (suction)	
LV compliance	
Mitral valve orifice area	

*Deceleration time of the A-wave in order to predict high diastolic pressures is low, and in general provides little information about LA function.

As diastolic dysfunction progresses, LA volume contributions to LV filling become different:

♦ In cases of abnormal LV relaxation (see ⮞ Chapter 9), a reduction in LA conduit volume and an enhancement of reservoir-pump complex take place.

♦ In cases of LVEDP elevation a progressive reduction in LA active contraction occurs. With sustained advanced degrees of diastolic dysfunction, LA contractility and reservoir

function are affected. The LA behaves mainly as a conduit. LA contribution to LV filling decreases (⮞ Fig. 10.9).

According to EAE/ASE recommendations for diastolic dysfunction, also the other secondary measurements of diastolic function (A-wave duration, A-wave velocity time integral [VTI], total mitral inflow VTI and atrial filling fraction, that is A-wave VTI/total mitral inflow VTI) may contain LA functional information (see ⮞ Chapter 9).

Main limitations of transmitral inflow Doppler analysis are:

♦ Tachycardia (merging of waves).

♦ Irregular rhythm (mainly atrial fibrillation).

♦ Mitral valve disease.

Assessment of pulmonary venous flow

The analysis of pulmonary vein flow, especially atrial velocity reversal and duration, is helpful for assessment of LA function and diastolic performance of the LV (see ⮞ Chapter 9).

The antegrade systolic period represents reservoir function, while the antegrade diastolic period represents conduit function and the atrial reversal wave indicates pump function (⮞ Figs. 10.10–10.12; ■10.4).

Mechanisms, determinants, and abnormalities of each phase have been summarized in ⮞ Tables 10.8 and 10.9.

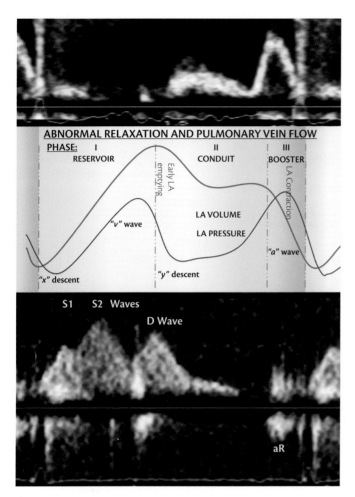

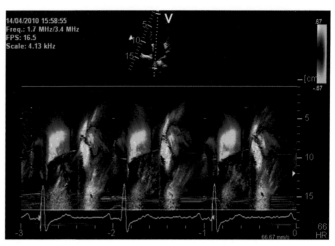

Figure 10.11 Colour Doppler M-mode for pulmonary vein flow assessment. Colour Doppler M-mode recorded from the pulmonary vein up to the LV in a normal subject. Pulmonary venous flow contribution to LA and LV filling is seen as flows coded in red crossing the LA. Small atrial contribution is represented by a small late A wave across the mitral valve.

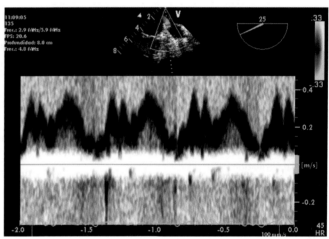

Figure 10.12 Transoesophageal echo during pulmonary vein ablation procedure for paroxysmal atrial fibrillation. PW Doppler recorded at the left superior pulmonary vein, first beats immediate post-recovery of sinus rhythm. S1, S2, and D waves are clearly seen; however, atrial reversal wave is not seen despite presence of P wave on the ECG (transient stunning).

Figure 10.9 Abnormal relaxation pattern. Upper panel: pulsed wave Doppler at the mitral inflow. Mid panel: changes in volume and pressure. Lower panel: pulmonary venous flow. The decrease in E velocity and prolonged decay (deceleration time) correlates with changes in D wave at the PV flow.

Tissue Doppler assessment of mitral annulus velocities

The two major components of mitral annulus motion diastolic waves, the mitral annular early diastolic (E′) and the late diastolic (A′), can be recorded and evaluated as representative of diastolic LV and LA function (see ➲ Chapter 9).

Low E′ peak velocity values are indicative of abnormal LV relaxation even with high LV filling pressures.

The lower the A′ peak-velocity, the greater the LVEDP. This parameter is determined mostly by haemodynamic parameters of LA function, such as LA contractility, pre- and afterload (➲ Fig. 10.13).

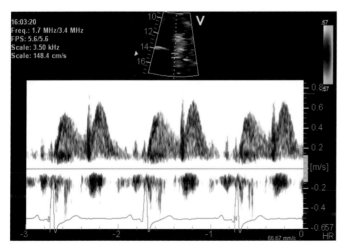

Figure 10.10 Pulmonary venous flow pattern. PW Doppler recorded at the right superior pulmonary vein. Normal LA and LV function.

Table 10.8 Pulmonary venous flow analysis mechanisms and determinants for the assessment of LA function

Antegrade systolic flow (S wave)	Antegrade diastolic flow (D wave)	Atrial reversal flow (aR wave)
LA expansion during LV systole. RESERVOIR	PV to LA gradient and PV to LV gradient. CONDUIT	Atrial contraction during LA systole. PUMP BOOSTER
This flow can be biphasic: S1: early peak systolic velocity due to atrial relaxation ('x' descent on the LA pressure curve). This component is better visualized in the presence of low filling pressures and lower heart rates S2: late systolic peak due to mitral annulus plane displacement	As LA is open to the LV during early diastole, both the peak velocity and the deceleration time of D wave are closely related to transmitral peak E velocity and deceleration time. Timing of peak D wave occurs a short time later than E wave (~50ms)	LA pump function causes both forward flow through the MV and reversed flow into the PV. The LA systolic pressure and the amount of forward flow are influenced by the end-diastolic pressure against which the LA must contract
1. Early systolic-LA relaxation: dependent on the previous LA contraction 2. Late-systolic mitral annular displacement: major determinant of LA filling 3. LA compliance: LA chamber stiffness 4. Right ventricular systole through PV flow 5. Mean LA pressure (LAP)	1. Early diastolic LA–LV pressure gradient 2. LV relaxation 3. LV compliance 4. Pulmonary venous flow 5. Mitral valve apparatus obstruction	1. LV compliance 2. LVEDP 3. LA contractility. 4. LA preload

Table 10.9 Pulmonary venous flow analysis abnormal patterns in LA and LV diastolic dysfunction

Antegrade systolic flow (S wave)	Antegrade diastolic flow (D wave)	Atrial reversal flow (aR wave)
1. **Abnormal LA relaxation:** ↓ S1 wave velocity. Related to the elastic energy stored in previous LA contraction. 2. **AV conduction block:** S1 due to atrial relaxation follows the P waves of the ECG, including those not conducted to the LV. 3. **Atrial fibrillation:** ↓ S1 wave velocity (due to atrial relaxation persists although at a reduced velocity) 4. **Increase in mean LA pressure (LAP):** ↓ S1, disappears if mean LAP is very ↑ 5. **LV ischaemia:** ↓ S2 as longitudinal LV myocardial shortening 6. **Decrease in LA compliance:** ↓ S2 as LA chamber stiffness increases: 7. **Mitral regurgitation:** ↓ S2 progressive decrease with complete reversal if regurgitation is very severe.	1. **Increase in LA–LV pressure gradient:** ↑ D wave velocity 2. **Prolonged LV relaxation:** ↓ D wave velocity due to lower LA–LV gradient 3. **Decreased LV compliance:** ↑ D wave as LA pressure increases 4. **Mid-diastolic forward flow:** In situations with high LV filling pressures. Concomitant with transmitral L wave 5. **Pulmonary venous obstruction:** ↑ D wave velocity > 1m/s (> 2m/s when severe) 6. **MV apparatus obstruction:** ↑ D wave velocity and prolonged decay 7. **Obstruction at the atrial level:** Masses, membranes (i.e. Cor triatriatum). ↑ D wave velocity and prolonged decay	1. **High LVEDP:** ↓ in forward flow into the LV and ↑ in velocity and duration of aR wave lasting 30ms more than antegrade A wave 2. **Increase in LA contractility:** ↑ in both forward and aR flow velocities.

Deformation imaging techniques for the assessment of left atrial mechanics and function: left atrial strain and strain rate

Global and segmental deformation analysis for the assessment of LA systolic and diastolic function is possible using deformation parameters obtained with either Doppler myocardial techniques (TD-derived) or with grey-scale derived algorithms (speckle tracking) (▣10.5) (see ➲ Chapter 6)

Strain and strain rate (SR) can be obtained during ventricular and atrial systole using sample volumes placed in the atrial myocardium.

During the reservoir phase, the atrial myocardium is pulled down by the systolic displacement of the LV annular plane. During this phase strain profile quantitates the relative amount of lengthening and stretching of LA walls. LA strain is strongly influenced by LV systolic function but passive atrial tissue properties also play a role.

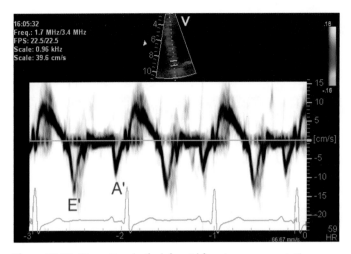

Figure 10.13 Tissue Doppler for left atrial function assessment. Tissue Doppler recorded at the annular level of the interventricular septum. Normal pattern with normal velocities.

LA strain during LA contraction appears to be a measure of LA systolic function, related to LVEDP, while SR better reflects atrial contractility and relaxation (➲ Figs. 10.14 and 10.15)

The advantages of deformation techniques for the evaluation of LA function are:

◆ Excellent temporal resolution, especially using TD.

◆ Possibility of assessing LA strain and SR in atrial fibrillation.

◆ Possibility of allowing global as well as regional assessment of intrinsic myocardial deformation properties (stretch of myocardium related to LA compliance, relaxation, and contractility) that might help to detect functional abnormalities in LA earlier than conventional echocardiographic parameters. However, to better define clinical applications, additional studies are needed.

Limitations of deformation techniques for the evaluation of LA function are:

◆ Angle-dependency of TD-derived deformation parameters, making the analysis of some regions of the LA wall very difficult. In contrast, methods based in grey-scale images provide angle-independent information.

◆ Complexity and time-consuming.

◆ Lower lateral resolution of LA walls located in the far-field in apical projections, in contrast to LV myocardium. Quantitative information is obtained from a relatively low number of stable patterns of speckles.

◆ Difficulty in tracing endocardial and tracking of speckles of LA thin wall.

◆ Possibility of analysing only the longitudinal component of deformation with current technology.

◆ Exclusion for analysis of interatrial septum should be recommended.

◆ Absence of software packages specifically designed for LA deformation evaluation.

Conclusions

The assessment of LA function is increasingly being used in various cardiovascular diseases because of its prognostic implications and the ability to detect changes induced by therapies.

Quantification of LA size is one of the mandatory items to be included, and should be reported in every echocardiographic study. Indexed volumes are preferred over linear dimension assessment because they better reflect severity and duration of LA pressure or volume overload, and also because it has shown

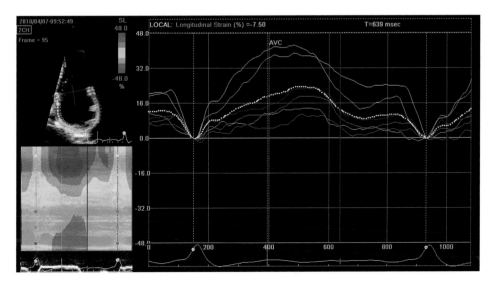

Figure 10.14 Longitudinal left atrial strain curves obtained with 2D speckle-tracking. Positive peak at end-systole represents maximal elongation caused by LV pull-down at the end of its ejective period.

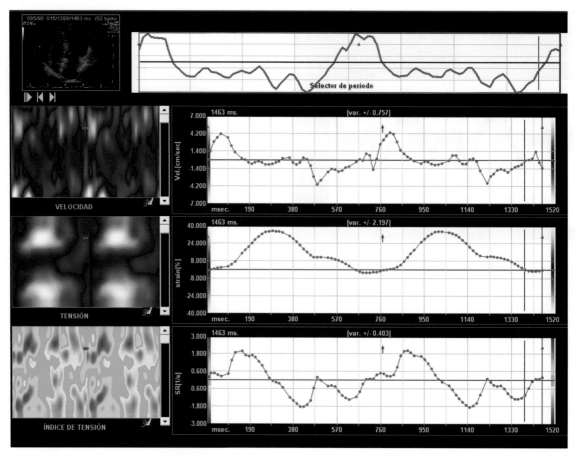

Figure 10.15 Algorithm for deformation analysis. la velocity (upper), strain (mid), and strain-rate (bottom) curves of two complete cardiac cycles obtained using VVI algorithm. It is noticeable how similar the strain curve is to that of volumetric changes.

to be an effective method for the early detection of subclinical abnormalities of LA function.

Phasic volumetric changes, and some traditional Doppler parameters, provide important clues, reflecting LA contribution and modulation of LV filling. However, many of these parameters directly affected by atrial function (transmitral A wave, atrial reversal flow at the pulmonary veins, Aa wave by TDI) present an important limitation: evaluation in subjects with atrial fibrillation is not possible. Some new appealing techniques, as the recently incorporated deformation parameters, might provide important information about the intrinsic mechanical properties of LA. However, extensive use, development of specific applications, and validation of some measurements are still required before their consolidation in the clinical scenario.

Personal perspective

A few years ago, echocardiographic assessment of LA was limited to a little more than the semiquantitative description of its enlargement.

Due to its prognostic implications, evaluation of LA has become an important part of every echocardiographic study. In addition, echocardiography has provided important physiological information, contributing to better understanding of LA function and its interaction with the LV during the complete cardiac cycle, not only during diastole.

Like other cardiac chambers, there is no single parameter to summarize LA function and multiple parameters determine the different phases of LA function.

Characterization of LA improves the evaluation of LV dysfunction, providing information about time of evolution (the past), the current haemodynamic situation (the present), and prognosis, regarding cardiovascular events, including death, in follow-up studies (the future). But, even in the absence of LV dysfunction, LA assessment is also of great value for suspecting a constellation of disturbances, categorized as pressure or volume LA overload or primary abnormalities in contractile function, which can be key factors for correct diagnosis of a previously unsuspected cardiac disease.

At the clinic, remember that echocardiography is the main method for LA functional assessment, and when at the echo lab, do not forget to assess the LA adequately.

References

1 Oh JK, Seward JB, Tajik AS (eds). *The Echo Manual*. 3rd ed. Philadelphia, PA: Lippincott Williams and Wilkins; (2007), pp.120–42.

2 Weyman AE. *Principles and Practice of Echocardiography*, 2nd ed. Philadelphia, PA: Lea and Febiger; (1994), pp.471–97.

3 Anwar AM, Geleiijnse ML, Soliman OII, Nemes A, Ten Cate FJ. Left atrial Frank-Starling law assessed by real-time, three-dimensional echocardiographic left atrial volume changes. *Heart* (2007); **93**:1393–7.

4 Barbier P, Solomon SB, Schiller NB, Glantz SA. Left atrial relaxation and left ventricular systolic function determine left atrial reservoir function. *Circulation* (1999); **100**:427–36.

5 Borg AN, Pearce KA, Williams SG, Ray SG. Left atrial function and deformation in chronic primary mitral regurgitation. *Eur J Echocardiogr* (2009); **10**:833–40.

6 Bukachi F, Waldenström A, Mörner S, Lindqvist P, Henein MY, Kazzam E. Pulmonary venous flow reversal and its relationship to atrial mechanical function in normal subjects – Umea general population heart study. *Eur J Echocardiogr* (2005); **6**:107–16.

7 De Marchi SF, Bondenmüller M, Lai DL, Seiler C. Pulmonary venous flow velocity patterns in 404 Individuals without cardiovascular disease. *Heart* (2001); **85**:23–9.

8 Gentile F, Mantero A, Lippolis A, Ornaghi M, Azzollini M, Barbier P, *et al.* Pulmonary venous flow velocity patterns in 143 normal subjects aged 20 to 80 years old. An echo 2D colour Doppler cooperative study. *Eur Heart J* (1997); **18**:148–64.

9 Ha JW, Ahn JA, Moon JY, Suh HS, Kang SM, Rim SJ, *et al.* Triphasic mitral inflow velocity with mid-diastolic flow: the presence of mid-diastolic mitral annular velocity indicates advanced diastolic dysfunction. *Eur J Echocardiogr* (2006); **7**:16–21.

10 Hoit BD, Gabel M. Influence of left ventricular dysfunction on the role of atrial contraction: an echocardiographic-hemodynamic study in dogs. *J Am Coll Cardiol* (2000); **36**: 1713–9.

11 Hoit BD. Assessing atrial mechanical remodelling and its consequences. *Circulation* (2005); **112**:304–6.

12 Kamohara K, Popovi ZB, Daimon M, Martin M, Ootaki Y, Akiyama M, *et al.* Impact of left atrial appendage exclusion on left atrial function. *J Thorac Cardiovasc Surg* (2007); **133**: 174–81.

13 Marino P, Faggian G, Bertolli P, Mazzucco A, Little W. Early mitral deceleration and left atrial stiffness. *Am J Physiol Heart Circ Physiol* (2004); **287**:H1172–78.

14 Nagueh SF, Sun H, Kopelen HA, Middleton KJ, Khoury DS. Hemodynamic determinants of the mitral annulus diastolic velocities by tissue Doppler. *J Am Coll Cardiol* (2001); **37**: 278–85.

15 Nishimura RA, Martin DA, Hatle LK, Tajik AJ. Relation of pulmonary vein to mitral flow velocities by transesophageal Doppler echocardiography. *Circulation* (1990); **81**:1488–97.

16 Okamatsu K, Takeuchi M, Nakai H, Nishikage T, Salgo IS, Husson S, *et al.* Effects of aging on left atrial function assessed by two-dimensional speckle tracking echocardiography. *J Am Soc Echocardiogr* (2009); **22**:70–5.

17 Ommen SR, Nishimura RA, Appleton CP, Miller FA, Oh JK, Redfield MM, *et al.* Clinical utility of Doppler echocardiography and tissue Doppler imaging in the estimation of left ventricular filling pressures. a comparative simultaneous Doppler-catheterization study. *Circulation* (2000); **102**:1788–94.

18 Ommen SR, Nishimura RA. A Clinical Approach to the assessment of left ventricular diastolic function by Doppler echocardiography: update (2003). *Heart* (2003); **89**(Suppl III):iii18–iii23.

19 Sanfilippo AJ, Abascal V, Sheehan M, Oertel LB, Harringan P, Hughes RA, *et al.* Atrial enlargement as a consequence of atrial fibrillation: a prospective echocardiographic study. *Circulation* (1990); **82**:792–7.

20 Sirbu C, Herbots L, D'hooge J, Claus P, Marciniak A, Langeland T, *et al.* Feasibility of strain and strain rate imaging for the assessment of regional left atrial deformation: a study in normal subjects. *Eur J Echocardiogr* (2006); **7**:199–208.

21 Spencer KT, Mor-Avi V, Gorcsan III J, De Maria A, Kimball TR, Monaghan MJ, *et al.* Effects of aging on left atrial reservoir, conduit, and booster pump function: a multi-institution acoustic qualification study. *Heart* (2001); **85**:272–7.

22 Suga H. Importance of atrial compliance in cardiac performance. *Circ Res* (1974); **35**:39–43.

23 Vianna-Pinton R, Moreno CA, Baxter CM, Lee KS, Tsang TS, Appleton CP. Two-dimensional speckle-tracking echocardiography of the left atrium: feasibility and regional contraction and relaxation differences in normal subjects. *J Am Soc Echocardiogr* (2009); **22**:299–305.

Further reading

Abhayaratna WP, Seward JB, Appleton CP, Douglas PS, Oh JK, Tajik J, *et al.* Left atrial size physiologic determinants and clinical applications. *J Am Coll Cardiol* (2006); **47**:2357–63.

Appleton CP, Kovács SJ. The role of left atrial function in diastolic heart failure. *Circ Cardiovasc Imaging* (2009); **2**: 6–9.

Evangelista A, Flachskampf F, Lancellotti P, Badano L, Aguilar R, Monaghan M, *et al.* European Association of Echocardiography recommendations for standardization of performance, digital storage and reporting of echocardiographic studies. *Eur J Echocardiogr* (2008); **9**:438–48.

Lang RM, Bierig M, Devereux RB, Flachskampf FA, Foster E, Pellikka PA, *et al.* Recommendations for chamber quantification. *Eur J Echocardiogr* (2006); **7**:79–108.

Nagueh SF, Appleton CP, Gillebert TC, Marino PN, Oh JK, Smiseth OA, *et al.* Recommendations for the evaluation of left ventricular diastolic function by echocardiography. *Eur J Echocardiogr* (2009); **10**:165–93.

Stefanadis C, Dernellis J, Toutouzas P. A clinical appraisal on left atrial function. *Eur Heart J* (2001); **22**:22–36.

Tsang TSM. Echocardiography in cardiovascular public health: The Feigenbaum Lecture (2008). *J Am Soc Echocardior* (2009); **22**: 649–56.

Additional DVD and online material

▣ 10.1 Left atrial expansion in superoinferior and anteroposterior directions.

▣ 10.2 3D echocardiographic image of left atrium and mitral valve.

▣ 10.3 Calculation left atrial volume by 3D echocardiography.

▣ 10.4 Systolic and diastolic period assessed by colour Doppler.

▣ 10.5 Assessment of systolic and diastolic LA function using deformation parameters.

⤵ For additional multimedia materials please visit the online version of the book (⌘ http://escecho.oxfordmedicine.com).

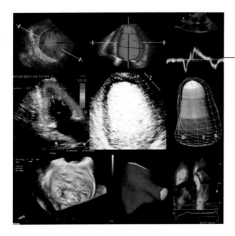

CHAPTER 11

Assessment of right heart function and haemodynamics

Luigi P. Badano and Denisa Muraru

Contents

Summary

Assessment of right ventricular (RV) size, function, and haemodynamics has been challenging because of its unique cavity geometry. Conventional two-dimensional assessment of RV function is often qualitative. Doppler methods involving tricuspid inflow and pulmonary artery flow velocities, which are influenced by changes in pre- and afterload conditions, may not provide robust prognostic information for clinical decision making. Recent advances in echocardiographic assessment of the RV include tissue Doppler imaging, speckle-tracking imaging, and volumetric three-dimensional imaging, but they need specific training, expensive dedicated equipment, and extensive clinical validation. However, assessment of RV function is crucial, especially in patients with signs of right-sided failure and those with congenital or mitral valve diseases. This chapter aims to address the role of the various echocardiographic modalities used to assess RV and pulmonary vascular bed function. Special emphasis has been placed on technical considerations, limitations, and pitfalls of image acquisition and analysis.

Introduction

An accurate assessment of right ventricular (RV) function is an essential part of any routine echocardiographic study, irrespective of the presence of left heart abnormalities. RV function may be impaired in pulmonary artery (PA) hypertension, acute and chronic pulmonary embolism, congenital heart diseases, valvular heart diseases, left ventricular (LV) dysfunction secondary to coronary artery disease, or cardiomyopathies (including arrhythmogenic RV cardiomyopathy), etc. In recent years, many studies have demonstrated the prognostic value of RV function in various cardiovascular diseases.

Echocardiography is the first-line imaging technique to screen for RV impairment, allowing a simultaneous, cheap, and non-invasive assessment of right chamber morphology, function, and haemodynamics. Unfortunately, RV function and geometry may be difficult to quantify by echocardiography, because of the RV complex geometry and poor endocardial definition, the characteristic pattern of myocardial contraction related to muscle fibre orientation, and RV anterior position within the chest, affecting its explorability and image quality. Therefore, when using conventional M-mode, two-dimensional (2D), and Doppler echocardiography to assess right heart function, a multiparameter approach is needed in clinical practice to compensate for the flaws of various methods. However, this approach is time-consuming and not routinely feasible, and new echocardiographic techniques like speckle-tracking deformation imaging and three-dimensional (3D) echocardiography are entering the clinical arena.[3,4]

The following sections will compare the strengths and weaknesses of the various echocardiographic parameters proposed for right heart geometry and function assessment, with a special emphasis on technical considerations,[6] limitations and pitfalls of image/tracing acquisition and analysis.

Right ventricular anatomy and physiology

The geometry of the normal RV is complex: its shape is almost triangular in frontal section and crescentic in transverse section (wrapping around the convex interventricular septum [IVS]). The RV is anatomically subdivided into three components.[7–9]

- The inflow tract (sinus), including the tricuspid valve (TV) apparatus.

- The outflow tract (infundibulum or conus) which corresponds to the smooth myocardium outflow region, separated from the inflow tract by crista supraventricularis (which is thought to aid RV free-wall contraction towards the IVS).

- The apical portion, heavily trabeculated and virtually immobile.

The RV wall is thinner (<5mm thick) and more compliant than the LV wall. It is composed mainly of circumferential fibres in the subepicardial layer and longitudinal fibres in the subendocardium. Spatially, RV wall deformation consists of three components (inward, longitudinal, and circumferential traction due to LV contraction), of which longitudinal shortening is the major contributor to the overall RV performance. Normal RV contraction acts in a sequential manner, as a peristaltic wave directed from inflow to infundibulum. RV free wall, and IVS contribute equally to RV performance. Functionally, the normal RV pumps the same stroke volume as the LV, but using only 25% of LV stroke-work, because of the low resistance of the pulmonary vasculature.

The RV is closely connected to LV: they share a wall (interventricular septum); the RV free wall is attached to the anterior and inferior IVS; they have mutually encircling epicardial fibres and share the same intrapericardial space. These explain an important aspect regarding RV physiology—*ventricular interdependence*—that may affect both RV and LV filling and systolic performance. During inspiration, transtricuspid flow

(RV preload) increases by approximately 20%, while transmitral flow is mildly decreased by approximately 10%, the process being reversed during expiration.

Imaging the right ventricle and assessing its geometry and function

Major challenges for RV assessment by conventional 2D echocardiography derive from:

- Complex asymmetric geometry.

- Anterior retrosternal position.

- Heavily trabeculated inner contour with poor endocardial definition.

- Separate inflow and outflow adequately visualized only from separate views. Thus, several views are needed for a comprehensive assessment of its geometry and function (→ Fig. 11.1, 11.1–11.6).

- Load-dependency and lower accuracy of most conventional echocardiographic parameters in comparison with invasive measures.

Qualitative assessment

A practical assessment of RV size is usually obtained by its comparison with the LV in apical four-chamber (A4C) view. Visually, the normal RV should be less than two-thirds of LV size. However, RV relative comparison to LV size may be misleading when LV dilation coexists.

A qualitative assessment of RV loading conditions can be performed by appreciating its shape from a parasternal short-axis (PSAX) view at LV papillary muscle level. An overloaded RV loses its normal crescentic shape, the IVS flattens, and the LV shape resembles the one of the letter 'D'. The IVS motion pattern during diastole and systole may help to distinguish between volume and pressure overload. In RV volume overload states, the septum flattens only in diastole, and regains its normal shape in systole (11.7). Conversely, in RV pressure overload states, the septum flattens in systole in early stages of the disease, while in more advanced stages it remains flattened throughout the entire cardiac cycle (11.8).

The qualitative assessment of a reduced RV free-wall excursion is usually the first sign indicating the need for a comprehensive echocardiographic examination of RV function. In addition, the detection of localized wall motion abnormalities may orientate the diagnosis and further work-up (e.g. localized hypokinesia or aneurysms in arrhythmogenic RV cardiomyopathy).

Right ventricular linear dimensions

RV free-wall thickness and linear dimensions can be easily measured from A4C or subcostal view at end-diastole, on

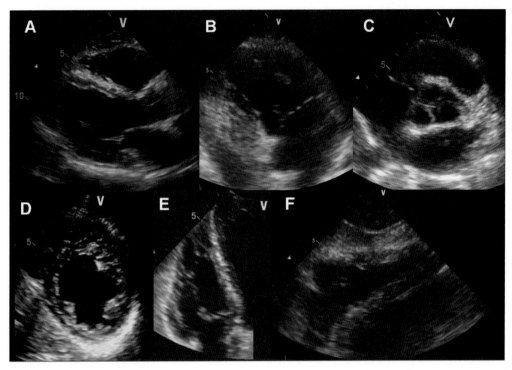

Figure 11.1 Echocardiographic views used to assess the right ventricle. A) Parasternal long-axis view which visualize the RV anterior wall. B) Long-axis view of the inflow tract which visualize the RV inferior (on the left) and anterior (on the right) walls. C) Parasternal short-axis view of right ventricular outflow tract. D) Parasternal short-axis view at the level of papillary muscles which visualizes the RV anterior, lateral, and inferior walls. E) apical four-chamber view which visualizes the RV lateral wall and interventricular septum. F) Subcostal view which visualize the RV inferior wall.

images obtained during quiet respiration or end-expiratory apnoea, using second-harmonic imaging, adjusting gain and compression to improve endocardial border definition (➲ Fig 11.2).[10] Cut-off values of RV diameters may identify RV dilation independently or relatively to LV size,[10] while RV free-wall thickness greater than 5mm indicates RV hypertrophy. However, RV diameters are inherently one-dimensional estimates and cannot by themselves describe the complex shape of the RV (➲ Fig. 11.3). Although linear measurements are time-saving, widely applicable, and practical, even for less experienced operators, they are highly dependent on image quality, insonation angle, and load. In addition, significant variability related to probe or patient position during examination renders them unreliable to identify mild RV abnormalities. For instance, simply rolling patient from supine to left lateral position increases measured RV diameter up to 40%.[11] Of note, progressive RV dilation is also accompanied by changes in heart position and by its rotation in the thorax, which impact on the interpretation of serial measurements. Diameter measurement inconsistency is even higher when performed regardless of the respiratory phase.

Eccentricity index

The eccentricity index is a relatively easy-to-use measure of septal shift towards LV in overloaded RV. Eccentricity index is calculated on routine 2D PSAX at papillary muscle level view,

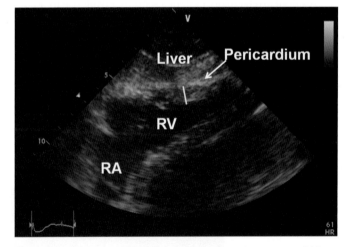

Figure 11.2 Right ventricular inferior wall thickness measurement. Right ventricular inferior wall thickness measurement is performed at end-diastole at the level of tricuspid valve chordae tendinae in the subcostal four-chamber view. Image optimized by decreasing depth. RA, right atrium; RV, right ventricle.

as the ratio of LV anteroposterior to septolateral diameter (➲ Fig. 11.4). It may be used to discriminate between RV volume overload and pressure overload states. Since normal LV is approximately circular in transverse section, the normal eccentricity index is close to 1 both in diastole and in systole.

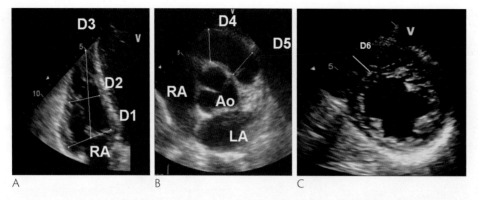

Figure 11.3 Linear measurements of the right ventricle A) modified apical 4-chamber view; B) parasternal short axis view at the great vessels level; C) parasternal short-axis view at papillary muscle level. D1, basal RV diameter; D2, mid-RV diameter; D3, base-to-apex length; D4, RV outflow tract diameter; D5, pulmonary annulus diameter; D6, latero-septal diameter; LA, left atrium; RA, Right atrium.

A value greater than 1 at end-diastole is indicative of RV volume overload, while a ratio greater than 1 both at end-diastole and end-systole is suggestive of an advanced RV pressure overload. A high eccentricity index is an important echocardiographic predictor of mortality in PA hypertension. Echocardiographic detection of a pressure overload pattern of a dilated RV with hypokinesia of the free wall sparing RV apex (*McConnell sign*), especially in patients with haemodynamic deterioration, is highly suggestive of acute pulmonary embolism, having an important value for risk stratification and therapeutic decisions. However, different short-axis level measurements impact on the accuracy of the results. In addition, slightly off-axis images can result in artefactually flattened septum, giving rise to incorrect eccentricity indexes.

Tricuspid annular plane systolic excursion

Tricuspid annular plane systolic excursion (TAPSE) is a simple M-mode measure of the longitudinal excursion of the lateral tricuspid annulus towards the RV apex, obtained from the A4C view (⮕ Fig. 11.5). TAPSE is obtained by positioning the M-mode scan line at the lateral tricuspid annulus from an A4C view and by measuring the distance from the lowest point to the highest point of the excursion curve. It is used as an estimate of RV systolic function, since, in normal ventricles, longitudinal displacement of RV base accounts for the greater proportion of total RV volume change in comparison with radial.[8] TAPSE has demonstrated prognostic value in patients with pulmonary hypertension or acute myocardial infarction involving the RV. A TAPSE value higher than 18–20mm is generally normal. A reasonable correlation between TAPSE and RV ejection fraction (RVEF) assessed by radionuclide angiography has been reported. However, TAPSE ignores the outflow tract and the septal contribution to RV ejection, which may become important to maintain overall RV function, especially in pathological conditions associated with impairment of longitudinal component.

Although simple, widely available, and feasible also in patients with poorly visualized RV endocardial borders, TAPSE is one-dimensional and angle-dependent. Regional RV myocardial abnormalities are also neglected when using TAPSE as a single measure of RV performance. Since it is measured with an external reference point, it also takes into account the overall heart motion and not only the longitudinal excursion of RV base. Moreover, its load dependency needs to be considered in cases

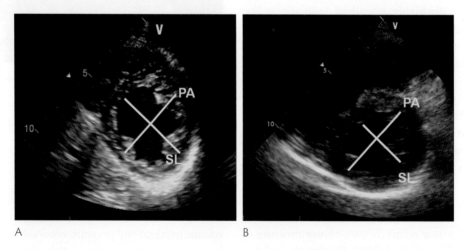

Figure 11.4 Measurement of eccentricity index. Parasternal short-axis views at papillary muscle level showing the measurement of postero-anterior (PA) and septolateral (SL) diameters for calculation of eccentricity index. In a normal subject (A) and in a patient with pulmonary hypertension (B).

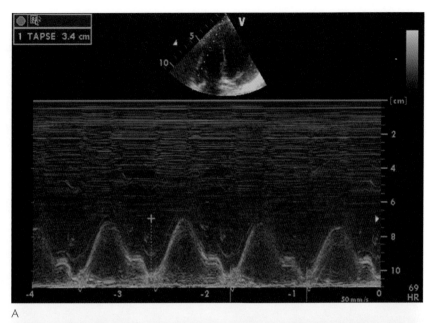

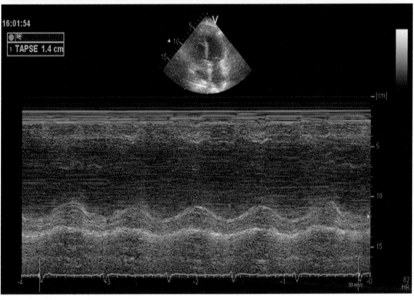

Figure 11.5 Tricuspid annular plane systolic excursion (TAPSE) measurement in a patient with normal right ventricular function (upper panel) and in a patient with moderate right ventricular dysfunction (lower panel).

of significant TR, when RV base active excursion may overestimate overall RV contractile function. Not only RV, but also LV systolic performance may influence TAPSE value due to ventricular interdependence.[12] In fact, in patients who underwent mitral valve repair surgery, TAPSE was discrepantly reduced in contrast with unchanged RVEF measured by 3D echocardiography, demonstrating its reduced accuracy to estimate true RV performance after cardiac surgery.[13]

Right ventricular quantitative systolic assessment

Right ventricular areas and fractional area change

Right ventricular areas and fractional area change (RVFAC) is a simple method, performed in the A4C view, representing an

indirect estimate of RVEF. It was shown to predict outcome in heart failure patients. RVFAC is calculated as the ratio of systolic area change to diastolic RV area, which means the percentage change in RV area measured in A4C view between end-diastole and end-systole (⊃ Fig. 11.6) as:

$$\text{RVFAC} = (\text{RV end-diastolic area} - \text{RV end-systolic area})/ \text{RV end-diastolic area}$$

(11.1)

The RVFAC is a rather simple method of assessing RV function and it has been shown to be the best correlate with RVEF by cardiac magnetic resonance, as compared with other 2D measures of RV systolic function (including TAPSE and transversal fractional shortening). Normal RVFAC is 32–60%,

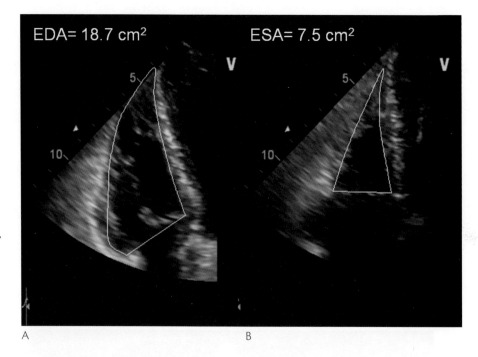

Figure 11.6 Right ventricular areas and fractional area change assessment. Right ventricular area measured at end-diastole (A) and end-systole (B). Both views are optimized by decreasing the depth, focusing on the right ventricle and adjusting gain and compression to optimize endocardial border detection. The calculated fractional area change is: (18.7 – 7.5)/18.7= 60%

mildly reduced is 25–31%, moderately reduced is 18–24%, and severely reduced if under 17%.

RV area measurements are grossly affected by inherent manual tracing pitfalls, particularly in patients with hypertrophied, heavily trabeculated RV. There is a significant overlap of the A4C view diameters and areas between normal and volume overloaded RV. In patients with a dilated RV, the A4C view often displays a foreshortened cavity, since it often fails defining anatomical landmarks for the RV and may not intersect the RV crescent at its maximal dimension. Finally, suboptimal RV endocardial definition, especially at the anterior RV wall, limits the accuracy and reproducibility of RVFAC.

Right ventricular ejection fraction and volumes

In clinical practice, the most intuitive parameters of RV size and pump function are RV volumes and RVEF, the same as for LV quantitation. RVEF is widely used as a non-invasive measure of RV performance, despite its well known load dependency. Depending on the type of echocardiographic modality used for its assessment, RVEF may range from 40–76%.

Several 2D methods have been proposed to calculate RV volumes. The most popular one uses the area and length from an A4C view and an outflow tract area view (⮕ Fig. 11.7). A prolate-ellipsoid shape assumption about RV is made and the two echocardiographic views are assumed to have an orthogonal relationship to each other. Unfortunately, the geometric assumption made does not accurately depict the actual shape of the RV. In order to acquire the two RV views, the transducer is moved from the apical position to the parasternal one based on operator's knowledge of anatomy. With this method, orthogonality is assumed, but not verified (no anatomical landmarks to refer to), and actually rarely satisfied. This explains the variable correlation of different RV models with angiographic or radionuclide studies. Difficulties in obtaining two standardized orthogonal RV views and failure to include the RV infundibulum (which

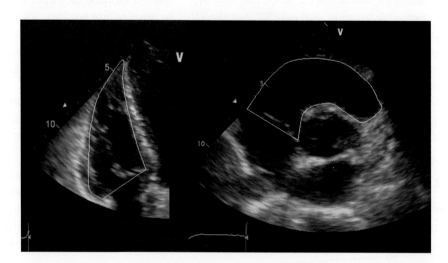

Figure 11.7 Right ventricular volume calculation. Two-dimensional apical four-chamber (left) and parasternal short-axis (right) views obtained to calculate right ventricular volume

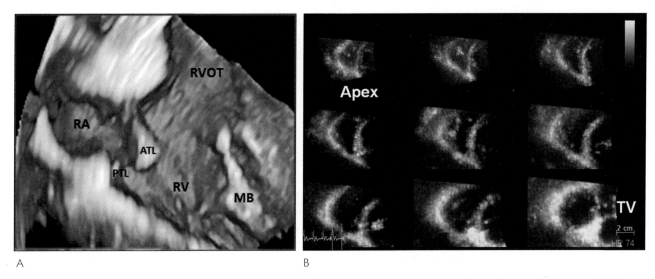

Figure 11. 8 Three-dimensional full-volume acquisition of a data set for the right ventricle. Volume rendered image showing simultaneously the three components of the right ventricle (inflow, outflow, and apex) (A) and multislice (nine transversal planes) of the right ventricle from the tricuspid valve in the right lower corner, to the apex, in the left upper corner (B). ATL, anterior tricuspid leaflet; MB, moderator band; PTL, posterior tricuspid leaflet; RA, right atrium; RV, right ventricle; RVOT, right ventricular outflow tract; TV, tricuspid valve

may account for up to 25% of RV volume)[11] are additional limitations of 2D echocardiography. Image quality and operator experience may further impact on the results.

Therefore, A4C RV area and maximal short-axis diameter offer the best estimation of RV volumes by 2D echocardiography. Cardiac magnetic resonance, which is the gold standard for calculating RV volumes and RVEF, has shown that normal RVEF is 61+7%, ranging from 47–76%.

However, complex anatomy is ideally displayed using volumetric acquisition by 3D echocardiography.[14] The assessment of RV volume and function for clinical use may represent the most justified application of 3D echocardiography. It provides accurate volume analysis independent of RV size and shape, without foreshortened views and geometric assumptions. Compared with cardiac magnetic resonance data, RV volumes calculated from 3D showed significantly better agreement and lower intra- and interobserver variability than 2D. Wide-angle full-volume acquisitions to accommodate enlarged RVs are presently feasible with good image quality in a time-saving manner. Full-volumetric data sets from four to seven EKG-triggered subvolumes (➲ Fig 11.8; ◪ 11.9 and 11.10). Then, post-processing analysis with electronic cropping, slicing, rotating, and translating tools allows the identification of pre-defined RV views to start quantitative analysis workflow.

Current semiautomated softwares for offline analysis of RV based on 3D data sets use border-detection algorithms to obtain a dynamic surface-rendered RV cast which enables the evaluation of RV geometry and contraction from any perspective (➲ Fig 11.9; ◪ 11.11). Qualitative assessment is complemented by time–volume curve display and a panel of quantitative data derived from actual volumetric measurements

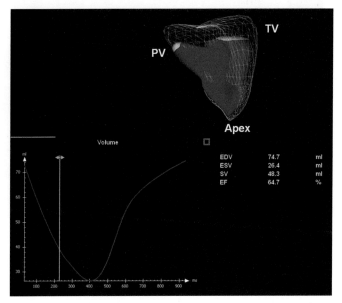

Figure 11.9 Surface rendering of the measured right ventricular volume. By adding a wire-frame rendering of the end-diastolic volume, the motion of the different components of the right ventricle is easily appreciated. The time volume curve of the right ventricle during the selected cardiac cycle is displayed below. PV, pulmonary valve; TV, tricuspid valve

and not simple calculations. Digitally archived 3D data sets may also be post-processed retrospectively for comparison during serial follow-up.

Yet, no imaging technique is ideal and 3D echocardiography makes no exception. Patients' inability to cooperate for breath-hold, arrhythmias, the large footprint and size of matrix-array transducer, dependence on optimal acoustic quality, and need for specific training are among the most incriminated drawbacks of this method. To date, limited data are available regarding normal reference values for RV volumes and EF using 3D echocardiography and further extensive studies are required in this area.

Right ventricular stroke volume

RV stroke volume may be easily estimated (see ➲ Chapter 5, 'Haemodynamic parameters'). A time velocity integral (TVI) less than12cm predicts a RV stroke volume less than 2.2l/min/ m². RV dP/dt can be readily measured by tricuspid regurgitant (TR) jet (see ➲ Chapter 5, 'Study of the intracardiac pressures'), but its utility was criticized for its high load-dependency.

Myocardial performance (Tei) index

Myocardial performance index is calculated from time intervals obtained from Doppler recordings of tricuspid and pulmonary flow. It is calculated as the ratio between total RV isovolumic time (both contraction and relaxation) divided by pulmonary ejection time (➲ Fig. 11.10). Since myocardial performance index incorporates both measures of systolic and diastolic

function, it represents an estimate of global RV performance independent of geometric assumptions. The normal value of this index for the RV is 0.28 ± 0.04 and it increases with decreasing RV function. A significant advantage is that myocardial performance index is relatively independent of RV loading conditions and heart rate. Moreover, its prognostic value was ascertained in pulmonary hypertensive patients, and its accuracy was also demonstrated in congenital heart disease, myocardial infarction, and chronic respiratory diseases. The calculation of this index is based on short intervals, requires very good quality Doppler tracings, and is adversely affected by rhythm and conduction disturbances. In addition, the myocardial performance index may suffer a 'pseudonormalization' effect due to a shortened isovolumic relaxation time when increased right atrial pressure coexists.

Tissue Doppler myocardial velocities

RV free-wall sampling using pulsed tissue Doppler (TD) imaging (see ➲ Chapter 6) may complement previous methods and allows quantitative assessment of both RV systolic and diastolic

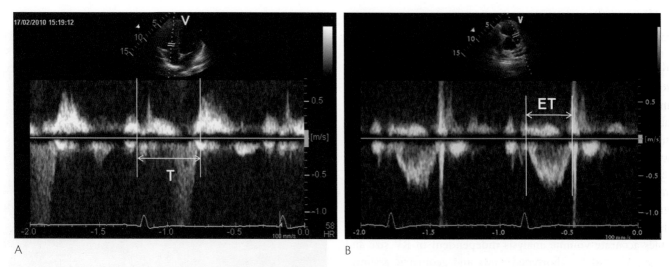

Figure 11.10 Myocardial performance (Tei) index calculation. Doppler tracings of antegrade pulmonary flow (B) and right ventricular filling (A) with the measurements needed to calculate the myocardial performance index (T – ET)/ET. ET, transpulmonary ejection time; T, time from cessation of transtricuspid A wave to the following E wave.

Figure 11.11 Tissue Doppler-derived right ventricular myocardial velocities obtained from lateral tricuspid annulus. A', velocity during atrial contraction; E', velocity during rapid right ventricular filling, ET, ejection time; ICT, isovolumic contraction time; IVRT, isovolumic relaxation time; S, systolic velocity. The myocardial performance index can be calculated as: (ICT – IVRT)/ET.

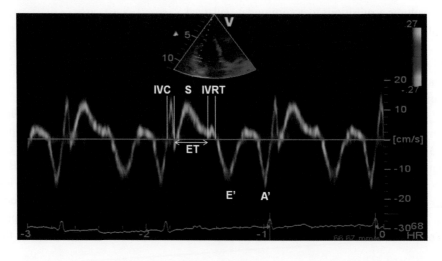

function in a less load-dependent way (➲ Fig. 11.11).[15] Myocardial systolic velocity (S) by TD is a relatively simple, reproducible and accurate non-invasive correlate of RV systolic function, and several cut-off values have been described to predict RV systolic dysfunction in various studies (<9.5–11.5cm/s). In some cohorts of patients, it was found that peak systolic values less than 11.5cm/s recognized the presence of RV systolic dysfunction with a sensitivity of 90% and specificity of 85%.[1,2]

Peak S-wave values with pulsed TD and with colour TD cannot be used interchangeably, since the former measures peak myocardial velocities, whereas the latter measures mean myocardial velocities, which are 20% lower. Colour TD may be useful to quantify RV dyssynchrony as the time delay between septal and RV free-wall contraction. TD imaging velocities may also be affected by overall cardiac motion and by tethering of the adjacent segments. Poor spatial resolution due to active systolic motion of RV base is problematic for the RV.

Isovolumic myocardial acceleration is a new TD-derived parameter of myocardial contractility, less affected by preload or afterload. It is calculated by dividing the maximal isovolumic myocardial velocity by the time-to-peak velocity (➲ Fig. 11.11). Further validation of this new index is warranted for clinical use.

Right ventricular deformation imaging

Right ventricular deformation can be quantitated by TDI as myocardial strain (see ➲ Chapter 6). Strain and strain-rate abnormalities of RV can be detected in pulmonary hypertension, as well as in amyloidosis, congenital heart diseases, and arrhythmogenic RV cardiomyopathy. Doppler-derived strain and strain-rate may identify subtle changes in response to vasodilator treatment and may outline early signs of RV involvement in the PA hypertension course. Colour TD imaging may facilitate simultaneous segmental recordings for comparative analysis of event timings.

Speckle-tracking echocardiography (see ➲ Chapter 6) has a great promise in assessing regional and global RV deformation in different directions, i.e. longitudinal, radial, and circumferential, in terms of both amplitude and timing (➲ Fig. 11.12). This new method is able to outline changes in RV systolic function, as assessed by 2D strain and strain-rate, in proportion to the severity of pulmonary pressure rise in PA hypertension patients.[3] Also, it is sensitive enough to detect early alterations of RV function in patients with systemic sclerosis and normal pulmonary pressures.

Right ventricular diastolic function

This is seldom considered as part of a routine RV examination, even though it may provide additional information in conditions evolving with altered RV compliance and relaxation, as pulmonary hypertension, pulmonary stenosis, constrictive pericarditis, or restrictive cardiomyopathies with RV involvement.

Various indices have been identified for this purpose (➲ Table 11.1), but several practical clues may indicate RV diastolic dysfunction in daily clinical practice:

◆ A dilated IVC with lack of respiratory variations and dilated RA in the presence of RV hypertrophy and no significant TV disease or atrial fibrillation.

◆ Slow upslope of TR Doppler signal (negative RV dP/dt).

◆ Rapid downslope of pulmonary regurgitation Doppler signal in the absence of significant regurgitation (PHT).

◆ Negative tricuspid E/A ratio with prolonged E wave deceleration time (excepting older subjects).

◆ Short E-wave deceleration time coexisting with RV systolic dysfunction, diastolic TR with no atrioventricular conduction abnormalities, short TDI-derived IVRT and high E/E′ ratio—suggestive of elevated RV filling pressures.

Imaging the right atrium

The RA area and volume can be easily measured in A4C view, as it is done for the LA.

Assessment of right ventricular haemodynamics

Pulmonary arterial pressure

The most common approach to estimate pulmonary arterial systolic pressure (PASP) (see also ➲ Chapter 5, 'Study of the intracardiac pressures') is to measure the peak velocity of a tricuspid regurgitant jet and apply the modified Bernoulli's equation (➲ Equation 5.3) (➲ Figs. 11.13 and 11.14). The proto- and end-diastolic gradients between the RV and the PA can be derived from the CW Doppler tracing of PR (➲ Fig. 11.15). In the absence of pulmonary stenosis or intracardiac shunts, pulmonary systolic, protodiastolic (considered to be representative of the mean pulmonary arterial pressure), and end-diastolic pressures can be calculated from these gradients by simply adding the estimated right atrial pressure to each. Pulmonary hypertension is unlikely if TR velocity is 2.8m/s or lower, and PASP is 36mmHg or lower, in the absence of other suggestive signs.

Avoidance of technical pitfalls in obtaining an adequate Doppler tracing of TR (e.g. malalignment, single view estimation, misinterpretation of aortic stenosis velocity jet or tricuspid valve closing click as TR signal, postextrasystolic or peak velocity measurement in irregular rhythms, etc.), is crucial for an accurate examination. In patients with inadequate Doppler tracings or undetectable TR (up to 20% of healthy subjects and up to 70% of patients suffering from chronic obstructive pulmonary disease), injection of agitated saline solution or

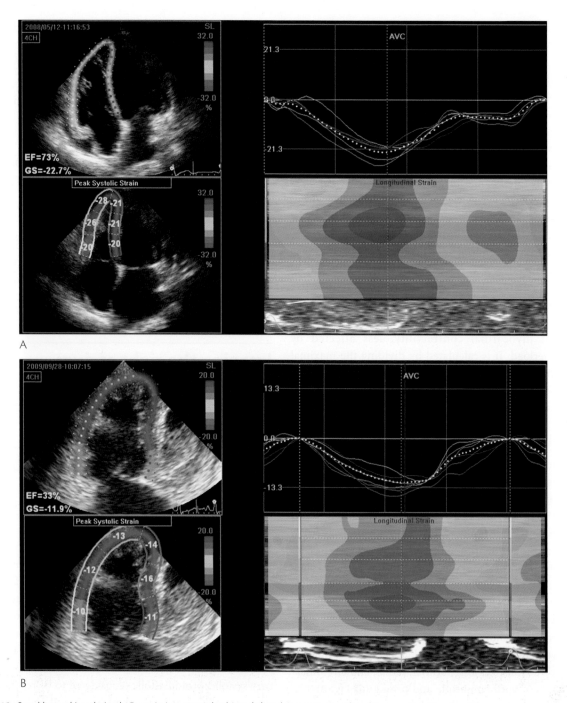

Figure 11.12 Speckle-tracking derived 2D strain in a normal subject (A) and in a patient with pulmonary hypertension (B).

contrast agents can be used to enhance the TR signal. However, several conditions preclude an accurate estimation of PASP on TR peak velocity:

◆ Severe (free) TR.

◆ Tricuspid stenosis or prosthetic valve.

◆ RV myocardial infarction or other causes of significant RV systolic dysfunction. In acute pulmonary embolism, the estimated pulmonary pressure usually does not exceed 40mmHg, due to an unadapted RV confronting a severe acute afterload rise.

A major variable in determining the RV systolic pressure (RVSP) is the method by which mean RA pressure is either assumed or calculated.

Mean right atrial pressure

RA pressure reflects both left- and right-sided cardiac function and chamber volumes, and thus carries diagnostic, therapeutic, and prognostic values for patients with cardiac and/or pulmonary diseases. In addition to guiding the management of the

Table 11.1 Proposed indices for echocardiographic evaluation of right ventricular function

- **RV global function:** myocardial performance index (Tei)
- **RV systolic function:**
  - RVEF (2D or 3D)
  - RVFAC
  - TAPSE
  - VTI of RVOT systolic flow; dp/dt of tricuspid regurgitation signal
  - TDI RV basal segment: S wave, IVA
  - STE: global longitudinal strain
- **RV regional systolic function:**
  - TDI: regional S wave, strain and strain-rate
  - STE: regional strain and strain-rate
- **RV diastolic function:**
  - RAsize; E/A and EDT of tricuspid PW recording; IVRT; negative dp/dt of tricuspid PW recording; PHT of pulmonary regurgitation CW signal; hepatic vein PW flow
- **TDI RV basal segment:**
  - E′, E/E′, E′/A′, IVRT

fluid status in patients with heart failure, elevated mean RA pressure is a marker for increased mortality in patients with primary pulmonary hypertension, probably because it reflects decompensation of ventricular systolic function after a long period of compensatory hypertrophy.

Many laboratories use a floating constant of 5mmHg, 10mmHg, or 15mmHg, based on size of the RA and the severity of TR:

- When TR is mild and the RA size is normal, an assumed RA pressure of 5mmHg is used.
- For moderate degrees of TR with mild or no RA enlargement, an assumed constant of 10mmHg can be used.

- If TR is severe in the presence of a dilated RA, an assumed constant of 15mmHg can be used.

An alternate approach is to use an assumed fixed constant in all patients. Typically, either 10mmHg or 14mmHg has been used. Although this approach provides excellent correlation over a broad range of RVSP, it will systematically overestimate the RVSP in the low ranges and potentially underestimate it in the high ranges in which the RA pressure could exceed 20mmHg.

Mean RA pressure is an important haemodynamic variable that aids optimal treatment of patients with cardiac and pulmonary disease.

Previous echocardiographic methods for measurement of RA pressure include the size and respiratory variation of the IVC by 2D imaging (see ➲ Chapter 2) and Doppler evaluation of hepatic venous flow velocities. The IVC changes shape and dimensions with changes in central venous pressure and with respiratory cycle (➲ Fig. 11.16). The size and respiratory variation of the IVC have been used to predict RA pressure according to the following principles:

- IVC dilation suggests increased central venous pressure and may accompany volume overload states.
- IVC diameter normally decreases more than 50% during inspiration.
- A blunted or absent inspiratory decrease of IVC diameter suggests increased RA pressure.

Based on such consideration, RA pressure is roughly estimated as follows:

- 5mmHg if IVC is normal.
- 5–10mmHg if IVC is normal and not collapsed.
- 10–15mmHg if IVC is dilated and collapsed.
- 15–20mmHg if IVC is dilated and not collapsed.

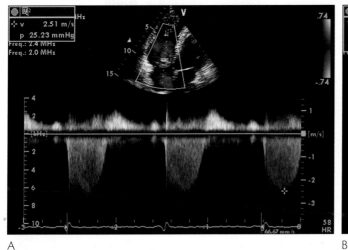
A

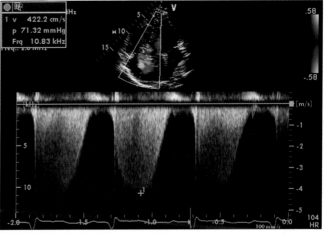
B

Figure 11.13 Continuous wave Doppler tracing of tricuspid regurgitant flow in a normal subject (A) and in a patient with severe pulmonary hypertension (B) ED, end-diastolic flow velocity.

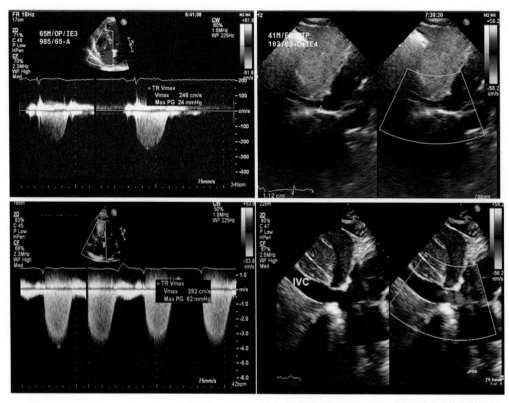

Figure 11.14 Assessment of pulmonary arterial systolic pressure. Assessment of PASP using the peak velocity of TR and IVC size and collapse. Example of normal subject (upper panel) and severe pulmonary hypertension (lower panel).

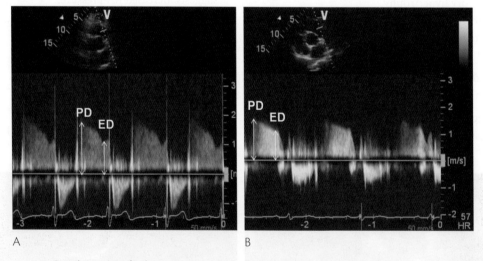

Figure 11.15 Continuous wave Doppler tracing of pulmonary regurgitation showing end-diastolic atrial contraction in a normal patient (A) and in a patient with a flat deceleration pattern (B) Measurements of proto- and end-diastolic gradients are shown. ED, end-diastolic flow velocity; PD, proto-diastolic flow velocity.

According to these principles a fairly accurate estimation of mean RAP can be obtained (➲ Table 11.2). However, respiratory IVC variability has also some limitations that should be taken into account:

◆ In patients who are mechanically ventilated, IVC size and respiratory response do not correlate well with mean RA pressure.

◆ In young individuals and athletes, the IVC may be dilated despite normal systemic venous pressure.

◆ IVC dilation may occur secondary to narrowing at the IVC–RA junction resulting from the presence of a web of tissue or due to a prominent Eustachian valve regardless of mean systemic venous pressure.

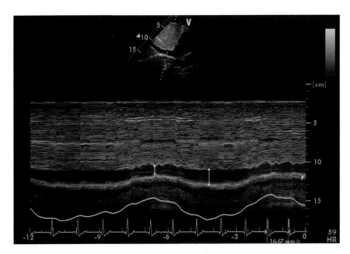

Figure 11.16 Measurements needed to obtain the inferior caval respiratory index.

Table 11.2 Estimation of right atrial pressure

IVC Diameter (cm)	Respiratory Change (%)	RA pressure (mm Hg)
<1.5	Collapse	0–5
1.5–2.5	>50%	5–10
1.5–2.5	<50%	10–15
>2.5	<50%	15–20
>2.5	No change	>20

◆ IVC changes during respiration may be altered by varying force of inspiratory effort and patient cooperation.

Doppler methods to confirm increased mean RA pressure

Due to the limitations of IVC evaluation, the finding of increased RA pressure should be confirmed using additional parameters.

Hepatic vein and IVC flow are similar and, because it is generally easier to align the Doppler signal with a hepatic vein, using the latter is both useful and practical. Antegrade flow (toward the RA) has two main components (➲ Fig. 11.17): a larger systolic wave and a slightly smaller diastolic wave. Between these two antegrade flow patterns, at end-systole, a small retrograde flow pattern may be recorded. Likewise, during atrial systole, some retrograde flow is also present.

Hepatic vein flow is respiratory cycle-dependent with increased flow velocity during inspiration and decreased flow velocity (and a greater degree of retrograde flow) during expiration. Any condition that affects either RA pressure or filling will alter hepatic vein flow velocity: increased RA pressure has been associated with a decrease in the systolic filling fraction of hepatic vein flow (calculated as the ratio between the TVI of the systolic component and sum of systolic and diastolic component TVIs). A systolic filling fraction less than 55% detects a RA pressure higher than 8mmHg.

The hepatic atrial reversal velocity also provides useful information. Hepatic vein atrial reversal velocity greater than antegrade systolic hepatic vein velocity predicts increased RA pressure: in severe TR, because the TR jet is transmitted retrograde into the RA, the normal antegrade systolic flow is replaced by a prominent retrograde wave.

Analysis of RA filling plays an important role in the assessment of different conditions:

◆ In the setting of atrial fibrillation, retrograde flow during atrial systole and the velocity of systolic antegrade flow are diminished, regardless of pressure.

◆ In patients with restrictive physiology and constrictive pericarditis (see ➲ Chapters 17 and 19).

◆ In patients with pulmonary hypertension. There is a prominent atrial flow reversal in the hepatic vein caused by increased diastolic pressure and decreased compliance of

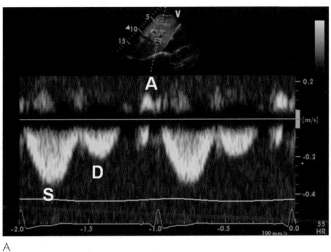
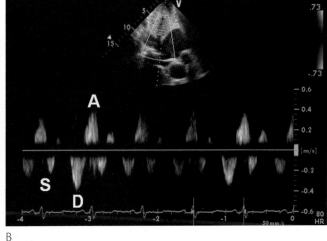

Figure 11.17 Hepatic vein Doppler flow tracing in a normal subject, with a prominent systolic component (A), and in a patient with increased right atrial pressure (B) S, systolic component; D, diastolic component; A, retrograde flow after right atrial contraction.

the RV. Conversely from what can be observed in restrictive or constrictive pericarditis, there is very little respiratory variation of atrial flow reversal in pulmonary hypertension.

The superior vena cava (SVC) can be visualized from the suprasternal notch as a vertical structure just to the right of the aortic arch, but is more readily evaluated using transoesophageal echocardiography. Doppler interrogation of flow velocities into the SVC in patients with congestive heart failure makes it possible to estimate the severity of the impairment of the right circulatory function. The venous flow velocity pattern (⇒ Fig. 11.18) was considered:

- Normal, when the systolic/diastolic ratio was ≥1 and ≤2.
- 'Predominant systolic wave', when the ratio was >2.
- 'Predominant diastolic wave', when the ratio was <1.

Patients showing a 'predominant systolic wave' pattern were characterized by RVEF less than 30% but RA pressure lower than 8mmHg.

TDI allows a one-step method for assessment of RA pressure, provides information independent from RV function, and is useful in mechanically ventilated patients. The ratio of tricuspid peak early inflow velocity (E), obtained by pulsed Doppler sampling the RV inflow to the tricuspid annular early diastolic velocity (E′) obtained by Doppler tissue imaging has been found to have a weak correlation with RAP, and requires two Doppler measurements.

Another method is the measurement of the time interval between the end of the systolic annular motion (S wave) to the onset of the E′ wave: RV isovolumic relaxation time (IVRT). RV IVRT is independent of RV end-diastolic or pulmonary artery pressure and thus it can be used as a non-invasive estimate of RA pressure. When the RA fails or is volume overloaded, RA pressure increases with an earlier TV opening, so

that RV IVRT shortens. Consequently, RV IVRT was found most useful in the stable paediatric congenital heart disease population to predict pulmonary artery systolic pressure, where compensatory RA hypertrophy would keep mean RA pressure normal, as compared to patients who are older or acutely ill, who tend to have more RV failure and higher RAP. In addition, RV IVRT identifies mean RA pressure in patients with suboptimal subcostal views.

Analysis of pulmonary Doppler flow tracing

In normal individuals, pulmonary flow tracing has a symmetric contour with a peak velocity occurring in mid-systole. As pulmonary pressure increases, peak velocity occurs earlier in systole and late systolic notching is often present (⇒ Fig. 11.19). With increased pulmonary pressure, the RV ejection pattern approximates more the left-sided one. The acceleration time (time from onset to peak flow velocity) can be measured and provides a rough estimate of the degree of increase in PA pressure. In normal individuals, acceleration time exceeds 140ms and progressively shortens with increasing degrees of pulmonary hypertension: at an acceleration time of less than 70–90ms, PASP exceeds 70mmHg.

The PA acceleration time is easily measured in most patients, including those with chronic lung disease. However, it has been replaced by the more direct Doppler assessment of RVSP from the TR signal, unless that is not measurable. Mahan's equation is a practical method for estimating mean PA pressure (MPAP) (⇒ Fig. 11.20):

$$MPAP = 79 - 0.45 \times PA \text{ acceleration time (ms)} \qquad (11.2)$$

Another method to calculate MPAP is described by the formula:

$$\text{Mean PAP} = 0.61 \times PASP + 2mmHg \qquad (11.3)$$

Acceleration time is dependent on cardiac output (CO) and heart rate (HR). With increased CO through the right side cardiac chambers (as in atrial septal defect), acceleration time may be normal even when PA pressure is increased. If the HR is slower than 60 beats per minute or more than 100 beats per minute, acceleration time needs to be corrected for HR. There is heavy dependence on the position of the Doppler sample volume because acceleration and velocities are higher along the inner edge of curvature of the PA: positioning of the sample volume in the middle of the vessel in the imaged plane may not avoid overestimation of velocity by sampling adjacent to the vessel wall in the orthogonal non-imaged plane.

RV ejection time shortens with increasing PA pressure. In contrast, the RV pre-ejection time lengthens with increasing

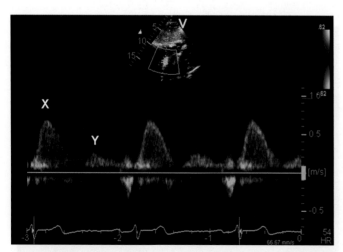

Figure 11.18 Superior vena cava Doppler flow tracing obtained from subcostal approach in a patient with right ventricular dysfunction and right atrial pressure <8mmHg (i.e. predominant systolic wave or X/Y > 2). X, systolic wave; Y, diastolic wave.

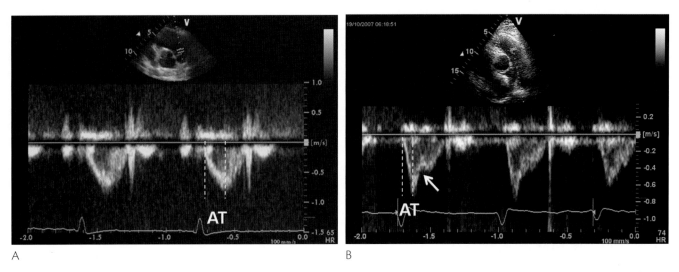

Figure 11.19 Right ventricular outflow tract flow pattern Doppler tracings in a normal subject (A) and in a patient with pulmonary hypertension (B). The triangular shape with rapid acceleration and mid-systolic cessation of flow (notching, arrow) are suggestive of sever pulmonary hypertension. AT, acceleration time.

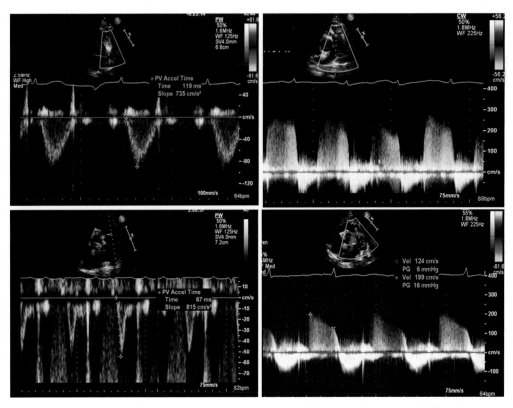

Figure 11.20 Estimation of pulmonary arterial pressure. PW and CW Doppler flow pattern in normal subject (upper normal) and in severe pulmonary hypertension (lower panel). Measurements of acceleration time of systolic flow, velocity and pressure gradient of pulmonary regurgitation helps in estimation of PAP.

PA pressure. The ratio of PA acceleration time to total RV ejection time or pre-ejection time can be used to estimate MPAP. However, the short values of these time intervals render them impractical for general clinical use.

With severe pulmonary hypertension, a mid-systolic notch may be present in the deceleration slope of the PA Doppler flow profile. This notch is analogous to the mid-systolic notch seen in

M-mode examination of the PV. The notch may be secondary to transient elevation of PA pressure above RV pressure, due to a decrease in PA compliance and an increase in main PA size, impedance, and transmission time of the velocity wave.

The mid-systolic notch in pulmonary flow profile may distinguish proximally located obstructions in the PA vasculature from distal obstructions. This notch occurs significantly later in systole in patients with primitive pulmonary hypertension than in those with proximal pulmonary embolism.

Pulmonary vascular resistance

Two methods have been proposed to assess PVR. The first one is described by ➲ Equation 5.22 (see ➲ Chapter 5, 'Study of the intracardiac pressures').

The second method is the ratio between the pre-ejection period time and the acceleration time of pulmonary systolic flow. This ratio greater than 2.6 predicts pulmonary vascular resistance greater than 2.5WU. When using the latter it should be noted that in the original paper the authors measured the pre-ejection period in an unconventional way starting from the onset of TR flow and not from the onset of QRS to compensate the intraventricular conduction delay of right heart failure.

Personal perspective

RV dysfunction and right heart haemodynamics are important predictors of survival and exercise capacity in cardiopulmonary diseases. Because of the complexity of the RV and the marked load dependence of its function and right heart haemodynamic parameters, the study of right heart function with conventional echocardiography remains challenging and requires integration of multiple parameters that can be obtained with several echo techniques. Future advances in echocardiography are expected in the field of 3D echocardiography, deformation imaging, and tissue characterization. This could lead to an easier, more comprehensive, and more reproducible way to assess right heart chamber function.

References

1 Voelkel NF, Quaife RA, Leinwand LA, Barst RJ, McGoon MD, Meldrum DR. et al. Right ventricular function and failure: report of a National Heart, Lung, and Blood Institute working group on cellular and molecular mechanisms of right heart failure. *Circulation* 2006; **114**:1883–91.

2 Haddad F, Doyle R, Murphy DJ, Hunt SA. Right ventricular function in cardiovascular disease, part II: pathophysiology, clinical importance, and management of right ventricular failure. *Circulation* 2008; **117**:1717–31.

3 Badano LP, Ginghina C, Easaw J, Muraru D, Grillo MT, Lancellotti P, et al. Right ventricle in pulmonary arterial hypertension: haemodynamics, structural changes, imaging, and proposal of a study protocol aimed to assess remodelling and treatment effects. *Eur J Echocardiogr* 2010; **11**:27–37.

4 Jurcut R, Giusca S, La Gerche A, Vasile S, Ginghina C, Voigt JU. The echocardiographic assessment of the right ventricle: what to do in (2010)? *Eur J Echocardiogr* 2010; **11**(2):81–96.

5 Selton-Suty C, Juilliere Y. Non-invasive investigations of the right heart: how and why? *Arch Cardiovasc Dis* 2009; **102**:219–32.

6 Horton KD, Meece RW, Hill JC. Assessment of the right ventricle by echocardiography: a primer for cardiac sonographers. *J Am Soc Echocardiogr* 2009; **22**:776–92.

7 Ho SY, Nihoyannopoulos P. Anatomy, echocardiography, and normal right ventricular dimensions. *Heart* 2006; **92**(Suppl 1):i2–13.

8 Haddad F, Hunt SA, Rosenthal DN, Murphy DJ. Right ventricular function in cardiovascular disease, part I: Anatomy, physiology, aging, and functional assessment of the right ventricle. *Circulation* 2008; **117**:1436–48.

9 Sheehan F, Redington A. The right ventricle: anatomy, physiology and clinical imaging. *Heart* 2008; **94**:1510–5.

10 Lang RM, Bierig M, Devereux RB, Flachskampf FA, Foster E, Pellikka PA, et al. Recommendations for chamber quantification. *Eur J Echocardiogr* 2006; **7**:79–108.

11 Jiang L, Levine RA, Weyman AE. Echocardiographic assessment of right ventricular volume and function. *Echocardiography* 1997; **14**:189–206.

12 Lopez-Candales A, Dohi K, Bazaz R, Edelman K. Relation of right ventricular free wall mechanical delay to right ventricular dysfunction as determined by tissue Doppler imaging. *Am J Cardiol* 2005; **96**:602–6.

13 Tamborini G, Muratori M, Brusoni D, Celeste F, Maffessanti F, Caiani EG, et al. Is right ventricular systolic function reduced after cardiac surgery? A two- and three-dimensional echocardiographic study. *Eur J Echocardiogr* 2009; **10**:630–4.

14 Shiota T. 3D echocardiography: evaluation of the right ventricle. *Curr Opin Cardiol* 2009; **24**:410–14.

15 Lindqvist P, Calcutteea A, Henein M. Echocardiography in the assessment of right heart function. *Eur J Echocardiogr* 2008; **9**:225–34.

16 Maslow AD, Regan MM, Panzica P, Heindel S, Mashikian J, Comunale ME. Precardiopulmonary bypass right ventricular function is associated with poor outcome after coronary artery bypass grafting in patients with severe left ventricular systolic dysfunction. *Anesth Analg* 2002; **95**:1507–18.

17 Jiang L. Right ventricle. In: Weyman AE (ed) *Principles and Practice of Echocardiography*. Baltimore, MD: Lippincott Williams & Wilkins; 1994, pp.901–21.

18 Sheehan F, Redington A. The right ventricle: anatomy, physiology and clinical imaging. *Heart* 2008; **94**(11):1510–15.

19 Eidem BW, Tei C, O'Leary PW, Cetta F, Seward JB. Nongeometric quantitative assessment of right and left ventricular function: myocardial performance index in normal children and patients with Ebstein anomaly. *J Am Soc Echocardiogr* 1998; **11**:849–56.

20 Yoshifuku S, Otsuji Y, Takasaki K, Yuge K, Kisanuki A, Toyonaga K, *et al*. Pseudonormalized Doppler total ejection isovolume (Tei) index in patients with right ventricular acute myocardial infarction. *Am J Cardiol* 2003; **91**:527–31.

Further reading

Haddad F, Hunt SA, Rosenthal DN, Murphy DJ. Right ventricular function in cardiovascular disease, part I: Anatomy, physiology, aging, and functional assessment of the right ventricle. *Circulation* 2008; **117**(11):1436–48.

Meluzin J, Spinarova L, Bakala J, Toman J, Krejci J, Hude P, *et al*. Pulsed Doppler tissue imaging of the velocity of tricuspid annular systolic motion: a new, rapid, and non-invasive method of evaluating right ventricular systolic function. *Eur Heart J* 2001; **22**(4):340–8.

Additional DVD and online material

- 11.1 Parasternal long-axis view of the right ventricle.
- 11.2 Long-axis view of the right ventricular inflow tract.
- 11.3 Parasternal short-axis view of right ventricular outflow tract.
- 11.4 Parasternal short-axis view at the level of papillary muscles.
- 11.5 Apical four-chamber view which visualizes the right ventricular lateral wall and interventricular septum.
- 11.6 Subcostal view which visualizes the right ventricular inferior wall.
- 11.7 Right ventricular volume overload.
- 11.8 Right ventricular pressure overload.
- 11.9 Volume rendered image of the right ventricle.
- 11.10 Multislice of the right ventricle.
- 11.11 Surface rendering of the measured right ventricular volume.

⟳ For additional multimedia materials please visit the online version of the book (http://escecho.oxfordmedicine.com).

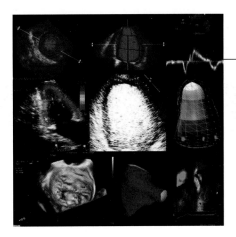

CHAPTER 12

Ischaemic heart disease

Petros Nihoyannopoulos
and Fausto Pinto

Contents

Summary

Echocardiography with its multiple modalities plays a central role in the evaluation of patients with known or suspected coronary artery disease, starting from the differential diagnosis of the patient presenting with acute chest pain. In the patient presenting with acute myocardial infarction (raised troponins) whether it is with ST-segment elevation or without, echocardiography is the first imaging modality used in order to ascertain the presence and extent of LV dysfunction and the presence of complications. In the absence of myocardial infarction (negative troponins), echocardiography will play an important diagnostic role in identifying the presence of reversible myocardial ischaemia. Stress echocardiography in many institutions is now the preferred stress modality associated with imaging as it is cost-effective and does not use ionizing radiation. Finally, echocardiography plays a pivotal role in the assessment of myocardial viability since the presence and extent of viable myocardium may guide therapeutic strategies. It has been stressed that laboratories and individuals need to have experience and be accredited by the authorities so that the results of echocardiographic investigations will be credible.

Introduction

Echocardiography has a central role in the diagnosis and management of patients with known or suspected coronary artery disease (CAD). Besides the fact that it plays a pivotal role in the differential diagnosis of patients presenting with chest pain in the emergency department and particularly in ruling out aortic dissection, echocardiography provides the possibility of performing a non-invasive haemodynamic and functional assessment of those patients.

Furthermore, echocardiography, by avoiding radiation, can be an alternative to other imaging modalities, often being more cost-effective. Therefore, it is necessary for practitioners to understand how echocardiography should be performed, its advantages and limitations, as well as the methods available to overcome those limitations.

In this chapter the spectrum of echocardiographic contributions in patients with ischaemic heart disease will be described.

Differential diagnosis in chest pain syndromes

Echocardiography plays an important role in the emergency department. Patients presenting to the emergency department complaining of acute chest pain often represent a diagnostic challenge. When a typical history of anginal pain is accompanied by ST-segment elevation, a diagnosis of evolving myocardial infarction can be made rapidly. Subarachnoid haemorrhage, acute pericarditis or myocarditis, hypertrophic cardiomyopathy, and aortic dissection may all mimic acute coronary syndromes, with potential catastrophic results for the patient as treatment for each of these conditions may be different. A potentially catastrophic scenario would be to give thrombolysis for suspected evolving myocardial infarction in a patient with aortic dissection or acute pericarditis. Conversely, not giving thrombolysis quickly in a patient with evolving myocardial infarction, because of a diagnostic uncertainty, may condemn the patient to sustain extensive myocardial damage. Echocardiography can readily recognize each of these clinical conditions and provide the precise diagnosis, allowing for appropriate and speedy intervention.

Acute myocardial infarction

Definition of myocardial infarction

Acute myocardial infarction is defined by the presence of acute chest pain or ischaemic equivalents associated to characteristic electrocardiographic (ECG) abnormalities lasting more than 20min and elevated myocardial necrosis biomarkers, such as troponin I, troponin T, creatine kinase-MB [CKMB], and myoglobin. According to specific ECG presentation, myocardial infarction is further divided into two categories: those with ST segment elevation (ST-elevation myocardial infarction, STEMI) and those without (non-ST-elevation myocardial infarction, NSTEMI). This early distinction is crucial as modern therapy greatly depends on it. Patients with STEMI should undergo primary angioplasty of the infarct-related artery, whereas patients with NSTEMI ought to be admitted and at first instance treated by medical therapy using acetylsalicylic acid, Clopidogrel, unfractionated heparin, nitrates and beta-blockers. If, however, they are at high risk (TIMI [Thrombolysis in Myocardial Infarction] risk score 5–7), coronary percutaneous intervention is recommended within 48 hours. If at intermediate risk (TIMI risk score 3–4), aggressive medical treatment followed by a provocative test is recommended.

Acute coronary artery occlusion leads to a rapid reduction in resting myocardial blood flow and hence cessation of muscular contraction in the area supplied. Relief of the occlusion, either spontaneously or by treatment resolves to recovery of regional wall function. The duration and severity of myocardial ischaemia determines the degree of wall motion abnormality (WMA): wall motion may not return to normal for several hours after the acute episode (*stunned myocardium*). The role of echocardiography in the setting of acute myocardial infarction is expressed by:

◆ The assessment of presence and extent of regional myocardial dysfunction.

◆ The assessment of presence of complications.

Assessment of left ventricular size and function

A standard protocol has been established, which requires at first the assessment of global size of the left ventricle (LV). Then, the overall LV function with an estimate of ejection fraction (EF) should be performed. Finally, the evaluation of the number of regional WMAs in a 16- or 17-segment model is strongly recommended.

Overall left ventricular size

Measurements of LV size are made from parasternal long-axis (PLAX) view at the tips of the mitral leaflets in diastole, as discussed in ➲ Chapter 2. There are two principles that need to be taken into account for this:

◆ Measurement of the LV sizes has to be performed perpendicularly to the septum and posterior wall.

◆ Good definition of the endocardium, particularly that of the posterior wall, is always required.

If either of those is not possible, then measurement should not be performed. It is important to emphasize that individuals who are performing and reporting echocardiographic studies need to be appropriately trained[1,2] and preferably the studies ought to be performed in an accredited laboratory.[3]

Global left ventricular function

There are several ways to assess global LV function (see ➲ Chapter 8). Historically, M-mode has been used to estimate LV function but this approach has inherent flaws as it only evaluates the most proximal portion of the ventricle, which, more often than not, is contracting well. Consequently, in the setting of acute myocardial infarction, M-mode echocardiography is not recommended to assess LV function.

The most widely used approach to assess global ventricular function is two-dimensional (2D) echocardiography and the recommended method is Simpson's apical biplane method[1] (see ➲ Chapter 8) (➲ Fig. 12.1). The average of volumes derived from the two apical views provides an accurate measurement of the overall LV function.

The prerequisite of accurate measurement of LV function is the ability to adequately visualize the endocardium. Unfortunately, this is not always possible: suboptimal visualization and

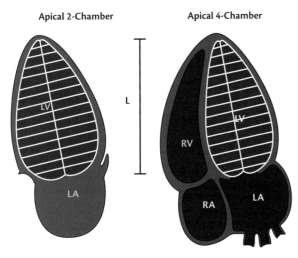

Figure 12.1 Modified Simpson's formula to calculate left ventricular volumes using the two standardized apical projections; the apical two-chamber view and the apical four-chamber view.

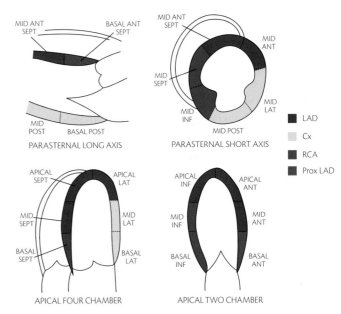

Figure 12.3 Coronary blood flow distribution. Regional distribution of coronary vascular beds from standardizsed parasternal (top) and apical (bottom) projections.

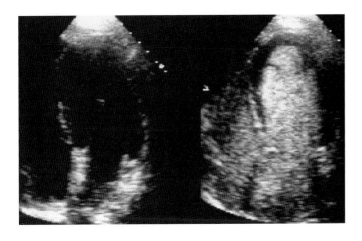

Figure 12.2 Endocardial border detection with ultrasound contrast agent. Apical four-chamber projections from a patient with sub-optimal endocardial visualizsation (left) improving dramatically after 0.3 mg of SonoVue® contrast injection (right).

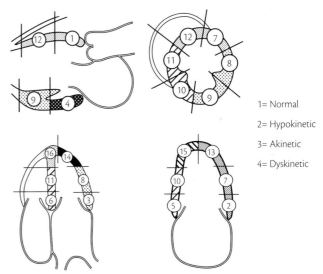

Figure 12.4 Regional wall motion assessment. Evaluation of regional wall motion score from two-dimensional echocardiography. Myocardial segments from 1 –16 indicate the regional segmentation of the left ventricle (see ➲ text).

consequently measurement of ejection fraction (EF) may lead to erroneous assessment of ventricular function. Although new imaging technologies using second harmonic imaging and other sophisticated post-processing methods has undoubtedly improved overall imaging, there are still a number of patients in which LV volumes cannot be evaluated. It is strongly recommended to use commercially available intravenous ultrasound contrast agents in order to improve endocardial border definition and consequently measure accurately LV volumes[4] (see ➲ Chapter 7) (➲ Fig. 12.2). With the use of ultrasound contrast agents, LV volumes assessment is comparable to that obtained with cardiac magnetic resonance (CMR).

The emergence of three-dimensional (3D) echocardiography is now able to assess LV volumes semi-automatically without making any geometric assumptions (see ➲ Chapters 3 and 8). The disadvantage of this imaging modality is that endocardial border delineation is still suboptimal and the ultrasound systems are not yet widely available, particularly in the acute setting.

Regional left ventricular function

This requires the evaluation of all 16 or 17 segments of the LV according to the American and European guidelines, as described in ➲ Chapter 8 (➲ Figs. 12.3 and 12.4).

Assessment of complications

Congestive heart failure

Following acute myocardial infarction, the LV undergoes a post-ischaemic remodelling, characterized by expansion of infarcted territory with wall thinning associated with compensatory ventricular hypertrophy in the non-infarcted territory. This ventricular remodelling may lead to heart failure (HF), particularly when the LAD territory is involved. This process can be followed over time by echocardiographic assessment.

Right ventricular infarction

This can cause a clinical scenario similar to LV heart failure with arterial hypotension. However, it necessitates fluid infusion rather than inotrope administration and is very difficult to diagnose clinically or by ECG alone. Conversely, the right ventricle (RV) can easily be described using echocardiography and, as for LV dysfunction, RV asynergy is a sensitive marker of myocardial infarction. The most commonly used views are the PLAX, short-axis (SAX), and apical two-chamber (A2C) views[5] (for assessment of RV function, see ⊃ Chapter 11).

Left ventricular wall rupture and ischaemic mitral regurgitation

Ventricular septal, free LV wall rupture, or papillary muscle dysfunction are difficult to clinically distinguish in a patient who develops a heart murmur, heart failure, or cardiogenic shock following acute myocardial infarction (⊃ Fig. 12.5).

Ventricular septal defect and LV free-wall rupture, usually at the apex or inferior segments, develop between day 1 and day 7 post-myocardial infarction and may easily be identified with 2D and colour flow imaging (for intracardiac shunt assessment, see ⊃ Chapter 5). Care must be taken to place the colour sector

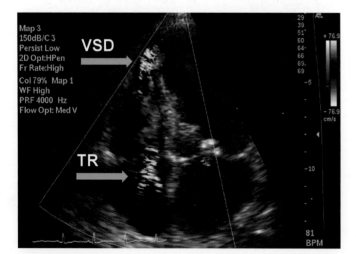

Figure 12.5 Left ventricular wall rupture. A patient with acute coronary syndrome 48h after admission. A systolic murmur was heard and an echocardiogram clearly showed the presence of an apical ventricular septal defect (VSD). Note the distinction between the VSD colour flow jet compared to the mild tricuspid regurgitant jet (TR).

across the ventricular septum both at the distal but also proximal part of the ventricular septum.

Occasionally, the free wall may not rupture into the pericardial sac, being enveloped by visceral pericardial layer and leading to a pseudoaneurysm. This needs to be distinguished from the more stable true aneurysm, because it is in danger of rupturing suddenly with catastrophic consequences. Again, echocardiography is ideally suited for the differential diagnosis at the bedside.

Ischaemic mitral regurgitation (MR) is one of the most frequent complications after myocardial infarction, accounting for 13–50% of patients included in large clinical trials. The incidence may rise up to 50–60%, if also transient MR is included. Such a complication seems to be associated with a poor outcome, as it independently predicts 1-year cardiovascular mortality and heart failure, particularly in patients with cardiogenic shock. Mechanisms underlying development of ischaemic MR may be:

◆ LV and mitral valve (MV) annulus dilation.

◆ Papillary muscle dysfunction or rupture.

◆ Acute systolic anterior motion of the MV.

Papillary muscle dysfunction and/or rupture can cause severe MR with pulmonary oedema and cardiogenic shock. Papillary muscle rupture is usually caused by a small myocardial infarct in the posterolateral wall, which is the territory of distribution of the right or circumflex coronary artery: as posterior papillary muscle is supplied by a single coronary artery, the incidence of its damage and rupture is 6–10 times higher than anterior papillary muscle, which receives two different vascularizations. Rupture of a papillary muscle can be partial or complete.

Recognition of the exact mechanism of ischaemic MR is mandatory in this clinical setting, because different therapeutic strategies have to be performed: papillary muscle rupture requires urgent MV replacement or repair, whereas ischaemic MR due to papillary muscle dysfunction or annulus dilation may improve with afterload reduction and coronary revascularization. Echocardiography with its fine spatial resolution can detect the underlying cardiac abnormality and assess the severity of MR (for MR assessment, see ⊃ Chapter 14b). Colour Doppler (CD) imaging is a useful tool in order to assess MR severity. As most patients present with haemodynamic instability, transoesophageal echocardiography (TOE) is necessary to achieve clear diagnosis. Echocardiographic imaging of papillary muscle rupture shows an echogenic mass attached to the MV or a mobile mass prolapsing into the LA during systole and moving back into the LV during diastole. In some patients, the ruptured papillary muscle head is not visualized to prolapse into the LA.

Left ventricular thrombus

This usually forms at the apex following acute anterior myocardial infarction. It may be difficult to detect particularly when the apex is imaged obliquely. Here the use of intravenous administration of ultrasound contrast agent will definitely confirm or refute the presence of thrombus[4] (see ➲ Chapter 7) (➲ Fig. 12.6).

Stable coronary artery disease

Diagnosis

There is a well-established parallel relationship between regional coronary blood flow and contractile function in the corresponding territory[6,7] (see ➲ Chapter 13).

In patients with a significant coronary artery stenosis (>70%), resting regional blood flow remains normal. When, however, oxygen demand increases, there is an inability to increase coronary perfusion to that area. This leads to a reduction of flow in the corresponding vascular territory leading to a reduction in wall thickening (hypokinesia). When oxygen demand is reduced with cessation of exercise, there is resolution of ischaemia and wall thickening returns to normal.[7]

Mechanism of reversible ischaemia

In chronic CAD, progressive reduction in myocardial blood flow due to the progression of CAD may result in downregulation of myocardial contractile function with preserved metabolic activity (*hibernating myocardium*). When myocardial blood flow is restored through revascularization of the stenotic arteries, contractile function is gradually restored. The detection of such regional LV dysfunction is important as it occurs early in the *ischaemic cascade* preceding ECG changes and symptoms.

Myocardial ischaemia is not the only cause of regional myocardial dysfunction (see ➲ Chapter 8). Distinction of non-ischaemic conditions from reversible ischaemia is mandatory in management of patients with chest pain.

Stress echo for ischaemia

Myocardial ischaemia is accompanied by characteristic mechanical, electrical, and perfusional abnormalities. Although coronary angiography is the gold standard for the diagnosis of CAD, the anatomical description alone does not indicate the physiological significance of stenosis. Exercise ECG, perfusion defects on technetium scans (single-photon emission computed tomography, SPECT), positron emission tomography (PET), or abnormalities of myocardial contractile reserve detected by stress echocardiography (or CMR) permit the assessment of the functional severity of coronary stenoses. Stress echocardiography has acquired an unquestioned clinical role as an accurate and inexpensive stress imaging technique[8] (➲ Figs. 12.7 and 12.8). For stress echocardiography principles and protocols, see ➲ Chapter 13.

Feasibility

The perceived disadvantage of stress echocardiography is its inability to obtain optimal imaging in all patients examined so that clear endocardial border delineation may not be possible. However, with the recent availability of intravenously administered ultrasound contrast agents worldwide, image quality is no longer an issue.[4] The use of ultrasound contrast agents during stress echocardiography is strongly recommended by the European Association of Echocardiography when more than two contiguous segments are not well visualized (➲ see Chapter 7).

Stress echocardiography, like all imaging techniques, is also an operator-dependent technique, both in respect to data acquisition and interpretation. Familiarity with all forms of

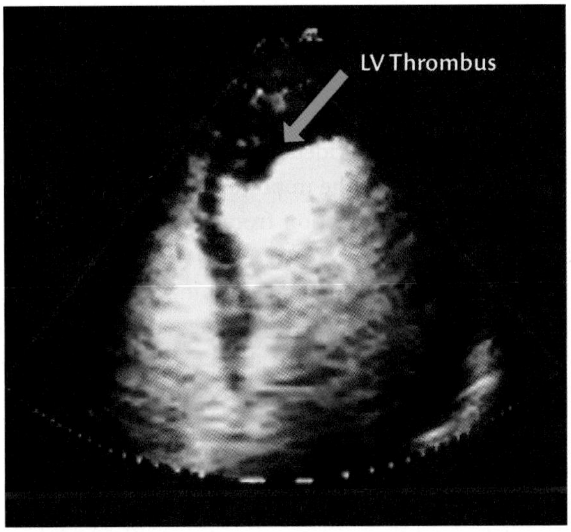

Figure 12.6 Left ventricular LV thrombus. Contrast echocardiography from apical four-chamber view in a patient with a 5-day post-myocardial infarction. Notice that at the apex there is a non-opacified longitudinal structure packing the apex, suggestive of an apical thrombus.

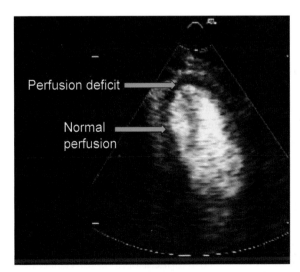

Figure 12.7 Myocardial perfusion defect. Stress test at maximum dobutamine dose (40mg/kg/min) from a patient referred with chest pain. From this apical four-chamber projection an apical hypoperfused area (arrow) is noted, while in the most proximal septal region the wall is normally opacified with contrast suggestive of normal perfusion.

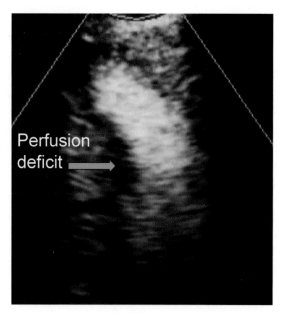

Figure 12.8 Myocardial perfusion defect. Another patient with chest pain. Apical two-chamber view demonstrating that the perfusion deficit now is in the inferior wall (arrow).

stress is an index of the quality of the echo laboratory. In this way, indications in the individual patient can be optimized, thereby avoiding the relative and absolute contraindications of each test. Proper training and experience is therefore pivotal, as for all imaging.[9] Finally, the use of contrast agents during stress echocardiography may also give important information about myocardial perfusion and further increases the diagnostic accuracy of the technique.[10]

Risk assessment

Stress echocardiography is an important test for screening high-risk patients before major peripheral vascular surgery or orthopaedic surgery, or in patients with chronic renal failure (➲ see Chapter 13).

A normal stress echocardiogram yields an annual risk of 0.4–0.9% based on a total of 9000 patients,[11] the same as for a normal stress myocardial perfusion scan. The positive and the negative response can be further stratified with interactions with clinical parameters (diabetes, renal dysfunction, and therapy at the time of test), resting echo (global LV function), and additive stress echo parameters (LV cavity dilation, coronary flow reserve, and previous revascularization).

Old myocardial infarction

CAD is responsible for almost two-thirds of cases of LV dysfunction. Established treatment options for ischaemic heart failure include medical therapy, revascularization, cardiac transplantation, and, more recently, cardiac resynchronization therapy (CRT).[12] Despite significant therapeutic advances, outcome of medical therapy in severe HF is still poor.[13,14] In specific

subsets of patients, the potential benefits of revascularization must be weighed against the potential high periprocedural risks, therefore it is crucial to correctly identify the group of those patients that will benefit from interventional procedures.

LV dysfunction due to CAD results from a combination of necrosis and scarring, as well as from functional and morphological adaptive abnormalities of the viable myocardium. The term *viability* has been used as a synonym of *contractile recovery*. So, in the setting of chronic LV dysfunction, this definition usually refers to the downregulation of contractile function in surviving myocardium in response to periodic or sustained reduction in coronary blood flow, which may be potentially reversed if normal blood flow is restored.

In the clinical setting, the individual patient can have various mixtures of stunned, hibernating, ischaemic, and fibrotic myocardium, in a variety of arrangements. As roughly 40% of myocardial segments with resting WMAs after acute myocardial infarction have viable tissue that may recover contractile function if revascularized, detection of viable myocardium is clinically relevant.

Myocardial stunning describes the post-ischaemic metabolic and contractile compromise in viable myocardium after a transient coronary occlusion (i.e. post-successful reperfusion in acute myocardial infarction). In stunned myocardium, blood flow has been restored but contraction has not returned to baseline. Dysfunction might persist from hours to weeks, but generally improves with time. An exception is repetitive stunning, defined as repeated episodes of ischaemia producing prolonged post-ischaemic contractile dysfunction,[15] which is similar to hibernation in that revascularization has the potential to improve contractile function.

Myocardial hibernation is a chronic state of impaired contractility at rest in non-infarcted myocardium as the result of persistently reduced blood flow, which has the potential to improve function after restoration of myocardial blood supply. The ability to recover systolic function after revascularization depends on the severity of structural abnormalities, i.e. the correction of cellular changes and the amount of tissue fibrosis.[16] These observations, and evidence that apoptosis is important in hibernation, underscore the importance of early revascularization in this dynamic transition from reversible to irreversible contractile dysfunction.[15,17]

Theoretically, hibernation and stunning are different pathophysiological states but, practically, they are often indistinct, appear to coexist in varying degrees in the same patient or myocardial region, and represent a continuum of the same process.[18] However, the timing of functional recovery after revascularization appears to differ between stunned and hibernating myocardium. Stunned myocardium recovery appears to be early after revascularization and more complete, while recovery of hibernating myocardium is late and often incomplete.[17]

Perioperative mortality rates for coronary artery bypass graft (CABG) surgery in LV systolic dysfunction vary widely, from approximately 5% in younger adults to more than 30% in order adults with more severe LV systolic dysfunction and comorbidities.[19] Similarly, percutaneous transluminal coronary angioplasty alone in LV systolic dysfunction is associated with a high periprocedural mortality of 2.5–5%. In a reported registry (before stents), 18.2% of patients with LVEF between 25–35% experienced nonfatal myocardial infarction and acute closure.[19]

Although published series allude to potential survival benefits of revascularization in ischaemic cardiomyopathy, limitations in study design and higher periprocedural risk have created uncertainty about the optimal treatment strategy. This has provided the rationale for non-invasive viability testing, which has potential value in moderate-to-severe ischaemic cardiomyopathy, identifying patients whose symptoms and natural history may potentially improve with revascularization.

Assessment of myocardial viability

The main goal of myocardial viability assessment is detecting dysfunctional myocardium that would improve in function once normal blood supply was restored. Several observational studies demonstrated that patients with ischaemic LV dysfunction with extensive areas of viable myocardium have lower perioperative mortality, greater regional and global LV function recovery, fewer HF symptoms, and improved survival after revascularization. After revascularization, the annual mortality rate in patients with viable myocardium was half as high as in patients without viable myocardium. Conversely, in those patients without significant myocardial viability, there was a trend toward a higher mortality following revascularization. So, it seems that survival benefit is obtained when the need of revascularization is guided by preoperative assessment of myocardial viability.

A number of non-invasive imaging procedures have been developed to evaluate myocardial viability and to identify markers of functional recovery, including dobutamine stress echocardiography, myocardial contrast echocardiography, SPECT, PET and CMR imaging. The currently available imaging techniques assess distinct characteristics of viable and dysfunctional myocardium, having different limitations and diagnostic accuracy. Comparison of the clinical utility of each in the assessment of myocardial viability is currently limited by the lack of randomized prospective trials. Besides, there is uncertainty about the best criteria to determine the clinical benefit of the assessment of myocardial viability, by which they should be compared. Several studies evaluated their accuracy for prediction of segmental improvement, but the global LV functional recovery after revascularization has greater clinical relevance. Theoretically, the best method should be the one with the optimal sensitivity and specificity for detection of viability. However, since the amount of hibernating myocardium is the critical determinant of global functional recovery, even methods with moderately high sensitivity may eventually identify those patients with great benefit. The precise extent of viability necessary to predict benefit from revascularization is unclear and may vary in different clinical circumstances. Most studies suggested that a substantial amount of viable myocardium (at least 20–30% of LV mass) is required for the improvement of LVEF. Hence, both identification and quantification of the extent of viable myocardium are required for a careful selection of patients who have a higher likelihood of benefit from revascularization. However, several authors showed that survival rates after CABG surgery were similar whether or not function improved after intervention, suggesting that relevant clinical benefits may occur even without LVEF recovery. Preservation of small viable areas may improve clinical outcome by reducing the risk of subsequent ischaemic events, improving LV remodelling processes, preventing additional LV dilation, promoting electrical stability, and eventually improving symptoms and functional capacity. So, large-scale prospective head-to-head comparisons of the available imaging modalities are needed to determine their independent value for detection of viable myocardium and to evaluate their accuracy in predicting patient response to therapy, regarding LV function recovery, symptoms, and survival.

Rest echocardiography

Resting echocardiographic examination is the single most useful test in the assessment of HF since structural abnormality, systolic dysfunction, diastolic dysfunction, or a combination of these abnormalities need to be obtained for the diagnosis of HF. Moreover, resting echocardiography provides valuable information that may guide the choice of imaging technique to use and assist in its interpretation. If there is adequate image quality, allowing full visualization of endocardial border and wall thickening in all myocardial segments, dobutamine stress echocardiography may be the test of choice. If the acoustic window is insufficient to provide a high degree of diagnostic certainty, despite contrast enhancement, another imaging approach should be used. Moreover, the wall motion score index (WMSI) and LVEF at rest differently affects accuracy of the several imaging methods used to assess viability.

The assessment of LV end-diastolic wall thickness can be used to obtain a first evaluation of myocardial viability: thinned (<6mm) and dense myocardial segments typically reflect scar tissue and have particularly low probability of improvement in function, while dysfunctional segments with preserved wall thickness (≥6mm) may be viable. The involvement of more than four ventricular wall segments by scarring is associated with low probability of global functional recovery after revascularization. Furthermore, the degree of LV remodelling and dilation may be an additional guide to predict functional recovery post revascularization. The likelihood of significant recovery of global LV function is inversely related to ventricular volume. LV end-diastolic volume (LVEDV) greater than 220mL is unlikely to show significant functional recovery, as the likelihood of significant scar tissue is high in the severely remodelled LV.

Until recently, resting echocardiography was considered of limited utility in discriminating viable from non-viable myocardium. However, myocardial velocity assessment with tissue Doppler (TD) imaging and speckle tracking-derived parameters may unmask viable myocardium.

TD imaging allows accurate assessment of regional myocardial function during all phases of the cardiac cycle. Experimental and clinical studies showed that TD-derived analysis of ejection systolic velocities, strain, and strain rate allows accurate definition of transmurality of myocardial infarction. TD-based longitudinal strain and strain rate are reduced in segments with subendocardial scarring, although the relationship is non-linear since subendocardium governs transmural contraction and longitudinal function. However, angle dependency (incapacity to assess shortening or thickening whenever the principal vector of contraction is not aligned with the ultrasound beam) significantly impairs their accuracy. Other TD-derived parameters may be useful to assess myocardial viability, particularly the detection of myocardial positive pre-ejection velocity occurring during isovolumic contraction. Penicka and co-workers[20] demonstrated high accuracy of TD-derived myocardial positive pre-ejection velocity qualitatively assessed by pulsed TD imaging to predict recovery of contractile function in patients with chronic CAD, WMAs, and global systolic dysfunction submitted to revascularization. The presence of positive pre-ejection velocity predicted improvement of regional function after revascularization (sensitivity 93%; specificity 77%), and the presence of positive pre-ejection velocity in five or more dysfunctional segments had a high accuracy to predict moderate (sensitivity 92%; specificity 79%) and marked (sensitivity 93%; specificity 60%) recovery of global systolic function.

Recently, Becker and co-workers[21] showed that myocardial deformation imaging in rest based on speckle tracking allows the assessment of transmurality since radial and circumferential strain impairment is proportional to the transmural scarring extent. Moreover, they also found that peak systolic radial strain identifies reversible myocardial dysfunction and predicts regional and global functional recovery at 9 ± 2 months of follow-up. Segments with functional recovery had significantly higher baseline peak systolic radial and circumferential strain values and a peak systolic strain greater than 17.2% predicted segmental functional recovery (sensitivity 70.2%; specificity 85.1%). Besides, a positive correlation was found between the number of segments with a peak systolic strain greater than 17.2% and LVEF improvement after surgical or percutaneous coronary revascularization. Moreover, the predictive value was similar to that achieved by contrast-enhanced CMR.[21]

Myocardial contrast echocardiography

Assessment of myocardial viability by myocardial contrast echocardiography (MCE) is based on the assumption that myocardial viability needs a preserved microvasculature. With its excellent spatial resolution (<1mm axially), MCE can accurately depict the presence of microvascular integrity (see ➲ Chapter 7). After a myocardial infarction, myocyte loss is associated with a loss of microvasculature; therefore absence of myocardial contrast enhancement on MCE should define regions that lack myocardial viability.[22] In patients with ischaemic cardiomyopathy undergoing coronary artery bypass grafting, Shimoni et al.[23] demonstrated an excellent correlation between contrast signal intensity and capillary density obtained from myocardial biopsies of the same region. Moreover, contrast signal intensity was inversely related to the extent of fibrosis. Peak contrast intensity has also been shown to correlate with the extent and severity of myocardial necrosis, as assessed by gadolinium-enhanced CMR imaging 7 days after acute myocardial infarction[24] (see ➲ Chapter 7).

MCE plays an important role in predicting the recovery of regional and global systolic function post-myocardial infarction. One month after myocardial infarction, patients with a patent infarct-related artery (IRA) and good contrast opacification demonstrated an improvement in contractile function compared with those patients with a poor or absent contrast opacification. Low-dose dobutamine echocardiography is widely used to assess myocardial viability. Huang et al.[25] found a good concordance between MCE and low-dose dobutamine echocardiography in predicting functional recovery after myocardial infarction. The presence of contrast enhancement even in segments that lack contractile response during dobutamine results in an improvement in regional function compared with those with no contrast enhancement.

Several MCE studies have demonstrated high sensitivity (75–90%) but poorer specificity (50–60%) in identifying the recovery of contractile function after myocardial infarction. The majority of the studies consisted of patients studied early after reperfusion and only assessed during rest. The combination of reactive hyperaemia, dynamic changes in the microcirculation early after myocardial infarction, and the fact that myocardial infarction involving more than 20% of the subendocardium can render the myocardium akinetic despite significant epicardial and mid-myocardial viability,[26] tend to make MCE less specific for the detection of myocardial viability if viability is defined in terms of the recovery of systolic function. Technical factors such as the inability to distinguish microbubble signature from the underlying tissue can also contribute to the low specificity of MCE. The key to improved accuracy for determining viability in a reperfused territory after myocardial infarction is to perform MCE at least 24h after reperfusion (➲ Fig. 12.9).

A combined assessment of perfusion and contractile reserve provides the most optimum sensitivity and specificity[27] (see ➲ Chapter 7).

Stress echocardiography

Infusions of low-dose dobutamine (see ➲ Chapter 13) increase contractility in dysfunctional but viable myocardium usually

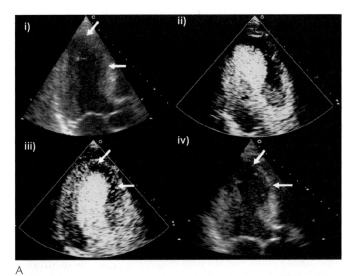

A

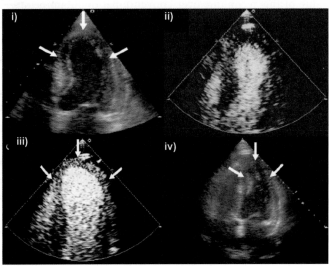

B

Figure 12.9 Viability assessment by MCE. A) End-systolic frames of the apical three-chamber view showing: i) akinetic mid-anterior septum and apex (arrows); ii) complete destruction of myocardial contrast immediately after a high mechanical index pulse on MCE; iii) lack of contrast opacification of the dyssynergic segments, even at 15 cycles (arrows); iv) lack of functional recovery at 12 weeks despite revascularizsation (arrows). B) End-systolic frames of the apical four-chamber view showing: i) akinetic mid-septum, apex, and mid-lateral segments (arrows); ii) complete destruction of myocardial contrast immediately after a high mechanical index pulse on MCE; iii) homogenous contrast opacification of the dyssynergic segments by 15 cardiac cycles (arrows); iv) functional recovery at 12 weeks after revascularizsation (arrows). Adapted from Cortez Dias N, Senior R, Pinto F. Iin *The ESC Textbook of Cardiovascular Medicine*, 2010.

without significant tachycardia. A combination of low and high doses has been shown to provide the greatest diagnostic information and accuracy for prediction of functional recovery after revascularization. This is ascribed to the ability of high-dose dobutamine infusion to recognize ischaemia with higher accuracy.

The pattern of response (see ➲ Chapter 13) is predictive of post-revascularization functional improvement. A biphasic response, indicating that the tissue is not only viable but also supplied by a stenosed artery, has greatest predictive accuracy for recovery. A uniphasic response with sustained improvement has limited specificity to predict functional recovery since augmentation alone may occur not only with non-jeopardized myocardium (stunned) but also in areas of non-transmural infarction without hibernating myocardium (subendocardial scar) or in remodelled myocardium. Finally, about 20–25% of viable segments do not improve functionally during inotropic stimulation since they have an almost exhausted blood flow reserve and extensive structural abnormalities. However, those viable segments without improvement with dobutamine stimulation usually do not recover contractile function after revascularization.

Various studies demonstrated that LVEF improved only in patients with substantial viability. A linear relation was present between the number of viable segments and the likelihood of recovery of overall LV function after revascularization, and the identification of four or more viable segments accurately predicted LVEF improvement (e.g. ≥5%) after revascularization, improvement in HF symptoms, and reduction of event-rate.[28]

Alternative protocols for echocardiographic assessment of myocardial viability include dipyridamole, low-level exercise (see ➲ Chapter 13) , and, more recently, levosimendan. Exercise, dobutamine, and dipyridamole show similar diagnostic accuracy in the induction of ischaemia. However, dobutamine stress echocardiography is the most extensively studied modality and the most widely used test for the assessment of myocardial viability. Cianfrocca and co-workers[29] compared the accuracy of levosimendan stress echocardiography with conventional dobutamine stress echocardiography. Levosimendan enhances cardiac contractility via Ca^{2+} sensitization without increasing myocardial oxygen consumption, and induces vasodilation through the activation of adenosine triphosphate-sensitive potassium channels. They found that levosimendan was more reliable than dobutamine in predicting reversible dysfunction, having higher sensitivity (75% vs. 59%; p = 0.026) and similar specificity (80%). Of note, a further improvement for prediction of functional recovery was found when wall motion response during levosimendan stress echocardiography was complemented by measurement of peak systolic strain rate based on TD imaging.

From experienced laboratories, visual wall motion assessment demonstrated a mean sensitivity of 85% and specificity of 79% in regional functional recovery prediction.[28] Inter- and intraobserver WMSI variability is even greater in those patients with previous myocardial infarction due to pre-existing WMAs and intraventricular conduction defects.

In recent years, quantitative parameters, such as acoustic quantification, colour kinesis, and TD myocardial velocity derived parameters (see ➲ Chapter 6), have been studied to provide objective and reproducible information on global and regional wall function during stress. Pre-ejection longitudinal tissue velocity change and peak systolic longitudinal velocity change assessed by pulsed-wave TD imaging during low-dose dobutamine are reliable parameters of myocardial viability, since their increase during the stress test strongly predicts recovery after revascularization. However, evaluation of myocardial velocities by pulsed-wave TD imaging during dobutamine stress echocardiography is a very time-consuming technique without proved incremental value, being impracticable in everyday practice. Strain and strain rate are less dependent on image quality and less subjective than the visual assessment of endocardial border motion (➲ Fig. 12.10). During dobutamine stress echocardiography, circumferential strain and strain rate are significantly lower in segments with myocardial infarction, compared to both subendocardial infarcts and

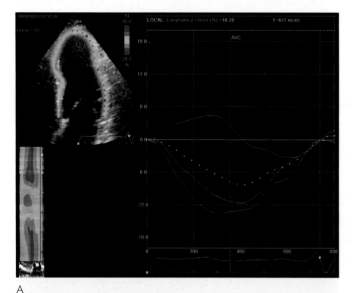

A

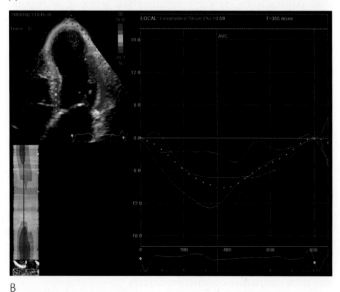

B

Figure 12.10 Strain and strain rate during stress echocardiography. Example of strain curves at rest (A) and with low-dose dobutamine (B) in a patient with previous antero-septal acute myocardial infarction, showing improvement in the distal septum segment demonstrating the presence of a viable segment.

normal myocardium, thus assessing the degree of transmurality. The assessment of strain rate imaging as an adjunct to routine visual wall-motion scoring during conventional dobutamine stress echocardiography provides incremental value to predict regional and global functional recovery following revascularization. A strain rate increment of 0.25/s during stress echo is the optimal cut-off for functional recovery prediction. Strain rate is a better quantitative parameter for the prediction of functional recovery compared to strain. Recent advances in this technology raised the prospect that strain rate imaging may become a routinely employed modality for quantitative assessment of viability during dobutamine stress echocardiography.

Finally, technological advances in transducer and computer technology led to introduction of real-time 3D echocardiography during stress but no data currently shows the additional value of this technique over conventional dobutamine stress echocardiography.

Ischaemic mitral regurgitation

As in the acute phase of myocardial infarction, chronic MR due to CAD shows prognostic implications, since it increases total and cardiovascular mortality. It has been demonstrated that an effective regurgitant orifice area (EROA) of 20mm² or more and a regurgitant volume (RVol) of 30mL or more were associated with increased mortality. EROA is mostly determined by MV deformation, which in turn is caused by apical and posterior displacement of the papillary muscles and contractile dysfunction of myocardial segments supporting papillary muscles and MV apparatus. Surgical treatment of such pathological condition has not been still demonstrated to improve patient outcome, because post-ischaemic cardiac remodelling also plays an important role in long-term prognosis.

Coronary artery anomalies

Coronary artery anomalies are congenital abnormalities of origin or course of coronary arteries. They occur in less than 1% of the general population, often in combination with other congenital heart disease. Although in many cases they do not cause symptoms, coronary artery anomalies are associated with increased risk of sudden death, particularly in athletes. Because these anomalies may be successfully treated by surgical approach, prompted recognition avoids unfavourable outcome.

Coronary artery anomalies most frequently associated with sudden cardiac death are those characterized by wrong aortic sinus origin (and course between the aorta and pulmonary trunk). These coronary anomalies include origin of the left main coronary artery from the right aortic sinus and origin of the right coronary artery from the left sinus.[30] Sudden death is mainly considered to be related to myocardial ischaemia episodes. Indeed, repetitive ischaemic episodes may result in patchy myocardial necrosis and fibrosis, which could predispose to lethal ventricular tachyarrhythmias by creating an electrically unstable myocardial substrate. Mechanisms, by which coronary artery anomalies determine myocardial ischaemia, may be different:

♦ The acute angle take-off and kinking of the coronary artery as it arises from the aorta.

♦ Flap-like closure of the abnormal slit-like coronary orifice.

♦ Compression of the anomalous coronary artery between the aorta and pulmonary trunk during exercise.

♦ Spasm of the anomalous coronary artery, possibly as a result of endothelial injury.

In some cases, the course of the proximal portion of the anomalous coronary artery is intramural, i.e. contained completely within the aortic wall, so that the coronary artery and the aorta share the same media without an interpositioned adventitia.[30]

The majority of athletes die during or after strenuous and prolonged exertion. Premonitory cardiovascular symptoms occur only in a few patients and usually consist in:

♦ Syncope episodes during exertion or in sedentary circumstances.

♦ Chest pain episodes (either typical or atypical of angina).

♦ Palpitations unrelated to physical activity.

Unfortunately, in these patients exercise stress test usually does not show electrocardiographic abnormalities suggestive for myocardial ischaemia.[30] Conversely, the anatomy of these malformations can be suspected or defined non-invasively by transthoracic echocardiography (TTE) or TOE, because echocardiography provides good anatomical definition of the ostium and proximal epicardial course of coronary arteries. In 1360 young athletes prospectively evaluated by echocardiography, the ostium and proximal epicardial course of left main coronary artery were visualized in 97% and right coronary artery in 80% of subjects.[31] Echocardiographic assessment of origin and course of coronary arteries, usually by PSAX view at the aortic level, is an efficient means to detect wrong sinus coronary malformations in a large population of children and adolescents: investigation of ostium and proximal course of coronary arteries should be a routine part of any echocardiographic study. When the origin of both coronary arteries cannot be identified by TTE, TOE is recommended. Colour flow imaging can further aid in the location of the origin and course of these abnormal vessels. Although TOE is able to visualize proximal coronary arteries and their abnormalities, some limitations exist. The position of the transducer, cardiac motion, and the curvilinear nature of the vessel along the epicardial surface impair the view of distal segments of coronary artery. Finally, if none of the non-invasive techniques are successful and suspicion for coronary artery anomalies is still high, coronary angiography is definitive.

Personal perspective

Echocardiography is the first imaging technique commonly used in evaluation of patients with suspected or known CAD. Knowledge of regional and global contractile function, as well as myocardial viability, is fundamental in establishing the diagnosis, management strategy, and prognosis of such patients, particularly because the treatment of myocardial infarction with thrombolysis and percutaneous coronary intervention has changed the natural history of the pathology. Exercise and pharmacological stress echocardiography have added relevant contributions to diagnostic process and prognostic stratification. Moreover, echocardiography plays a crucial role in clinical management of patients with acute coronary syndromes which occur in the absence of clear electrocardiographic abnormalities, allowing the formulation of differential diagnosis between cardiac and extracardiac causes of chest pain and to detect coronary artery abnormalities associated with a high risk of sudden death. Finally, both TTE and TOE provide a great advantage in identifying most, if not all, mechanical complications of acute and chronic myocardial infarction. Novel echocardiographic techniques will have further increasing importance in management of ischaemic heart diseases.

References

1 Popescu BA, Andrade MJ, Badano LP, Fox KF, Flachskampf FA, Lancellotti P, *et al.* European Association of Echocardiography recommendations for training, competence, and quality improvement in echocardiography. *Eur J Echocardiogr* 2009; **10**:893–905.

2 British Society of Echocardiography Guidelines. Training in echocardiography. *Br Heart J* 1994; **71**:2–5.

3 Nihoyannopoulos P, Fox K, Fraser A, Pinto F. EAE laboratory standards and accreditation. *Eur J Echocardiogr* 2007; **8**:80–7.

4 Senior R, Becher H, Monaghan M, Agati L, Zamorano J, Vanoverschelde JL, *et al.* Contrast echocardiography: evidence-based recommendations by European Association of Echocardiography. *Eur J Echocardiogr* 2009; **10**:194–212.

5 Foale RA, Nihoyannopoulos P, McKenna WJ, Kleinebenne A, Nadazdin A, Rowland E, *et al.* The echocardiographic measurements of the normal adult right ventricle. *Br Heart J* 1986; **56**:33.

6 Tennant R, Wiggers CJ. The effect of coronary artery occlusion on myocardial contraction. *Am J Physiol* 1935; **12**:351.

7 Gallagher KP, Matsuzaki M, Osakada G, Kemper S, Ross J Jr. Effect of exercise on the relationship between myocardial blood flow and systolic wall thickening in dogs with acute coronary stenosis. *Circ Res* 1983; **52**:716–29.

8 Sicari R, Nihoyannopoulos P, Evangelista A, Kasprzak J, Lancellotti P, Poldermans D, *et al.* Stress echocardiography expert consensus statement European Association of Echocardiography (EAE). *Eur J Echocardiogr* 2008; **9**:415–37.

9 Pamela S. Douglas. Appropriateness criteria for stress echocardiography. *J Am Coll Cardiol* 2008; **51**:1127–47.

10 Elhendy A, O'Leary EL, Xie F, McGrain AC, Anderson JR, Porter TR. Comparative accuracy of real-time myocardial contrast perfusion imaging and all motion analysis during dobutamine stress echocardiography for the diagnosis of coronary artery disease. *J Am Coll Cardiol* 2004; **44**:2185–91.

11 Metz LD, Beattie M, Hom R, Redberg RF, Grády D, Fleischmann KE. The prognostic value of normal exercise myocardial perfusion imaging and exercise echocardiography: a meta-analysis. *J Am Coll Cardiol* 2007; **49**:227–37.

12 Melo LG, Pachori AS, Kong D, Gnecchi M, Wang K, Pratt RE, *et al.* Molecular and cell-based therapies for protection, rescue, and repair of ischemic myocardium: reasons for cautious optimism. *Circulation* 2004; **109**(20):2386–93.

13 Bax JJ, van der Wall EE, Harbinson M. Radionuclide techniques for the assessment of myocardial viability and hibernation. *Heart* 2004; **90**(Suppl 5):v26–33.:v26–v33.

14 Cleland JG, Pennell DJ, Ray SG, Coats AJ, Macfarlane PW, Murray GD, *et al.* Myocardial viability as a determinant of the ejection fraction response to carvedilol in patients with heart failure (CHRISTMAS trial): randomised controlled trial. *Lancet* 2003; **362**(9377):14–21.

15 Dispersyn GD, Borgers M, Flameng W. Apoptosis in chronic hibernating myocardium: sleeping to death? *Cardiovasc Res* 2000; **45**(3):696–703.

16 Bax JJ, Visser FC, Poldermans D, Elhendy A, Cornel JH, Boersma E, *et al.* Time course of functional recovery of stunned and hibernating segments after surgical revascularization. *Circulation* 2001; **104**(12 Suppl 1):I314–I318.

17 Beanlands RS, Hendry PJ, Masters RG, deKemp RA, Woodend K, Ruddy TD. Delay in revascularization is associated with increased mortality rate in patients with severe left ventricular dysfunction and viable myocardium on fluorine 18-fluorodeoxyglucose positron emission tomography imaging. *Circulation* 1998; **98**(19 Suppl):II51–II56.

18 Senior R, Lahiri A. Dobutamine echocardiography predicts functional outcome after revascularisation in patients with dysfunctional myocardium irrespective of the perfusion pattern on resting thallium-201 imaging. *Heart* 1999; **82**(6):668–73.

19 Alderman EL, Fisher LD, Litwin P, Kaiser GC, Myers WO, Maynard C, *et al.* Results of coronary artery surgery in patients with poor left ventricular function (CASS). *Circulation* 1983; **68**(4):785–95.

20 Penicka M, Tousek P, De Bruyne B, Wijns W, Lang O, Madaric J, *et al.* Myocardial positive pre-ejection velocity accurately detects presence of viable myocardium, predicts recovery of left ventricular function and bears a prognostic value after surgical revascularization. *Eur Heart J* 2007; **28**(11):1366–73.

21 Becker M, Lenzen A, Ocklenburg C, Stempel K, Kuhl H, Neizel M, *et al.* Myocardial deformation imaging based on ultrasonic pixel tracking to identify reversible myocardial dysfunction. *J Am Coll Cardiol* 2008; **51**(15):1473–81.

22 Senior R, Swinburn JM. Incremental value of myocardial contrast echocardiography for the prediction of recovery of function in dobutamine nonresponsive myocardium early after acute myocardial infarction. *Am J Cardiol* 2003; **91**:397–402.

23 Shimoni S, Frangogiannis NG, Aggeli CJ, Shan K, Quinones MA, Espada R, *et al.* Microvascular structural correlates of myocardial contrast echocardiography in patients with coronary artery disease and left ventricular dysfunction: implications for the assessment of myocardial hibernation. *Circulation* 2002; **106**:950–6.

24 Janardhanan R, Moon JC, Pennell DJ, Senior R. Myocardial contrast echocardiography accurately reflects transmurality of myocardial necrosis and predicts contractile reserve after acute myocardial infarction. *Am Heart J* 2005; **149**(2):355–62.

25 Huang WC, Chiou KR, Liu CP, Lin SL, Lee D, Mar GY, *et al.* Comparison of real-time contrast echocardiography and low-dose dobutamine stress echocardiography in predicting the left ventricular functional recovery in patients after acute myocardial infarction under different therapeutic intervention. *Int J Cardiol* 2005; **104**:81–91.

26 Myers JH, Stirling MC, Choy M, Buda AJ, Gallagher KP. Direct measurement of inner and outer wall thickening dynamics with epicardial echocardiography. *Circulation* 1986; **74**:164–72.

27 Meza MF, Ramee S, Collins T, Stapleton D, Milani RV, Murgo JP, *et al.* Knowledge of perfusion and contractile reserve improves the predictive value of recovery of regional myocardial function post revascularization: a study using the combination of myocardial contrast echocardiography and dobutamine echocardiography. *Circulation* 1997; **96**:3459–65.

28 Rizzello V, Poldermans D, Bax JJ. Assessment of myocardial viability in chronic ischemic heart disease: current status. *Q J Nucl Med Mol Imaging* 2005; **49**(1):81–96.

29 Cianfrocca C, Pelliccia F, Pasceri V, Auriti A, Guido V, Mercuro G, *et al.* Strain rate analysis and levosimendan improve detection of myocardial viability by dobutamine echocardiography in patients with post-infarction left ventricular dysfunction: a pilot study. *J Am Soc Echocardiogr* 2008; **21**(9):1068–74.

30 Basso C, Maron B J, Corrado D, Thiene G. Clinical profile of congenital coronary artery anomalies with origin from the wrong aortic sinus leading to sudden death in young competitive athletes. *J Am Coll Cardiol* 2000; **35**:1493–501.

31 Pelliccia A, Spataro A, Maron BJ. Prospective echocardiographic screening for coronary artery anomalies in 1,360 elite competitive athletes. *Am J Cardiol* 1993; **72**:978–9.

Further reading

Balcells E, Powers ER, Lepper W, Belcik T, Wei K, Ragosta M, *et al.* Detection of myocardial viability by contrast echocardiography in acute infarction predicts recovery of resting function and contractile reserve. *J Am Coll Cardiol* 2003; **41**:827–33.

Cobb FR, Bache RJ, Rivas F, Greenfield JC, Jr. Local effects of acute cellular injury on regional myocardial blood flow. *J Clin Invest* 1976; **57**(5):1359–68.

Coggins MP, Sklenar J, Le DE, Wei K, Lindner JR, Kaul S. Noninvasive prediction of ultimate infarct size at the time of acute coronary occlusion based on the extent and magnitude of collateral-derived myocardial blood flow. *Circulation* 2001; **104**:2471–7.

deFilippi CR, Willett DL, Irani WN, Eichhorn EJ, Velasco CE, Grayburn PA. Comparison of myocardial contrast echocardiography and low-dose dobutamine stress echocardiography in predicting recovery of left ventricular function after coronary revascularization in chronic ischemic heart disease. *Circulation* 1995; **92**:2863–8.

Dwivedi G, Janardhananan R, Hayat SA, Swinburn JM, Senior R. Prognostic value of myocardial viability detected by myocardial contrast echocardiography early after acute myocardial infarction. *J Am Coll Cardiol* 2007; **50**(4): 327–34.

Holmes DR, Jr., Detre KM, Williams DO, Kent KM, King SB, III, Yeh W *et al.* Long-term outcome of patients with depressed left ventricular function undergoing percutaneous transluminal coronary angioplasty. The NHLBI PTCA Registry. *Circulation* 1993; **87**(1):21–9.

Kaul S, Jayaweera AR. Coronary and myocardial blood volumes: noninvasive tools to assess the coronary microcirculation? *Circulation* 1997; **96**(3):719–24.

Linka AZ, Sklenar J, Wei K, Jayaweera AR, Skyba DM, Kaul S. Assessment of transmural distribution of myocardial perfusion with contrast echocardiography. *Circulation* 1998; **98**(18): 1912–20.

Main ML, Magalski A, Chee NK, Coen MM, Skolnick DG, Good TH. Full-motion pulse inversion power Doppler contrast echocardiography differentiates stunning from necrosis and predicts recovery of left ventricular function after acute myocardial infarction. *J Am Coll Cardiol* 2001; **38**:1390–4.

Marwick TH, Nemec JJ, Pashkow FJ, Stewart WJ, Salcedo EE. Accuracy and limitations of exercise echocardiography in a routine clinical setting. *J Am Coll Cardiol* 1992; **19**:74–81.

Nagueh SF, Vaduganathan P, Ali N, Blaustein A, Verani MS, Winters WL Jr, *et al.* Identification of hibernating myocardium: comparative accuracy of myocardial contrast echocardiography, rest-redistribution thallium-201 tomography and dobutamine echocardiography. *J Am Coll Cardiol* 1997; **29**:985–993.

Sabia P, Afrookteh A, Touchstone DA, Keller MW, Esquivel L, Kaul S. Value of regional wall motion abnormality in the emergency room diagnosis of acute myocardial infarction. A prospective study using two-dimensional echocardiography. *Circulation* 1991; **84** (3 Suppl):185–92.

Sawada SG, Ryan T, Conley MJ, Corya BC, Feigenbaum H, Armstrong WF. Prognostic value of a normal exercise echocardiogram. *Am Heart J* 1990; **120**:49–55.

Shimoni S, Frangogiannis NG, Aggeli CJ, Shan K, Verani MS, Quinones MA, *et al.* Identification of hibernating myocardium with quantitative intravenous myocardial contrast echocardiography: comparison with dobutamine echocardiography and thallium-201 scintigraphy. *Circulation* 2003; **107**:538–44.

Swinburn JM, Senior R. Real time contrast echocardiography – a new bedside technique to predict contractile reserve early after acute myocardial infarction. *Eur J Echocardiogr* 2002; **3**:95–9.

Wei K, Jayaweera AR, Firoozan S, Linka A, Skyba DM, Kaul S. Basis for detection of stenosis using venous administration of microbubbles during myocardial contrast echocardiography: bolus or continuous infusion? *J Am Coll Cardiol* 1998; **32**(1):252–60.

Wei K, Jayaweera AR, Firoozan S, Linka A, Skyba DM, Kaul S. Quantification of myocardial blood flow with ultrasound-induced destruction of microbubbles administered as a constant venous infusion. *Circulation* 1998; **97**(5):473–83.

➲   For additional multimedia materials please visit the online version of the book (✎ http://escecho.oxfordmedicine.com).

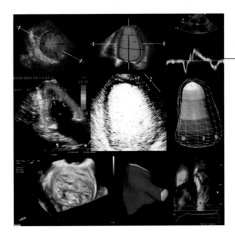

CHAPTER 13

Stress echocardiography

Lauro Cortigiani and Eugenio Picano

Contents

Summary

Stress echocardiography is a widely used method for assessing coronary artery disease, due to the high diagnostic and prognostic value. While inducible ischaemia predicts an unfavourable outcome, its absence is associated with a low risk of future events. The evaluation of coronary flow reserve by Doppler adds prognostic information to that of standard stress test. Stress echocardiography is indicated in cases when exercise testing is unfeasible, uninterpretable, or gives ambiguous result, and when ischaemia during the test is frequently a false positive response, as in hypertensives, women and patients with left ventricular hypertrophy. Viability detection represents another application of stress echocardiography. The documentation of viable myocardium predicts an improved outcome following revascularization in ischaemic and following resynchronization therapy in idiopathic cardiomyopathy. Moreover, stress echocardiography can aid significantly in clinical decision making in patients with valvular heart disease through dynamic assessment of mitral insufficiency, transvalvular gradients and pulmonary artery systolic pressure. Among the various stress modalities, exercise is safer than pharmacologic stress, in which major complications are three times more frequent with dobutamine than with dipyridamole. Stress echocardiography provides similar accuracy than perfusion scintigraphy but a substantially lower cost, without environmental impact and with no radiation biohazards for the patient.

Introduction

Stress echocardiography combines two-dimensional (2D) echocardiography with a physical, pharmacological, or electrical stress for assessing the presence, localization, and extent of myocardial ischaemia. Stress-induced wall motion abnormality (WMA) is the early and specific marker of ischaemia. Identification of viable myocardium and evaluation of severity of valvular heart disease are additional recognized applications of stress echocardiography. The wide availability of echocardiographic equipment in all medical centres has been a factor of paramount importance for the diffusion of the technique, especially in light of its limited costs and resource consumption.

Pathophysiology

Effects of ischaemia

Coronary flow reserve (CFR) is the ability of coronary arteriolar bed to dilate in response to increased metabolic demand. In normal conditions, arteriolar vasodilation can determine a four-to sixfold increment of coronary blood flow, leading to global increase in left ventricular (LV) contractility. In the presence of coronary stenosis of 75–95%, CFR reduces progressively,[1] and a transient imbalance between oxygen demand and supply occurs. This results in a typical *cascade* of ischaemic events in which the various markers are ranked in a well-defined temporal sequence. Regional malperfusion is the forerunner of ischaemia, followed by regional systolic dysfunction, and only at a later stage by electrocardiographic (ECG) changes and angina.[1] Ischaemia tends to propagate centrifugally with respect to the ventricular cavity, involving primarily the subendocardial layer, whereas the subepicardial layer is affected only at a later stage if ischaemia persists. In fact, extravascular pressure is higher in the subendocardial than in the subepicardial layer; this provokes a higher metabolic demand (wall tension being among the main determinants of myocardial oxygen consumption) and an increased resistance to flow. The impairment of systolic function correlates with the severity of flow reduction. In fact, a 20% reduction in subendocardial flow produces a 15–20% decrease in LV wall thickening; a 50% reduction in subendocardial flow decreases regional wall thickening by about 40%, and when subendocardial flow is reduced by 80%, akinesia occurs. When the flow deficit is extended to the subepicardial layer, dyskinesia appears.[2]

Mechanisms of ischaemia

Cardiovascular stress can induce ischaemia by means of different mechanisms that may either act by enhancing myocardial oxygen consumption, or by reducing oxygen supply, through an inappropriate arteriolar vasodilation, with subsequent flow maldistribution, or coronary artery spasm.

Increased demand

In resting conditions, myocardial oxygen consumption is dependent mainly on heart rate, inotropic state, and the LV wall stress (which is proportional to the systolic blood pressure, SBP). During exercise, the increase in heart rate (HR), blood pressure, and inotropic state accounts for the overall increase in myocardial oxygen consumption.[2] To a lesser degree, pacing and dobutamine also increase myocardial oxygen demand. During pacing, the increase is mainly due to the increased HR.[2] Dobutamine stimulates adrenoreceptors markedly increasing contractility and HR[2] (◑ Table 13.1). Following dipyridamole or adenosine administration, only a mild increase in myocardial oxygen consumption, due to a slight increase in contractility

Table 13.1 Pharmacodynamics of dobutamine

	Receptor populations		
	α_1	β_1	β_1
Myocardium	Increased inotropy	Increased chronotropy	
		Increased inotropy	
Vasculature	Vasoconstriction		Vasodilation

and HR, can be observed. Greater myocardial oxygen consumption due to HR increase occurs with coadministration of atropine with dobutamine and dipyridamole.[2]

Flow maldistribution

In the presence of a fixed coronary stenosis, arteriolar dilation can paradoxically exert detrimental effects on regional myocardial perfusion, causing overperfusion of myocardial layers or regions already well perfused in resting conditions at the expense of layers or regions with a precarious flow balance in resting conditions.[2] In *vertical steal* the anatomical requisite is the presence of an epicardial coronary stenosis and the subepicardium *steals* blood from the subendocardial layers. In fact, the administration of a coronary vasodilator causes a fall in poststenotic pressure, and therefore a critical fall in subendocardial perfusion pressure, which in turn provokes a fall in absolute subendocardial flow, even with subepicardial overperfusion. Regional thickening is closely related to subendocardial rather than transmural flow, and this explains the apparent paradox of a regional asynergy, with ischaemia despite a regionally increased transmural flow.[2] *Horizontal steal* requires the presence of collateral circulation between two vascular beds; the victim of the steal is the myocardium fed by the more stenotic vessel. After vasodilation, the flow in the collateral circulation is reduced relative to resting conditions, since the arteriolar bed of the donor vessel competes with the arteriolar bed of the receiving vessel, whose vasodilatory reserve was already exhausted in resting conditions.[2] The biochemical effector of this haemodynamic mechanism is the inappropriate accumulation of adenosine, which is the main physiological modulator of arteriolar vasodilation by stimulating A_2a adenosinergic receptors present on the endothelial and smooth muscle cells of coronary arterioles (◑ Table 13.2). Flow maldistribution plays a key role in myocardial ischaemia induced by adenosine or dipyridamole (which acts by blocking the uptake of endogenous adenosine into the cells), while it is likely to have a minor role in exercise- or pacing-induced ischaemia.

Vasospasm

The mechanisms of coronary spasm are still unclear. The smooth muscle cell in the medial layer of coronary epicardial arteries reacts to several vasoconstrictive stimuli, coming from the adventitial layer (such as α-mediated vasoconstriction) or centrifugally from the intima–blood interface (such as

Table 13.2 Pharmacodynamics of adenosine and dipyridamole

	Receptor populations			
	A_1	A_2a	A_2b	A_3
Myocardium	Decreased chronotropy			
	Decreased dromotropy			
	Chest pain?			
Vasculature		Coronary arteriolar vasodilation	Conductance vessel vasodilation	
Mast cells				Bronchospasm?
				Hypotension
				Preconditioning?

endothelin and serotonin). Clinically, coronary vasospasm can be elicited by ergonovine, which exerts a direct constrictive effect on vascular smooth muscle by stimulating both alpha-adrenergic (nonbeta-adrenergic) and serotoninergic receptors. Exercise and dobutamine can also induce an increase in coronary tone, up to complete vasospasm, through α-adrenergic stimulation.[1] Interruption of dipyridamole test by aminophylline (blocking adenosine receptors but also stimulating α-adrenoreceptors) can evoke vasospasm in one-third of patients with variant angina.[1]

Diagnostic criteria

All stress echocardiographic diagnoses can be summarized into four equations centred on regional wall function and describing the fundamental response patterns: normal, ischaemic, necrotic, and viable (◗ Fig. 13.1).

◆ Normal response: a segment is normokinetic at rest and normal or hyperkinetic during stress.

◆ Ischaemic response: the function of a segment worsens during stress from normokinesia to hypokinesia (decrease of endocardial movement and systolic thickening), akinesia (absence of endocardial movement and systolic thickening), or dyskinesia (paradoxical outward movement and possible systolic thinning). However, a resting akinesia becoming dyskinesia during stress reflects purely passive phenomenon of increased intraventricular pressure developed by normally contracting walls and should not be considered a true active ischaemia.[1]

◆ Necrotic response: a segment with resting dysfunction remains fixed during stress.

◆ Viability response: a segment with resting dysfunction may show either a sustained improvement during stress indicating a non-jeopardized myocardium (stunned) or improve during early stress with subsequent deterioration at peak

(biphasic response). The biphasic response is suggestive of viability and ischaemia, with jeopardized myocardium fed by a critical coronary stenosis.[1]

Methodology

General test protocol

During stress echo, a 12-lead ECG and cuff blood pressure are recorded in resting condition and each minute throughout the examination. Echocardiographic imaging is performed from the standard parasternal and apical views. Images are recorded in resting condition from all views and captured digitally.[3] A quad-screen format is used for comparative analysis. Echocardiography is then continuously monitored and intermittently stored. In the presence of dyssynergy, a complete echo examination is performed and recorded from all employed approaches to allow optimal documentation of the presence and extent of myocardial ischaemia.[3] The same projections are obtained and recorded during the recovery phase, after cessation of stress (exercise or pacing) or administration of the antidote (aminophylline for dipyridamole, beta-blocker for dobutamine, nitroglycerine for ergonovine). Analysis of the study is usually performed using a 16- or 17-segment model of the left ventricle[3] (see ◗ Chapter 8).

Diagnostic endpoints of stress echocardiography include:

◆ Maximum workload (for exercise testing).

◆ Maximum dose (pharmacological).

◆ Achievement of target HR.

◆ Echocardiographic positivity (akinesis of two or more LV segments).

◆ Severe chest pain.

◆ ECG positivity (>2mV ST-segment shift).

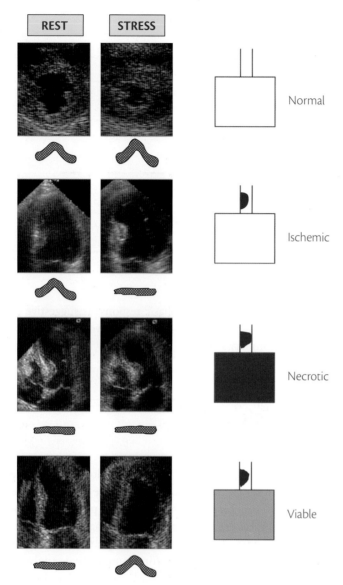

Figure 13.1 Fundamental pattern of response to stress echo. Echocardiographic examples of normal (upper row), ischaemic (second row), necrotic (third row), and viable (fourth row) response. On the left side, the end-systolic frames of a rest (left part) and stress (right part) study are shown. On the right site, the corresponding schemes of the coronary artery (parallel lines) and the myocardium (box) are shown. A normal myocardium is represented as a white box; a necrotic myocardium as a black box; a viable myocardium as a grey box. In a normal segment fed by a normal coronary artery, the segment is normokinetic at rest and normal-hyperkinetic during stress (upper row). In a normal myocardium fed by a critically stenosed coronary artery, the segment is normokinetic at rest and hypo, a- or dyskinetic during stress (second row). A necrotic segment shows a fixed wall motion abnormality at rest and during stress (third row). A viable segment is akinetic at rest and normal during stress (fourth row). Modified from Picano E. *Stress Echocardiography*, 5th ed. Heidelberg: Springer-Verlag, 2009.

Submaximal non-diagnostic endpoints are:

◆ Non-tolerable symptoms.

◆ Asymptomatic side effects such as hypertension (SBP >220mmHg or diastolic blood pressure [DPB] >120mmHg), symptomatic hypotension (>40mmHg drop in blood pressure), supraventricular arrhythmias (supraventricular tachycardia or atrial fibrillation), and complex ventricular arrhythmias (ventricular tachycardia or frequent, polymorphic premature ventricular beats).

Specific test protocols

Exercise, dobutamine, and dipyridamole are the most frequently used stressors for echocardiographic testing. There are distinct advantages and disadvantages to exercise versus pharmacological stress, which are outlined in ➲ Table 13.3.

Exercise

Exercise echocardiography can be performed using either a treadmill or bicycle protocol. When a treadmill test is performed, scanning during exercise is not feasible, so most protocols rely on post-exercise imaging. It is imperative to complete post-exercise imaging as soon as possible. To accomplish this, the patient is moved immediately from the treadmill to an imaging table so that imaging may be completed within 1–2min. This technique assumes that regional WMAs will persist long enough into recovery to be detected. When abnormalities recover rapidly, false-negative results occur.[3] Information on exercise capacity, HR response, and rhythm and blood pressure changes are analysed and, together with wall motion (WM) analysis, become part of the final interpretation.[3] Bicycle exercise echocardiography is performed during either an upright or a recumbent posture. Unlike treadmill test, bicycle exercise allows images to be obtained during the various levels of exercise. The patient pedals against an increasing workload (escalated in a stepwise fashion) while imaging is performed.

Table 13.3 Exercise versus pharmacological stress

Parameter	Exercise	Pharmacological
Intravenous line required	No	Yes
Diagnostic utility of heart rate and blood pressure response	Yes	No
Use in deconditioned patients	No	Yes
Use in physically limited patients	No	Yes
Level of echocardiography imaging difficulty	High	Low
Safety profile	High	Moderate
Clinical role in valvular disease	Yes	Minor
Clinical role in pulmonary hypertension	Yes	No
Fatigue and dyspnoea evaluation	Yes	No

In the supine posture, it is relatively easy to record images from multiple views during graded exercise. In the upright posture, imaging is generally limited to apical views.[2]

Dobutamine

The standard dobutamine stress protocol consists of continuous intravenous infusion of dobutamine in 3-min increments, starting with 5mcg/kg/min and increasing to 10, 20, 30, and 40mcg/kg/min. If no endpoint is reached, atropine (up to 1mg) is added to the 40mcg/kg/min dobutamine infusion.[3]

Dipyridamole

The standard dipyridamole protocol consists of an intravenous infusion of 0.84mg/kg over 10min, in two separate infusions: 0.56mg/kg over 4min, followed by 4min of no dose and, if still negative, an additional 0.28mg/kg over 2min. If no endpoint is reached, atropine (up to 1mg) is added. The same overall dose of 0.84mg/kg can be given over 6min.[3] Aminophylline should be available for immediate use in case an adverse dipyridamole-related event occurs and routinely infused at the end of the test independently of the result.

Adenosine

Adenosine is usually infused at a maximum dose of 140mcg/kg/min over 6min.[3] When side effects are intolerable, downtitration of the dose is also possible.

Pacing

The presence of a permanent pacemaker can be exploited to conduct a pacing stress test in a totally non-invasive manner by externally programming the pacemaker to increasing frequencies. Pacing is started at 100 beats per minutes (bpm) and increased every 2min by 10bpm until the target heart rate or other standard endpoints are achieved.[3] A limiting factor is, however, that several pacemakers cannot be programmed to the target HR.

Ergonovine

A bolus injection of ergonovine (5mcg) is administered intravenously at 5-min intervals until a positive response is obtained or a total dose of 0.35mg is reached.[3] Positive criteria for the test include the appearance of ST-segment elevation or depression greater than 0.1mV (ECG criteria) or WMA (echocardiographic criteria). An intravenous bolus injection of nitroglycerin is administered as soon as an abnormal response is detected; sublingual nifedipine is also recommended to counter the possible delayed effects of ergonovine.[3]

Diagnostic value

The accuracy of stress echocardiography for the detection of angiographically significant coronary artery disease (CAD) is high, regardless of the stress employed: exercise, dobutamine, dipyridamole, and adenosine echocardiography show a sensitivity, respectively, of 83%, 81%, 72%, and 79%, and a specificity of 84%, 84%, 95%, and 91%.[4] In head-to-head comparison, dipyridamole and dobutamine have identical sensitivity and comparable specificity (92% vs 87%)[5] (➲ Fig. 13.2). Good diagnostic

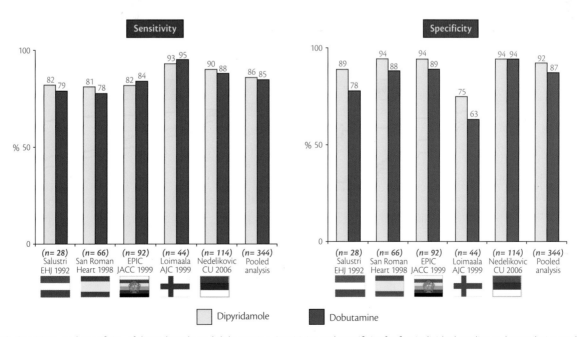

Figure 13.2 Sensitivity and specificity of dipyridamole and dobutamine. Sensitivity and specificity for five individual studies and cumulative analysis of dipyridamole vs dobutamine state-of-the-art protocols. Reproduced from Picano E, Molinaro S, Pasanisi E. The diagnostic accuracy of pharmacological stress echocardiography for the assessment of coronary artery disease: a meta-analysis. *Cardiovasc Ultrasound* 2008; **6**:30. Copyright 2008, Picano *et al*; licensee BioMed Central Ltd.

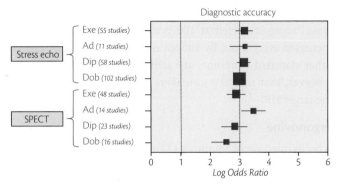

Figure 13.3 The diagnostic accuracy of stress echocardiography versus single-photon emission tomography (SPECT). The value of the log odds ratio is a measure of overall diagnostic accuracy. The size of the box is smaller for smaller sizes, with high confidence intervals. Ad, adenosine; Dip, dipyridamole; Dob, dobutamine; Exe, exercise. Modified from Heijenbrok-Kal MH, Fleischmann KE, Hunink MG. Stress echocardiography, stress single-photon-emission computed tomography and electron beam computed tomography for the assessment of coronary artery disease: a meta-analysis of diagnostic performance. *Am Heart J* 2007; **154**:415–23, with permission from Elsevier.

results have also been reported with pacing stress echocardiography (70% sensitivity, 90% specificity).[6] Ergonovine stress echocardiography provides greater than 90% sensitivity and specificity for assessing variant angina.[7]

Anti-ischaemic therapy lowers sensitivity of either exercise[8] and pharmacological stress echocardiography.[8,9] However, therapy lowers the sensitivity of dipyridamole more than that of dobutamine.[8] Additionally, beta-blockers are more effective than calcium antagonists and long-acting nitrates in decreasing test sensitivity[9].

When compared to standard exercise ECG, stress echocardiography has a particularly impressive advantage in terms of specificity.[10] Compared to nuclear perfusion imaging, stress echocardiography at least has similar accuracy (➲ Fig. 13.3), with a moderate sensitivity gap that is more than balanced by a markedly higher specificity.[4]

Prognostic value

It has been demonstrated that exercise[11–13] or pharmacological stress echocardiography[13–17] are capable to allow effective risk assessment in patients with known or suspected CAD. While the ischaemic or necrotic pattern is associated with markedly increased risk of death or myocardial infarction, a normal test is predictive of a generally favourable outcome particularly in non-diabetic patients[17] (➲ Fig. 13.4). The ischaemic response can be further stratified with additive stress echo parameters, such as the extent of inducible WMAs and the workload/dose. The higher the WM score index (see ➲ Chapter 8) and the shorter the ischaemia-free stress time are, the lower is the survival rate[11,16] (➲ Fig. 13.5). Particularly appealing is the very high negative predictive value of the test in patients with suspected CAD: a normal exercise echo yields 0.5% yearly hard event-rate.[18]

Stress echocardiography result can therefore heavily impact on the decision-making process, allowing a selective use of invasive procedures, with economical and logistic consequences potentially favourable. Stress echocardiography maintains a high prognostic value also in an angiographically benign subset such as that of single-vessel disease.[19] Furthermore, the result of the test has shown the capability to predict which patient can obtain the maximal beneficial effect by coronary revascularization. In fact, ischaemia at stress echo was the only independent prognostic indicator in medically treated patients among clinical, angiographic, and echocardiographic parameters. Moreover, coronary revascularization was effective in improving

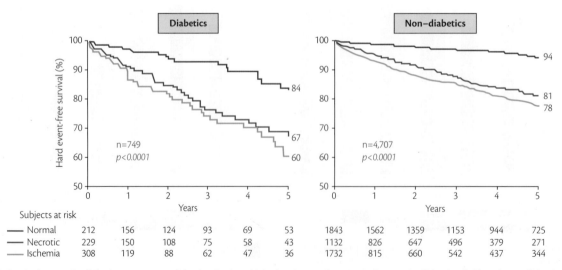

Subjects at risk												
—— Normal	212	156	124	93	69	53	1843	1562	1359	1153	944	725
—— Necrotic	229	150	108	75	58	43	1132	826	647	496	379	271
—— Ischemia	308	119	88	62	47	36	1732	815	660	542	437	344

Figure 13.4 Survival curves in diabetics versus non-diabetics. Kaplan–Meier hard event-free survival curves in diabetics (left) and non-diabetics (right). In patients with normal test result the prognosis is excellent in non-diabetics, but still poor in diabetics in whom a better stratification is needed. Modified from Cortigiani L, Bigi R, Sicari R, Landi P, Bovenzi F, Picano E. Prognostic value of pharmacological stress echocardiography in diabetic and non-diabetic patients with known or suspected coronary artery disease. *J Am Coll Cardiol* 2006; **47**:605–10.

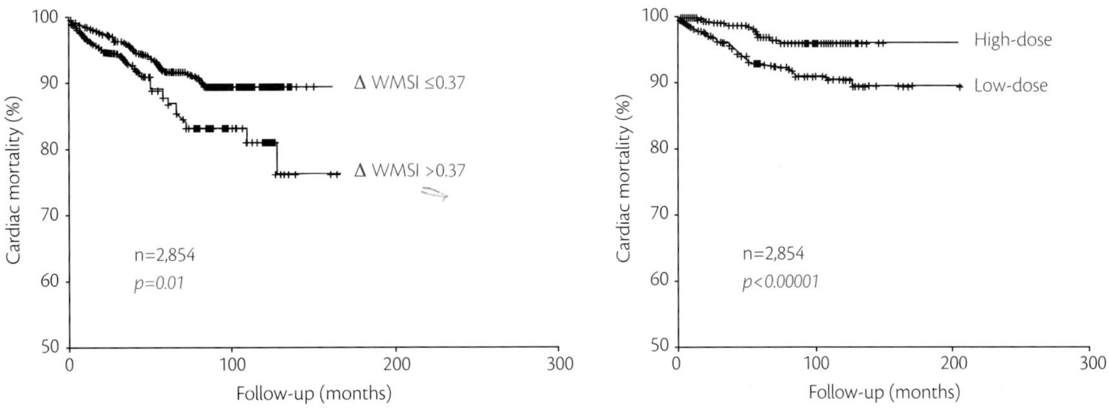

Figure 13.5 Kaplan–Meier survival curves in patients with inducible ischaemia at pharmacological stress echocardiography. Survival is worst in patients with higher rest-stress wall motion score index (left) and in those with ischaemia at low-dose (right). Modified from Sicari R, Pasanisi E, Venneri L, Landi P, Cortigiani L, Picano E. Stress echo results predict mortality: a large scale multicenter prospective international study. *J Am Coll Cardiol* 2003; **41**:589–95.

the infarction-free survival in subjects with ischaemia but not in those without ischaemia.[19] As for the prognostic implication of the different pharmacological stress modalities, a similar prognostic value has been reported for dobutamine and dipyridamole testing.[20] Anti-ischaemic therapy heavily modulates the prognostic impact of pharmacological stress echocardiography.[21] Inducible myocardial ischaemia in patients on medical therapy identifies the subset of patients at highest risk of death. Conversely, the incidence of death in patients with a negative test off therapy is very low. At intermediate risk are those patients with a negative test on medical therapy or a positive test off medical therapy[21] (➲ Fig. 13.6). ➲ Tables 13.4 and 13.5 summarize the established prognostic parameters of a stress echocardiography test that is positive or negative for ischaemia.

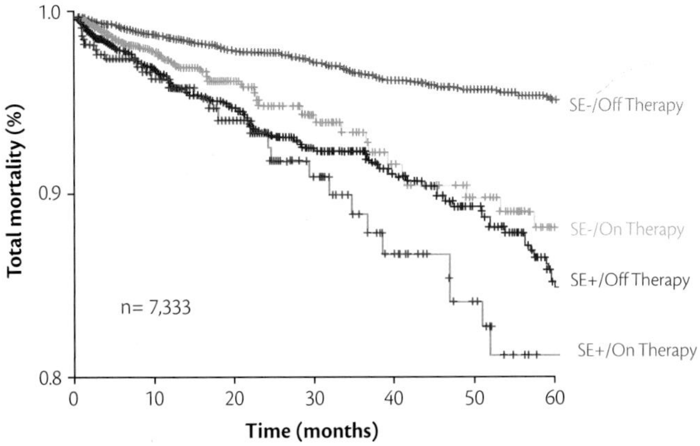

Figure 13.6 Kaplan–Meier survival curves in patients stratified according to presence (SE+) or absence (SE–) of myocardial ischaemia at pharmacological stress echocardiography on and off antianginal medical therapy. Best survival is observed in patients with no inducible ischaemia off therapy; worst survival is seen in patients with inducible ischaemia on therapy. Modified from Sicari R, Cortigiani L, Bigi R, Landi P, Raciti M, Picano E. The prognostic value of pharmacologic stress echo is affected by concomitant anti-ischemic therapy at the time of testing. *Circulation* 2004; **109**:1428–31.

Table 13.4 Stress echocardiography risk titration of a positive test result

1-year risk (hard events)	Intermediate (1–3% year)	High (>10% year)
Dose/workload	High	Low
Resting EF	>50%	<40%
Anti-ischemic therapy	Off	On
Coronary territory	RCA/LCx	LAD
Peak WMSI	Low	High
Recovery	Fast	Slow
Positivity or baseline dyssynergy	Homozonal	Heterozonal
CFR	>2.0	<2.0

CFR, coronary flow reserve; EF, ejection fraction; LAD, left anterior coronary artery; LCx, left circumflex coronary artery; RCA, right coronary artery; WMSI, wall motion score index.

Table 13.5 Stress echocardiography risk titration of a negative test result

1-year risk (hard events)	Very low (<0.5% year)	Low (1–3% year)
Stress	Maximal	Submaximal
Resting EF	>50%	<40%
Anti-ischaemic therapy	Off	On
CFR	>2.0	<2.0

CFR, coronary flow reserve; EF, ejection fraction.

Stress echo in special subsets of patients

Hypertensive patients

Arterial hypertension can provoke a reduction in CFR through several mechanisms, which may overlap in the individual patient: CAD, left ventricular hypertrophy, and microvascular disease.[22] The diagnostic value of exercise ECG and nuclear techniques has been very disappointing in the hypertensive population, due to high rate of false-positive responses.[22] Reduced CFR in the absence of organic CAD accounts for this false-positivity.[22] In hypertensive patients, stress echocardiography provides superior diagnostic specificity than exercise ECG with no differences in sensitivity.[23–25] Moreover, dipyridamole stress echocardiography is most accurate than perfusion scintigraphy to assess CAD in patients with exercise ECG positive for ischaemia[26] (➲ Fig. 13.7). The prognostic value of stress-induced WMAs is strong and extensively documented in hypertensive patients with suspected CAD[27] as well as in consecutive cohorts of hypertensive patients.[28] The incremental prognostic value of stress-induced WMAs over clinical and exercise ECG findings has also been proven.[29]

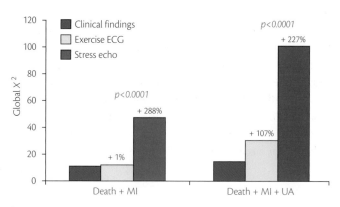

Figure 13.8 Incremental prognostic value of stress echocardiography to clinical and exercise electrocardiography data, as determined by the comparison of the global chi-square at each step. MI, myocardial infarction; UA, unstable angina. Modified from Dodi C, Cortigiani L, Masini M, Olivotto I, Azzarelli A, Nannini E. The incremental prognostic value of stress echo over exercise electrocardiography in women with chest pain of unknown origin. *Eur Heart J* 2001; **22**:145–52.

Women

The diagnostic specificity of exercise ECG and myocardial perfusion scintigraphy is definitely lower in women than in men. Explanations for this include reduction of CFR in syndrome X (mostly affecting female patients), hormonal influences for exercise testing, and breast attenuation for nuclear technique. In contrast, echocardiography combined with exercise or pharmacological agents provides similar sensitivity but a better specificity as compared to exercise ECG[30,31] and perfusion scintigraphy.[32] In women the prognostic value of stress echocardiography is high, similar to that in men.[12,13,33] In patients with chest pain of unknown origin, a normal test is associated with lower than 1% event-rate at 3 years of follow-up, while an ischaemic test is a strong and independent predictor of future events.[34] Moreover, stress-induced ischaemia adds prognostic information on top of clinical and exercise ECG data[35] (➲ Fig. 13.8).

Diabetic patients

Exercise ECG is of limited value in diabetic patients because exercise capacity is often impaired by peripheral vascular disease, neuropathic disease, and obesity. In addition, test specificity on ECG criteria is less than ideal due to high prevalence of hypertension and microvascular disease. Stress echocardiography can play a key role in the optimal identification of high-risk diabetic patients, providing similar diagnostic,[36] and prognostic information in patients with and without diabetes (➲ Fig. 13.4), independently of age.[17] Moreover, stress echocardiography allows effective risk assessment both in diabetics and non-diabetics with intermediate- to high-threshold ischaemic exercise ECG.[37] Nevertheless, the normal test result predicts a less favourable outcome in the diabetic population.[17,37]

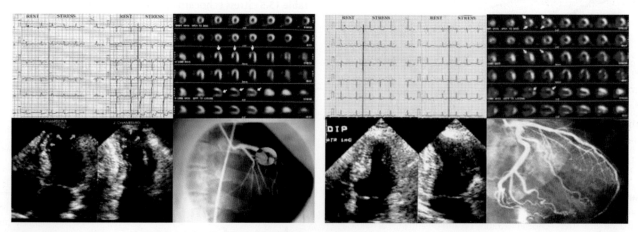

Figure 13.7 Diagnosis of myocardial ischaemia in CAD and hypertensive patient. On the left a positive ECG response is shown (left upper panel), positive thallium scan (right upper panel), apical four- and two-chamber view of end-systolic frames at peak stress with apical akinesia (indicated by arrows, left lower panel) of a hypertensive patient with significant left descending coronary artery stenosis (right lower panel). On the right a positive ECG response is shown (left upper panel), positive thallium scan (right upper panel), apical four- and two-chamber view of end-systolic frames at peak stress with normal left ventricular motion (left lower panel) of a hypertensive patient without significant coronary artery disease (right lower panel). Modified from Picano E. *Stress Echocardiography*, 5th ed. Heidelberg: Springer-Verlag, 2009.

Left bundle branch block

The presence of left bundle branch block makes the ECG uninterpretable for ischaemia and, therefore, a stress imaging is necessary. The abnormal sequence of LV activation determines increased diastolic extravascular resistance, with lower and slower diastolic coronary flow, accounting for the stress-induced defect often observed by perfusion imaging in patients with normal coronary arteries.[38] In spite of the difficulty posed by abnormal WM, stress echocardiography is the best diagnostic option in patients with left bundle branch block. It is more specific than perfusion imaging,[38] and its sensitivity is good, albeit reduced in the left anterior descending territory in the presence of a dyskinetic septum in resting conditions.[39] Moreover, myocardial ischaemia by pharmacological stress echo has a strong and independent power in the prediction of future hard events in left bundle branch block patients, providing a prognostic contribution that is incremental to that of clinical and resting echo findings in the group without previous myocardial infarction.[40]

Non-cardiac vascular surgery

CAD is the leading cause of perioperative morbidity and mortality following vascular surgery. Thus, risk stratification before surgery is a major issue, and pharmacological stress echocardiography appears to be the ideal first choice being more feasible than exercise ECG, and less expensive and safer than nuclear scintigraphy. The experience with either dipyridamole or dobutamine indicates that these tests have a very high and comparable negative predictive value (90–100%), allowing a safe surgical procedure.[41] To date, it appears reasonable to perform coronary revascularization before peripheral vascular surgery in the presence of a markedly positive result of stress echocardiography. A more conservative approach, including watchful cardiological surveillance coupled with cardioprotection with beta-blockers, can be adopted in patients with less severe ischaemic response during stress.[42] Risk stratification with stress echocardiography should be probably targeted to patients over 70 years, with current or prior angina, and previous myocardial infarction and heart failure. In other patients, the event rate under beta-blocker therapy is so low that an indiscriminate risk stratification policy with stress echocardiography is probably untenable. Interestingly, inappropriate indications for perioperative risk stratification before non-cardiac surgery account for 25% of all inappropriate testing in large-volume stress echocardiography laboratories.[43]

Coronary flow reserve

In recent years the evaluation of CFR by combining transthoracic Doppler assessment of coronary flow velocities with vasodilator stress has entered the echo lab as an effective modality for both diagnostic and prognostic purposes.

Methodology

The coronary flow velocity profile recorded with pulsed wave Doppler shows a high peak mostly during diastole. In fact, the myocardial extravascular resistance is lower in diastole due to the effect of myocardial relaxation. The flow velocity variations are proportional to the total blood flow if the vessel lumen is kept constant. This assumption is reasonable with vasodilators such as adenosine or dipyridamole,[1] and less valid with dobutamine. The coronary flow velocity variation between baseline and peak effect of a coronary vasodilator makes it possible to derive an index of CFR. Peak diastolic flow is the simplest and the easiest parameter to obtain (➲ Fig. 13.9). Moreover, it is the most reproducible and the one with the closest correlation to coronary perfusion reserve measured with Doppler flow wire[44] and positron emission tomography.[45] After stress, the balance between exercise, dobutamine, and vasodilators clearly goes in the direction of vasodilators, which fully recruit CFR and minimize the factors polluting image quality. Among vasodilators, dipyridamole is better tolerated subjectively than adenosine, induces less hyperventilation (which may pollute echocardiographic images), costs much less in most countries, and has a longer-lasting vasodilatory effect, which is more convenient for dual flow and function imaging.

A broadband transducer (2–7MHz) or two transducers (with low-frequency imaging of WM and high-frequency imaging of left anterior descending artery flow) must be used, allowing an intermittent imaging of coronary flow and wall motion[46] (➲ Fig. 13.10). Coronary flow in the mid-distal portion of left anterior descending artery is searched from a modified apical three-chamber view under the guidance of colour Doppler (CD) flow mapping, with about 95% feasibility.[46] The posterior descending coronary artery can also be imaged using a modified apical two-chamber view, but with greater difficulty and a success rate of about 60%.[47] A value of CFR less than or equal to 2 is generally considered abnormal[46] (➲ Fig. 13.9).

Stress contrast echocardiography

Evaluation of CFR and stress-induced perfusion abnormalities is significantly improved by the use of ultrasound contrast agents (see ➲ Chapter 7). Assessment of myocardial blood flow (MBF) at myocardial contrast echocardiography (MCE) during hyperaemia provides an accurate measurement of CFR, as compared to positron emission tomography, and allows detection of both presence and severity of a flow-limiting coronary stenosis. Stress contrast echocardiography can be performed by both high and low mechanical index contrast imaging modes. During myocardial replenishment phase, MBF can be calculated as the product of peak contrast intensity and myocardial flow velocity, within several myocardial segments, both at rest and during pharmacological vasodilation (see ➲ Chapter 7).

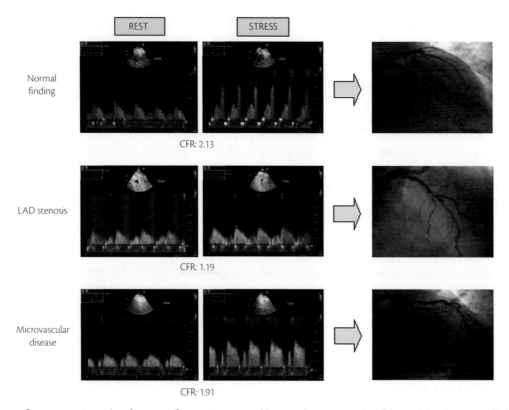

Figure 13.9 Coronary flow reserve. Examples of coronary flow reserve assessed by transthoracic Doppler of the mid-distal portion of left anterior descending artery. Coronary flow reserve is calculated as the ratio between peak diastolic coronary flow velocity at hyperaemia and its value in resting condition. The normal finding is characterized by coronary flow reserve >2.0 associated with angiographically normal coronary arteries (upper row). In the presence of significant stenosis of the left anterior descending artery, coronary flow reserve is <2.0 (second row). Coronary flow reserve can be <2.0 also in the presence of normal coronary anatomy, indicating underlying microvascular disease (third row).

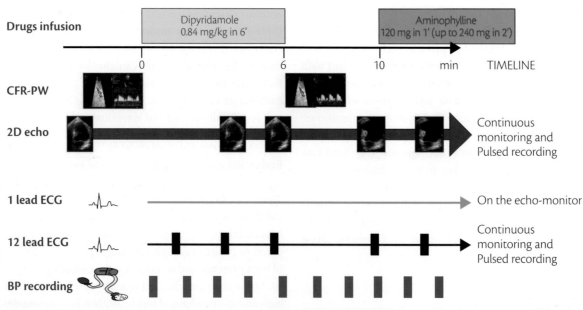

Figure 13.10 Dipyridamole stress echo for wall motion and coronary flow assessment. The state-of-the-art protocol of high-dose, fast dipyridamole stress echocardiography with dual imaging (wall motion and coronary flow reserve on the left anterior descending artery). BP, blood pressure; CFR-PW, coronary flow reserve-pulsed wave; ECG, electrocardiogram. Modified from Cortigiani L, Rigo F, Gherardi S, Sicari R, Galderisi M, Bovenzi F, Picano E. Additional prognostic value of coronary flow reserve in diabetic and nondiabetic patients with negative dipyridamole stress echocardiography by wall motion criteria. *J Am Coll Cardiol* 2007; **50**:1354–61, with permission from Elsevier.

Diagnostic value

The use of CFR as a stand-alone diagnostic criterion suffers from two main limitations. In fact, only the left anterior descending artery is sampled with a very high success rate. Moreover, CFR cannot distinguish between microvascular and macrovascular coronary disease. Therefore it is much more interesting to assess the additional diagnostic value over conventional WM analysis. By adding evaluation of CFR to WM analysis, the sensitivity of the test is significantly increased with only a modest loss of specificity:[48] test sensitivity improves from 67% to 90% after the addition of flow information, while specificity is reduced from 93% to 86%.[48] The superior sensitivity of CFR compared to WM analysis can be attributed to two main causes. First, a coronary stenosis can reduce flow reserve producing, however, no effect on systolic function. In fact, the detection of a regional dysfunction by 2D echocardiography requires a critical ischaemic mass of at least 20% of transmural wall thickness and about 5% of the total myocardial mass.[1] Second, the flow information is relatively unaffected by anti-ischaemic therapy,[49] which markedly reduces sensitivity of ischaemia-dependent regional WMA.[8, 9]

Prognostic value

With the advent of CFR in the stress echocardiography laboratory, within a few years a striking amount of information has became available through multicentre studies, showing the impressive prognostic value of CFR. In fact, CFR on the left anterior descending artery has shown to provide additional prognostic value over stress echo result in patients with known or suspected CAD,[50] and allows effective risk stratification in diabetic patients with unchanged WM during stress[46] (➲ Fig. 13.11), in patients with intermediate coronary stenosis,[51] and in patients with normal or near normal coronary arteries.[52] A CFR of 2.0 or lower is an additional parameter of ischaemia

severity in the risk stratification of the stress echocardiographic response whereas patients with a negative test for WM criteria and CFR greater than 2.0 have a favourable outcome during dipyridamole stress echocardiography (➲ Fig. 13.12). However, the spectrum of prognostic stratification is expanded if the response is titrated according to a continuous scale rather than artificially dichotomized. Indeed, the analysis of quartiles of CFR has revealed that a value of 1.80 or lower is a strong and independent predictor of death or myocardial infarction in patients with known or suspected CAD, while a value of 1.81–2.16 is associated with intermediate risk, and a value greater than or equal to 2.17 is predictive of a better prognosis[53] (➲ Fig. 13.13). A similar prognostication is obtained also when the group with no stress-induced ischaemia is separately analyzed[53] (➲ Fig. 13.13). Moreover, an even more effective prognostication in patients with no stress-induced ischaemia has been obtained by the combined evaluation of CFR in both the left anterior descending artery and the right coronary artery. In particular, a normal CFR in the two vascular territories is predictive of excellent survival, with only 0.7% yearly hard event-rate[47] (➲ Fig. 13.14). Anti-ischaemic medication at the time of testing does not modulate the prognostic value of CFR, which is per se a prognostic marker independent of therapy.[49]

Diagnostic flowcharts

Exercise ECG still remains the first-line tool for screening patients with known or suspected CAD due to the high feasibility, excellent safety, ease of application, low cost, and high negative predictive value, similar to that of stress echocardiography.[10,29,35] Accordingly, no further imaging test is warranted in low-risk patients with a maximal negative exercise ECG test result (➲ Fig. 13.15). At the other end of the spectrum, a high-risk ischaemic response at exercise ECG (i.e. positivity

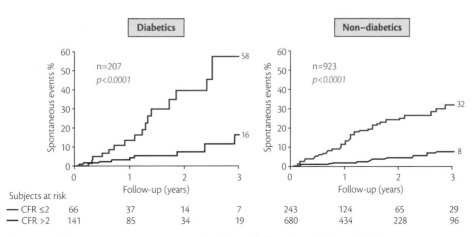

Figure 13.11 Risk stratification in diabetic patients. Hard event-rate for diabetic (left) and non-diabetic (right) patients with coronary flow reserve (CFR) > or ≤2.0 and negative stress echocardiography for wall motion criteria. Modified from Cortigiani L, Rigo F, Gherardi S, Sicari R, Galderisi M, Bovenzi F, Picano E. Additional prognostic value of coronary flow reserve in diabetic and nondiabetic patients with negative dipyridamole stress echocardiography by wall motion criteria. *J Am Coll Cardiol* 2007; **50**:1354–61, with permission from Elsevier.

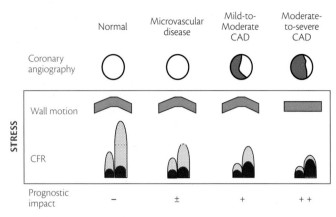

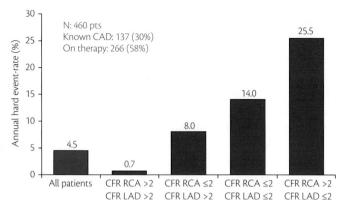

Figure 13.12 Different wall motion and CFR responses during stress echo. A synthetic view of the different coronary anatomic (first row) and prognostic CFR conditions (last row) underlying wall motion and CFR response during stress (framed). In normal conditions (left), there is normal coronary anatomy (upper row), normal wall motion response (second row), and normal CFR response (third row), with threefold increase in peak diastolic flow velocity during stress (dotted) versus baseline (full profile). An abnormal CFR with normal wall motion response can be found in presence of prognostically meaningful microvascular disease (second column from left) or mild-to-moderate epicardial stenosis (third column from left). With more advanced epicardial coronary artery stenosis (far right column), the reduction of CFR is consistently associated with wall motion abnormalities of obvious unfavorable prognostic impact (− = good prognosis; ± = possibly unfavourable prognosis; + = unfavourable prognosis; ++ = very unfavourable prognosis). CAD, coronary artery disease. Modified from Cortigiani L, Rigo F, Gherardi S, Sicari R, Galderisi M, Bovenzi F, Picano E. Additional prognostic value of coronary flow reserve in diabetic and nondiabetic patients with negative dipyridamole stress echocardiography by wall motion criteria. *J Am Coll Cardiol* 2007; **50**:1354–61, with permission from Elsevier.

Figure 13.14 Survival rate with normal CFR. Annual definite event rate in patients with stress echo negative for wall motion criteria separated in the different subgroups according to CFR >2.0 or ≤2.0 in left anterior descending (LAD) and posterior right coronary artery (RCA). Modified from Cortigiani L, Rigo F, Sicari R, Gherardi S, Bovenzi F, Picano E. Prognostic correlates of combined coronary flow reserve assessment on left anterior descending and right coronary artery in patients with negative stress echocardiography by wall motion criteria. *Heart* 2009; **95**:1423–8, with permission from BMJ Publishing Group Ltd.

with an exercise time <4min, positivity with recovery >8min, >3mm of ST-segment depression, ST-segment elevation in the absence of Q waves, global ST-segment changes, associated hypotension, malignant arrhythmias) warrants direct coronary angiography without any further investigations (➲ Fig. 13.15). In patients unable to exercise, with negative exercise testing at a submaximal workload or with uninterpretable or ambiguous ECG as those with left bundle branch block or paced rhythm, and those with ST-segment depression greater than 1mm, an

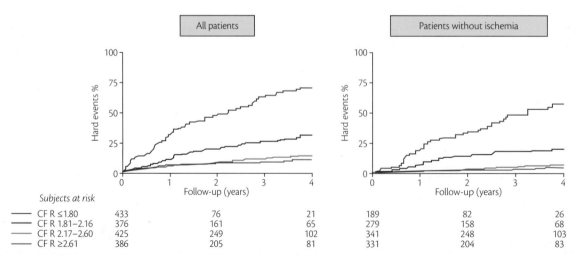

Figure 13.13 Hard event-rate according to quartiles of CFR in the entire study population (left) and in the group with no ischaemia at stress echocardiography (right). Modified from Cortigiani L, Rigo F, Gherardi S, Bovenzi F, Picano E, Sicari R. Prognostic implication of the continuous sprectrum of doppler echocardiographic derived coronary flow reserve on left anterior descending artery. *Am J Cardiol* 2010; **105**:158–62, with permission from Elsevier.

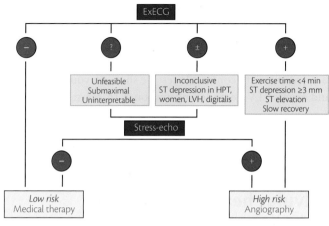

Figure 13.15 Diagnostic flowcharts. In stable patients with known or suspected CAD, the diagnostic algorithm should start with the exercise electrocardiography test. This remains the first non-invasive test to be done and often the last one: a negative test result is associated with an extremely good prognosis; at the other end of the spectrum, a response of severe ischaemia warrants coronary angiography without further investigations. In patients unable to exercise or with ambiguous or uninterpretable results during exercise electrocardiography or patients in whom exercise is contraindicated or submaximal, stress echocardiography is an excellent choice. A normal stress echocardiography identifies a low-risk group. A positive finding on stress echocardiography warrants a more aggressive therapeutic approach. ExECG, exercise electrocardiography; HPT, hypertensives; LVH, left ventricular hypertrophy. Modified from Picano E. *Stress Echocardiography*, 5th ed. Heidelberg: Springer-Verlag, 2009.

imaging technique is indicated and stress echocardiography has to be preferred for logistic and economic reasons (➔ Fig. 13.15). Stress echocardiography is also indicated in patients with exercise ECG positivity at intermediate to high load,[37] patients with negativity in the presence of chest pain, and patients in whom ST-segment changes during exercise can often occur in the absence of true ischaemia, such as women,[30,31] hypertensive patients,[23–25] patients with left ventricular hypertrophy,[22] and those taking digitalis. Stress echocardiography test positivity identifies a group of patients at higher risk in whom coronary angiography is warranted (➔ Fig. 13.15). Stress echocardiography test negativity makes the presence of prognostically important organic coronary disease unlike and identifies a group of patients at low-risk[11–17,27–29,33–35] (➔ Fig. 13.15). In these patients, a further effective prognostication can derive from the analysis of CFR in the left anterior descending artery[46] (➔ Table 13.5).

Myocardial viability

Pathophysiology

When the local supply–demand balance of the cell is critically endangered, the cell minimizes expenditure of energy used for the development of contractile force and utilizes whatever is left for the maintenance of cellular integrity. The echocardiographic counterpart of this cellular strategic choice is the regional asynergy of viable segments. Both viable and necrotic segments show a depressed resting function, but the segmental dysfunction of viable regions can be transiently normalized by inotropic stimulus. Hibernation and stunning are the two pathophysiological forms of viable myocardium which may be detected, respectively, in ischaemic cardiomyopathy and acute coronary syndromes. In the hibernating myocardium, myocardial perfusion is chronically reduced (for months or years), although remains beyond the critical threshold indispensable to keep the tissue viable, and recovery of function occurs after revascularization.[1] In the stunned myocardium, persistent but reversible ischaemia causes a metabolic alteration and imbalance between energy supply and work produced; recovery of function occurs spontaneously within hours, days, and even weeks after restoration of flow.[1]

Dobutamine stress echocardiography

In patients with dysfunctional but viable myocardium, regional function can be improved by the inotropic effect of low-dose (5–10mcg/kg/min) dobutamine stress echocardiography.[3] Sensitivity and specificity of low-dose dobutamine test are, respectively, 86% and 90% for predicting spontaneous functional recovery after an acute myocardial infarction (*stunning*),[54] and 84% and 81% for predicting functional recovery following revascularization in patients with chronic CAD (*hibernation*).[55] Compared to nuclear techniques, dobutamine stress echocardiography has lower sensitivity, but higher specificity, with similar overall accuracy regarding recovery of function[55] (➔ Fig. 13.16). In quantitative terms, contractile reserve evidenced by a positive dobutamine requires at least 50% viable myocytes in a given segment, whereas scintigraphic methods

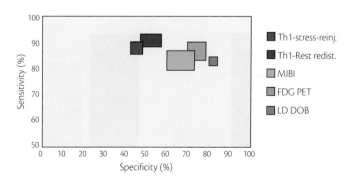

Figure 13.16 Prediction of functional recovery after revascularization. Sensitivity and specificity of nuclear techniques and low-dose dobutamine stress echocardiography in predicting functional recovery after revascularization in patients with ischaemic cardiomyopathy. Dobutamine stress echocardiography has a clearly better specificity and slightly lower sensitivity than nuclear techniques. FDG PET, fluorodeoxyglucose positron emission tomography; LD DOB, low-dose dobutamine. Modified from Bax JJ, Wijns W, Cornel JH, Visser FC, Boersma E, Fioretti PM. Accuracy of currently available techniques for prediction of functional recovery after revascularization in patients with left ventricular dysfunction due to chronic coronary artery disease: comparison of pooled data. *J Am Coll Cardiol* 1997; **30**:1451–60, with permission from Elsevier.

also identify segments with less viable myocytes.[56] Minor levels of viability, characterized by scintigraphic positivity and dobutamine echocardiography negativity, are often unable to translate into functional recovery. This explains the different diagnostic performance of the two methods, where post-revascularization functional recovery is considered as gold-standard of viability.

Prognostic value

In conservatively managed myocardial infarction the prognostic significance of tissue viability detected by dobutamine stress echocardiography depends on the characteristics of the study population. In patients with depressed LV function, the presence of substantial contractile reserve is associated with significantly better survival compared to patients with smaller or absent myocardial viability.[57] On the other hand, viability has no impact on survival in patients with preserved or just moderately depressed LV function; in this case, it can predict the occurrence of acute coronary events, representing a substrate for unstable ischaemic episodes.[58]

In patients with markedly reduced resting function (ejection fraction <35%) and chronic CAD, the stress echocardiography documentation of a large amount of viable myocardium (at least four segments or 20% of the total LV) is associated with a much lower mortality rate in revascularized patients than in medically treated patients[59–62] (➡ Fig. 13.17). Viability at dobutamine stress echocardiography predicts an improved outcome following revascularization both in diabetic and non-diabetic patients with ischaemic cardiomyopathy.[62] No measurable performance difference for predicting revascularization

benefit between stress echocardiography and nuclear methods has been reported.[63]

The documentation of viable myocardium at dobutamine test also predicts responders to resynchronization therapy. In fact, patients with contractile reserve show a favourable clinical and reverse LV remodelling response to resynchronization therapy.[64]

Stress echocardiography in valvular heart disease

Stress echocardiography has an established role in the evaluation of patients with valvular heart disease that can aid significantly in clinical decision making.

Aortic stenosis

Patients with severe aortic stenosis and LV systolic dysfunction often present with a relatively low-pressure mean gradient (see ➡ Chapter 14a). This entity represents a diagnostic challenge because it is difficult to differentiate between patients having true severe aortic stenosis from those having pseudosevere aortic stenosis.[65] In these patients it may be useful to determine the transvalvular pressure gradient and to calculate aortic valve area in resting condition and again during low-dose dobutamine stress. Patients who have pseudosevere aortic stenosis will show an increase in the aortic valve area and little change in gradient in response to the increase in transvalvular flow rate, while those with severe aortic stenosis will have a fixed valve area with an increase in stroke volume and in gradient[65–67] (for details, see ➡ Chapter 14a).

Mitral stenosis

A resting echocardiogram is usually sufficient to guide management in asymptomatic patients with mild to moderate mitral stenosis and in symptomatic patients with severe mitral stenosis who are candidates for mitral valve (MV) repair. In asymptomatic patients with severe mitral stenosis (mean gradient >10mmHg and mitral valve area, MVA, <1.0cm^2), or symptomatic patients with moderate stenosis (with mean gradient of 5–10mmHg and MVA of 1.0–1.5cm^2), a peak pulmonary artery pressures higher than 60mmHg or a mean transmitral pressure gradient greater than 15mmHg during exercise are cut-off values above which valvuloplasty or valve replacement is recommended.[68]

Mitral regurgitation

Degenerative mitral regurgitation

In symptomatic patients with mild mitral regurgitation (MR), exercise echocardiography may be useful in elucidating the cause of symptoms by determining whether the severity of MR

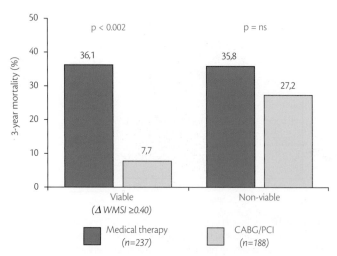

Figure 13.17 Death rates for patients with and without myocardial viability treated by revascularization or medical therapy. There was a 79% reduction in cardiac mortality for patients with viability treated by revascularization. In patients without myocardial viability, there was no significant difference in mortality with revascularization compared with medical therapy. Modified from Sicari R, Picano E, Cortigiani L, Borges A, Varga A, Palagi C, Bigi R, Rossini R, Pasanisi E. Prognostic value of myocardial viability recognized by low-dose dobutamine echocardiography in chronic ischemic left ventricular dysfunction. *Am J Cardiol* 2003; **92**:1263–6.

increases or pulmonary arterial hypertension develops during exercise.[65] In asymptomatic patients with severe MR, exercise stress echocardiography may help identify patients with subclinical latent LV dysfunction and poor clinical outcome.[65] Worsening of MR severity, a marked increase in pulmonary arterial pressure, impaired exercise capacity, and the occurrence of symptoms during exercise echocardiography can be useful findings for identifying the subset of high-risk patients who may benefit from surgery.[68] A pulmonary artery systolic pressure greater than 60mmHg during exercise has been suggested as a threshold value above which asymptomatic patients with severe MR might be referred for surgical valve repair.[68]

Ischaemic mitral regurgitation

The magnitude of ischaemic MR varies dynamically in accordance with changes in loading conditions, annular size, and the balance of tethering versus closing forces applied on the MV leaflets. Hence the severity of MR assessed by resting echocardiography does not necessarily reflect the severity under exercise conditions.[65] Exercise stress echocardiography is able to unmask haemodynamically significant MR, identifying patients at higher risk for heart failure and death.[69,70] An increase in the effective regurgitant orifice area (EROA) of 13mm² of more or an increase in the systolic pulmonary arterial pressure of 60mmHg or more at peak exercise is predictive of increased morbidity and mortality[69] (🔿 Fig. 13.18).

Exercise stress echocardiography in patients with ischaemic MR can provide useful information in the following situations:

- Patients with exertional dyspnoea out of proportion to the severity of resting LV dysfunction or MR.

- Patients in whom acute pulmonary oedema occurs without an obvious cause.

- Patients with moderate MR before surgical revascularization.[70]

Feasibility and safety

Exercise

The safety of exercise stress is witnessed by decades of experience with ECG testing and stress imaging. Also in stress echocardiography registries, exercise was safer than pharmacological stress.[71] Death occurs at an average of 1 in 10,000 tests, according to the American Heart Association statements on exercise testing based on a review of more than 1000 studies on millions of patients.[72] Major life-threatening effects, including myocardial infarction, ventricular fibrillation, sustained ventricular tachycardia, and stroke, were reported in about 1 in 6000 patients with exercise in the international stress echocardiography registry.[71]

Dobutamine

Minor but limiting side effects preclude the achievement of maximal dobutamine stress in about 10% of patients.[73] The history of systemic hypertension is an independent predictor of cumulative adverse effects, lowering test feasibility.[73] In order of frequency, limiting side effects during dobutamine stress include complex ventricular tachyarrhythmias, hypotension,

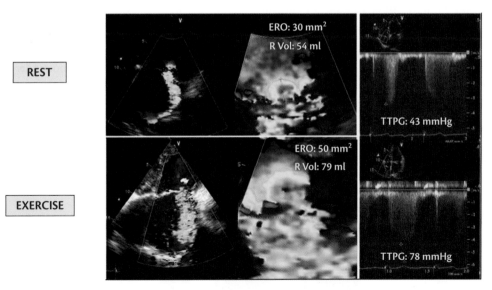

Figure 13.18 Ischaemic mitral regurgitation. Apical four-chamber views of colour-flow Doppler and proximal flow-convergence region (left panels) are shown in a patient with ischaemic mitral regurgitation along with the systolic tricuspid regurgitation velocity (right panel). With exercise, there is a major increase in both the severity of mitral regurgitation and the estimated pulmonary artery systolic pressure. ERO, effective regurgitant orifice measured by the proximal isovelocity surface area; R Vol, regurgitant volume; TTPG, systolic transtricuspid pressure gradient. Modified from Picano E, Pibarot P, Lancellotti P, Monin JL, Bonow RO. The emerging role of exercise testing and stress echocardiography in valvular heart disease. *J Am Coll Cardiol* 2009; **54**:2251–60, with permission from Elsevier.

atrial fibrillation, hypertension, and bradyarrhythmia[73] (⊃ Fig. 13.19). Both the patients and the physician should be aware of the rate of major complications that may occur in 1 of 300 cases during dobutamine stress.[71–74] Tachyarrhythmias are the most frequent complications, which are independent of ischaemia in many cases and can also develop at low-dose dobutamine regimen. The mechanism of their onset can be attributed to the direct adrenergic arrhythmogenic effect of dobutamine, through myocardial β-receptor stimulation.[1] Significant hypotension, sometimes associated with bradyarrhythmias, including asystole, is another frequent adverse reaction during dobutamine echocardiography. In some cases this findings has been attributed to dynamic intraventricular obstruction provoked by inotropic action of dobutamine, especially in hypertrophic hearts.[1] A vasodepressor reflex triggered by LV mechanoreceptors stimulation (*Bezold–Jarish reflex*) due to excessive inotropic stimulation may be an alternative mechanism.[1] Late and long-lasting transmural myocardial ischaemia, with persistent ST-elevation, is probably due to the coronary vasoconstrictive effect of dobutamine, through α-receptor stimulation.

Dipyridamole

Limiting side effects occur in 3% of patients tested with dipyridamole.[73] In order of frequency, they include hypotension, supraventricular tachycardia, general malaise, headache, dyspnoea, and atrial fibrillation.[73] Major life-threatening complications, such as myocardial infarction, third-degree atrioventricular block, cardiac asystole, sustained ventricular tachycardia, or pulmonary oedema, occur in about 1 in 1000 cases with high-dose dipyridamole stress.[71] Accordingly, the test induces major complications three times less frequently than dobutamine.

Adenosine

Side effects are very frequent and are limiting in up to 20% of patients investigated with adenosine stress echocardiography.[75]

They include high-degree atrioventricular block, hypotension, intolerable chest pain (possibly induced for direct stimulation of myocardial A1 adenosine receptors), shortness of breath, flushing, and headache. Although side effects are frequent, the incidence of life-threatening complications, such as myocardial infarction, ventricular tachycardia, and shock, has been shown to be very low, with only one fatal myocardial infarction in approximately 10,000 cases.[75] Among pharmacological stress tests, adenosine is probably the least well tolerated subjectively, but at the same time possibly the safest.

Contraindications

Exercise

Contraindications to exercise stress echocardiography include unstable haemodynamic conditions or severe, uncontrolled hypertension.[3] Additional relative contraindications are inability to exercise adequately, and a difficult resting echocardiogram.

Dobutamine

Patients with a history of complex atrial (paroxysmal atrial fibrillation, paroxysmal supraventricular tachycardia) or ventricular arrhythmias (sustained ventricular tachycardia or ventricular fibrillation) or with moderate to severe hypertension should not undergo dobutamine stress echocardiography and be referred for safer vasodilator stress.[3]

Dipyridamole

Patients with second- or third-degree atrioventricular block, sick sinus syndrome, bronchial asthma, or a tendency to bronchospasm should not receive dipyridamole.[3] Patients using dipyridamole chronically should not undergo adenosine testing for at least 24h after withdrawal of therapy, because their blood levels of adenosine could be unpredictably high.

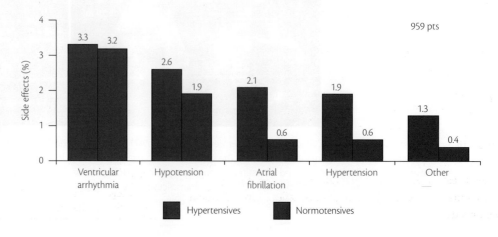

Figure 13.19 Safety and tolerability profile of dobutamine stress echocardiography in hypertensive and normotensive patients. All side effects are more frequent in hypertensive subjects. Modified from Cortigiani L, Zanetti L, Bigi R, Desideri A, Fiorentini C, Nannini E. Safety and feasibility of dobutamine and dipyridamole stress echocardiography in hypertensive patients. *J Hypertens* 2002; **20**:1423–9.

Appropriateness

An appropriate imaging study is one in which the expected incremental information, combined with clinical judgement, exceeds any expected negative consequences by a sufficiently wide margin for a specific indication that the procedure is generally considered acceptable care and a reasonable approach for the indication.[76] Negative consequences include the risks of the procedure itself (i.e. radiation) and the downstream impact of poor performance such as delay in diagnosis (*false-negative results*) or inappropriate diagnosis (*false-positive results*). According to recent estimates, more that 30% of cardiac stress imaging studies, including stress echocardiography, are unnecessary. This implies potential harm for patients undergoing imaging (who takes the risks of the technique without a commensurate benefit), excessive delay in the waiting lists for other patients needing the examination, and an exorbitant cost for society. Every test has a cost and a risk. Compared with the treadmill exercise test, the cost of stress echocardiography is 2.1 times higher, myocardial perfusion imaging is 5.7 times higher, and coronary angiography is 21.7 times higher.[77]

All forms of stress echocardiography are inappropriately applied as a first-line test in lieu of exercise electrocardiography. As a rule, the less informative the exercise testing is, the stricter the indication to stress echocardiography.

Indications for stress echocardiography can be grouped in very broad categories, which encompass the majority of patients:[78]

♦ Diagnosis of CAD in patients in whom exercise ECG is contraindicated, not feasible, uninterpretable, non-diagnostic, or gives an ambiguous result.

♦ Risk stratification in patients with established diagnosis.

♦ Preoperative risk assessment (high-risk non-emergent, poor exercise tolerance).

♦ Evaluation after revascularization (not in the early post-procedure period, with change in symptoms).

♦ Search for viability in patients with ischaemic cardiomyopathy eligible for revascularization.

♦ CAD of unclear significance at angiography or computed tomography.

♦ Evaluation of valvular heart disease severity.

Pharmacological stress echocardiography is the choice for patients in whom exercise is unfeasible or contraindicated. The choice of dobutamine or dipyridamole should depend on specific contraindications of either drug, patient characteristics, local drug cost, and the physician's preference. It is important for all stress echocardiography laboratories to become familiar with all stresses to achieve a flexible and versatile diagnostic approach that enables the best stress to be tailored to individual patient needs.

Competence

Interpretation of stress echocardiography requires extensive experience in echocardiography and should be performed only by physicians with specific training in the technique.[3] The basic skills required for imaging the heart under resting conditions are not substantially different from those required for imaging the same heart during stress. Furthermore, the echocardiographic signs of ischaemia are basically the same as those during myocardial infarction. The diagnostic accuracy of an experienced echocardiographer who is an absolute beginner in stress echocardiography is equivalent to that achieved by tossing a coin.[79] However, 100 stress echocardiography studies are sufficient to build the individual learning curve and reach the plateau of diagnostic accuracy.[79] After 15–30 days of exposure to a high-volume stress echocardiography laboratory, the physician begin to accumulate his or her own experience with a stepwise approach, starting from more innocuous and simple stresses (such as vasodilator tests) and moving up to more technically demanding ones (such as dobutamine and exercise). Maintenance of competence requires at least 15 stress echo exams per month.[80] The use of stresses is associated with the possibility of life-threatening complications. Therefore, the cardiologist and the attendant nurse should be certified in Basic and Advanced Life Support[80] (➲ Table 13.6).

Comparison with other imaging techniques

When compared with perfusion scintigraphy, stress echocardiography has an advantage in terms of specificity, versatility, cost, and risk.[3] The advantages of stress perfusion imaging include less operator-dependence, higher technical success rate, higher sensitivity, better accuracy when multiple resting LV WMAs are present, and a more extensive database for the evaluation of prognosis.[3] The European Society of Cardiology guidelines on stable angina conclude that 'On the whole, stress

Table 13.6 Additive skills necessary to perform, interpret, and report pharmacological stress echocardiography

1. Knowledge of advantages and disadvantages of the different agents
2. Knowledge of the pharmacokinetics and the physiological response to the different agents
3. Knowledge of the contraindications to the different agents
4. Knowledge of the side effects and complications of the different agents and how to manage them
5. Competence in cardiopulmonary resuscitation
6. Knowledge of the end points of pharmacological stress and indications for termination the test

Table 13.7 Head-to-head comparison between myocardial perfusion scintigraphy and stress echocardiography

	Scintigraphy	Stress echocardiography
Diagnostic parameter	Perfusion	Wall motion
Relative cost	3	1
Sensitivity	Higher	High
Specificity	Moderate	High
Radiation burden (CXr)	500–1000	0
Patient friendliness	Low	High
Operator friendly	Low	High
Environment friendly	Low	High

CXr, X-ray

echocardiography and stress perfusion scintigraphy, whether using exercise or pharmacological stress (inotropic or vasodilator), have very similar applications. The choice as to which is employed depends largely on local facilities and expertise. Advantages of stress echocardiography include its being free of radiation'[81] (➲ Table 13.7). On the basis of the large body of evidence assessing the comparable accuracy of stress echocardiography and perfusion scintigraphy, the choice of one test over

the other will depend on the overall biological risk related to the use of radiations.[3] The European law (Euratom directive 97/43) states that a radiological (and medico-nuclear) examination can be performed only 'when it cannot be replaced by other techniques that do not employ ionising radiation' and it should always be justified (article 3: 'if an exposure cannot be justified it should be prohibited'). At patient level, the effective dose of a single nuclear cardiology stress imaging ranges from 10mSv (corresponding to 500 chest X-rays) for a technetium-MBI scan to 25mSv (corresponding to 1250 chest X-rays) from a thallium scan.[82] According to the latest estimation of BEIR VII (2006), this exposure corresponds to an extra-lifetime risk of cancer per examination ranging from 1 in 1000 (sestamibi) to 1 in 500 (thallium).[83] The risk is greatest in special subsets particularly vulnerable to the damaging effects of ionizing radiation, such as women of reproductive age and children[84] (➲ Fig. 13.20). Therefore, in an integrated risk–benefit balance, stress echocardiography has advantages when compared with perfusion scintigraphy and should be preferred.

Cardiac magnetic resonance has higher costs, higher time of image acquisition, and lower availability when compared with echocardiography. Therefore, it represents an excellent option only when stress echocardiography is inconclusive or not feasible.[3]

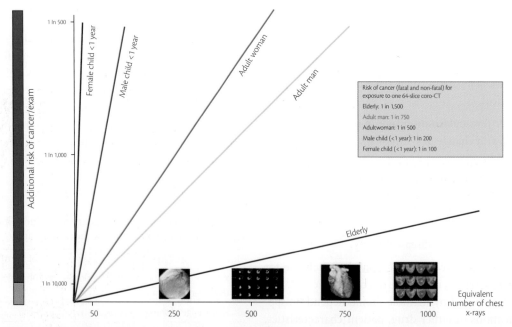

Figure 13.20 Biological risk of imaging modalities. Simplified effective dose ranges of some common medical procedures involving exposure to ionizing radiations in diagnostic nuclear medicine and radiological procedures. The reference unit is one chest X-ray (postero-anterior projection), equal to an effective dose of 0.02mSv. There is a linear relation between dose (x-axis) and risk (y-axis), with no safe dose (the risk line starts from zero). Ultrasound and magnetic resonance imaging have zero dose and zero risk. Modified from Picano E. Informed consent and communication of risk from radiological and nuclear medicine examinations: how to escape from a communication inferno. Education and debate. *BMJ* 2004; **329**:849–851.

Personal perspective

The state-of-the-art diagnosis of ischaemia in stress echocardiography was, 30 years ago, and still is today, the visual interpretation of black-and-white regional WM. The future issues in stress echo will be the possibility of obtaining quantitative information translating the current qualitative assessment of regional wall motion into a number. Real-time 3D echo, 2D-strain, and perfusion imaging with microbubbles are all candidates, providing exciting potential to describe clinically pathophysiological parameters located upstream in the ischaemic cascade when compared with regional WMAs. However, none of these methods is currently available for advantageous routine clinical application. These are *hot topics* for the researchers but at present are mostly confounding noise for the practising clinician. A second key issue in stress echocardiography is the combination of WM and CFR, assessed in the left anterior descending artery, into a single test. The improvement of technology and in imaging quality will make this approach more and more feasible. In coming years, obvious cost–benefit and risk–benefit assessment applied to stress imaging will reduce the role of nuclear medicine in favour of stress echocardiography due to the need to minimize the global radiological warming and associated cancer risk at the individual patient and population level.

References

1 Picano E. *Stress Echocardiography*, 5th ed. Heidelberg: Springer-Verlag, 2009.

2 Picano E. Stress echocardiography: from pathophysiological toy to diagnostic tool. Point of view. *Circulation* 1992; **85**: 1604–12.

3 Sicari R, Nihoyannopoulos P, Evangelista A, Kasprzak J, Lancellotti P, Poldermans D, et al. Stress echocardiography expert consensus statement. *Eur J Echocardiogr* 2008; **9**:415–37.

4 Heijenbrok-Kal MH, Fleischmann KE, Hunink MG. Stress echocardiography, stress single-photon-emission computed tomography and electron beam computed tomography for the assessment of coronary artery disease: a meta-analysis of diagnostic performance. *Am Heart J* 2007; **154**:415–23.

5 Picano E, Molinaro S, Pasanisi E. The diagnostic accuracy of pharmacological stress echocardiography for the assessment of coronary artery disease: a meta-analysis. *Cardiovasc Ultrasound* 2008; **6**:30.

6 Picano E, Alaimo A, Chubuchny V, Plonska E, Baldo V, Baldini U, et al. Noninvasive pacemaker stress echocardiography for diagnosis of coronary artery disease: a multicenter study. *J Am Coll Cardiol* 2002; **40**:1305–10.

7 Song JK, Lee SJ, Kang DH, Cheong SS, Hong MK, Kim JJ, et al. Ergonovine echocardiography as a screening test for diagnosis of vasospastic angina before coronary angiography. *J Am Coll Cardiol* 1996; **27**:1156–61.

8 San Roman JA, Vilacosta I, Castillo JA, Rollan MJ, Peral V, Sanchez-Harguindey L, et al. Dipyridamole and dobutamine-atropine stress echocardiography in the diagnosis of coronary artery disease. Comparison with exercise stress test, analysis of agreement, and impact of antianginal treatment. *Chest* 1996; **110**:1248–54.

9 Lattanzi F, Picano E, Bolognese L, Piccinino C, Sarasso G, Orlandini A, et al. Inhibition of dipyridamole-induced ischemia by antianginal therapy in humans. Correlation with exercise electrocardiography. *Circulation* 1991; **83**:1256–62.

10 Severi S, Picano E, Michelassi C, Lattanzi F, Landi P, Distante A, et al. Diagnostic and prognostic value of dipyridamole echocardiography in patients with suspected coronary artery disease. Comparison with exercise electrocardiography. *Circulation* 1994; **89**:1160–73.

11 Marwick TH, Case C, Vasey C, Allen S, Short L, Thomas JD. Prediction of mortality by exercise echocardiography: a strategy for combination with the duke treadmill score. *Circulation* 2001; **103**:2566–71.

12 Arruda-Olson AM, Juracan EM, Mahoney DW, McCully RB, Roger VL, Pellikka PA. Prognostic value of exercise echocardiography in 5,798 patients: is there a gender difference? *J Am Coll Cardiol* 2002; **39**:625–31.

13 Shaw LJ, Vasey C, Sawada S, Rimmerman C, Marwick TH. Impact of gender on risk stratification by exercise and dobutamine stress echocardiography: long-term mortality in 4234 women and 6898 men. *Eur Heart J* 2005; **26**:447–56.

14 Picano E, Severi S, Michelassi C, Lattanzi F, Masini M, Orsini E, et al. Prognostic importance of dipyridamole-echocardiography test in coronary artery disease. *Circulation* 1989; **80**:450–9.

15 Poldermans D, Fioretti PM, Boersma E, Bax JJ, Thomson IR, Roelandt JR, et al. Long-term prognostic value of dobutamine-atropine stress echocardiography in 1737 patients with known or suspected coronary artery disease: A single-center experience. *Circulation* 1999; **99**:757–62.

16 Sicari R, Pasanisi E, Venneri L, Landi P, Cortigiani L., Picano E. Stress echo results predict mortality: a large scale multicenter prospective international study. *J Am Coll Cardiol* 2003; **41**: 589–95.

17 Cortigiani L, Bigi R, Sicari R, Landi P, Bovenzi F, Picano E. Prognostic value of pharmacological stress echocardiography in diabetic and mondiabetic patients with known or suspected coronary artery disease. *J Am Coll Cardiol* 2006; **47**:605–10.

18 Metz LD, Beattie M, Hom R, Redberg RF, Grady D, Fleischmann KE. The prognostic value of normal exercise myocardial perfusion imaging and exercise echocardiography: a meta-analysis. *J Am Coll Cardiol* 2007; **49**:227–37.

19 Cortigiani L, Picano E, Landi P, Previtali M, Pirelli S, Bellotti P, et al. Value of pharmacologic stress echocardiography in risk stratification of patients with single-vessel disease: a report from the Echo-Persantine and Echo-Dobutamine International Cooperative Studies. *J Am Coll Cardiol* 1998; **32**:69–74.

20 Pingitore A, Picano E, Varga A, Gigli G, Cortigiani L, Previtali M, et al. Prognostic value of pharmacological stress echocardiography in patients with known or suspected coronary artery disease: a prospective, large scale, multicenter, head-to-head comparison between dipyridamole and dobutamine test. J Am Coll Cardiol 1999; 34:1769–77.

21 Sicari R, Cortigiani L, Bigi R, Landi P, Raciti M, Picano E. The prognostic value of pharmacologic stress echo is affected by concomitant anti-ischemic therapy at the time of testing. Circulation 2004; 109·1428–31.

22 Picano E, Pálinkás A, Amyot R. Diagnosis of myocardial ischemia in hypertensive patients. J Hypertens 2001; 19:1177–83.

23 Picano E, Lucarini AR, Lattanzi F, Distante A, Di Legge V, Salvetti A, et al. Dipyridamole-echocardiography test in essential hypertensives with chest pain. Hypertension 1988; 12:238–43.

24 Cortigiani L, Bigi R, Rigo F, Landi P, Baldini U, Mariani PR, Picano E. Diagnostic value of exercise electrocardiography and dipyridamole stress echocardiography in hypertensive and normotensive chest pain patients with right bundle branch block. J Hypertens 2003; 21:2189–94.

25 Senior R, Basu S, Handler C, Raftery EB, Lahiri A. Diagnostic accuracy of dobutamine stress echocardiography for detection of coronary heart disease in hypertensive patients. Eur Heart J 1996; 17:289–95.

26 Astarita C, Palinkas A, Nicolai E, Maresca FS, Varga A, Picano E. Dipyridamole-atropine stress echocardiography versus exercise SPECT scintigraphy for detection of coronary artery disease in hypertensives with positive exercise test. J Hypertens 2001; 19:495–502.

27 Cortigiani L, Paolini EA, Nannini E. Dipyridamole stress echocardiography for risk stratification in hypertensive patients with chest pain. Circulation 1998; 98:2855–9.

28 Marwick TH, Case C, Sawada S, Vasey C, Thomas JD. Prediction of outcomes in hypertensive patients with suspected coronary disease. Hypertension 2002; 39:1113–8.

29 Cortigiani L, Coletta C, Bigi R, Amici E, Desideri A, Odoguardi L. Clinical, exercise electrocardiographic, and pharmacologic stress echocardiographic findings for risk stratification of hypertensive patients with chest pain. Am J Cardiol 2003; 9:941–5.

30 Masini M, Picano E, Lattanzi F, Distante A, L'Abbate A. High-dose dipyridamole echocardiography test in women: correlation with exercise-electrocardiography test and coronary arteriography. J Am Coll Cardiol 1988; 12:682–5.

31 Marwick TH, Anderson T, Williams MJ, Haluska B, Melin JA, Pashkow F, et al. Exercise echocardiography is an accurate and cost-efficient technique for detection of coronary artery disease in women. J Am Coll Cardiol 1995; 26:335–41.

32 Elhendy A, van Domburg RT, Bax JJ, Nierop PR, Geleijnse ML, Ibrahim MM, et al. Noninvasive diagnosis of coronary artery stenosis in women with limited exercise capacity: comparison of dobutamine stress echocardiography and 99mTc sestamibi single-photon emission CT. Chest 1998; 114:1097–104.

33 Cortigiani L, Sicari R, Bigi R, Landi P, Bovenzi F, Picano E. Impact of gender on risk stratification by stress echocardiography. Am J Med 2009; 122:301–9.

34 Cortigiani L, Dodi C, Paolini EA, Bernardi D, Bruno G, Nannini E. Prognostic value of pharmacological stress echocardiography in women with chest pain and unknown coronary artery disease. J Am Coll Cardiol 1998; 32:1975–81.

35 Dodi C, Cortigiani L, Masini M, Olivotto I, Azzarelli A, Nannini E. The incremental prognostic value of stress echo over exercise electrocardiography in women with chest pain of unknown origin. Eur Heart J 2001; 22:145–52.

36 Elhendy A, van Domburg RT, Poldermans D, Bax JJ, Nierop PR, Geleijnse ML, et al. Safety and feasibility of dobutamine-atropine stress echocardiography for the diagnosis of coronary artery disease in diabetic patients unable to perform an exercise stress test. Diabetes Care 1998; 21:1797–802.

37 Cortigiani L, Bigi R, Sicari R, Rigo F, Bovenzi F, Picano E. Comparison of the prognostic value of pharmacologic stress echocardiography in chest pain patients with versus without diabetes mellitus and positive exercise electrocardiography. Am J Cardiol 2007; 100:1744–9.

38 Mairesse GH, Marwick TH, Arnese M, Vanoverschelde JL, Cornel JH, Detry JM, et al. Improved identification of coronary artery disease in patients with left bundle branch block by the use of dobutamine stress echocardiography and comparison with myocardial perfusion tomography. Am J Cardiol 1995; 76:321–5.

39 Geleijnse ML, Vigna G, Kasprzak JD, Rambaldi R, Salvatori MP, Elhendy A, et al. Usefulness and limitations of dobutamine-atropine stress echocardiography for the diagnosis of coronary artery disease in patients with left bundle branch block. Eur Heart J 2000; 21:1666–73.

40 Cortigiani L, Picano E, Vigna C, Lattanzi F, Coletta C, Mariotti E, et al. Prognostic value of pharmacologic stress echocardiography in patients with left bundle branch block. Am J Med 2001; 110:361–9.

41 Beattie WS, Abdelnaem E, Wijeysundera DN, Buckley DN. A meta-analytic comparison of preoperative stress echocardiography and nuclear scintigraphy imaging. Anesth Analg 2006; 102:8–16.

42 Boersma E, Poldermans D, Bax JJ, Steyerberg EW, Thomson IR, Banga JD, et al.; DECREASE Study Group (Dutch Echocardiographic Cardiac Risk Evaluation Applying Stress Echocardiogrpahy). Predictors of cardiac events after major vascular surgery: Role of clinical characteristics, dobutamine echocardiography, and beta-blocker therapy. JAMA 2001; 285:1865–73.

43 Picano E, Pasanisi E, Brown J, Marwick TH. A gatekeeper for the gatekeeper: inappropriate referrals to stress echocardiography. Am Heart J 2007; 154:285–90.

44 Caiati C, Montaldo C, Zedda N, Bina A, Iliceto S. New noninvasive method for coronary flow reserve assessment: contrast-enhanced transthoracic second harmonic echo Doppler. Circulation 1999; 99:771–8.

45 Radvan J, Marwick TH, Williams MJ, Camici PG. Evaluation of the extent and timing of the coronary hyperemic response to dipyridamole: a study with transesophageal echocardiography and positron emission tomography with oxygen 15 water. J Am Soc Echocardiogr 1995; 8:864–73.

46 Cortigiani L, Rigo F, Gherardi S, Sicari R, Galderisi M, Bovenzi F, Picano E. Additional prognostic value of coronary flow reserve in diabetic and nondiabetic patients with negative dipyridamole stress echocardiography by wall motion criteria. J Am Coll Cardiol 2007; 50:1354–61.

47 Cortigiani L, Rigo F, Sicari R, Gherardi S, Bovenzi F, Picano E. Prognostic correlates of combined coronary flow reserve assessment on left anterior descending and right coronary artery in patients with negative stress echocardiography by wall motion criteria. Heart 2009; 95:1423–8.

48 Rigo F, Gherardi S, Galderisi M, Cortigiani L. Coronary flow reserve evaluation in stress-echo lab. *J Cardiovasc Med* 2006; **7**:472–9.

49 Sicari R, Rigo F, Gherardi S, Galderisi M, Cortigiani L, Picano E. The prognostic value of Doppler echocardiographic-derived coronary flow reserve is not affected by concomitant antiischemic therapy at the time of testing. *Am Heart J* 2008; **156**:573–9.

50 Rigo F, Sicari R, Gherardi S, Djordjevic-Dikic A, Cortigiani L, Picano E. The additive prognostic value of wall motion abnormalities and coronary flow reserve during dipyridamole stress echo. *Eur Heart J* 2008; **29**:79–88.

51 Rigo F, Sicari R, Gherardi S, Djordjevic-Dikic A, Cortigiani L, Picano E. Prognostic value of coronary flow reserve in medically treated patients with left anterior descending coronary disease with stenosis 51%-75% in diameter. *Am J Cardiol* 2007; **100**:1527–31.

52 Sicari R, Rigo F, Cortigiani L, Gherardi S, Galderisi M, Picano E. Long-term survival of patients with chest pain syndrome and angiographically normal or near normal coronary arteries: the additional prognostic value of coronary flow reserve. *Am J Cardiol* 2009; **103**:626–31.

53 Cortigiani L, Rigo F, Gherardi S, Bovenzi F, Picano E, Sicari R. Prognostic implication of the continuous sprectrum of doppler echocardiographic derived coronary flow reserve on left anterior descending artery. *Am J Cardiol* 2010; **105**:158–62.

54 Smart SC, Sawada S, Ryan T, Segar D, Atherton L, Berkovitz K, et al. Low-dose dobutamine echocardiography detects reversible dysfunction after thrombolytic therapy of acute myocardial infarction. *Circulation* 1993; **88**:405–15.

55 Bax JJ, Wijns W, Cornel JH, Visser FC, Boersma E, Fioretti PM. Accuracy of currently available techniques for prediction of functional recovery after revascularization in patients with left ventricular dysfunction due to chronic coronary artery disease: comparison of pooled data. *J Am Coll Cardiol* 1997; **30**:1451–60.

56 Baumgartner H, Porenta G, Lau YK, Wutte M, Klaar U, Mehrabi M, et al. Assessment of myocardial viability by dobutamine echocardiography, positron emission tomography and thallium-201 SPECT: correlation with histopathology in explanted hearts. *J Am Coll Cardiol* 1998; **32**:1701–8.

57 Picano E, Sicari R, Landi P, Cortigiani L, Bigi R, Coletta C, et al. The prognostic value of myocardial viability in medically treated patients with global ventricular dysfunction early after an acute uncomplicated myocardial infarction: a dobutamine stress echocardiographic study. *Circulation* 1998; **98**:1078–84.

58 Sicari R, Picano E, Landi P, Pingitore A, Bigi R, Coletta C, et al. Prognostic value of dobutamine-atropine stress echocardiography early after acute myocardial infarction. *J Am Coll Cardiol* 1997; **29**:54–60.

59 Meluzin J, Cerny J, Frelich M, Stetka F, Spinarova L, Popelova J, Stipal R. Prognostic value of the amount of dysfunctional but viable myocardium in revascularized patients with coronary artery disease and left ventricular dysfunction. Investigators of this Multicenter Study. *J Am Coll Cardiol* 1998; **32**:912–20.

60 Senior R, Kaul S, Lahiri A. Myocardial viability on echocardiography predicts long-term survival after revascularization in patients with ischemic congestive heart failure. *J Am Coll Cardiol* 1999; **33**:1848–54.

61 Sicari R, Picano E, Cortigiani L, Borges A, Varga A, Palagi C, et al. Prognostic value of myocardial viability recognized by low-dose dobutamine echocardiography in chronic ischemic left ventricular dysfunction. *Am J Cardiol* 2003; **92**:1263–6.

62 Cortigiani L, Sicari R, Desideri A, Bigi R, Bovenzi F, Picano E. Dobutamine stress echocardiography and the effect of revascularization on outcome of diabetic and nondiabetic patients with chronic ischemic left ventricular dysfunction. *Eur J Heart Fail* 2007; **9**:1138–43.

63 Allman KC, Shaw LJ, Hachamovitch R, Udelson JE. Myocardial viability testing and impact of revascularization on prognosis in patients with coronary artery disease and left ventricular dysfunction: a meta-analysis. *J Am Coll Cardiol* 2002; **39**:1151–8.

64 Ciampi Q, Pratali L, Citro R, Piacenti M, Villari B, Picano E. Identification of responders to cardiac resynchronization therapy by contractile reserve during stress echocardiography. *Eur J Heart Fail* 2009; **11**:489–96.

65 Picano E, Pibarot P, Lancellotti P, Monin JL, Bonow RO. The emerging role of exercise testing and stress echocardiography in valvular heart disease. *J Am Coll Cardiol* 2009; **54**:2251–60.

66 Monin JL, Monchi M, Gest V, Duval-Moulin AM, Dubois-Rande JL, Gueret P. Aortic stenosis with severe left ventricular dysfunction and low transvalvular pressure gradients: risk stratification by low dose dobutamine echocardiography. *J Am Coll Cardiol* 2001; **37**:2101–7.

67 Quere JP, Monin JL, Levy F, Petit H, Baleynaud S, Chauvel C, et al. Influence of preoperative left ventricular contractile reserve on postoperative ejection fraction in low-gradient aortic stenosis. *Circulation* 2006; **113**:1738–44.

68 Bonow RO, Carabello BA, Chatterjee K, de Leon AC Jr, Faxon DP, Freed MD, et al. ACC/AHA (2006) guidelines for the management of patients with valvular heart disease: a report of the American College of Cardiology/American Heart Association Task Force on Practice Guidelines (writing Committee to Revise the (1998) guidelines for the management of patients with valvular heart disease) developed in collaboration with the Society of Cardiovascular Anesthesiologists endorsed by the Society for Cardiovascular Angiography and Interventions and the Society of Thoracic Surgeons. *J Am Coll Cardiol* 2006; **48**:e1–148.

69 Pierard LA, Lancellotti P. The role of ischemic mitral regurgitation in the pathogenesis of acute pulmonary edema. *N Engl J Med* 2004; **351**:1627–34.

70 Lancellotti P, Gérard P, Piérard LA. Long term outcome of patients with heart failure and dynamic mitral regurgitation. *Eur Heart J* 2005; **26**:1528–32.

71 Varga A, Garcia MA, Picano E. Safety of stress echocardiography (from the International Stress Echo Complication Registry). *Am J Cardiol* 2006; **98**:541–3.

72 Fletcher GF, Balady GJ, Amsterdam EA, Chaitman B, Eckel R, Fleg J, et al. Exercise standards for testing and training: a statement for healthcare professionals from the American Heart Association. *Circulation* 2001; **104**:1694–740.

73 Cortigiani L, Zanetti L, Bigi R, Desideri A, Fiorentini C, Nannini E. Safety and feasibility of dobutamine and dipyridamole stress echocardiography in hypertensive patients. *J Hypertens* 2002; **20**:1423–9.

74 Picano E, Mathias W Jr, Pingitore A, Bigi R, Previtali M, on behalf of the EDIC study group. Safety and tolerability of dobutamine-atropine stress echocardiography: a prospective, large scale, multicenter trial. *Lancet* 1994; **344**:1190–2.

75 Cerqueira MD, Verani MS, Schwaiger M, Heo J, Iskandrian AS. Safety profile of adenosine stress perfusion imaging: results from the Adenoscan Multicenter Trial Registry. *J Am Coll Cardiol* 1994; **23**:384–9.

76 Patel MR, Spertus JA, Brindis RG, Hendel RC, Douglas PS, Peterson ED, *et al.*; American College of Cardiology Foundation. ACCF proposed method for evaluating the appropriateness of cardiovascular imaging. *J Am Coll Cardiol* 2005; **46**:1606–13.

77 Gibbons RJ, Abrams J, Chatterjee K, Daley J, Deedwania PC, Douglas JS, *et al.*; American College of Cardiology; American Heart Association Task Force on practice guidelines (Committee on the Management of Patients With Chronic Stable Angina). ACC/AHA (2002) guideline update for the management of patients with chronic stable angina–summary article: a report of the American College of Cardiology/American Heart Association Task Force on practice guidelines (Committee on the Management of Patients With Chronic Stable Angina). *J Am Coll Cardiol* 2003; **41**:159–68.

78 Douglas PS, Khandheria B, Stainback RF, Weissman NJ, Peterson ED, Hendel RC, *et al.* ACCF/ASE/ACEP/AHA/ASNC/SCAI/SCCT/SCMR (2008) appropriateness criteria for stress echocardiography: a report of the American College of Cardiology Foundation Appropriateness Criteria Task Force, American Society of Echocardiography, American College of Emergency Physicians, American Heart Association, American Society of Nuclear Cardiology, Society for Cardiovascular Angiography and Interventions, Society of Cardiovascular Computed Tomography, and Society for Cardiovascular Magnetic Resonance: endorsed by the Heart Rhythm Society and the Society of Critical Care Medicine. *Circulation* 2008; **117**:1478–97.

79 Picano E, Lattanzi F, Orlandini A, Marini C, L'Abbate A. Stress echocardiography and the human factor: the importance of being expert. *J Am Coll Cardiol* 1991; **17**:666–9.

80 Popp R, Agatston A, Armstrong W, Nanda N, Pearlman A, Rakowski H, *et al.* Recommendations for training in performance and interpretation of stress echocardiography. Committee on Physician Training and Education of the American Society of Echocardiography. *J Am Soc Echocardiogr* 1998; **11**:95–6.

81 Fox K, Garcia MA, Ardissino D, Buszman P, Camici PG, Crea F, *et al.*; Task Force on the Management of Stable Angina Pectoris of the European Society of Cardiology; ESC Committee for Practice Guidelines (CPG). Guidelines on the management of stable angina pectoris: executive summary: The Task Force on the Management of Stable Angina Pectoris of the European Society of Cardiology. *Eur Heart J* 2006; **27**:1341–81.

82 Picano E. Stress echocardiography: a historical perspective. Special article. *Am J Med* 2003; **114**: 126–30.

83 Picano E. Informed consent and communication of risk from radiological and nuclear medicine examinations: how to escape from a communication inferno. Education and debate. *BMJ* 2004; **329**:849–851.

84 Picano E. Sustainability of medical imaging. Education and debate. *BMJ* 2004; **328**:578–80.

Fleisher LA, Beckman JA, Brown KA, Calkins H, Chaikof EL, Fleischmann KE, *et al.* ACC/AHA (2007) Guidelines on Perioperative Cardiovascular Evaluation and Care for Noncardiac Surgery: Executive Summary: A Report of the American College of Cardiology/American Heart Association Task Force on Practice Guidelines (Writing Committee to Revise the (2002) Guidelines on Perioperative Cardiovascular Evaluation for Noncardiac Surgery) Developed in Collaboration With the American Society of Echocardiography, American Society of Nuclear Cardiology, Heart Rhythm Society, Society of Cardiovascular Anesthesiologists, Society for Cardiovascular Angiography and Interventions, Society for Vascular Medicine and Biology, and Society for Vascular Surgery. *J Am Coll Cardiol* 2007; **50**:1707–32.

Gerber TC, Carr JJ, Arai AE, Dixon RL, Ferrari VA, Gomes AS, Heller GV, McCollough CH, McNitt-Gray MF, Mettler FA, Mieres JH, Morin RL, Yester MV. Ionizing radiation in cardiac imaging: a science advisory from the American Heart Association Committee on Cardiac Imaging of the Council on Clinical Cardiology and Committee on Cardiovascular Imaging and Intervention of the Council on Cardiovascular Radiology and Intervention. *Circulation* 2009; **119**:1056–65.

Lang RM, Bierig M, Devereux RB, Flachskampf FA, Foster E, Pellikka PA, *et al.* Chamber Quantification Writing Group; American Society of Echocardiography's Guidelines and Standards Committee; European Association of Echocardiography. Recommendations for chamber quantification: a report from the American Society of Echocardiography's Guidelines and Standards Committee and the Chamber Quantification Writing Group, developed in conjunction with the European Association of Echocardiography, a branch of the European Society of Cardiology. *J Am Soc Echocardiogr* 2005; **18**:1440–63.

Patel MR, Spertus JA, Brindis RG, Hendel RC, Douglas PS, Peterson ED, *et al.*; American College of Cardiology Foundation. ACCF proposed method for evaluating the appropriateness of cardiovascular imaging. *J Am Coll Cardiol* 2005; **46**: 1606–13.

Pellikka PA, Nagueh SF, Elhendy AA, Kuehl CA, Sawada SG; American Society of Echocardiography. American Society of Echocardiography recommendations for performance, interpretation, and application of stress echocardiography. *J Am Soc Echocardiogr* 2007; **20**:1021–41.

President's Cancer Panel: Environmentally caused cancers are 'grossly underestimated' and 'needlessly devastate American lives'. http://www.environmentalhealthnews.org/ehs/news/presidents-cancer-panel

⮡ For additional multimedia materials please visit the online version of the book (🔖 http://escecho.oxfordmedicine.com).

Further reading

Brindis R, Douglas PS. President's page: The ACC encourages multi-pronged approach to radiation safety. *J Am Coll Cardiol* 2010; **56**:522–4.

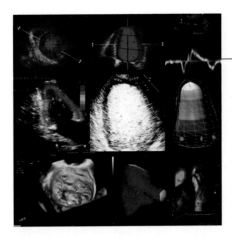

CHAPTER 14A

Aortic valve disease

Raphael Rosenhek, Robert Feneck, and Fabio Guarracino

Contents

Summary

Echocardiography is the gold standard for the assessment of patients with aortic valve (AoV) disease. It allows a detailed morphological assessment of the AoV and thereby makes determination of the aetiology possible. In general, the quantification of aortic stenosis is based on the measurement of transaortic jet velocities and the calculation of AoV area, thus combining a flow-dependent and a flow-independent variable. In the setting of low-flow low-gradient AS, dobutamine echocardiography is of particular diagnostic and prognostic importance. The quantification of aortic regurgitation is based on qualitative and quantitative parameters. Awareness of potential pitfalls is fundamental. Haemodynamic consequences of AoV disease on left ventricular size, hypertrophy, and function as well as potentially coexisting valve lesions can be assessed simultaneously. In patients with AoV disease, predictors of outcome and indications for surgery are substantially defined by echocardiography.

Introduction

Aortic stenosis (AS) is increasingly diagnosed in developed countries due to an ageing population but also to more widely available diagnostic methods. The presentation encompasses the spectrum from asymptomatic patients in different disease stages to symptomatic patients who may present with preserved or already depressed ventricular function. Echocardiography is the method of choice permitting a comprehensive non-invasive diagnostic work-up of these patients.

Aortic stenosis

Assessment of aortic stenosis morphology

Differential diagnosis of left ventricular outflow obstruction

Valvular AS is the most frequent heart valve disease and also the most common form of left ventricular (LV) outflow obstruction. Yet, possible differential diagnoses need to be considered when outflow obstruction is present.

Subvalvular AS consists of a fixed obstruction below the AoV level in the LV outflow tract (LVOT) and may be due to a membrane or a fibromuscular ridge or narrowing (➲ Fig. 14a.1).

Hypertrophic obstructive cardiomyopathy results in a dynamic obstruction that is most accentuated in mid-systole.

Supravalvular AS is a rare congenital lesion in which the ascending aorta is narrowed (➲ Fig. 14a.2).

The differential diagnosis is based on the morphologic localization as well as the site and pattern of flow acceleration.

Aetiology of aortic stenosis

The most detailed morphological assessment of the AoV is performed in a parasternal short-axis (PSAX) view. Additional information on AoV morphology and mobility can be obtained from the parasternal long-axis (PLAX), the apical three-chamber (A3C) and five-chamber (A5C) views.[1]

Congenital aortic stenosis

Congenital AS is typically encountered in the form of a bicuspid AoV (➲ Fig. 14a.3A), although unicuspid, tricuspid, and

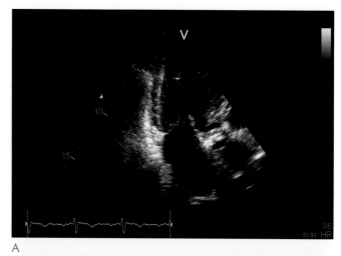

A

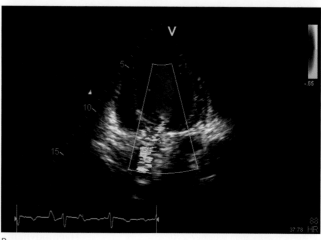

B

Figure 14a.2 Example of supravalvular stenosis. A) Three-chamber view of a patient with supravalvular stenosis. An obstruction is recognizable in the ascending aorta at the level of the sinotubular junction. B) Colour flow image of the same patient in a five-chamber view.

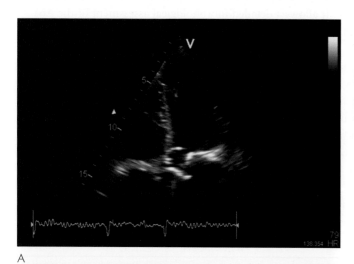

A

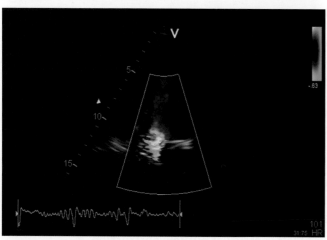

B

Figure 14a.1 Example of subaortic stenosis. A) Five-chamber view of a patient with subaortic stenosis. The subaortic membrane can be seen in the outflow tract. B) Colour flow image of a five-chamber view of the same patient. Flow convergence can be seen in before the subvalvular membrane

quadricuspid forms are encountered. The most common type of bicuspidity is a fusion between the right and left coronary cusps (approximately 90%), followed in incidence by a fusion of the right and the non-coronary cusps (approximately 9%), while a fusion between the left and the non-coronary cusps is rare (approximately 1%). A raphe, which corresponds to an area of thickening at the site of the fused leaflets, may be present. The distinction between a tricuspid and a bicuspid aortic valve with a raphe is not always unequivocal. Suggestive signs of a bicuspid aortic valve are a sigmoid shape of the AoV in the PLAX view or an eccentric closure line in the M-mode.

Rheumatic aortic stenosis

Rheumatic AS (➲ Fig. 14a.3B) is nowadays rarely encountered in the developed world but is still a major health issue in developing countries. The valve is characterized by thickening at the leaflet borders and commissural fusion. Frequently, concomitant aortic regurgitation (AR) is present and in most cases also the mitral valve (MV) is affected.

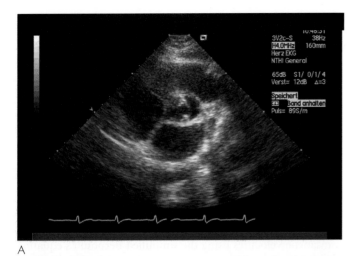

A

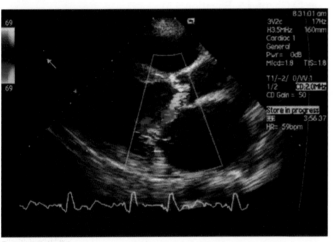

B

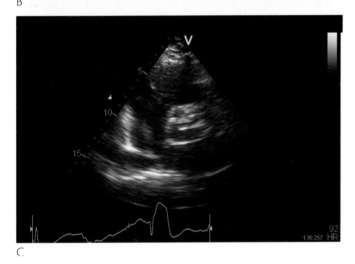

C

Figure 14a.3 Aetiologies of aortic stenosis. A) PSAX view of a bicuspid aortic valve with minimal calcification. B) PLAX colour flow view of a rheumatically affected aortic valve with AS and concomitant regurgitation. Predominant thickening of the cusp edges and affection of the mitral valve can be observed. C) PSAX view of a calcific aortic stenosis with thickened and calcified cusps

Calcific aortic stenosis

Calcific AS (➲ Fig. 14a.3C) is the most common form of AS observed in adult patients and is characterized by thickened and calcified aortic leaflets with reduced motion. Echocardiographically, echodense zones, which correspond to zones of calcification, are visualized. This entity used to be denominated *degenerative aortic stenosis* as it was thought to be a degenerative process. However, it has been demonstrated that the underlying disease process is active and ultimately leading to valve calcification: *calcific aortic stenosis* is thus the more appropriate term. It is of note that also bicuspid aortic valves tend to calcify and that the distinction between a bi- and tricuspid valve may be difficult when extensive calcification is present.

Aortic valve calcification

Echocardiography is an excellent semiquantitative tool to assess AoV calcification by description of echodense zones. For this purpose, the AoV is best viewed in a PSAX view, although the PLAX and the A3C and A5C views are also helpful. The following classification has been proposed:

- Mild calcification: isolated, small echodense spots (➲ Fig. 14a.4A).
- Moderate calcification: multiple bigger spots (➲ Fig. 14a.4B).
- Severe calcification: extensive thickening and calcification of all cusps (➲ Fig. 14a.4C).[2]

For prognostic purposes, the differentiation between no or mild calcification on one side and moderate or severe calcification on the other side is essential.

Assessment of the ascending aorta

The ascending aorta should be routinely assessed in patients with AS since a dilation of the ascending aorta is frequently observed. In particular, patients with bicuspid but also those with unicuspid AoVs tend to have associated aortic aneurysms. The assessment is performed in a PLAX view and includes measurements at the levels of the aortic annulus, the sinuses of Valsalva, the sinotubular junction, and the ascending aorta. While the aortic annulus is measured as an inner diameter, the other measures of the ascending aorta are measured from leading edge to leading edge. The assessment of the ascending aorta and of the aortic annulus is of critical importance in the patient screening process for percutaneous AoV therapies. Transoesophageal echocardiography (TOE) is of additional diagnostic value in selected cases and is now routinely used in the assessment of potential candidates for percutaneous valve implantation.

When an ascending aneurysm is detected by echocardiography or when the echocardiographic visualization is insufficient, additional imaging methods, such as cardiac magnetic resonance (CMR) or computed tomography (CT) may be indicated.

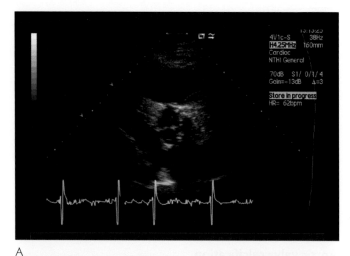

A

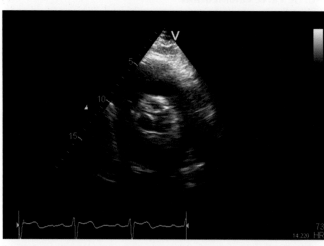

B

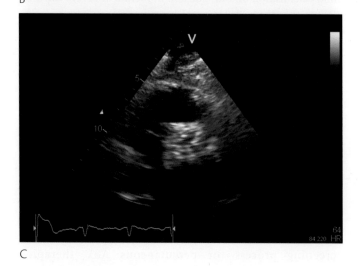

C

Figure 14a.4 Degree of aortic valve calcification. A) PSAX view of a bicuspid aortic stenosis with mild calcification. B) PSAX view of a stenotic aortic valve with moderate calcification. C) PSAX view of a stenotic aortic valve with severe calcification of all cusps.

Quantification of aortic stenosis severity

The normal AoV area is in the range of 3–4cm². Under normal conditions, the transvalvular flow is laminar with a peak transaortic jet velocity typically less than 2m/s. With narrowing of the AoV, the transaortic jet velocities increase, the velocity increase being most significant in the presence of severe stenosis.[3–5]

Transaortic jet velocities and pressure gradients

Transaortic jet velocities are measured by recording the maximal transaortic flow signal using a continuous wave (CW) Doppler mode.[6] Transaortic gradients can be derived from transaortic velocities using the simplified Bernoulli's equation (see ➲ Chapter 5, Equation 5.3).

With increasing AS severity, the peak of the transaortic gradient is reached later during systole (➲ Fig. 14a.5).

The mean gradient can be determined by integrating the gradient over the entire systole (see ➲ Chapter 5, 'Haemodynamic parameters' and 'Study of valvular stenosis'): this feature is included in all commercially available echo machines. Overall a good correlation is observed between peak and mean gradients assessed by echocardiography.

In AS, the value of pressure gradients obtained with invasive haemodynamic procedures is different from that calculated with echocardiography: the catheter-determined peak-to-peak gradient and the peak instantaneous gradient that is measured by echocardiography are not identical. The peak-to-peak gradient is calculated by measuring the pressure difference between systolic LV pressure and systolic aortic pressure. This measurement is not performed instantaneously, as is the case for echocardiography. The maximal systolic ventricular pressure is determined first and, after having pulledback the catheter into the ascending aorta, the aortic peak pressure is measured. Since the two pressure peaks do not occur simultaneously, the measured gradient does not correspond to a physiological value. In contrast, the maximal instantaneous echocardiographic gradient represents the difference of pressure at the same time point of the curve of ventricular and aortic systolic pressure. The maximal instantaneous echocardiographic gradient is higher than the peak-to-peak one. In case of severe AS, the difference between both gradients decreases. The mean gradients measured by echo or by catheterization are comparable (➲ Fig. 14a.6).

Pitfalls of aortic velocity measurement

Recording of the peak transaortic velocity

For an accurate measurement of the transaortic jet velocity, the Doppler beam needs to be aligned with the stenotic aortic jet. Alignment errors lead to an underestimation of the true velocity, and consequently to a potential underestimation of AS severity. Consequently, a meticulous search of the peak signal is

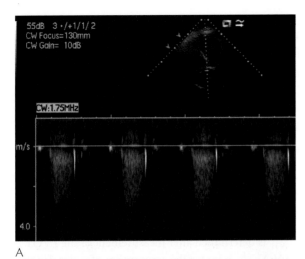

A

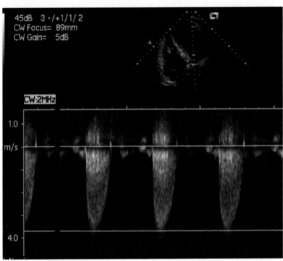

B

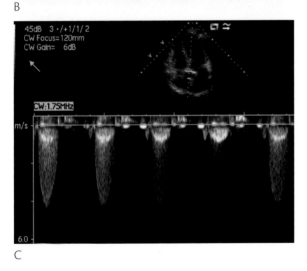

C

Figure 14a.5 Continuous-wave Doppler spectrums showing the velocity peaks. A) Mild AS with immediate peak. B) Moderate AS with early peak. C) Severe AS with mid-systolic peak.

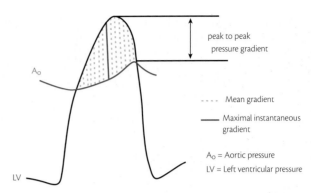

Figure 14a.6 Aortic pressure gradients. Schema of the aortic pressure gradient measured by echocardiography and its comparison with peak-to-peak gradient.

mandatory. In clinical routine, aortic jet velocity is typically recorded using the CW Doppler mode from an apical transducer position. In some cases a more lateral transducer position may lead to a better alignment with the stenotic jet. A comprehensive assessment includes the search of the peak velocity through additional acoustic windows including right parasternal intercostal spaces, suprasternal and subcostal approaches using a small, dedicated CW Doppler transducer (*pencil probe*). It is not rare, that significantly higher aortic jet velocities can be recorded from these image windows (➲ Fig. 14a.7). Particularly, in symptomatic patients in whom initially measured velocities would correspond to moderate stenosis, it is essential to assert that stenosis severity is not underestimated.

Confusion with other signals

Another possible pitfall is to confound the AS CW Doppler signal with a mitral regurgitation (MR) or even a tricuspid regurgitation (TR) signal. When hypertrophic cardiomyopathy is coexisting, the differentiation of the two components of obstruction leading to increased outflow tract velocities may be difficult: the typical shape of the signal in hypertrophic obstructive cardiomyopathy and the two-dimensional (2D) colour Doppler (CD) view may be of help to distinguish the signals.

Arrhythmia

In the presence of arrhythmia, the gradients vary between the beats. In particular, atrial fibrillation is not uncommonly encountered in patients with AS. In this setting, gradient and velocity measurements of 5–10 beats should be averaged.

Pressure recovery

Pressure recovery may explain some discordance between echocardiographically and invasively determined transaortic gradients. From a haemodynamic perspective, flow accelerates across the stenotic AoV to a maximum at the level of maximal flow contraction, which is called the vena contracta. After this point flow decelerates and part of the kinetic energy is reconverted into pressure downstream from the stenotic orifice in the ascending aorta. Since echocardiography measures the peak velocity (occurring at the level of the vena contracta), the Doppler gradient may be

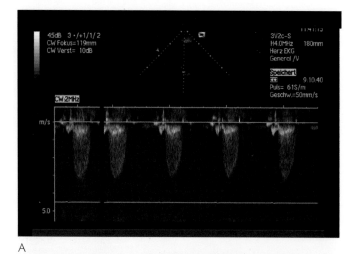

A

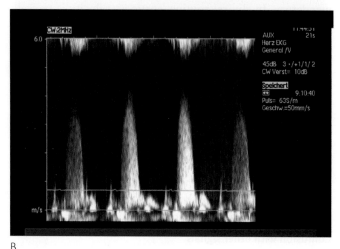

B

Figure 14a.7 Severe aortic stenosis. CW Doppler recordings in the same patient as ➲ Fig. 14a.6 from the: A) apical window AV-Vel 3.3m/s corresponding to moderate AS; B) and from the right parasternal window (AV-Vel 4.6m/s) corresponding with severe AS.

higher than an invasively measured gradient. While the phenomenon of pressure recovery is of negligible magnitude in most cases encountered in clinical practice, it is most accentuated in the presence of a small ascending aorta and when AS is less severe.[7] In this latter setting, higher transaortic gradients may be recorded echocardiographically than invasively.

Flow dependence

Transaortic jet velocities are flow-dependent. In the presence of high output states such as anaemia, hyperthyroidism, or in patients with arteriovenous shunts, transaortic velocities may be increased. On the other hand, a low cardiac output may result in relatively low velocities (see later).

Assessment of valve area by continuity equation

Aortic valve area (AVA) is a flow independent variable that is calculated using the continuity equation (see ➲ Chapter 5, 'Study of the intracardiac pressures'), since the same stroke

volume flows through the LVOT and through the stenotic AoV (➲ Fig. 14a.8).[8]

By applying ➲ Equation 5.18 to study of LVOT and AoV, the stroke volume at the level of LVOT is calculated by multiplying the cross-sectional area (CSA_{LVOT}) by the VTI_{LVOT}. Similarly, the stroke volume at the level of the stenotic valve is defined as the product of AVA and VTI_{AS}:

$$CSA_{LVOT} \times VTI_{LVOT} = AVA \times VTI_{AS}$$

Thus aortic valve is calculated as follows:

$$AVA = (CSA_{LVOT} \times VTI_{LVOT})/VTI_{AS} \qquad (14a.1)$$

CSA_{LVOT} is determined after measurement of the LVOT diameter ($LVOT_{Diam}$), under the assumption of a circular shape of the latter:

$$CSA_{LVOT} = \pi (LVOT_{Diam}/2)^2 \qquad (14a.2)$$

$LVOT_{Diam}$ is measured as an inner diameter proximally to the AoV in mid-systole and is best visualized in a PLAX view, ideally after zooming in on the area of interest. In practice, confirmation of the diameter from an A5C view is recommendable.

VTI_{LVOT} is measured with pulsed wave (PW) Doppler proximally to the AoV from an A5C view, prior to the AoV, and VTI_{AS} is determined from the CW peak transaortic velocity signal.

In clinical practice, a simplified form of the continuity equation, in which velocities are used instead of velocity time integrals, can be used:

$$AVA = (CSA_{LVOT} \times Vel_{LVOT})/Vel_{AS}$$

The assumptions of a circular outflow tract and of a laminar flow profile as well as measurement errors will result in some degree of imprecision of AVA calculations.

Velocity ratio

Since the determination of LVOT is prone to sources of error, another flow independent variable, the velocity ratio, which is defined as the ratio of velocities in the LVOT and across the AoV was proposed.

$$\text{Velocity ratio} = Vel_{LVOT}/Vel_{AS} \quad \text{or}$$
$$\text{Velocity ratio} = VTI_{LVOT}/VTI_{AS} \qquad (14a.3)$$

Severe stenosis is defined by velocity ratio less than 0.25.

Definition of aortic stenosis severity

AS severity encompasses a continuous spectrum of disease, ranging from aortic sclerosis without haemodynamic obstruction to very severe AS. In context, the measures of disease severity need to be viewed in a continuous way. Definition of grades of severity of AS is consequently to some extent arbitrary. In clinical practice, peak transaortic jet velocities, mean gradients

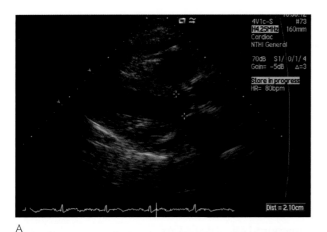

A

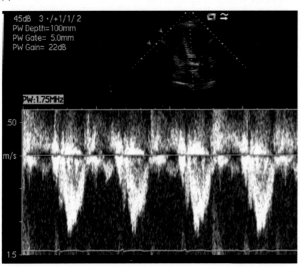

B

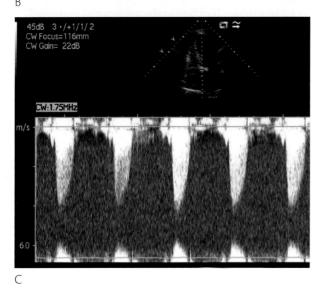

C

Figure 14a.8 Measurements for the continuity equation.
A) Measurement of the LVOT diameter in a PLAX view. B) Measurement of the LVOT velocity by PW Doppler from an A5C view. C) Measurement of the peak aortic jet velocity by CW Doppler from an A5C view

and valve areas (calculated with the continuity equation) should be considered and the findings are ideally concordant (➲ Table 14a.1). The prognostic importance of peak aortic jet velocity across the whole spectrum of AS and even beyond the threshold of severe stenosis has been demonstrated. It should be recognized that in clinical practice, a relatively large variability in AoV area measurements for a given peak aortic jet velocity has been reported.[9]

♦ Aortic sclerosis: is defined as the presence of calcific changes at the AoV level without haemodynamic obstruction to blood flow.

♦ Mild AS: is characterized by beginning outflow tract obstruction with peak transaortic jet velocity superior to 2.0m/s and an AVA that is larger than 1.5m/s.

♦ Moderate AS: is defined by a peak aortic jet velocity comprised between 3.0–4.0m/s and a AVA between 1.5–1.0cm^2.

♦ Severe AS: because of the poor outcome of symptomatic patients with severe AS, the threshold characterizing severe AS is the most relevant, clinically. an AVA less than 1.0cm^2 and a peak aortic jet velocity greater than 4.0m/s define severe AS according to both the European Society of cardiology (ESC) and the American College of Cardiology/ American Heart Association (ACC/AHA) guidelines.

There is a slight discrepancy between the guidelines with regard to the mean gradient: a mean gradient greater than 50mmHg is proposed by the ESC guidelines, whereas a mean gradient greater than 40mmHg is suggested by the ACC/AHA guidelines. Considering that symptom onset occurs with variable interindividual characteristics, that a variability of measurements is documented and knowing the poor outcome of symptomatic patients with severe AS, a valve should be considered as being significantly stenotic in this intermediate zone in symptomatic patients. In the asymptomatic patient, the prognostic consequences are of lesser magnitude and the difference is rather of semantic nature. Patient stature should also be considered. An AVA indexed to body surface area (BSA) of less than 0.6cm^2/m^2, has been proposed as a threshold for severe AS. However, this value may not be valid in tall and very obese or very slim and small patients in whom the indexed AVA may lead to a misinterpretation of true AS severity.

Recent prognostic data, seem to justify the definition of *very severe* stenosis,[10] based on a peak aortic jet velocity greater than 5m/s, a mean gradient less than 60mmHg, and a AVA less than 0.9cm^2.

Assessment of aortic stenosis progression

AS progression should be routinely assessed in clinical practice. Changes in peak aortic jet velocity, mean gradient, and AVA can be determined between two exams. Haemodynamic progression can be expressed as an annualized progression rate. It is advisable to use examinations that are separated by 6–12 months. AS progression is most sensitively recorded by changes in peak aortic jet velocity, while AVA is less sensitive to detect

Table 14a.1 Quantification of aortic stenosis severity[4,5,10]

	Aortic sclerosis	Mild aortic stenosis	Moderate aortic stenosis	Severe aortic stenosis	Very severe aortic stenosis***
Peak aortic jet velocity (m/s)	≤2.5	2.5–3.0	3.0–4.0	>4.0	>5.0***
Mean gradient (mmHg)		<30*	30–50*	>50*	>60***
		<25**	25–40**	>40**	
Aortic valve area (cm²)		>1.5	1.0–1.5	<1.0	<0.9

* ESC Guidelines, ** AHA/ACC Guidelines, ***According to Reference 10.

Table 14a.2 Requirement of a standard echocardiographic report of a patient with aortic stenosis

Aetiology of aortic stenosis
Morphology of the aortic valve and degree of valve calcification
Quantification of stenosis severity including the following measurements:
Peak aortic jet velocity
Mean transaortic gradient
Aortic valve area
Specification of the echocardiographic window used to measure the velocity
Left ventricular function and hypertrophy
Associated valve lesions

small changes in AS severity due to imprecision involved in its calculation. The assessment of changes in aortic jet velocity is only reliable when the velocity measurements are performed from the same echocardiographic window, which should therefore be mentioned in the echocardiographic report. Furthermore, a change in ventricular function needs to be excluded when using flow dependent measures to assess haemodynamic progression

Other measures of severity

Aortic valve area planimetry

Due to the complex orientation of the stenotic AoV orifice, adjusting the exact plane for valve area planimetry is technically difficult and imprecise, particularly in the presence of extensive valve calcification. AS planimetry is therefore not used in clinical routine. However, recent advances in 3D echocardiography and in particular of 3D-TOE may make this method more attractive in selected cases when other measures are not concordant or for patients being in an intensive care setting when an adequate acquisition of Doppler signals is not feasible.

Aortic valve resistance

Valve resistance (R; in dynes·s·cm⁻⁵) is calculated using the following formula:

$$R = (\Delta P_{mean}/Q_{mean}) \times 1333 \qquad (14a.4)$$

where ΔP_{mean} is the mean transaortic gradient (in mmHg) and Q_{mean} is the mean flow rate (in mL/s). From some observations,

it appears that valve resistance is not flow independent and thus not superior to calculated AVAs.

These and other measures of AS severity such as stroke work loss which corresponds to the amount of work required to maintain the flow through the stenotic AoV in relation to the total systolic work have been proposed but have not found an established place in clinical practice, in particular due to an unconfirmed clinical prognostic value.

Low cardiac output

While transaortic jet velocities correlate with AS severity, they have the potential limitation of being flow-dependent. Thus, they may be lower than expected when stroke volume is reduced. In the presence of LV dysfunction, peak jet velocities smaller than 4.0m/s do not systematically rule out the presence of significant AS and the measurements need to be interpreted with caution (⊃ Fig. 14a.9).

Reduced ventricular function in the presence of preserved transaortic gradients

Some patients with impaired LV function may still present with elevated transaortic gradients and small, calculated valve areas corresponding to severe AS. Even patients with markedly depressed ventricular function may have preserved gradients. In this setting the quantification of stenosis severity may thus be unequivocal.

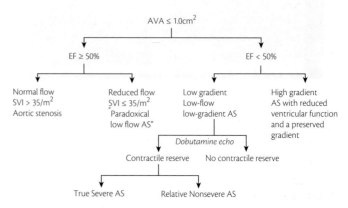

Figure 14a.9 Classification of AS with a calculated valve area ≤1.0cm² according ventricular function, transvalvular gradients, and flow.

Low-flow low-gradient aortic stenosis

Low-flow low-gradient AS is characterized by a small calculated AVA corresponding to severe stenosis ($<1.0cm^2$) and a low transvalvular gradient (mean gradient $<30–40mmHg$) in the presence of a depressed ventricular function. This situation may either be the consequence of true severe AS with consequently depressed LV function or of moderate AS with an independent reason of LV dysfunction such as ischaemic heart disease or a primary cardiomyopathy. From a diagnostic point of view, the work-up of these patients may be challenging. A dobutamine stress echocardiography may provide additional information and help to differentiate between these two entities (➲ Fig. 14a.9).

To avoid potential adverse reactions, a low-dose dobutamine echocardiography protocol is used starting with a dose of 2.5–5.0mcg/kg/min and gradually increasing the dose to a maximum of 20mcg/kg/min. Among the potential complications, arrhythmias may arise due to the induction of ischaemia or due to adrenergic stimulation. The dobutamine echocardiographic exam should be performed by an experienced echocardiographer. It should be terminated in the following conditions:

- A heart rate >100bpm.
- A blood pressure drop.
- The occurrence of symptoms or arrhythmias.

At each stage ventricular function (including ejection fraction [EF], transaortic velocities, and AVAs) should be determined. Ideally the different stages are reviewed side by side—this functionality is routinely included in newer echocardiographic machines and image storing software packages.

In the setting of a low-flow low-gradient AS, the dobutamine echocardiographic exam allows identification of the presence or absence of contractile reserve, which is defined as an increase in stroke volume of 20% or more during stress. In the absence of contractile reserve, the explanatory power of the exam is limited and no conclusions can be inferred on the severity of AS. In contrast, in the presence of a contractile reserve, differential diagnosis between true severe and relative, non-severe stenosis may be possible.[11]

In patients with *true severe AS*, a significant increase in transaortic gradients with increasing flow is observed whereas the calculated valve area remains small. In the case of a *relative, non-severe stenosis*, gradients typically remain low, while the calculated valve area is increasing (➲ Fig. 14a.9): in particular, a true severe AS corresponds to a final AVA less than $1cm^2$ with a stress induced jet velocity greater than 4m/s or a mean pressure gradient greater than 40mmHg. Because this is the result of an increasing opening force on the AoV, which then opens to a greater extent with increasing flow, one of the most important role of dobutamine stress in these patients is to assess the *contractile or inotropic reserve*, defined as an increase of transaortic pressure gradient or stroke volume by at least 20% with dobutamine.

Inotropic reserve correlates with perioperative mortality and prognosis (see later).

Additional information permitting differentiation between these true severe and relative AS can be obtained by assessing the extent of AoV calcification—extensive calcification being suggestive of severe stenosis. Furthermore planimetry may be of help in selected cases.

'Paradoxical low flow aortic stenosis'

Recently the concept of 'paradoxical low flow AS' has been proposed. It is defined by a small calculated AVA, while the measured transaortic gradients correspond to a non-severe stenosis.[12] In contrast to low-flow low-gradient AS, these patients have a normal EF, but nevertheless a reduced stroke volume (a stroke volume index of $\leq35mL/m^2$ has been proposed to define a low stroke volume). This situation may be observed in the presence of a severely hypertrophied LV with a small LV cavity, leading to a reduced stroke volume. Prior to diagnosing paradoxical low flow AS, it is important to rule out both, an underestimation of peak aortic jet velocity and a potential measurement error of LVOT area, both of which may also lead to a similar constellation of measurements.

Left ventricular response

Diastolic filling abnormalities are already present early in the disease course. Chronic pressure overload in AS leads to concentric LV hypertrophy, which is an adaptive mechanism to the increased LV pressure. It is a compensatory mechanism permitting the maintenance of a normal wall stress. Phenotypically, the extent of LV hypertrophy is variable between individuals. While some patients with severe AS may present with extensive hypertrophy, others may only have mild hypertrophy or even a normal wall thickness. The exact prognostic value of LV hypertrophy in AS remains to be determined. The concomitant presence of a hypertrophic cardiomyopathy, of a hypertensive cardiomyopathy, or of an infiltrative myocardial disease should be considered when hypertrophy is excessive. While LV hypertrophy can be assessed by the measurement of LV wall thickness in routine clinical practice, the calculation of LV mass is more exact.

Concomitant valve lesions

Aortic regurgitation

Coexisting AR leads to higher forward flow across the AoV and consequently to an increase in transaortic gradients. This should be considered when defining AS severity. At the same time, the calculation of AVA, which is a flow independent measure, should not be affected by the presence of AR.

Mitral regurgitation

When MR is severe it may lead to a reduction in transaortic flow and as a consequence also of transaortic jet velocities. When MR is present, it is important to assess the mechanism. When an organic lesion is present, correction of significant MR at the moment of AoV surgery is warranted. At the same time, controversy exists with regard to concomitant MV surgery in the setting of secondary MR. Without MV surgery an improvement of MR has been reported in about half of the patients after AoV surgery.

Risk stratification by echocardiography and clinical implications: timing of surgery in aortic stenosis and scheduling follow-up intervals

An essential criterion indicating the need for AoV replacement surgery is the onset of symptoms since the outcome is very poor after this moment with a very high mortality. Earlier elective valve replacement surgery may be useful in selected patients who are still asymptomatic. In this decision-making process, pros (avoidance of waiting lists for surgery, lower operative risk for less symptomatic patients) and cons (immediate surgical risk, prosthesis-associated morbidity and mortality) have to be individually weighed and echocardiography allows the identification of high-risk patients having a high likelihood of becoming symptomatic in the short term. In addition risk-stratification permits to optimize the scheduling of follow-up intervals in these patients.

Aortic valve calcification

The presence of moderate-to-severe AoV calcification is an important predictor of outcome in patients with mild-to-moderate AS ($\bigcirc$ Fig. 14a.10A).[13] In patients with severe AS, the presence of a moderately-to-severely calcified AoV identifies

a patient group in whom an 80% event-rate can be expected within 4 years, whereas no or mild AoV calcification is associated with a significantly better prognosis ($\bigcirc$ Fig. 14a.10B).[2] AoV calcification also identifies patients who are likely to have a haemodynamic progression to significant stenosis in the near future and who thus need more frequent control exams.

Haemodynamic progression

Rapid haemodynamic progression is associated with a high event-rate. From a haemodynamic point of view this is due to the increase in the degree of AS severity. Among patients with severe AS, a rapid haemodynamic progression (defined as an increase in peak aortic jet velocity of >0.3m/s within 12 months) in the presence of a moderately-to-severely calcified AoV identifies high-risk patients with a very high event-rate ($\bigcirc$ Fig. 14a.10C).[2]

Peak aortic jet velocity

In the presence of a preserved LV function, peak aortic jet velocity is directly related to AS severity. Based on peak aortic jet velocity, increasing event-rates for patients with mild, moderate, and severe AS have been defined ($\bigcirc$ Fig. 14a.11).[14] Also among patients with severe AS, aortic jet velocity allows a further risk stratification and patients having very severe stenosis with velocities ≥5m/s and ≥5.5m/s have incrementally higher event rates ($\bigcirc$ Fig. 14a.12).[10] These findings emphasize that AS severity should be viewed as a continuum.

Exercise haemodynamics

In an exercise-echocardiographic study, it was shown that patients who have an increase of the mean transaortic gradient

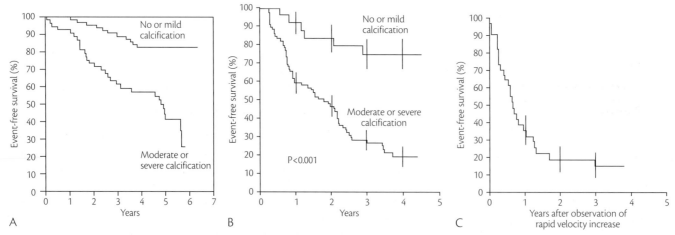

Figure 14a.10 Prognosis of mild to moderate AS. A) Kaplan–Meier analysis of event-free survival for patients with mild or moderate AS having no or mild calcification compared with patients having moderate or severe aortic valve calcification (p = 0.0001). Modified from Rosenhek R, Klaar U, Schemper M, Scholten C, Heger M, Gabriel H, *et al.* Mild and moderate aortic stenosis; Natural history and risk stratification by echocardiography. *Eur Heart J* 2004; 25:199–205. B) Kaplan–Meier analysis of event-free survival for patients with severe AS jet velocity of at least 4m/s at study entry) having no or mild aortic valve calcification compared with patients having moderate or severe calcification (p <0.001). The vertical bars indicate standard errors. C) Kaplan–Meier analysis of event-free survival patients with moderate or severe calcification of their aortic valve and a rapid increase in aortic jet velocity (at least 0.3m/s within 1 year). In this analysis, follow-up started with the visit at which the rapid increase was identified. The vertical bars indicate standard errors. B) and C) Reproduced with permission from Rosenhek R, Binder T, Porenta G, Lang I, Christ G, Schemper M, Maurer G, Baumgartner H. Predictors of outcome in severe, asymptomatic aortic stenosis. N Engl J Med. 2000;343:611–617. Copyright 2000 Massachusetts Medical Society. All rights reserved.

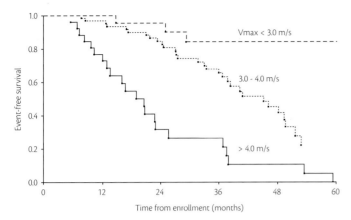

Figure 14a.11 Event-free survival in asymptomatic patients. Cox regression analysis showing event-free survival in 123 initially asymptomatic adults with aortic stenosis, defined by aortic jet velocity at entry (p <0.0001 by log rank test). Reproduced with permission from Otto CM, Burwash IG, Legget ME, Munt BI, Fujioka M, Healy NL, Kraft CD, Miyake-Hull CY, Schwaegler RG. Prospective study of asymptomatic valvular aortic stenosis. Clinical, echocardiographic, and exercise predictors of outcome. *Circulation* 1997; **95**:2262–70.

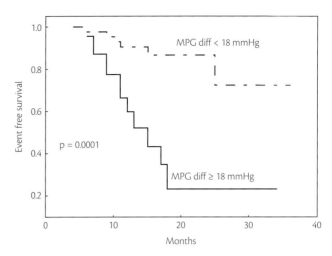

Figure 14a.13 Event-free survival according to exercise haemodynamics. Event-free survival curves according to exercise-induced changes in mean transaortic pressure gradient (MPG) in 69 consecutive patients with severe aortic stenosis (p = 0.0001). Reproduced with permission from Lancellotti P, Lebois F, Simon M, Tombeux C, Chauvel C, Pierard LA. Prognostic importance of quantitative exercise Doppler echocardiography in asymptomatic valvular aortic stenosis. *Circulation* 2005; **112**:1377–382.

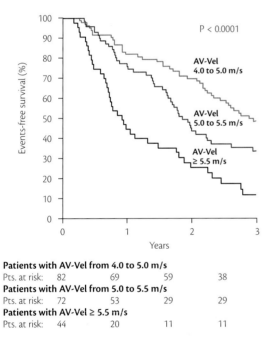

Figure 14a.12 Event-free survival for patients with different peak aortic jet velocity. Kaplan–Meier event-free survival rate for patients with a peak aortic jet velocity (AV–Vel) between 4.0–5.0m/s (light grey line; n = 82) vs between 5.0–5.5m/s (dark grey line; n = 72) vs ≥5.5m/s (black line; n = 44). Reproduced with permission from Rosenhek R, Zilberszac R, Schemper M, Czerny M, Mundigler G, Graf S, Bergler-Klein J, Grimm M, Gabriel H, Maurer G. Natural history of very severe aortic stenosis. *Circulation* 2010; **121**:151–6.

of more than 18mmHg during exercise have a significantly higher event-rate (➲ Fig. 14a.13).[15]

The factors mentioned previously permit the identification of high-risk patients. This information may be included in the management decisions concerning the timing of surgery. Presently, the presence of a calcified AoV in combination with a

rapid haemodynamic progression is recognized as an indication for elective valve surgery according to ESC guidelines. In addition of being helpful in the optimization of the timing of AoV surgery, these factors also permit an individualized scheduling of control intervals.

Decision making in patients with impaired ventricular function

Impaired ventricular function in the presence of a preserved transaortic gradient

Patients with reduced ventricular function who still have 'high' transaortic gradients corresponding to severe AS generally benefit from AoV surgery and an improvement in ventricular function and symptoms can be expected.

Low-flow low-gradient aortic stenosis

Decision making in patients with low-flow low-gradient AS is particularly difficult since these patients have a poor outcome when untreated and a high operative risk. Assessment of these patients involves assessment of coronary morphology and risk stratification is performed using dobutamine echocardiography (see earlier).

When these patients have a contractile reserve and true severe AS, AoV replacement is associated with an improved long-term outcome, although the operative risk is non-negligible (➲ Fig. 14a.14).[11]

In the presence of relative, non-severe stenosis and ventricular impairment related to another reason, surgery is not indicated.

In the absence of contractile reserve, dobutamine echocardiography does not permit the differentiation between true severe

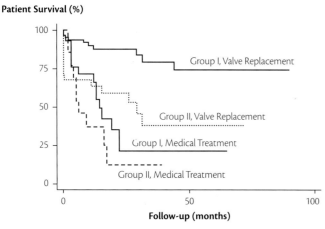

Figure 14a.14 Survival rates in patients with low-flow low-gradient AS. Kaplan–Meier survival estimates of 136 consecutive patients with low-flow low-gradient AS. Group I (n = 92) represents patients with contractile reserve determined by low-dose dobutamine echocardiography, Group II represents the group of patients with absent contractile reserve (n = 44). Survival estimates are represented according to contractile reserve and treatment strategy (aortic valve replacement versus medical therapy). Reproduced with permission from Monin JL, Quere JP, Monchi M, Petit H, Baleynaud S, Chauvel C, Pop C, Ohlmann P, Lelguen C, Dehant P, Tribouilloy C, Gueret P. Low-gradient aortic stenosis: operative risk stratification and predictors for long-term outcome: a multicenter study using dobutamine stress hemodynamics. *Circulation* 2003; **108**:319–24.

and relative (non-severe) stenosis. These patients have a particularly poor outcome and a very high operative risk. Nevertheless some of these patients may benefit from valve replacement surgery, which should thus not be systematically precluded.

Coincidental aortic valve disease in the cardiac surgery patient

With aging of the coronary artery bypass graft (CABG) population, a substantial number of patients present with asymptomatic mild to moderate AS which may be detected during pre-operative testing. The immediate operative risk has been reported to increase from 1–3% with isolated CABG to 6–7% with combined AoV replacement and CABG. The progression of AS is about 0.1cm^2 decrease of AVA per year or an increase of 5–10mmHg in transvalvular gradient per year. Haemodynamic progression is faster in older patients, when the valve is calcified and when the initial degree of stenosis is higher.

In patients who are scheduled for CABG surgery, AoV replacement is recommended for those with either severe or moderate AS, but not mild AS unless there is significant suspicion of an accelerated stenotic process such as significant calcification. Although the level of evidence is currently weak, both American and European guidelines currently give strong consideration to the advisability of AoV replacement in such patients who are already undergoing CABG surgery.

Proponents of AoV replacement at the time of CABG argue that it will avoid the need for reoperation when or if the patient becomes symptomatic and that one should not miss an optimal *window of opportunity* before LV dysfunction appears. Opponents will point to the increased risk of a combined procedure, and the late morbidity, including endocarditis, embolism, and haemorrhage, and the mortality associated with valve prostheses.

Aortic regurgitation

Aortic regurgitation aetiology

AoV morphology is ideally assessed in a PSAX view as detailed earlier the section relating to AS. Morphological differentiation between the different aetiologies is based on the same features as in AS. Because of the frequent association with aortic disease, the ascending aorta should be routinely assessed in patients with AR (see earlier). AR may be the result of a valvular lesion or may be of functional origin in pathologies involving the aortic root. In the assessment of patients with AR, the fact that AoV surgery may ultimately be indicated due to reasons related directly to the valve or to reasons related to aortic root pathologies, should be considered.[16]

Aortic valve leaflet pathologies

The most frequent aetiology of AR is bicuspid AoV disease. Other aetiologies include rheumatic AR, endocarditis, and also degenerative forms. Patients with Marfan syndrome who have a typical appearance of their AoV have a high likelihood of developing AR.

Aortic root pathologies with functional aortic regurgitation

A direct anatomical relationship is present between the AoV and the aortic root. Pathologies of the latter in the form of an aneurysm or of an aortic dissection may cause the apparition of secondary or functional AR. The following forms of functional AR can be differentiated:

- Sinotubular junction dilation: this results from a dilation of the sinotubular junction relative to the annulus and involves leaflet tethering.

- Aortic leaflet prolapse: an aortic dissection extending into the aortic root may cause a disruption of the normal leaflet attachment and thereby cause an aortic leaflet prolapse resulting in AR.

- Dissection flap prolapse: in the presence of an aortic dissection, a dissection flap may prolapse through intrinsically normal leaflets thereby leading to AR despite an anatomically normal AoV.

Functional classification of aortic regurgitation

A correct assessment of the mechanism of AR is important, particularly when aortic repair procedures are considered. In analogy to the Carpentier classification proposed for MR, a functional classification has been proposed for AR:[17]

◆ Type 1: enlargement of the aortic root with normal cusps.

◆ Type 2: cusp prolapse or fenestration.

◆ Type 3: poor cusp tissue quality or quantity.

The extent of AoV calcification can be quantified as in AS (see earlier).

Left ventricular response to aortic regurgitation

In AR, the LV is subject to volume overload that is a direct result of regurgitant flow. In addition, the ejection of a larger stroke volume into the aorta results in pressure overload. In chronic AR, the LV dilates and develops eccentric hypertrophy, as an adaptive response. This compensatory mechanism permits the maintenance of a normal wall stress and systolic function. In acute regurgitation, compensatory mechanisms are absent.

The assessment of LV function and size is an integrative component of the echocardiographic exam. EF should be routinely determined in patients with severe AR. It is recognized that EF is an imperfect measure of LV systolic function, in particular in regurgitant lesions. Nevertheless it has been shown to be of important prognostic value and thus should be an integral part of the echocardiographic assessment of patients with AR. LV diameters should be measured in 2D and M-mode echocardiography and values of diameters indexed to BSA should be reported.

Quantification of aortic regurgitation severity

Quantification of AR severity should be based on an integrative approach of qualitative and quantitative parameters using colour-flow, PW, and CW Doppler imaging[18,19] (◯ Table 14a.3).

Colour flow Doppler

Jet size

Regurgitant flow can be directly visualized by CD imaging. *Regurgitant jet length and area* depend on the pressure difference between the aorta and the LV as well as on LV compliance and are only poorly related with AR severity—hence their use for quantification of regurgitation severity is discouraged. The *proximal jet width or CSA* are measured just below the AoV. It is

Table 14a.3 Quantification of aortic regurgitation severity

	Mild	Moderate	Severe
Qualitative structural and Doppler parameters			
Valve morphology (2D/3D)	Normal or abnormal	Normal or abnormal	Abnormal / flail or coaptation defect
Jet width (colour flow)	Small	Intermediate	Large (central jets), Variable (eccentric jets)
Jet density (CW)	Faint	Dense	Dense
Diastolic flow reversal in descending aorta (PW)	Early diastolic	Intermediate	Holodiastolic
Indirect quantitative parameters			
Pressure half-time, ms (CW)	>500	200–500	<200
Vena contracta width, mm (colour flow)	<3	3–6	>6
Quantitative parameters			
EROA, cm^2	<10	10–30	≥30
Regurgitant volume, mL	<30	30–60	≥60
Regurgitant fraction, %	<30	30–50	≥50

CW, continuous wave Doppler; EROA, effective regurgitant orifice area; PW, pulsed wave Doppler.

Modified from References 18 and 19

Table 14a.4 Requirement of a standard echocardiographic report of a patient with aortic regurgitation

Aetiology of aortic regurgitation
Morphology of the aortic valve and degree of valve calcification
Quantification of stenosis severity including the following measurements based on qualitative and quantitative parameters
Left ventricular function and size
Size of the ascending aorta
Associated valve lesions

recommended to calculate the ratio between the proximal jet width and the LVOT or the ratios between the jet CSA and the LVOT CSA: ratios of 65% and 60% are suggestive of severe AR. A limitation of this measure is the potential underestimation of eccentric jets and the overestimation of central jets, which expand fully.

Vena contracta

The vena contracta width represents the narrowest regurgitant jet width and is measured at the level of the AoV in the PLAX view (➲ Fig. 14a.15). For an accurate assessment of the vena contracta, the three jet components should all be visualized: flow convergence, vena contracta and regurgitant jet. A vena contracta of less than 3mm width is compatible with mild, a vena contracta of 3–6mm is suggestive of moderate, and a vena contracta of more than 6mm has the highest specificity and sensitivity for the diagnosis of severe AR. The vena contracta is not reliable in the presence of multiple regurgitant jets.

Flow convergence

The flow convergence zone can be visualized from apical imaging windows, the PLAX, or an upper right-parasternal view.

It is important to zoom on the area of interest and to adjust the Nyquist limit so as to obtain a round and defined PISA radius (see ➲ Chapter 5). After measuring the peak regurgitant velocity and the VTI from a CW Doppler recording, the EROA and the RVol can be calculated. Severe AR is defined by an EROA of $0.30cm^2$ or higher, and a RVol of 60mL or more. In AR, the PISA (proximal surface isovelocity area) method is only reliably performable in a limited number of patients due to technical and anatomical limitations resulting in suboptimal visualization of the flow convergence zone. A planar convergence zone is mandatory since the method is based on the assumption of a hemispheric flow convergence. Furthermore, AR severity may be underestimated in the presence of an aortic aneurysm.

Pulsed wave Doppler

Diastolic aortic flow reversal

The flow in the descending aorta can be measured from a suprasternal approach using a PW Doppler mode (➲ Fig. 14a.16). A prominent holodiastolic flow reversal is suggestive of severe AR. Measurement of holodiastolic flow reversal in the abdominal aorta is an even more specific indicator of severe AR. A mild flow reversal early in diastole is not a pathological finding. Of note, flow reversal may be extended when aortic compliance is reduced in the presence of a stiff aorta.

Calculation of volume flow

Stroke volume can be determined across the AoV and across the MV (in the absence of relevant MR) or the pulmonary valve

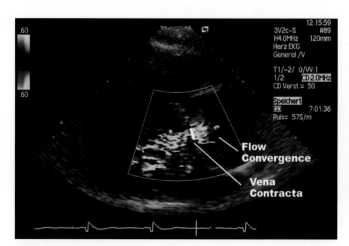

Figure 14a.15 Vena contracta width in severe aortic regurgitation. Colour flow imaging in a PLAX view in a patient with severe aortic regurgitation. The flow convergence zone and the vena contracta width are indicated.

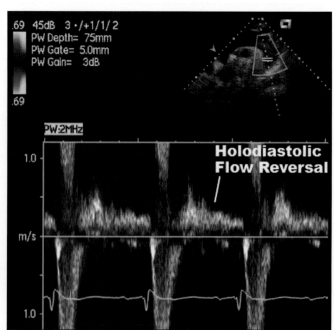

Figure 14a.16 Holodiastolic flow reversal in descending aorta. PW Doppler imaging in the descending aorta: the holodiastolic flow reversal is indicative of severe aortic regurgitation.

as measures of systemic stroke volume (see ➲ Chapter 5). A regurgitant fraction of more than 50% is compatible with severe AR. Aortic RVol may also be calculated as the difference of transaortic and transmitral flow.

Continuous wave Doppler

Diastolic jet deceleration: pressure half-time

The pressure half-time (PHT) is determined by measuring the diastolic flow deceleration across the AoV on a CW Doppler recording (see ➲ Chapter 5, 'Study of valvular insufficiency') (➲ Fig. 14a.17). For an accurate recording, the CW beam needs to be aligned with the regurgitant jet. If aortic insufficiency is mild, the pressure gradient decreases during a long time lapse. As AR progresses up to a severe degree, a rapid fall of aortic diastolic pressure and rise of intraventricular pressure occur: then, pressure gradient tends to decrease more rapidly. A PHT of less than 200ms corresponds to severe AR and a PHT of more than 500ms to mild regurgitation. However, the PHT is not independent of LV compliance and aortic pressure. An elevated LVFP may lead to a shortening, whereas chronic changes of LV compliance due to AR may lead to a lengthening of the PHT.

Signal density of the CW Doppler signal

The CW Doppler signal of AR can be measured from an A5C view, although in eccentric jets, the signal may be more reliably recorded from a parasternal window. The density of the CW Doppler signal is usually weak in the presence of mild AR. At the same time it does not have a significant discriminatory power to distinguish between moderate and severe regurgitation and is thus of limited use in clinical practice.

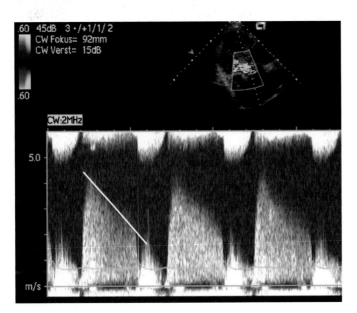

Figure 14a.17 Deceleration slope in aortic regurgitation. CW Doppler recording showing the deceleration slope in a patient with aortic regurgitation.

Risk stratification by echocardiography and clinical implications: timing of surgery in aortic regurgitation

Many of the criteria that define the timing of AoV surgery were identified in studies assessing the prognostic value of preoperative variables on postoperative survival. Long-term outcome after AoV surgery is significantly better in patients who are operated in an asymptomatic or mildly symptomatic stage (New York Heart Association [NYHA] classes I or II) as compared to severely symptomatic patients (NYHA classes III or IV) (➲ Fig. 14a.18).[20] A preoperative LVESD of more than 55mm is associated with a poor long-term outcome.[21] Furthermore, a preoperative impairment of LV function of less than 50% is associated with a reduced outcome (➲ Fig. 14a.19).[22] The necessity of surgery indicated by the development of symptoms or LV dysfunction is predicted by the presence of LV dilation with an LVESD greater than 50mm and an LVEDD greater than 70mm (➲ Fig. 14a.20).[23] These criteria are incorporated into current ESC practice guidelines,[5] which recommend surgery in patients with severe AR who are symptomatic or present with an impaired LV fraction (≤50%) or with LVESD and LVEDD of more than 50mm (or >25mm/m² indexed to BSA) and 70mm, respectively. A severely regurgitant AoV should be operated when surgery of the aorta or other heart surgery is performed: in this setting, replacement of a moderately regurgitant valve may be considered but constitutes only a class IIb indication according to ESC guidelines.

Once the criteria indicating AoV surgery, as defined in current guidelines, are reached, surgery should no longer be postponed, since more advanced symptoms, LV enlargement or dysfunction are associated with worse long-term postoperative outcome as compared to patients being operated *early* according to the guidelines (Fig. 14a.21).[24]

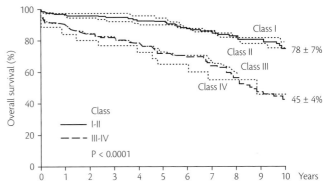

Figure 14a.18 Preoperative symptoms and survival after aortic valve replacement. Long-term postoperative survival after aortic valve replacement in patients with severe aortic regurgitation stratified according to preoperative symptoms. Patients in NYHA functional classes III or IV (n = 128) had a significantly worse outcome than patients in classes I or II (n = 161). Reproduced from Klodas E, Enriquez-Sarano M, Tajik AJ, Mullany CJ, Bailey KR, Seward JB. Optimizing timing of surgical correction in patients with severe aortic regurgitation: role of symptoms. *J Am Coll Cardiol* 1997; **30**:746–52, with permission from Elsevier.

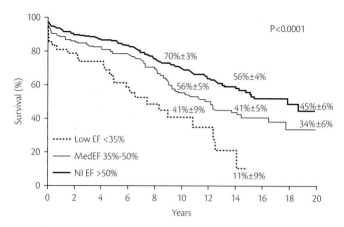

Figure 14a.19 Ejection fraction and survival after aortic valve replacement. Survival after aortic valve replacement in patients with severe aortic regurgitation stratified according to ejection fraction (n = 450). Patients with markedly low ejection fraction had significantly lower survival rates than those with normal EF and moderately reduced ejection fraction before aortic valve replacement. Reproduced with permission from Chaliki HP, Mohty D, Avierinos JF, Scott CG, Schaff HV, Tajik AJ, Enriquez-Sarano M. Outcomes after aortic valve replacement in patients with severe aortic regurgitation and markedly reduced left ventricular function. *Circulation* 2002; **106**:2687–93.

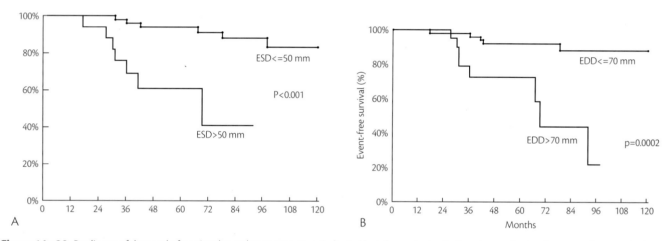

Figure 14a.20 Predictors of the need of aortic valve replacement surgery indicated by left ventricular dysfunction or the development of symptoms in patients with severe aortic regurgitation (n = 101). The need of subsequent surgery was predicted by a left ventricular end-systolic diameter >50mm (A) and an end-diastolic diameter >70mm (B). Reproduced from Tornos MP, Olona M, Permanyer-Miralda G, Herrejon MP, Camprecios M, Evangelista A, Garcia del Castillo H, Candell J, Soler-Soler J. Clinical outcome of severe asymptomatic chronic aortic regurgitation: a long-term prospective follow-up study. *Am Heart J* 1995; **130**:333–9, with permission from Elsevier.

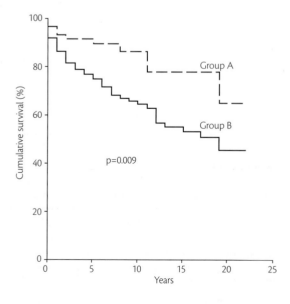

Figure 14a.21 Survival after aortic valve replacement in patients with severe aortic regurgitation operated according to a guidelines-based strategy. Patients operated 'early' according to the guidelines (n = 60, NYHA I–II, EF 45–50%, LVESD 50–55mm) had a significantly better survival than those operated 'late' according to the guidelines (n = 110, NYHA III–IV, EF <45%, LVESD >55mm). Reproduced from Tornos P, Sambola A, Permanyer-Miralda G, Evangelista A, Gomez Z, Soler-Soler J. Long-term outcome of surgically treated aortic regurgitation: influence of guideline adherence toward early surgery. *J Am Coll Cardiol* 2006; **47**:1012–17, with permission from Elsevier.

Personal perspective

Echocardiography is the gold standard for the diagnosis, quantification, and risk stratification of patients with AoV disease. Apart from symptomatic status, the majority of indications for AoV surgery are defined by echocardiography, both in AR and in AS. Nevertheless quantification of AoV disease may be challenging and the currently used parameters also have their pitfalls leading to problems of under- and overestimation of disease severity. Also, intrinsic myocardial function is not optimally assessed with conventional parameters. Advances in the fields of 3D echocardiography and of speckle tracking imaging may prove helpful in the future, possibly in combination with stress echocardiography. Theoretically speckle flow-imaging could be realizable and could become an angle-independent measure of velocities. At the same time echocardiographic assessment may be complemented by other imaging techniques and novel biomarkers. In any case, the currently used variables are here to stay, at least for the next decades.

References

1 Roberts WC, Ko JM. Frequency by decades of unicuspid, bicuspid, and tricuspid aortic valves in adults having isolated aortic valve replacement for aortic stenosis, with or without associated aortic regurgitation. *Circulation* (2005); **111**:920–5.

2 Rosenhek R, Binder T, Porenta G, Lang I, Christ G, Schemper M, *et al*. Predictors of outcome in severe, asymptomatic aortic stenosis. *N Engl J Med* (2000); **343**:611–17.

3 Baumgartner H, Hung J, Bermejo J, Chambers JB, Evangelista A, Griffin BP, *et al*. Echocardiographic assessment of valve stenosis: EAE/ASE recommendations for clinical practice. *Eur J Echocardiogr* (2009); **10**:1–25.

4 Bonow RO, Carabello BA, Chatterjee K, de Leon AC, Jr., Faxon DP, Freed MD, *et al*. (2008) focused update incorporated into the ACC/AHA (2006) guidelines for the management of patients with valvular heart disease: a report of the American College of Cardiology/American Heart Association Task Force on Practice Guidelines (Writing Committee to revise the (1998) guidelines for the management of patients with valvular heart disease). Endorsed by the Society of Cardiovascular Anesthesiologists, Society for Cardiovascular Angiography and Interventions, and Society of Thoracic Surgeons. *J Am Coll Cardiol* (2008); **52**:e1–142.

5 Vahanian A, Baumgartner H, Bax J, Butchart E, Dion R, Filippatos G, *et al*. Guidelines on the management of valvular heart disease: The Task Force on the Management of Valvular Heart Disease of the European Society of Cardiology. *Eur Heart J* (2007); **28**:230–68.

6 Currie PJ, Seward JB, Reeder GS, Vlietstra RE, Bresnahan DR, Bresnahan JF, *et al*. Continuous-wave Doppler echocardiographic assessment of severity of calcific aortic stenosis: a simultaneous Doppler-catheter correlative study in 100 adult patients. *Circulation* (1985); **71**:1162–9.

7 Baumgartner H, Stefenelli T, Niederberger J, Schima H, Maurer G. 'Overestimation' of catheter gradients by Doppler ultrasound in patients with aortic stenosis: a predictable manifestation of pressure recovery. *J Am Coll Cardiol* (1999); **33**:1655–61.

8 Otto CM, Pearlman AS, Comess KA, Reamer RP, Janko CL, Huntsman LL. Determination of the stenotic aortic valve area in adults using Doppler echocardiography. *J Am Coll Cardiol* (1986); **7**:509–17.

9 Minners J, Allgeier M, Gohlke-Baerwolf C, Kienzle RP, Neumann FJ, Jander N. Inconsistencies of echocardiographic criteria for the grading of aortic valve stenosis. *Eur Heart J* (2008); **29**:1043–8.

10 Rosenhek R, Zilberszac R, Schemper M, Czerny M, Mundigler G, Graf S, *et al*. Natural history of very severe aortic stenosis. *Circulation* (2010); **121**:151–6.

11 Monin JL, Quere JP, Monchi M, Petit H, Baleynaud S, Chauvel C, *et al*. Low-gradient aortic stenosis: operative risk stratification and predictors for long-term outcome: a multicenter study using dobutamine stress hemodynamics. *Circulation* (2003); **108**:319–24.

12 Hachicha Z, Dumesnil JG, Bogaty P, Pibarot P. Paradoxical low-flow, low-gradient severe aortic stenosis despite preserved ejection fraction is associated with higher afterload and reduced survival. *Circulation* (2007); **115**:2856–64.

13 Rosenhek R, Klaar U, Schemper M, Scholten C, Heger M, Gabriel H, *et al*. Mild and moderate aortic stenosis; Natural history and risk stratification by echocardiography. *Eur Heart J* (2004); **25**:199–205.

14 Otto CM, Burwash IG, Legget ME, Munt BI, Fujioka M, Healy NL, *et al*. Prospective study of asymptomatic valvular aortic stenosis. Clinical, echocardiographic, and exercise predictors of outcome. *Circulation* (1997); **95**:2262–70.

15 Lancellotti P, Lebois F, Simon M, Tombeux C, Chauvel C, Pierard LA. Prognostic importance of quantitative exercise Doppler echocardiography in asymptomatic valvular aortic stenosis. *Circulation* (2005); **112**:I377–382.

16 Roberts WC, Ko JM, Moore TR, Jones WH, 3rd. Causes of pure aortic regurgitation in patients having isolated aortic valve replacement at a single US tertiary hospital (1993 to (2005)). *Circulation* (2006); **114**:422–9.

17 le Polain de Waroux JB, Pouleur AC, Goffinet C, Vancraeynest D, Van Dyck M, Robert A, *et al*. Functional anatomy of aortic regurgitation: accuracy, prediction of surgical repairability, and outcome implications of transesophageal echocardiography. *Circulation* (2007); **116**:I264–269.

18 Zoghbi WA, Enriquez-Sarano M, Foster E, Grayburn PA, Kraft CD, Levine RA, *et al*. Recommendations for evaluation of the severity of native valvular regurgitation with two-dimensional and Doppler echocardiography. *J Am Soc Echocardiogr* (2003); **16**:777–802.

19 Lancellotti P, Tribouilloy C, Hagendorff A, Moura L, Popescu BA, Agricola E, *et al*. European Association of Echocardiography

recommendations for the assessment of valvular regurgitation. Part 1: aortic and pulmonary regurgitation (native valve disease). *Eur J Echocardiogr* (2010); **11**:223–44.

20 Klodas E, Enriquez-Sarano M, Tajik AJ, Mullany CJ, Bailey KR, Seward JB. Optimizing timing of surgical correction in patients with severe aortic regurgitation: role of symptoms. *J Am Coll Cardiol* (1997); **30**:746–52.

21 Bonow RO, Rosing DR, Kent KM, Epstein SE. Timing of operation for chronic aortic regurgitation. *Am J Cardiol* (1982); **50**:325–36.

22 Chaliki HP, Mohty D, Avierinos JF, Scott CG, Schaff HV, Tajik AJ, *et al.* Outcomes after aortic valve replacement in patients with severe aortic regurgitation and markedly reduced left ventricular function. *Circulation* (2002); **106**:2687–93.

23 Tornos MP, Olona M, Permanyer-Miralda G, Herrejon MP, Camprecios M, Evangelista A, *et al.* Clinical outcome of severe asymptomatic chronic aortic regurgitation: a long-term prospective follow-up study. *Am Heart J* (1995); **130**:333–9.

24 Tornos P, Sambola A, Permanyer-Miralda G, Evangelista A, Gomez Z, Soler-Soler J. Long-term outcome of surgically treated aortic regurgitation: influence of guideline adherence toward early surgery. *J Am Coll Cardiol* (2006); **47**:1012–17.

Further reading

Bonow RO, Carabello BA, Chatterjee K, de Leon AC Jr, Faxon DP, Freed MD, *et al.* (2008) Focused update incorporated into the ACC/AHA (2006) guidelines for the management of patients with valvular heart disease: a report of the American College of Cardiology/American Heart Association Task Force on Practice Guidelines. *Circulation.* (2008); **118**:523–661.

Dal-Bianco JP, Khandheria BK, Mookadam F, Gentile F, and Sengupta PP, *et al.* Management of asymptomatic severe aortic stenosis. *J Am Coll Cardiol* (2008); **52**:1279–92.

Filsoufi F, Aklog L, Adams DH, Byrne JG. Management of mild to moderate aortic stenosis at the time of coronary artery bypass grafting. *J Heart Valve Dis* (2002); **11**(Suppl 1):S45–9.

Vahanian A, Baumgartner H, Bax J, Butchart E, Dion R, Filippatos G, *et al.* Guidelines on the management of valvular heart disease: The Task Force on the Management of Valvular Heart Disease of the European Society of Cardiology. *Eur Heart J* (2007); **28**: 230–68.

➲ For additional multimedia materials please visit the online version of the book (http://escecho.oxfordmedicine.com).

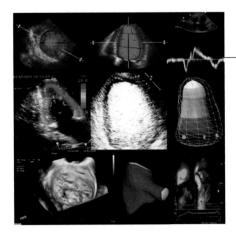

Mitral valve disease

Patrizio Lancellotti, Julien Magne, Kim
O'Connor, and Luc A. Pierard

Contents

Summary

Native mitral valve disease is the second valvular heart disease after aortic valve disease. For the last few decades, two-dimensional Doppler echocardiography was the cornerstone technique for evaluating patients with mitral valve disease. Besides aetiological information, echocardiography allows the description of valve anatomy, the assessment of disease severity, and the description of the associated lesions.

This chapter will address the echocardiographic evaluation of mitral regurgitation (MR) and mitral stenosis (MS).

In MR, the following findings should be assessed:

1. Aetiology.

2. Type and extent of anatomical lesions and mechanisms of regurgitation.

3. The possibility of mitral valve repair.

4. Quantification of MR severity.

5. Quantification of MR repercussions.

In MS, the following findings should be assessed:

1. Aetiology.

2. Type and extent of anatomical lesions.

3. Quantification of MS severity.

4. Quantification of MS repercussions.

5. Wilkins or Cormier scores for the possibility of percutaneous mitral commissuroplasty.

Management of patients with mitral valve disease is currently based on symptoms and on echocardiographic evaluation at rest. Therefore, knowing how to assess the severity of valve diseases as well as the pitfalls and the limitations of each echocardiographic method is of primary importance.

Mitral regurgitation

Aetiology

Mitral regurgitation (MR) is roughly classified as organic (primary) or functional (secondary). Organic MR is due to intrinsic valvular disease whereas functional MR is caused by regional and/or global left ventricular (LV) remodelling without structural abnormalities of the mitral valve (MV).

Causes of primary MR include most commonly degenerative disease (Barlow, fibroelastic degeneration, Marfan, Ehlers–Danlos, annular calcification), rheumatic disease, and endocarditis. Ruptured papillary muscle secondary to myocardial infarction is defined as organic ischaemic MR.

Causes of secondary MR include ischaemic heart disease and dilated cardiomyopathy.

Mechanisms

Functional classification of Carpentier

Precise determination of the mechanism of MR is an essential component of the echocardiographic examination, in particular when MV repair is considered. Carpentier's functional classification is often used (➲ Fig. 14b.1):

◆ Type I: normal leaflet mobility MR is determined by leaflet perforation (infective endocarditis) or more frequently by annular dilation.

◆ Type II: excessive leaflet mobility accompanied by displacement of the free edge of one or both leaflets beyond the mitral annular plane (mitral valve prolapse).

◆ Type III: type III is subdivided into type IIIa implying restricted leaflet motion during both diastole and systole due to shortening of the chordae and/or leaflet thickening such as in rheumatic disease, and type IIIb when leaflet motion is restricted only during systole such as in ischaemic or non-ischaemic cardiomyopathy

Specific mechanisms

Mechanisms of MR are varied. Both organic and functional MR can be generated by ischaemic or non-ischaemic pathological conditions.

Organic ischaemic MR is mainly represented by papillary muscle rupture, which is a rare and dramatic complication of acute myocardial infarction requiring emergency surgery: if the rupture is complete, a mass attached to flail segments of anterior and posterior leaflets is seen in the left atrium (LA) in systole and in LV in diastole. If the rupture is incomplete, it is possible to see a thin, excessively mobile papillary muscle.

Organic non-ischaemic MR occurs in pathological conditions characterized by congenital or acquired structural abnormalities of mitral leaflets or subvalvular apparatus, such as MV prolapse, chordal elongation, myxomatous disease, rheumatic disease, endocarditis, Marfan syndrome, infiltrative disorders, and systemic inflammatory disease. In these cases, leaflets and chordate can be irregular, thickened, redundant, fused, shortened, perforated or deformed, resulting in their inadequate coaptation or displacement into the LA. Also, mitral annular calcification (MAC), which occurs in the elderly and in younger

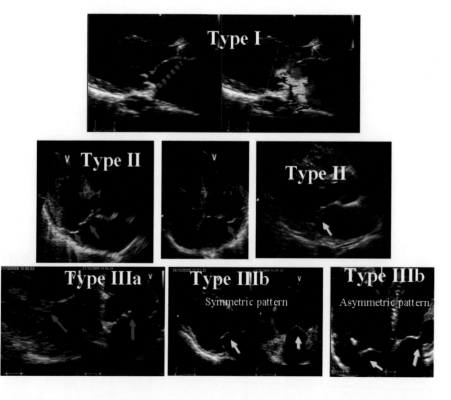

Figure 14b.1 Carpentier's functional classification. Mechanisms of mitral regurgitation according to the Carpentier's functional classification.

people with renal failure and arterial hypertension, can be considered as an organic non-ischaemic cause of MR, since it impairs systolic contraction of MV annulus. Increased leaflet rigidity, leaflet retraction, and calcifications may limit the possibility of valve repair.

Functional MR due to ischaemic condition may occur in the presence of LV dysfunction with abnormal contraction of papillary muscles or underlying ventricular wall. MR can be persistent, when dysfunctional myocardial wall is replaced by scar, or intermittent, if MR only appears during ischaemia and can be unmasked by stress echocardiography. Moreover, LV dilation due to post-ischaemic remodelling causes MV annulus dilation and papillary muscle displacement, finally resulting in MR. Thus, functional MR results from an imbalance between tethering forces—annular dilation, LV dilation, papillary muscles displacement, LV sphericity—and closing forces—reduction of LV contractility, global LV dyssynchrony, papillary muscle dyssynchrony.

Functional MR due to non-ischaemic conditions occurs in the presence of dilated cardiomyopathy or MV annular enlargement secondary to LA dilation in patients with chronic atrial fibrillation.

Two main patterns of mechanisms of leaflet tethering involved in functional ischaemic and non-ischaemic MR are described:

◆ Asymmetric tethering is characterized by a regional LV remodelling with displacement of the posteromedial papillary muscle, causing posterior leaflet restriction.

◆ Symmetric tethering generally results from global LV remodelling with a displacement of both anterolateral and posteromedial papillary muscles.

Jet direction as a clue to mechanism

MR jet direction evaluated using both transthoracic (TTE) or transoesophageal (TOE) echocardiography may be used to accurately identify the mechanisms of valvular lesion. Indeed, MR jet can be eccentric or central and is generally related to the leaflet motion.

Eccentric MR jet occurs:

◆ In mitral valve prolapse (MR jet is oriented in opposition to the lesion, i.e. a posterior leaflet prolapse produces an anteriorly oriented jet. When prolapse arises on both anterior and posterior leaflets, MR jet is often complex).

◆ In patients with functional ischaemic MR associated to an asymmetric pattern of tethering (MR jet is oriented toward the posterior wall of the LA).

Central MR jet usually occurs:

◆ In patients with functional ischaemic MR associated with a symmetric pattern of tethering.

◆ In patients with functional non-ischaemic MR.

Mitral valve prolapse evaluation

Concomitantly to the finding of mid-to late systolic click and late systolic murmur on auscultation, echocardiographic visualization of thickened leaflets with marked systolic displacement into the LA, often in association with MR, are the key features for the diagnosis of MV prolapse. Historically, the presence of MV prolapse was diagnosed by M-mode criteria: late or holosystolic bowing of a leaflet below the C-D line (see ⊃ Chapter 2). Two-dimensional (2D) echocardiography, allowing the real-time visualization of MV motion, is now the preferred tool to detect MV prolapse. In parasternal long-axis (PLAX) view, the systolic displacement of one or both leaflets into the LA, below the mitral annulus plane, is a criterion of choice. A flail leaflet, usually a consequence of ruptured chordae, is present when the free edge of a leaflet is completely eversed in the LA. The diagnosis appear more certain if the leaflets are thickened (>5mm) or myxomatous. The main echocardiographic findings in association with MV prolapse, especially in the presence of related significant MR, are leaflet thickening and redundancy, mitral annulus enlargement, elongated or ruptured chordae tendinae, and eccentric MR jet.

Indirect signs of mitral regurgitation

The haemodynamic and physiological consequences of MR intervene in both systemic and pulmonary circulations.

Left ventricular and left atrial consequences

In a chronic situation, the increased volume load is accompanied by a progressive increase in end-diastolic volume and eccentric hypertrophy to maintain forward stroke volume. Note that preload is increased whereas the afterload is normal or occasionally decreased in such a way that the ventricular emptying is facilitated. In the compensated phase, often asymptomatic, the forward stroke volume is maintained through an increase in LV ejection fraction (LVEF) resulting in apparent normal or supranormal LVEF (>65%). Even in the acute stage, the LVEF increases in response to the increased preload. In the chronic decompensated phase (the patient could still be asymptomatic or may fail to recognize deterioration in clinical status), the forward stroke volume decreases and the LA pressure increases significantly. The LV contractility can thus decrease silently and irreversibly. Nonetheless, the LVEF may remain in low normal range and mask subclinical LV dysfunction and substantial myocardial alteration.

The LA dilates in response to chronic volume and pressure overload (LA volume index > 40mL/m^2). A normal sized LA is not normally associated with significant MR unless it is acute, in which case the valve appearance is likely to be grossly abnormal. The excess regurgitant blood entering in the LA may induce acutely or chronically a progressive rise in pulmonary arterial pressure. Mitral valve repair is recommended when pulmonary arterial systolic pressure (PASP) is higher than 50mm Hg at rest.

Severity of mitral regurgitation: qualitative assessment

Colour flow imaging

The regurgitant jet area is frequently measured by planimetry. However, as this method is a source of many errors, it is not recommended to quantify MR severity. Nevertheless, the detection of a large eccentric jet adhering, swirling, and reaching the posterior wall of the LA is in favour of significant MR. Conversely, small thin jets that appear just beyond the mitral leaflets usually indicate mild MR (➲ Fig. 14b.2).

Continuous wave Doppler signal intensity

The signal intensity (jet density) of the continuous wave (CW) Doppler envelope of the MR jet can be a qualitative guide to MR severity. A dense MR signal with a full envelope indicates more severe MR than a faint signal. The CW Doppler envelope may be truncated (notch) with a triangular contour and an early peak velocity (blunt). This indicates elevated LA pressure or a prominent regurgitant pressure wave in the LA due to severe MR (➲ Fig. 14b.3). In eccentric MR, it may be difficult to record the full CW envelope of the jet because of its eccentricity, while the signal intensity shows dense features.

Severity of mitral regurgitation: semiquantitative assessment

Anterograde velocity of mitral inflow: mitral to aortic TVI ratio

Pulsed wave (PW) Doppler mitral inflow pattern can be a supportive sign to evaluate the severity of MR. In the absence of mitral stenosis, a E-wave velocity exceeding 1.5m/s suggests severe MR. Conversely, a dominant A wave basically excludes severe MR.

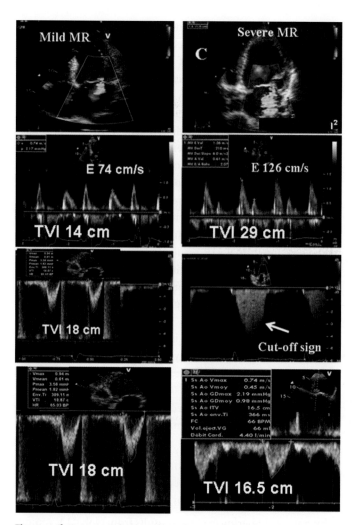

Figure 14b.3 Various degrees of MR. Two examples of various degrees of MR, mild (left), and severe (right) are provided. The regurgitant jet as well as the mitral E wave velocity increase with the severity of MR. In severe MR, the continuous wave Doppler signal of the regurgitant jet is truncated, triangular, and intense. Notching of the continuous wave envelope (cut-off sign) can occur in severe MR. TVI: time-velocity integral.

The PW Doppler mitral to aortic TVI ratio is also used as an easily measured index for the quantification of isolated pure organic MR. Mitral inflow Doppler tracings are obtained at the mitral leaflet tips and aortic flow at the annulus level in the apical three-chamber view. A TVI ratio more than 1.4 strongly suggests severe MR whereas a TVI ratio less than 1 is in favour of mild MR (➲ Fig 14b.3). Moderate MR could not be accurately distinguished with such parameters.

Systolic flow reversal in pulmonary veins

PW Doppler evaluation of pulmonary venous flow pattern is a useful adjunct to evaluate the haemodynamic consequences and for grading the severity of MR. In severe MR, the systolic component (S wave) of pulmonary flow becomes frankly reversed if the jet is directed into the sampled vein (➲ Fig 14b.4). Atrial fibrillation and elevated LA pressure from any cause can blunt forward systolic pulmonary vein flow. Nevertheless, the

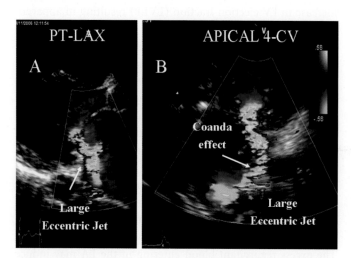

Figure 14b.2 Colour-flow imaging of mitral regurgitant jet. Visual assessment of mitral regurgitant jet using colour-flow imaging. Examples of two patients with severe mitral regurgitation and large eccentric jet with a clear Coanda effect.

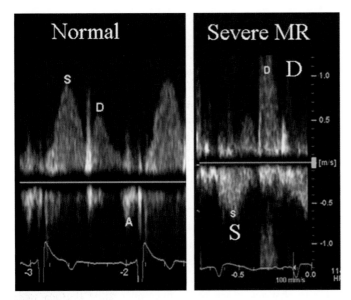

Figure 14b.4 Pulmonary vein flow pattern. A) Normal pulmonary vein flow pattern. B) Reversed systolic pulmonary flow in a patient with severe MR. D, diastolic wave; S, systolic wave.

finding of systolic flow reversal in more than one pulmonary vein is specific but not sensitive to identify severe MR.

Vena contracta width

The vena contracta is the narrowest portion of the regurgitant jet downstream from the regurgitant orifice. It is slightly smaller than the anatomical regurgitant orifice due to boundary effects. To properly identify the vena contracta, a scan plane that clearly shows the three components of the regurgitant jet has to be selected. In some cases, it may be necessary to angulate the transducer out of the normal echocardiographic imaging planes to separate the area of proximal flow acceleration, the vena contracta, and the downstream expansion of the jet. The colour sector size and imaging depth are reduced as narrow as possible to maximize lateral and temporal resolution. Visualization is optimized by expanding the selected zone. The selected cineloop is reviewed frame by frame to find the best frame for measurement (➲ Fig. 14b.5). The largest diameter of a clearly defined

vena contracta is thus measured. Averaging measurements over at least two to three beats and using two orthogonal planes whenever possible are recommended. A vena contracta less than 3mm indicates mild MR while a width of 7mm or more defines severe MR. Intermediate values are not accurate for distinguishing moderate from mild or severe MR (large overlap); they require the use of another method for confirmation. To note, this approach is not valid for multiple jets or in case of non-circular orifice and is affected by systolic changes in regurgitant flow.

Severity of mitral regurgitation: quantitative assessment

Quantitative assessment of the severity of the regurgitation using TTE is the cornerstone in the management and risk stratification of patients with MR. Both the effective regurgitant orifice area (EROA) and the regurgitant volume (RVol) are estimated.

Doppler volumetric method

In the absence of significant aortic regurgitation, mitral RVol may be assumed as the difference between mitral antegrade stroke volume and LV outflow tract (LVOT) stroke volume, so it may be calculated by the ➲ Equation 5.11 (see Chapter 5, 'Study of valvular insufficiency') (➲ Fig. 14b.6). This approach can be used as an additive or alternative method, especially when the proximal isovelocity surface area (PISA) and the vena contracta are not accurate or not applicable. This approach is time consuming and is associated with several drawbacks. The most common limitation relies to the measurement of the mitral annulus (error is squared in the equation).

PISA method

This is considered the most recommended quantitative approach whenever feasible. The apical four-chamber (A4C) view is classically recommended for optimal visualization of the PISA. However, the PLAX or PSAX views are often useful for visualization of the PISA in case of anterior MV prolapse.

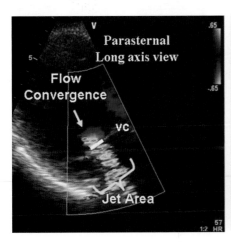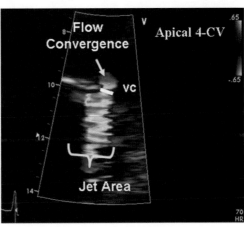

Figure 14b.5 Vena contracta width. Semiquantitative assessment of MR severity using the vena contracta width (VC). The three components of the regurgitant jet (flow convergence zone, vena contracta, jet turbulence) are obtained. CV, chamber view.

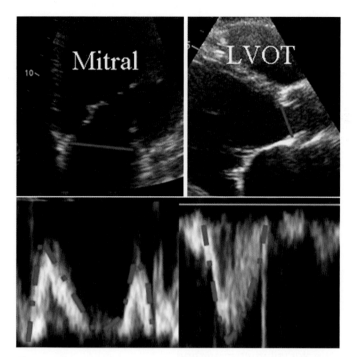

Figure 14b.6 Doppler volumetric method for assessment of mitral regurgitation severity. The quantitative assessment of mitral regurgitation severity by the Doppler volumetric method requires the measurement of the left ventricular outflow tract diameter (LVOT), the mitral annulus diameter and of two pulse wave velocity profiles (outflow tract and mitral inflow velocities). TVI, time-velocity integral.

Principles and technical aspects of PISA method are described in ⊃ Chapter 5, 'Study of valvular insufficiency'. EROA may accurately be quantified using ⊃ Equations 5.16 and 5.17; then RVol is obtained by multiplying EROA and VTI of the regurgitant flow (⊃ Figs. 14b.7 and 14b.8).

Qualitatively, the presence of flow convergence at a Nyquist limit of 50–60cm/s should be an alert to the presence of significant MR. Grading of severity of organic MR classifies regurgitation as mild, moderate, or severe, and subclassifies the moderate regurgitation group into *mild-to-moderate* (EROA of 20–29mm or a RVol of 30–44mL) and *moderate-to-severe* (EROA of 30–39mm^2 or a RVol of 45–59mL). Quantitatively, organic MR is considered severe if EROA is 40mm^2 or more and RVol is 60mL or above (⊃ Table 14b.1). In ischaemic MR, the thresholds of severity, which are of prognostic value, are 20 mm^2 and 30mL, respectively.

The aetiology of MR or the presence of concomitant valvular disease does not affect the EROA calculation. Although less accurate, this method can still be used in eccentric jet without significant distortion in the isovelocity contours (⊃ Fig. 14b.9). The configuration or shape of PISA changes as the aliasing velocity changes, since the convergence zone flattens with higher aliasing velocities and become more elliptical with lower aliasing velocities. Variation in the regurgitant orifice during the cardiac cycle is particularly important in mitral valve prolapse where the regurgitation is often confined to the latter half of systole (⊃ Fig. 14b.10). The precise location of the regurgitant orifice can be difficult to judge, which may cause an error in the measurement of the PISA radius. A more important limitation is the distortion of the isovelocity contours by encroachment of proximal structures on the flow field. In this situation, an angle correction for wall constraint has been proposed but it is difficult in practice and thus not recommended. Three-dimensional (3D) echocardiography has been shown to overcome some of these limitations. Although promising, further 3D experience remains still required.

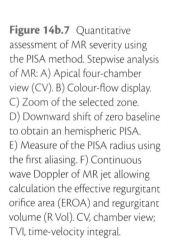

Figure 14b.7 Quantitative assessment of MR severity using the PISA method. Stepwise analysis of MR: A) Apical four-chamber view (CV). B) Colour-flow display. C) Zoom of the selected zone. D) Downward shift of zero baseline to obtain an hemispheric PISA. E) Measure of the PISA radius using the first aliasing. F) Continuous wave Doppler of MR jet allowing calculation the effective regurgitant orifice area (EROA) and regurgitant volume (R Vol). CV, chamber view; TVI, time-velocity integral.

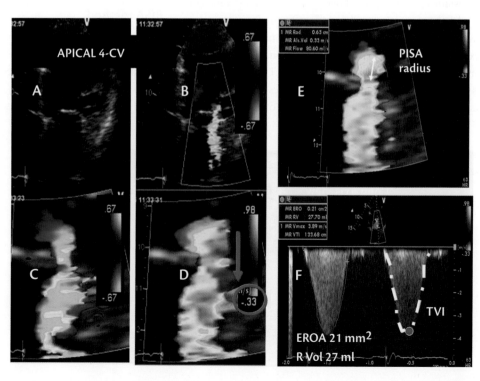

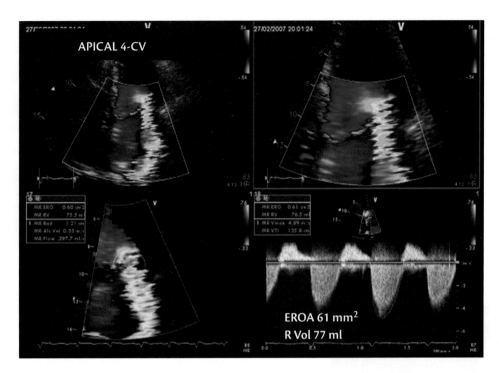

Figure 14b.8 Severe mitral regurgitation assessed by the PISA method. Quantitative assessment of MR severity using the PISA method in a patient with severe mitral regurgitation. CV, chamber view.

Table 14b.1 Grading the severity of organic MR

Parameters	Mild	Moderate	Severe
Qualitative:			
MV morphology	Normal/abnormal	Normal/abnormal	Flail leaflet/ruptured PMs
Colour flow MR jet	Small, central	Intermediate	Very large central jet or eccentric jet adhering, swirling and reaching the posterior wall of the LA
Flow convergence zone[a]	No or small	Intermediate	Large
CW signal of MR jet	Faint/parabolic	Dense/parabolic	Dense/triangular
Semi-quantitative:			
VC width (mm)	<3	Intermediate	≥7 (>8 for biplane) [b]
Pulmonary vein flow	Systolic dominance	Systolic blunting	Systolic flow reversal[c]
Mitral inflow	A wave dominant*	Variable	E wave dominant (>1.5cm/s)**
TVI mit /TVI Ao	<1	Intermediate	>1.4
Quantitative:			
EROA (mm²)	<20	20–29; 30–39!	≥40
RVol (mL)	<30	30–44; 45–59!	≥60
		+ LV and LA size and the systolic pulmonary pressure §	

CW, continuous-wave; EROA, effective regurgitant orifice area; LA, left atrium, LV, left ventricle; MR, mitral regurgitation; RVol, regurgitant volume; VC, vena contracta. [a]At a Nyquist limit of 50–60cm/s; [b]or average between apical 4-and 2-chamber views; [c]Unless other reasons of systolic blunting (atrial fibrillation, elevated LA pressure); *Usually after 50 years of age; ** In the absence of other causes of elevated LA pressure and of mitral stenosis. § Unless for other reasons, the LA and LV size and the pulmonary pressure are usually normal in patients with mild MR. In acute severe MR, the pulmonary pressures are usually elevated while the LV size is still often normal. **Accepted cut-off values for non-significant left-sided chambers enlargement**: LA volume <36ml/m², LV end-diastolic diameter <56mm, LV end-diastolic volume <82mL/m², LV end-systolic diameter <40mm, LV end-systolic volume <30mL/m², LA diameter <39mm, LA volume <29mL/m².! Grading of severity of organic MR classifies regurgitation as mild, moderate or severe, and sub-classifies the moderate regurgitation group into 'mild-to-moderate' (EROA of 20–29mm or a RVol of 30–44mL) and 'moderate-to-severe' (EROA of 30–39mm² or a RVol of 45–59mL).

Adapted from Lancellotti P, *et al.* on behalf of the European Association of Echocardiography. European Association of Echocardiography Recommendations for the Assessment of Valvular Regurgitation. Part 2: Mitral and Tricuspid Regurgitation. *Eur J Echocardiogr* 2010; **11**(4):307–332.

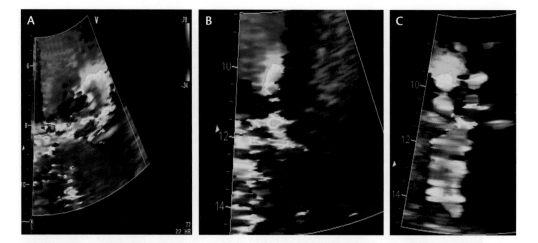

Figure 14b.9 Pitfalls with the PISA method. A) and B) distorted and constrained flow convergence zone by the lateral myocardial wall. C) Presence of two jets

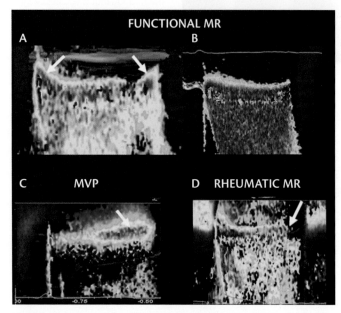

Figure 14b.10 Flow convergence zone changes. Four examples of flow convergence zone changes during systole using colour M-mode. A) and B) Functional MR (A: early and late peaks and mid-systolic decreases; B: early systolic peak). C) Mitral valve prolapse (late systolic enhancement). D) Rheumatic MR with an end-systolic decrease in flow convergence zone.

Chronic versus acute mitral regurgitation

In the chronic compensated phase of MR, LA pressure is often normal due to an increase in LA compliance, with absence of v-wave. Pulmonary pressure remains in the normal range, precluding pulmonary congestion. Nevertheless, LV and LA size increase progressively. Hence, symptoms are extremely rare in this setting. When chronic MR becomes decompensated, LA pressure tends to increase and a v-wave may occur. The LV eccentric hypertrophy arises and patients gradually develop symptoms, firstly dyspnoea on exertion and then even at rest. In contrast, the acute onset of MR or sudden major worsening of chronic MR causes a severe elevation of LA pressure due to

the abrupt increase in RVol. Usually, LA and LV sizes are normal and acute MR is often associated with LA v-wave. In this context, LA compliance is low, leading to a rapid increase in LA pressure, progressive increase in LA wall thickness, and pulmonary vascular resistance. Acute pulmonary oedema, abrupt congestive heart failure (HF), or cardiogenic shock, are frequently observed in acute MR.

Sequential evaluation of chronic asymptomatic mitral regurgitation

Recommended follow-up

Following the assessment of clinical history, risk factors, and physical examination, non-invasive evaluation is decisive for risk stratification and management of patients with significant MR. Typically, TTE is the preferred method for periodic evaluation in order to evaluate LA and LV size and function changes and to estimate pulmonary pressure. Initial comprehensive echocardiographic exam defining the mechanisms and severity of MR and the consequences of MR on LV and LA, is mandatory. Secondly, repeated examinations can focus on LV size and function, LA enlargement and pulmonary pressure. In the presence of significant changes in clinical status, more complete examination is required. Whenever the optimal timing for sequential echocardiographic examination remains unclear in the literature, a second time point evaluation, following the initial complete echocardiography identifying the presence of significant MR, is useful to determine if the previous findings are stable or if the disease rapidly progresses. The timing of repeated examinations should be adapted to the specific clinical situation. Asymptomatic patient with chronic MR and no LV dilation may be examined annually without jeopardizing the patient's prognosis. On the other hand, follow-up could be shortened to 6 or 3 months when LVEF or diameter is close to guideline thresholds (LVEF 60%, LV end-systolic diameter 45mm) or in cases of increasing pulmonary pressure.

Role of Doppler echocardiography in timing of surgery

Current European Society of Cardiology (ESC) guidelines recommend mitral valve surgery when severe MR is associated with symptoms and/or LV dysfunction (LVEF <60%; LV end-systolic diameter >45mm). In asymptomatic patients with preserved LV function, surgery is deemed reasonable in the presence of atrial fibrillation, with resting pulmonary hypertension (>50mmHg). Furthermore, severe MR may also be considered as the sole and sufficient indication for surgery when the likelihood of repair is high and operative risk is low.

Echocardiographic predictors of outcome

Several Doppler echocardiographic parameters have been shown to predict the outcome in asymptomatic patients with organic MR. In patients with preserved LVEF, an EROA of 40mm^2 or more, a LA diameter greater than 40–50mm or LA volume index greater than 40mL/m^2, an end-systolic diameter larger than 22mm/m^2, are associated independently with a worse outcome. New parameters are currently available for a better assessment of LV function and could help for risk stratification. A systolic tissue Doppler velocity measured at the lateral annulus less than 10.5cm/s, a resting longitudinal strain rate value less than 1.07/s (average of 12 basal and mid segments) by using tissue Doppler imaging, a global longitudinal strain less than 18.1% by using 2D speckle tracking have been shown to identify subclinical LV dysfunction.

Feasibility of mitral valve repair

In organic MR, numerous studies reported the superiority of MV repair over replacement in term of both short- and long-term postoperative survival. The preoperative prediction of performing MV repair is based on surgeon skills and experience, and on the localization and the type of aetiology involved in MR. Some predictors of unsuccessful repair have been reported: the presence of a large central regurgitant jet, severe annular dilation (>50mm), involvement of three or more scallops especially if the anterior leaflet is involved, and extensive valve calcification. The quality of valve tissue also affects the possibility of repair. Severe valve retraction usually precludes repair (➲ Table 14b.2).

In ischaemic MR, the superiority of MV repair over replacement is not clearly recognized. Although the MV and subvalvular apparatus are normal, underlying mechanisms may preclude optimal surgical repair and, thus, require MV replacement. Undersized MV annuloplasty is currently the most frequently used technique for the surgical management of patients with severe ischaemic MR. However, this procedure is associated with substantial rates of residual/recurrent MR following surgery, essentially due to continued global and/or localized adverse LV remodelling. Pre-operatively (TTE), a coaptation distance greater than 1cm (distance between the leaflet coaptation point and the mitral annulus plane in the A4C view), a systolic tenting area greater than 2.5cm^2 (the area enclosed between the annular plane and mitral leaflets in the PLAX view), a posterior leaflet angle larger than 45°, a large central regurgitant jet, the presence of complex jets originating centrally and posteromedially, and a severe LV enlargement (end-systolic diameter >51mm) increase the risk of MV repair failure. In patients with ischaemic MR and in whom preoperative echocardiography indicates a high risk of suboptimal results following valve repair, alternative or concomitant surgical approach could be recommended.

Role of exercise stress echocardiography

In the management of patients with ischaemic MR, the role of stress echocardiography is well established. Exercise stress echocardiography may identify the dynamic component of ischaemic MR and predict its clinical outcome. Given that the exercise-induced changes in MR severity are not related to the resting MR severity, stress echocardiography may therefore provide major important incremental information for the assessment of MR severity and thus for clinical decision making.

Table 14b.2 Probability of successful mitral valve repair in organic MR based on echo findings

Aetiology	Dysfunction	Calcification	Mitral annulus dilation	Probability of repair
Degenerative	II: Localized prolapse (P2 and/or A2)	No/localized	Mild/moderate	**Feasible**
Ischaemic/functional	I or IIIb	No	Moderate	
Barlow	II: Extensive prolapse (≥3 scallops, posterior commissure)	Localized (annulus)	Moderate	**Difficult**
Rheumatic	IIIa but pliable anterior leaflet	Localized	Moderate	
Severe Barlow	II: Extensive prolapse (≥ 3 scallops, anterior commissure)	Extensive (annulus + leaflets)	Severe	**Unlikely**
Endocarditis	II: Prolapse but destructive lesions	No	No/Mild	
Rheumatic	IIIa but stiff anterior leaflet	Extensive (annulus + leaflets)	Moderate/Severe	
Ischaemic/Functional	IIIb but severe valvular deformation	No	No or Severe	

Adapted from Lancellotti P, et al. on behalf of the European Association of Echocardiography. European Association of Echocardiography Recommendations for the Assessment of Valvular Regurgitation. Part 2: Mitral and Tricuspid Regurgitation. Eur J Echocardiogr 2010; **11**(4):307–332.

A 13mm^2 or more increase in EROA during exercise characterizes patients at increased risk of events.

Stress echocardiography is thus recommended:

- In patients with LV dysfunction who present exertional dyspnoea out of proportion to the severity of resting dysfunction or MR.
- In patients in whom acute pulmonary oedema occurs without any obvious cause to unmask patients at high risk of mortality and HF.
- Before surgical revascularization in patients with moderate MR.

In degenerative mitral disease, patients with MV prolapse but no or mild MR at rest frequently develop significant regurgitation during exercise. Marked exercise-induced changes in MR severity is also frequent in chronic asymptomatic degenerative MR (>30%) and is unrelated to resting MR severity. In addition, the extent of changes in MR severity quantified during stress echocardiography is correlated with exercise-induced changes in PASP and is associated with reduced symptom-free survival. Consequently, exercise stress echocardiography may be useful in the management of asymptomatic degenerative MR and could be considered to improve the timing of surgery.

Mitral stenosis

Aetiology

Rheumatic fever is the leading cause for mitral stenosis (MS) worldwide, even in industrialized countries. The second cause of MS in developed countries is degenerative MS or calcific MS. Other causes are rare and include congenital anomalies (parachute valve, cor triatriatum), infiltrative diseases, inflammatory diseases (erythematous lupus or rheumatoid arthritis), carcinoid disease, or tumours (myxoma).

Two-dimensional echo findings of the mitral valve

Echo findings are closely related to the aetiology of MS. In rheumatic disease, the classical finding is commissural fusion with a classic fish-mouth orifice in PSAX view. With the evolution of the disease there is a fusion and shortening of the subvalvular apparatus. At later stages, occurrence of superimposed calcification beginning at the tips of the leaflet restricts the motion of the MV. Classically, the anterior leaflet has a restricted motion in diastole with a hockey-stick appearance or a doming pattern (◐ Fig.14b.11) that can be best appreciated in PLAX view.

In degenerative disease, the mitral annulus is predominantly involved by the calcification process. Most of the time no stenosis results from this process unless the leaflets and the subvalvular apparatus are also affected. The absence of commissural fusion and the predominance of calcification at the base instead of leaflets tips help to differentiate degenerative MS from rheumatic disease.

Quantitation of mitral stenosis

Pressure gradient

Transmitral pressure gradient is obtained by tracing the CW Doppler transmitral flow velocity curve in A4C view (see ◐ Chapter 5). Pressure gradients are calculated using the simplified Bernoulli's equation (◐ Chapter 5, Equation 5.3). The mean transmitral gradient is the most relevant haemodynamic finding whereas maximal gradient is modified by LA compliance, LV function, and the concomitant presence of MR.

The use of colour Doppler may be useful to identify the highest diastolic flow velocity that may be sometimes eccentric. In patients with atrial fibrillation, averaged measurements of five cycles should be performed. Mean transmitral pressure gradient is largely modified by heart rate, rhythm, cardiac output, and the presence of MR. For these reasons, the assessment of mitral valve area is the best marker of MS severity.

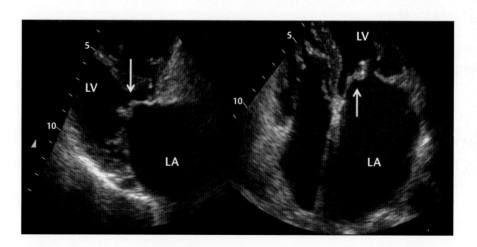

Figure 14b.11 Hockey-stick appearance of the anterior leaflet. Restriction of the anterior leaflet in diastole with a hockey-stick appearance which is a classic characteristic of rheumatic mitral stenosis.

Mitral valve area

Planimetry

Planimetry is considered as the method of reference to measure mitral valve area (MVA) as it is a direct measurement, theoretically independent of loading conditions. Previous study has demonstrated that planimetry of MV has the best correlation with anatomical valve area assessed on explanted valves. On a zoomed PSAX view, a direct tracing of the mitral orifice is performed (➲ Fig. 14b.12). The optimal timing for measurement is at mid-diastole and should include commissural opening when it is possible. Attention should be focused on adequately aligning the plane of the valve at the leaflet tips by carefully scanning the ventricle from the base to the apex to select the narrowest orifice.

In rheumatic disease, MV has an elliptical shape. Gain setting should be adjusted to avoid underestimation of valve area in patients with dense and severe calcification. An average of several measures is recommended, particularly in patients with atrial fibrillation or just after commissurotomy since flow conditions can have a slight impact on valve opening.

Planimetry of MVA is not possible in around 5% of patients with MS because of inappropriate acoustic window or intense shadowing by severe calcification. Correct assessment of MVA by planimetry has also been demonstrated to be dependant on technical expertise and experience of the observer. In these situations, the use of real-time 3D echo or 3D-guided biplane imaging may be more accurate than 2D echocardiography by providing an optimal plan positioning of the MV orifice (➲ Fig.14b.13).

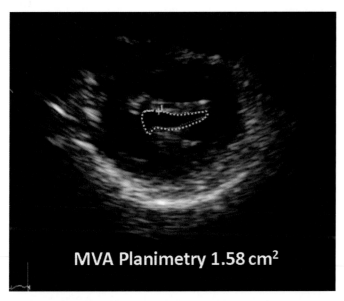

Figure 14b.12 Short-axis view displaying a planimetry of mitral valve area. Commissural opening is included in the measurement. In this example, mitral valve area is 1.58cm² which defines moderate stenosis.

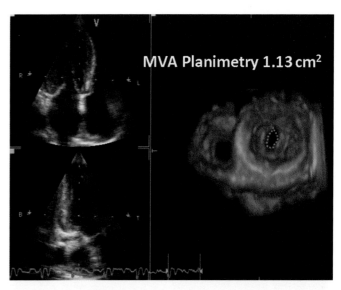

Figure 14b.13 3D-echo of planimetry of mitral valve area. This is an example of planimetry of mitral valve area assessed by 3D-echo in a patient with a significant mitral stenosis. The measurement is performed with an optimal alignment at the tips of the mitral leaflets.

Pressure half-time method

Basic principles and technical aspects of the PHT method are defined in ➲ Chapter 5. PHT is calculated by ➲ Equation 5.19 (➲ Fig.14b.14).

Despite its simplicity and its widespread use in clinical practice, the PHT method has only a fair correlation with planimetry, especially in patients with atrial fibrillation or advanced age. The deceleration slope of the mitral E-wave is also highly dependent on mitral gradient in early diastole and on LA and LV compliances. For these reasons, PHT is not accurate and cannot be used in patients with aortic regurgitation greater than moderate or during the first 24–72 hours after percutaneous mitral valve commissurotomy (PMC). In fact, early after mitral valvuloplasty, despite relief of stenosis, pressure gradients between LA and LV are not yet equilibrated and PHT is not accurate for the measurement of MVA. Subsequently, fall of LA pressure and increase of LV filling tend to stabilize gradients and PHT becomes useful again.

Continuity equation

The continuity equation can be used to assess MVA, stating that mitral stroke volume is equal to aortic stroke volume (see ➲ Chapter 5). It is easily calculated by using ➲ Equation 5.18. When applied to MS assessment, it becomes:

$$\text{MVA} = (D^2 \times 0.785)_{\text{LVOT}} \times (\text{TVI}_{\text{LVOT}} / \text{TVI}_{\text{MV}}) \qquad (14b.1)$$

where D is the LVOT diameter. The pulmonary stroke volume may also be used instead of the aortic stroke volume but is rarely performed. Generally, MVA measured by the continuity equation is *smaller* than the MVA obtained by planimetry (functional vs. anatomical surface area).

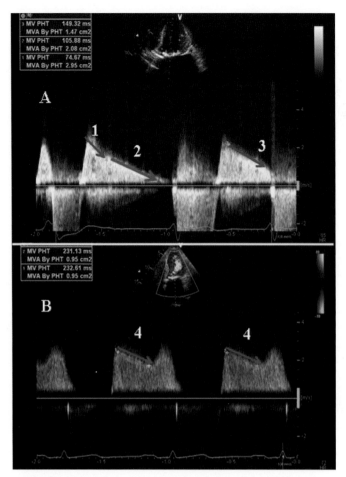

Figure 14b.14 PHT measurement in MS. Examples of mitral valve area (MVA) assessed by the pressure half-time (PHT) measurement. A) A patient with moderate mitral stenosis and atrial fibrillation. Arrow 1: the PHT is taken at the more abrupt part of the E wave which overestimates MVA (MVA 2.95cm²). Arrow 2: PHT is measured at the longer portion of the cycle and still results in an overestimation of MVA because of a long atrial fibrillation cycle (MVA 2.08cm²). Arrow 3 represents an average of the measurements performed in this patient (MVA 1.47cm²). Planimetry of this patient demonstrates a MVA of 1.52cm². B) This figure illustrates the MVA (Arrow 4, MVA 0.95cm²) assessed accurately by PHT method in a patient in sinus rhythm and no other cardiac disease.

The accuracy and the reproducibility of the continuity equation are limited by the fact that many measurements with an inherent degree of error need to be performed and are not acquired simultaneously. In addition, the continuity equation is invalidated when significant MR (underestimation of MVA) or aortic regurgitation (overestimation of MVA) are present. Finally, because stroke volumes vary from cycle to cycle, it should be avoided in patients with atrial fibrillation.

PISA method

Similarly to MR, in MS the PISA method is based on consideration that diastolic flow converges towards stenotic MV orifice, producing multiple shells of isovelocity hemispheric shape on the atrial side of the MV (➲ Fig. 14b.15). It is sometimes the only method available to assess MVA. In fact, the PISA method

offers the advantage of being still accurate in case of MR or aortic regurgitation.

MVA can be calculated by using this formula:

$$MVA = 6.28 \times r^2 \times \frac{\text{aliasing velocity}}{\text{Peak mitral stenosis velocity}} \times \frac{\propto^\circ}{180^\circ} \quad (14b.2)$$

where r is the radius of the convergence flow (in cm) and $\propto$ is the opening angle of mitral leaflets relative to flow direction. Technical attention is required for using the PISA method in the assessment of MS: the baseline velocity should be shifted up to an aliasing velocity of 20–45cm/s, the radius ideally should be measured at the same time of transmitral velocity and the angle between two mitral leaflets at the atrial surface should be determined. Measurement of the opening angle is performed off-line which is quite demanding. On the other hand, it has been demonstrated that there is only slight change of angle between patients and the use of fixed angle of 100 degrees provides accurate estimation of MVA. Colour M-mode PISA may also be useful by simultaneously recording measurement of flow and velocity and improves accuracy of the PISA method.

Consecutive changes and associated lesions

Left atrial dilation

Significant MS induces a chronic increase of LA pressure that consequently induces progressive LA enlargement (➲ Fig. 14b.16). LA volume should be assessed instead of LA size as LA enlarges mostly following an inferior-to-superior axis. Few studies have evaluated the prognosis impact of LA size or volume in MS. However, it has been demonstrated that the presence of spontaneous echo contrast is associated with increased LA size and thus, thrombus formation and/or embolic event. When present, LA thrombi are usually located in the LA appendage and diagnosis is obtained by using TOE. The sensitivity and specificity of TOE to detect LA thrombus are well known. Ruling out LA thrombus before PMC is the main indication of performing TOE in MS. The presence of spontaneous echo contrast is not a contraindication to perform PMC; conversely, it may be an indication for PMC in asymptomatic patients with MVA less than 1.5cm² and suitable characteristics.

Pulmonary hypertension, tricuspid regurgitation, and right ventricle

The estimation of pulmonary pressure is usually obtained from the tricuspid regurgitant velocity, using the modified Bernouilli's equation (see ➲ Chapter 5). ESC guidelines recommend PMC in patients with PASP higher than 50mmHg at rest. Incidence of pulmonary hypertension in MS depends on population studied and on severity of MS. There is a wide range of pulmonary arterial pressure (PAP) for a given valve area and PMC has variable effect on residual PAP. Moderate-to-severe TR may be observed up to one-third of patients with MS preceding PMC.

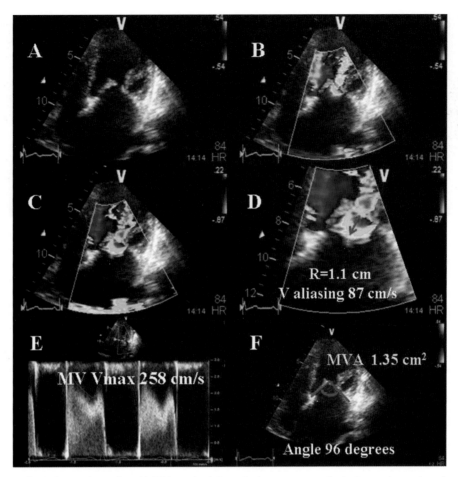

Figure 14b.15 Assessment of mitral stenosis severity with PISA method. Quantitative assessment of mitral stenosis severity using the PISA method. Stepwise analysis: A) Apical four-chamber view (CV). B) Colour-flow display. C) Upward shift of zero baseline to obtain a hemispheric PISA area. D) Zoom of the selected zone and measure of the PISA radius using the first aliasing. E) Continuous wave Doppler of mitral inflow jet velocity allowing calculation of maximal velocity (V max). F) Angle is measured offline. Mitral valve area (MVA) is 1.35cm^2. R, radius of PISA; V aliasing, aliasing velocity.

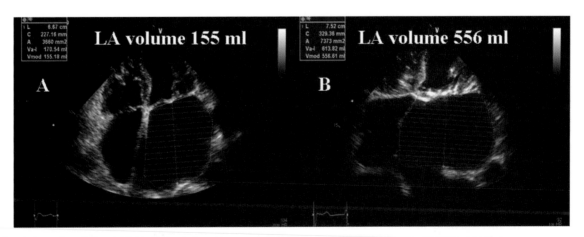

Figure 14b.16 Examples of left atrial (LA) dilation induced by severe mitral stenosis. A) Severe LA dilation. B) A huge LA dilation.

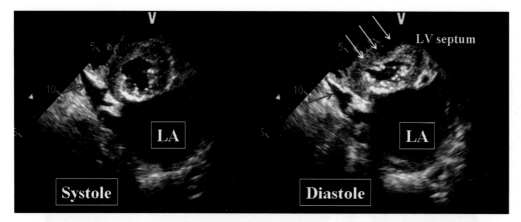

Figure 14b.17 Mitral stenosis and pulmonary hypertension. Example of a patient with severe mitral stenosis and pulmonary hypertension. There is a classical D-shape of the left ventricle (LV) septum in diastole (white arrows), illustrating the increased right ventricular afterload. Of note, there is also a severe left atrial (LA) dilation and a pericardial effusion (red arrow).

It can be the consequence of rheumatic disease or, most of the time, it is a functional TR related to pulmonary hypertension. In the latter case, concomitant RV dilation may also occur (➲ Fig.14b.17).

Other valve diseases

Rheumatic MR is frequently associated with MS. Description and quantitation of MR in this situation is of crucial importance for guiding the choice of intervention. In fact, patients with MR greater than mild have a relative contraindication to PMC. The mechanism of MR in rheumatic fever is mostly restriction of leaflet motion. Coaptation defect induced by calcification of the valve may also explain MR. After PMC, the occurrence or the worsening of MR may result from leaflet tearing during the procedure. Patients with traumatic MR may be considered earlier for a surgical intervention.

Rheumatic fever may induce other cardiac valves disorders that are, in order: aortic (regurgitation <stenosis), tricuspid (functional regurgitation >stenosis), and, rarely, pulmonary involvement. Looking at other valves in patients with MS is an essential part of the echocardiographic examination because mixed valvular diseases are commonly seen. Symptomatology and management of these patients may differ from patients with isolated valve diseases.

Classification of MS severity

Echocardiography is a key tool for diagnosis and assessment of MS severity (➲ Table 14b.3). The severity of MS should primarily rely on MVA, preferably assessed by planimetry and should be validated with another method in case of discrepancy (➲ Fig. 14b.18; ➲ Table 14b.4). Normal valve area is 4–6cm^2 and patients with MVA greater than 1.5cm^2 are rarely symptomatic. When MS becomes tighter, the mitral valve behaves like

Table 14b.3 Assessment of mitral valve stenosis

Mean transmitral gradient with CWD in four-chamber view
Mitral valve area:
A) Planimetry of MVA in short-axis view
B) Pressure half-time
C) Continuity equation
D) PISA method
Estimation of systolic pulmonary pressure from the transtricuspid regurgitant velocity
Left atrial volume
Right ventricular dilation and function
Other valve lesions (concomitant mitral regurgitation, aortic stenosis or regurgitation, functional tricuspid regurgitation or stenosis)
Wilkins score or Cormier score before PMC
TOE to rule out LA thrombus before PMC

Table 14b.4 Recommendations for classification of MS according to echocardiographic criteria

	Mild	Moderate	Severe
Specific findings:			
Valve area (cm^2)	>1.5	1.0–1.5	<1.0
Supportive findings:	<5	5–10	>10
Mean gradients (mmHg)*	<30	30–50	>50
Pulmonary artery pressure (mmHg)			

At heart rates of 60–80bpm and in sinus rhythm.

Adapted from Baumgartner H, Hung J, Bermejo J, Chambers JB, Evangelista A, Griffin BP, *et al*. Echocardiographic assessment of valve stenosis: EAE/ASE recommendations for clinical practice. *Eur J Echocardiogr* 2009; **10**:1–25.

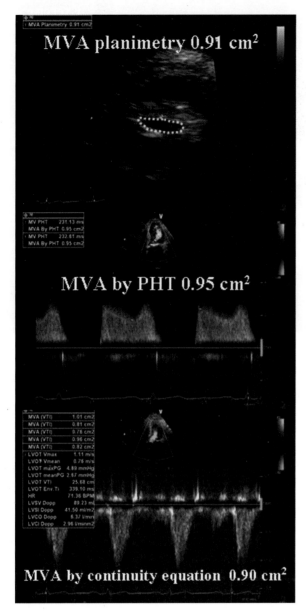

Figure 14b.18 Assessment of mitral valve area with three different methods. Example of three different methods used in the same patient to assess mitral valve area. In this case, all methods gave a similar result which is not always the case, especially in patients with atrial fibrillation. MVA, mitral valve area; PHT, pressure half-time.

a fixed orifice, cardiac output (CO) becomes subnormal, and there is little mitral functional reserve at exercise. This is why current guidelines consider significant MS when MVA is less than 1.5cm².

Role of haemodynamic stress testing

The ESC guidelines on valvular heart diseases recommend exercise stress testing in asymptomatic patients without high risk of embolism and/or haemodynamic decompensation to unmask symptoms and assess exercise capacity. Exercise is thus recommended when there is a discrepancy between symptoms,

clinical evaluation, and echocardiographic findings at rest. Patients with a PASP higher than 60mmHg at exercise may be considered for PMC when mitral valve characteristics are suitable (➲ Fig 14b.19). Mean transmitral gradient greater than 15mmHg at exercise echocardiography or greater than 18mmHg at dobutamine stress echocardiography have also been proposed as criteria to predict the occurrence of symptoms or to indicate PMC.

Exercise Doppler echocardiography is a more physiological test than dobutamine stress echocardiography in MS. In the latter, the interpretation of PAP is confounded by the preload and afterload reductions induced by dobutamine. Stress echocardiography testing data are limited in MS. The prognostic importance and the additive value of stress echocardiography need to be prospectively validated regarding these criteria, especially according to the cut-off value of PAP at exercise relying on low level of evidence.

Role of echo in percutaneous mitral valve commissurotomy/plasty

2D echocardiography of MV is essential before performing PMC. The evaluation of valve morphology by looking carefully at chordal shortening and thickening, the extent of subvalvular disease, the degree of leaflet mobility, and the amount of calcification is of primary importance when considering PMC. Calcification of commissural areas should receive special attention as it is an important criterion for successful PMC. Several scoring systems have been proposed, the so-called Wilkins score being used more frequently worldwide (➲ Table 14b.5) and the Cormier score (➲ Table 14b.6), which has the advantage of its simplicity. A Wilkins score higher than 8 reflects an unsuitable anatomy and predicts a lower success rate of PMC. No proposed scores have proven their superiority over the others as no randomized comparison trials have been undertaken in this regard. Patients should not be refused for PMC based solely on score systems because patients may achieve good results with PMC even with unfavourable mitral anatomy, as long-term outcome depends also on clinical (age, heart rhythm, New York Heart Association class) and echocardiographic data (MVA, commissural calcification).

Several contraindications to perform PMC should be acknowledged (➲ Table 14b.7). During the procedure, echo-guiding is necessary for the transseptal puncture and balloon positioning. The use of real-time 3D TOE is a novel method to facilitate and improve the success rate of PMC. During and after the procedure, few complications may occur and should rapidly be identified given their high rate of mortality. Procedural mortality of PMC is 0–3% and is mostly the result of tamponade or acute severe MR. Other complications include haemopericardium, embolism, and significant atrial septal defect after transseptal puncture.

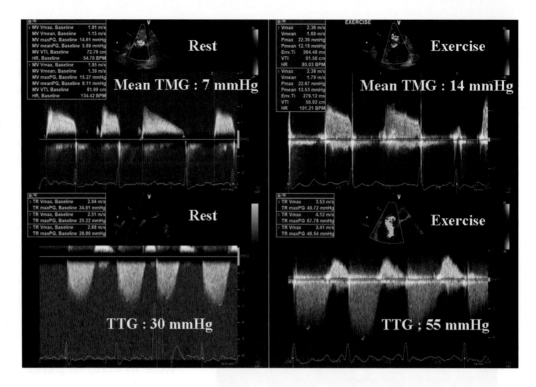

Figure 14b.19 Haemodynamic stress testing. Exercise stress testing results in a patient with moderate mitral stenosis (1.4cm²) and well controlled atrial fibrillation. He described a slight decrease of exercise capacity in the last few weeks. Left panel: measurements of mean transmitral gradient (TMG) and transtricuspid pressure gradient (TTG) at rest; Right panel: a significant increase of mean TMG and TTG at exercise is demonstrated. In this patient, knowing he had a favourable anatomy and systolic pulmonary pressure >60mmHg, a percutaneous mitral commissuroplasty was performed.

Table 14b.5 Assessment of mitral valve anatomy according to the Wilkins score

Grade	Mobility	Thickening	Calcification	Subvalvular thickening
1	Highly mobile valve with only leaflet tips restricted	Leaflets near normal in thickness (4–5mm)	A single area of increased echo brightness	Minimal thickening just below the mitral leaflets
2	Leaflet mid and base portions have normal mobility	Mid-leaflets normal, considerable thickening of margins (5–8mm)	Scattered areas of brightness confined to leaflet margins	Thickening of chordal structures extending to one-third of the chordal length
3	Valve continues to move forward in diastole, mainly from the base	Thickening extending through the entire leaflet (5–8mm)	Brightness extending into the mid-portions of the leaflets	Thickening extended to distal third of the chords
4	No or minimal forward movement of the leaflets in diastole	Considerable thickening of all leaflet tissue (>8–10mm)	Extensive brightness throughout much of the leaflet tissue	Extensive thickening and shortening of all chordal structures extending down to the papillary muscles

The total score is the sum of the four items and ranges from 4–16.

Adapted from Wilkins GT, Weyman AE, Abascal VM, Block PC, Palacios IF. Percutaneous balloon dilation of the mitral valve: an analysis of echocardiographic variables related to outcome and the mechanism of dilation. *Br Heart J* 1988; **60**:299–308.

Table 14b.6 Assessment of mitral valve anatomy according to the Cormier score

Echocardiographic group	Mitral valve anatomy
Group 1	Pliable non-calcified anterior mitral leaflet and mild subvalvular disease (i.e. thin chordae ≥10mm long)
Group 2	Pliable non-calcified anterior mitral leaflet and severe subvalvular disease (i.e. thickened chordae <10mm long)
Group 3	Calcification of mitral valve of any extent, as assessed by fluoroscopy, whatever the state of subvalvular apparatus

Adapted from Iung B, Cormier B, Ducimetière P, Porte JM, Nallet O, Michel PL, *et al.* Immediate results of percutaneous mitral commissurotomy. A predictive model on a series of 1514 patients. *Circulation* 1996; **94**:2124–30.

Table 14b.7 Contraindications to percutaneous mitral valve commissurotomy

Mitral valve area ≥1.5cm²
Left atrial thrombus
Mitral regurgitation that is more than mild
Severe or bicommissural calcification
Absence of commissural fusion
Severe concomitant aortic valve disease or severe combined tricuspid stenosis and tricuspid regurgitation
Concomitant coronary artery disease requiring bypass surgery

Personal perspective

The evaluation and the management of mitral valve diseases will improve considerably in the next decades. Nowadays, MS remains a serious burden in undeveloped countries and although its prevalence tends to substantially decrease in Western countries, MR frequency progressively increases and, thus, maintains such pathologies in the most prevalent cardiac diseases.

The development of tissue Doppler imaging and specifically of 2D speckle-tracking may noticeably enhance the evaluation of the function of each cardiac chamber. Consequently, the impact of MR or MS on LV and LA will be more accurately assessed. The management of patients with MR is strongly dependent on the consequences of the disease on left-sided cavities. The longitudinal, radial, and circumferential myocardial functions assessed with new echocardiographic modalities allow the identification of subclinical and latent dysfunctions, even in asymptomatic patients. Recent advances have highlighted the use of tissue Doppler imaging to evaluate the LA function and not only the geometry. Such improvement may also be helpful to quantify the impact of volume or pressure overload on LA and on pulmonary circulation.

Real-time 3D imaging is a growing tool truly useful to appraise the complex configuration, morphology, and dynamics of mitral subvalvular apparatus, leaflets, and annulus. Indeed, due to its 3D shape, mitral valve could, theoretically, be more precisely explored by 3D rather than 2D echocardiography. Furthermore, recent development of the 3D-TOE probe provides an accurate description of the mechanism of MR and of the leaflet/scallop involved in the disease which the surgeon should target. Preoperative strategies and surgical results may, thus, be refining by the common use of 3D echocardiography. This tool gives a fascinating impetus toward a better synergy between cardiological and surgical teams.

Meanwhile the universal use of these new echocardiographic techniques, further studies and data are required to evaluate whether the use of such tools may optimize the management of mitral valve diseases.

Further reading

Baumgartner H, Hung J, Bermejo J, Chambers JB, Evangelista A, Griffin BP, *et al.* Echocardiographic assessment of valve stenosis: EAE/ASE recommendations for clinical practice. *Eur J Echocardiogr* 2009; **10**:1–25.

Iung B, Cormier B, Ducimetière P, Porte JM, Nallet O, Michel PL, *et al.* Immediate results of percutaneous mitral commissurotomy. A predictive model on a series of 1514 patients. *Circulation* 1996; **94**:2124–30.

Lancellotti P, Pasquet A, Cosyns B, Unger P, Paelinck B, Voigt J, *et al.* (eds). *The Echo Pocket-Book*. Belgian Working Group of Non Invasive Cardiac Imaging, 2008.

Lancellotti P, Moura L, Pierard LA, Agricola E, Popescu BA, Tribouilloy C, *et al.* on behalf of the European Association of Echocardiography. European Association of Echocardiography Recommendations for the Assessment of Valvular Regurgitation. Part 2: Mitral and Tricuspid Regurgitation. *Eur J Echocardiogr* 2010; **11**(4):307–32.

Papers of interest on echocardiography by the European Association of Echocardiography.

Pierard LA, Lancellotti P. Stress testing in valve disease. *Heart* 2007; **93**:766–72.

Wilkins GT, Weyman AE, Abascal VM, Block PC, Palacios IF. Percutaneous balloon dilation of the mitral valve: an analysis of echocardiographic variables related to outcome and the mechanism of dilation. *Br Heart J* 1988; **60**:299–308.

⊃ For additional multimedia materials please visit the online version of the book (⌂ http://escecho.oxfordmedicine.com).

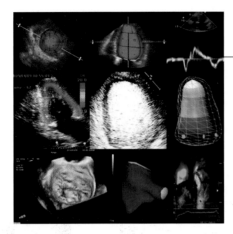

CHAPTER 14C

Tricuspid and pulmonary valves

Ashraf M. Anwar and Folkert Jan ten Cate

Contents

Summary

Right-sided heart valves are complex anatomical structures. Studies describing the morphological and functional assessment of both valves are lacking. Most echocardiographic modalities provide a qualitative rather than quantitative approach.

Echocardiography has a central role in the assessment of tricuspid regurgitation through estimation of severity, understanding the mechanism, assessment of pulmonary artery pressure, evaluation of right ventricular function, guidance towards surgery versus medical therapy, and assessment of valve competence after surgery.

Transoesophageal echocardiography is an accurate method providing a qualitative assessment of right-sided heart valves. However, the lack of good validation makes it difficult to recommend its use for a quantitative approach. Hopefully, the future will provide refinements in instrumentation and techniques leading to increased accuracy in reporting and cost-effectiveness in making clinical decisions.

Tricuspid valve

Background

The tricuspid valve (TV) apparatus includes leaflets, chordae, papillary muscles, and annulus. The TV has three distinct leaflets (septal, anterior, and posterior) attached by chordae to papillary muscles. The septal and the anterior leaflets are larger than the posterior leaflet. There are three sets of smaller papillary muscles, each set composed of up to three muscles. The chordae tendineae arising from each set are inserted into two adjacent leaflets. Thus, the anterior set chordae insert into half of septal and half of anterior leaflets. The medial and posterior sets are similarly related to adjacent valve leaflets.[1] The annulus is oval in shape and becomes more circular when dilated. The annulus expands in diastole and constricts in mid-systole. The proper function of TV requires the coordination of right ventricle (RV), right atrium (RA), papillary muscles, chordate, and both interatrial and interventricular septae.

Tricuspid stenosis

Organic tricuspid stenosis (TS) is an unusual finding. Rheumatic heart disease is the commonest cause, accounting for over 90% and is usually associated with mitral and/or aortic valve affection. Rheumatic TV inflammation causes scarring and fibrosis of TV leaflets, fusion of commissures, and shortening of chordae resulting in reduced valve area. Other causes include carcinoid disease, obstruction by RA myxoma, and a rare congenital malformation. Careful echocardiographic examination of TV should be performed in patients presenting with rheumatic aortic and/or mitral valve disease.

Tricuspid regurgitation

Nearly 50–60% of young adults exhibit mild tricuspid regurgitation (TR) and its prevalence increases with age. Up to 15% of normals have moderate TR. Moderate and severe TR is usually associated with abnormalities in one or more of the TV apparatus:

- Leaflet abnormalities (intrinsic): thickening, fibrosis, and /or calcification (rheumatic, carcinoid, infective endocarditis, trauma, and degeneration) may lead to malcoaptation of leaflets. Tethering of leaflets due to RV segmental dysfunction and prolapse of TV leaflets can contribute.

- Annulus abnormalities (functional): annular dilation is the commonest mechanism of non-organic TR secondary to RV dilation, RV dysfunction, and pulmonary hypertension (PH).

- Diastolic TR: this can occur in certain conditions, e.g. heart block, atrial flutter, severe pulmonary regurgitation, and restrictive cardiomyopathy, due to reversal of pressure gradient between RA and RV during diastole (RV >RA).

Assessment with two-dimensional transthoracic echocardiography

Views

2D TTE assessment of TV can be performed by standard and modified views (➲ Fig. 14c.1) (for details, see also ➲ Chapter 2, 'Two-dimensional echocardiography'):

- Parasternal RV inflow view: with medial angulation, septal and anterior leaflets are seen (▣ 14c.1)

- Parasternal short-axis (PSAX) view at great vessel level: this view provides the best visualization of TV, where the anterior leaflet is seen attached to RV free wall. The other leaflet adjacent to aorta is either the posterior (in 52%) or septal (in 48%) depending on the cut plane.[2]

- Apical four-chamber (A4C) view: in this view, the septal and anterior leaflets are seen (▣ 14c.2).

- Subcostal view: both four-chamber and short axis display the same leaflets, visualized in parasternal and apical views

- Parasternal short axis midway between papillary and mitral level: in this modified view, the three TV leaflets may be seen especially with dilated RV.

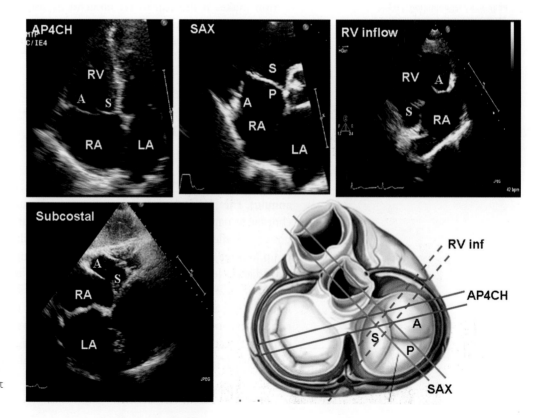

Figure 14c.1 Standard views by 2D TTE show the distribution of TV leaflets (A: anterior, S: septal, and P: posterior) in each view. The schematic diagram showed the cut plane direction of each view.

Qualitative and quantitative data

In standard 2D TTE report both qualitative features and quantitative data regarding TV should be included. Accurate description of TV morphology should include leaflet position, mobility, thickness, calcification, tethering, and coaptation.

Quantitative evaluation of TV encompasses measurement of sizes and function, which can particularly be performed by assessing:

◆ Tricuspid annulus diameter, that is better obtained from A4C view (➲ Fig. 14c.2).

◆ Annulus deformation (reduction during systole), that can be calculated as follow:

$$\text{(End-systolic diameter} - \text{end-diastolic diameter)}/ \text{end-systolic diameter} \tag{14c.1}$$

Similarly to mitral valve stenosis, assessment of TS severity requires measurement of transvalvular peak and mean diastolic pressure gradients, using continuous wave (CW) Doppler mode (➲ Fig. 14c.3), whereas calculation of TV area by pressure half-time (PHT) is used uncommonly in clinical practice. However, it is obtained by the following formula:

$$\text{TV area} = 190/\text{PHT} \tag{14c.2}$$

The presence of TR and its severity degree are easily assessed by colour Doppler (CD) mode (➲ Fig. 14c.4, ▤ 14c.3). Moreover, TR peak velocity, measured by CW Doppler mode, is representative of pressure gradient existing between RV and RA during systole. High values indicate either pulmonary stenosis (PS) or PH (see also ➲ Chapter 5 and 11).

Furthermore, at the level of TV, it is possible to perform other measurements which could be used as markers of RV systolic and diastolic function (for details, see also ➲ Chapter 11):

◆ Tricuspid annulus peak systolic excursion (TAPSE), obtained by aligning M-mode scan line through the plane of systolic motion of anterior leaflet from A4C or PSAX view (➲ Fig. 14c.2).

◆ Tricuspid annulus peak systolic velocity, obtained by tissue Doppler signal (➲ Fig. 14c.5). Lower values confer poor prognostic implications.

◆ PW Doppler pattern of TV inflow, that is the same of that recorded at the level of mitral valve but shows lower velocities than the left-sided heart chambers. In particular, it is of note that in normal condition E/A ratio is greater than 1 and E wave velocity increases of 14% during inspiration.

Technical considerations and limitations

Some technical considerations and limitations have to be known in order to improve acquisition and interpretation of TV echocardiographic images:

◆ Visualization of the stenotic TV orifice by 2D echocardiography is cumbersome and therefore the measurement of TV area by planimetry is difficult.

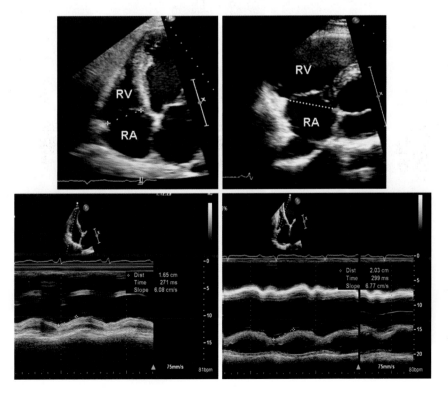

Figure 14c.2 Tricuspid annulus diameter measurements by 2D TTE in apical 4-chamber and short-axis views (upper panel). TAPSE in patient with normal and impaired RV function (lower panel).

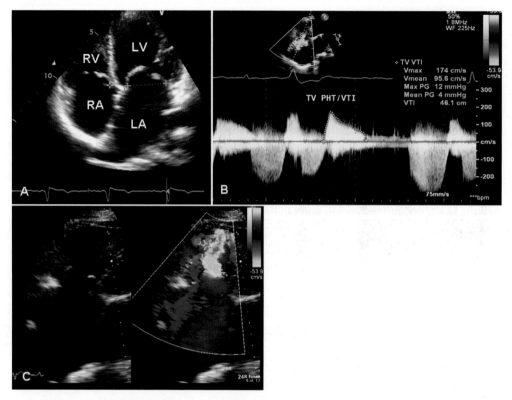

Figure 14c.3 Rheumatic tricuspid stenosis. Example of 2D TTE morphology of rheumatic TS associated with mitral stenosis (A), CW Doppler measuring the peak and mean diastolic gradient across it (B), and diastolic colour flow of TS (C).

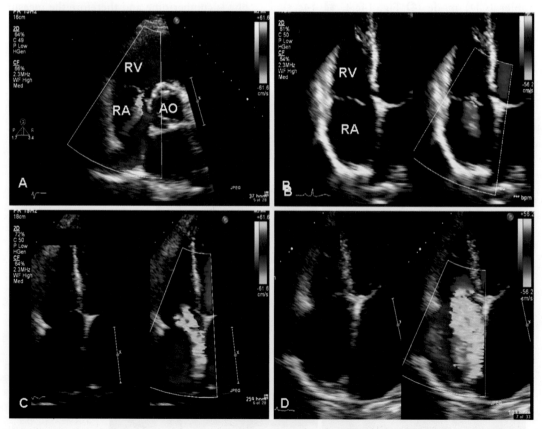

Figure 14c.4 Colour flow Doppler pattern of tricuspid regurgitation. Colour flow Doppler pattern of different grades of TR, mild physiological TR (A,B), moderate TR (C), and severe TR (D).

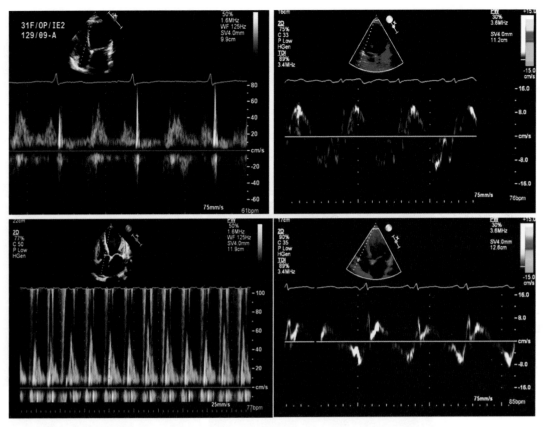

Figure 14c.5 PW and TDI of TV flow pattern in normal (upper panel) and impaired RV function (lower panel).

◆ In PS, the RV systolic pressure is not equal to pulmonary arterial systolic pressure (PASP), so calculation of PASP by TR velocity is not accurate.

◆ M-mode plays a small role in identification of TV leaflets pathology because it can demonstrate a two-phase opening pattern of one leaflet regardless of its view.

◆ In advanced cases of PH and impaired RV systolic function, the RV and RA pressures are nearly equal. So, the regurgitation velocity may be less than 2.0m/s. Other markers are beneficial, e.g. RV dimension, and TV annulus size.

◆ High velocity TR does not indicate severity of TR but indicates severity of PH. For example, severe TR with normal RV systolic pressure has low peak velocity, while mild TR with high RV systolic pressure has higher peak velocity.

◆ Tricuspid annulus velocity by TDI is an indicator of RV systolic function but can not be used in evaluating the severity of RV dysfunction.

◆ Doppler velocity and gradient measurements are affected by heart rate (HR) and respiration, so proper measurement should be obtained at end-expiration with HR 70–80 beats per minute

◆ TV area by continuity equation is not accurate in the presence of moderate to severe TR.

◆ In combined lesion (TS and TR), the CW Doppler assessment is not ideal due to opposite effects of both lesions on

the velocity and pressure gradient. In such case, CD is accurate for the assessment of TR

◆ Mild to moderate TR is usually direct towards the interatrial septum. Careful discrimination between TR and other flow, e.g. atrial septal defect or caval flow, is essential.

Assessment with two-dimensional transoesophageal echocardiography

Views

2D TOE evaluation of TV morphology and function can be obtained by the following standard and modified views (see also ➔ Chapter 4) (➔ Figs. 14c.6 and 14c.7):

◆ The four-chamber view (standard) at mid oesophageal level 0–20 degrees. In this view, the anterior and septal leaflets are seen. With probe retroflexion it is sometimes possible to see the posterior leaflet instead of the anterior leaflet to the left of the image. This imaging plane provides adequate orientation for color flow mapping and conventional Doppler interrogation for the evaluation of TS and TR.[3]

◆ At mid-oesophageal level 30–80 degrees with clockwise rotation of the probe to the right, the short-axis or (RV inflow–outflow) view becomes visible. In this view, the posterior leaflet is seen to the left and the anterior or septal leaflet (50:50 in the general population) to the right of the image.

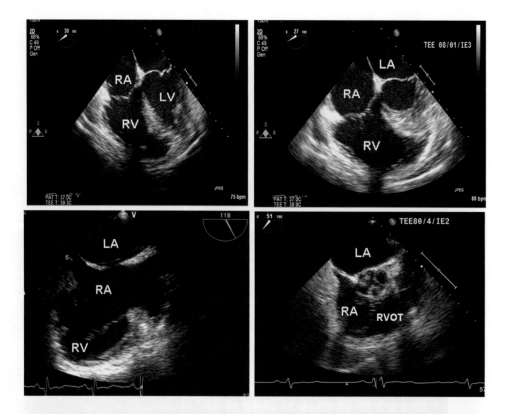

Figure 14c.6 Standard views of TV by 2D TOE, mid-oesophageal level at different angles.

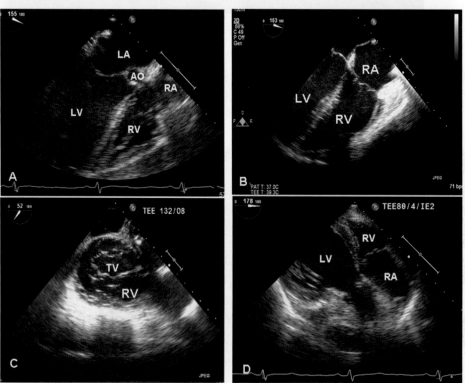

Figure 14c.7 Mid-oesophageal and transgastric views of TV. Standard views of TV by 2D TOE, mid-oesophageal (A, B) and transgastric (C, D) levels at different angles. In (C), TV is shown in short axis.

- Between 80–120 degrees with lateral flexion (RV two-chamber view) demonstrates the TV anterior and posterior leaflets.

- At 120 degrees, rightward rotation of the probe shaft yields the long-axis RV inflow view which demonstrates the TV anterior and posterior leaflets.

- Transitional (or gastro-oesophageal) view from the mid-oesophageal to transgastric at 0 degrees at the level of the coronary sinus displays the TV posterior and septal leaflets.

- A deeper transgastric view at 120 degrees allows further visualization of the TV anterior and posterior leaflets and the subvalvar apparatus.

◆ Transgastric view at 0–40 degrees with tilting to the right (modified): The three leaflets of the TV can be seen 'en face' when the RV is markedly dilated. In this cross-section the anterior TV leaflet is to the left in the far field, the posterior leaflet is to the left in the near field, and the septal leaflet is to the right side of the display.

Measurements and technical considerations

The application of 2D-TOE for assessment of TV is used for morphological description but is less useful for Doppler measurements. Tricuspid annulus diameter is best measured in four-chamber view with care to avoid apical foreshortening. It measures 28 ± 5mm or 16 ± 3mm/m². Conversely, the assessment of tricuspid flow is often hindered by its perpendicular direction to the ultrasound beam as well as occasional shadowing by the left-sided valves and the septum. For this reason, underestimation of the severity of TS and TR is common due to misalignment of Doppler beam to the flow direction. Thus, the assessment of TR severity by 2D-TOE has not been standardized.

Assessment with real-time three-dimensional echocardiography

Because of its peculiar features, 3D TV qualitative and quantitative assessment requires being performed specifically in TTE and TOE (➲ Fig. 14c.8).

Qualitative assessment

Acquisition of real-time 3D TTE imaging of TV can be obtained optimally from the apical and/or PSAX views. Visualization of all three TV leaflets simultaneously in one cross-sectional view is possible with the ability to distinguish each leaflet separately.[4] The new real-time 3D TOE probe is expected to achieve easier analysis in a higher percentage of patients than real-time 3D TTE, but has not been studied extensively. There is no standard view for optimal visualization of TV but this can be achieved from mid-oesophageal level at 0–20 degrees in most patients. Use of zoom mode helps in rapid and actual real-time assessment of the valve morphology. Probe manipulation may be needed to clarify suboptimal visualization of one of the valve leaflets or commissures because the three leaflets and commissures are not at the same level. The acquisition and analysis of full volume images obtained by both probes are the same.

Quantitative assessment

Quantitative assessment of TV by real-time 3D echocardiography relies on the calculation of TV area and annulus size and on estimation of some parameters derived by TR jet:

◆ TV area: measurement of the triangular TV area and the width of the three commissures between leaflets are valuable for diagnosis, follow-up, and selection of therapeutic modality of TS (➲ Fig. 14c.9). The three commissures are not at the same cut planes, so modification of the cut plane is needed to depict the optimal width of each commissure (normally: 4–6mm). The same measurements can be obtained by real-time 3D TOE.[2]

◆ TV annulus: measurement of TV annulus (diameter, circumference and area) is best obtained from apical window acquisition (➲ Fig. 14c.10; ▪ 14c.4).

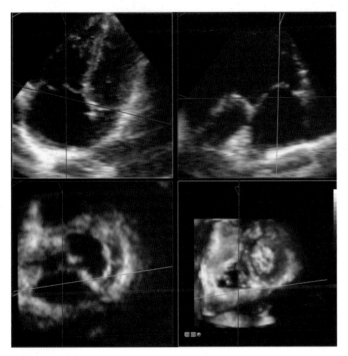

Figure 14c.8 Full volume real-time 3D TTE image of TV in patient with TS showing narrowed orifice and fused commissures

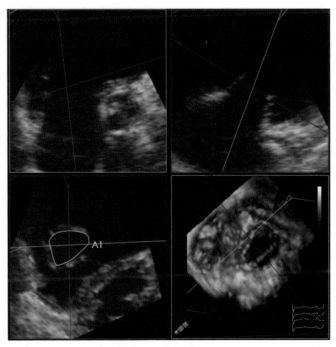

Figure 14c.9 3D TTE measurement of TV area. Measurement of normal TV area using crop function of full volume real-time 3D TTE image.

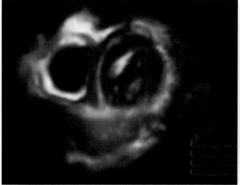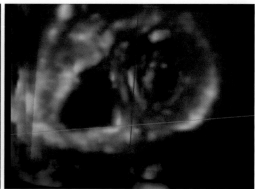

Figure 14c.10 3D TTE en face view of TV annulus. Real-time 3D-TTE enface view from ventricular aspect showing the oval shaped normal (left), and dilated TV annulus (right).

◆ Measurements obtained from the regurgitant colour jet, such as vena contracta, jet area, and jet volume (➲ Fig. 14c.11; 🎞 14c.5): unfortunately, the role of these parameters in definition and grading of TR severity is not established.

Clinical applications

➲ Table 14c.1 shows echo parameters regarding TV structure and function, obtained by different modalities in normal subjects, associated with possible clinical applications.

On the other hand, the assessment of TV disease is based on the following findings:

Assessment of severity of tricuspid stenosis

Markers for TS are thickened leaflets with restricted mobility, short and thickened chordae, increased peak and mean gradients across the valve, and reduced TV area and width of commissures.

Criteria for diagnosis of severe TS are:

◆ Mean diastolic gradient ≥5mmHg.

◆ PHT of tricuspid flow ≥190ms.

◆ TV area by continuity equation ≤1cm².

◆ Other indirect markers, e.g. dilated RA and inferior vena cava (IVC).

Assessment of mechanism and severity of tricuspid regurgitation

In most patients, 2D echocardiography helps in differentiation between primary (due to valve pathology) and secondary (due to annular dilation) TR. 3D echocardiography is superior to 2D for the measurement of annulus and descriptive morphology of leaflets. Meticulous assessment of TR is important especially in patients planned for mitral valve surgery.

In clinical practice, the definition of severe TR still depends on 2D measurements which include:[6]

◆ Colour flow regurgitant jet area ≥30% of RA area.

◆ Annulus dilation (≥4cm) or inadequate cusp coaptation.

◆ Late systolic concave configuration of the CW signal.

◆ Late systolic flow reversals in the hepatic vein.

◆ EROA ≥0.4cm².

◆ Regurgitant volume (RVol) ≥45mL.

◆ Width of vena contracta ≥6.5mm.

◆ Dense signal of CW Doppler with early peaking.

Miscellaneous conditions

Carcinoid heart disease

Carcinoid heart disease occurs in over 50% of patients with metastatic carcinoid syndrome, and may be the initial presentation of carcinoid disease. Deposition of a matrix-like material on the PV and TV results in retraction, fixation of their leaflets, reduced leaflet motion, and lack of central coaptation (➲ Fig. 14c.12A). The echocardiographic features include

Figure 14c.11 3D colour images of severe TR. Real-time 3DE colour images in patients with severe TR with measurement of irregular shaped vena contracta. Quantification of regurgitant volume can also be obtained

Table 14c.1 Echo parameters obtained by different modalities in normal subjects and their values in clinical application

Parameter	Normal value	Clinical application
2D measurements		
Annulus diameter (cm)	3–3.5	Dilated annulus is the commonest cause of TR
		Surgical repair if >21mm/m² or ≥3.5cm
Leaflet thickness (mm)	3	≥5mm indicating abnormal affection
M-mode measurements		
TAPSE (cm)	>2.0	<1.5 indicates RV dysfunction and poor prognosis
Doppler measurements		
Systolic velocity of TR (m/s)	2.0–2.5	3.0–3.9m/s indicates moderate PH, and ≥4.0m/s indicates severe
Diastolic E velocity (m/s)	0.50 (0.3–0.7)	≥1.0m/s indicate TS
Mean diastolic gradient (mmHg)	<2	≥5mmHg indicates severe TS
RV systolic pressure (mmHg)	≤25	25–40 mild PH; 40–60 moderate PH; and >60 : severe
TDI velocity of S' at annulus (cm/s)	4.95 ± 6.17	Reliable marker for RV function. Cutoff value of 9.5cm/s is valuable in detecting RV dysfunction.
Real-time 3DE measurements		
TV area (cm²)	4.8 ± 1.6	Reduced in TS
Commissural width (mm)	5.2 ± 1.5	Marker of organic TS (rheumatic).
Annulus area (cm²)	10.0 ± 2.9	As in 2DE
Annulus diameter (cm)	4.0 ± 0.7	As in 2DE

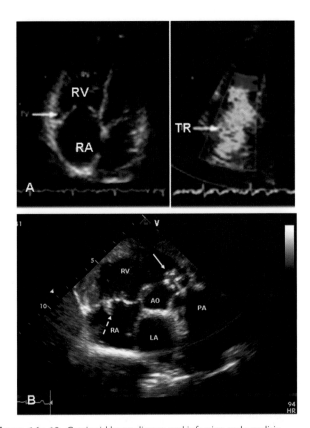

Figure 14c.12 Carcinoid heart disease and infective endocarditis. A) 2D TTE of TV morphology in carcinoid heart disease: both leaflets are thickened and restricted with severe TR. B) In infective endocarditis, vegetations are attached to atrial surface of TV and ventricular surface of PV (arrows).

thickening and retraction of immobile TV leaflets with associated severe TR (common) and TS (less common). Other findings are progressive RV dilation, high RV diastolic pressure, pericardial effusions, left-sided valvular affection (10%), and myocardial metastases (5%).

Endocardial fibroelastosis

Endocardial fibrosis can occur due to hypereosinophilia syndrome and tropical forms of endocardial fibroelastosis. The underlying pathology is a marked inflammatory response leading to diffuse endocardial thickening that extends to the chordae and papillary muscles. The leaflets will be restricted and the annulus dilates which leads to non-coaptation and severe TR. The RV apex is often obliterated due to inflammatory tissue and secondary thrombosis.

Tricuspid valve prolapse

TV prolapse is an incidental finding in 30–40% of patients with mitral valve prolapse. Echocardiography reveals billowing of septal and anterior leaflets above the plane of TV annulus. The associated TR is generally mild. Rarely, spontaneous chordae rupture may result in severe regurgitation. Severe mitral regurgitation with degenerative mitral valve disease can occur with moderate or severe TR and TV annulus dilation.

Tricuspid valve endocarditis

Endocarditis is a common problem in intravenous drug abuse. TV affection can be manifested by chaotically mobile vegetation attached to its atrial aspect, leaflet destruction or perforation, chordal or papillary muscle rupture, and abscess (➲ Fig. 14c.12B). The sensitivity of TTE and TOE for TV endocarditis is similar. TOE provides a superior characterization of vegetation size and extent as well as a greater specificity for endocarditis. A vegetation size of 10mm or above is associated with an increased likelihood of pulmonary emboli.

Tricuspid annular calcification

TV annular calcification is relatively rare and its clinical significance is not well studied. It appears as intense echo-producing mass in the myocardium at the base of TV leaflets associated with acoustic shadowing.

Pulmonary valve

Background

The PV consists of cusps, annulus, and commissures. Behind each cusp is an outpouching of the arterial root, known as a sinus. There are three semilunar cusps, two posterior cusps (right and left), and one anterior cusp in mirror image to the aortic cusp which project into the pulmonary trunk. The cusps are usually similar in size, although minor variations are commonly observed. Proper PV function requires normal leaflet anatomy and support from the pulmonary artery and right ventricular outflow tract (RVOT). During closure, the apposing cusps contact one another forming a competent seal. Diseases that increase cusp rigidity by fibrosis or calcification, or lead to commissural fusion such as rheumatic valvulitis produce stenosis. If the line between commissures straightens such as arterial root dilation or rheumatic retraction of cusps, pulmonary regurgitation (PR) occurs.

Pulmonary stenosis

Congenital PS is a common anomaly accounting for 7–12 % of congenital heart disease and is usually isolated. The valve may be bicuspid (20%), unicuspid (%), or dysplastic (10–13%). Rheumatic affection is rare and usually associated with other valves involvement. Extrinsic obstruction of the PV may be produced by cardiac tumours or by aneurysm of the sinus of Valsalva. In moderate to severe PS, the commissures became fused and the PV is effectively converted to a unicuspid or bicuspid funnel-shaped valve. This results in restriction of the orifice at the distal portion of the valve. The severity of stenosis ranges from mild to severe. In severe RV hypertrophy also subpulmonic stenosis might be present.

Aetiology

Aetiologies of PS can be distinguished into two groups:

* Congenital: valvular, infundibular, supravalvular, or distal branch stenosis. It can be isolated or as a part of complex congenital heart defects.

* Acquired (uncommon): rheumatic, infective endocarditis, carcinoid, pulmonary hypertension, and iatrogenic as following Ross operation.

Pulmonary regurgitation

Mild PR has been reported in 40–78% with normal PV and no structural heart disease. Acquired mild to moderate PR is seen often with PH due to annulus dilation. Severe PR is uncommon and usually observed with PV anatomical abnormalities or post-valvulotomy.

Aetiology

Aetiologies of PR can be distinguished into two groups:

* Most common causes: dilated valve ring secondary to PH (of any aetiology), dilated pulmonary artery, either idiopathic or consequent to a connective tissue disorder such as Marfan syndrome and infective endocarditis.

* Less frequent causes: iatrogenic after surgical or balloon treatment of congenital PS or tetralogy of Fallot, congenital malformations, such as absent, malformed, fenestrated, or supernumerary leaflets. These anomalies may occur as isolated lesions but more often are associated with other congenital anomalies.

* Rare causes: trauma, carcinoid syndrome, rheumatic involvement, endocarditis, and injury by a pulmonary artery flow-directed catheter.

Assessment with two-dimensional transthoracic echocardiography

Views

Evaluation of PV should be performed in conjunction with the RVOT, including an assessment of the degree of hypertrophy in the outflow tract. 2D TTE standard and modified views, usually used to assess PV, are (➲ Fig. 14c.13) (see also ➲ Chapter 2):

* PSAX view, with transducer position at the base of the heart where the bifurcation of the pulmonary artery is also visualized (◧ 14c.6).

* Long-axis projection of the RVOT and PV, obtained by rotating the transducer approximately 90 degrees with angulation toward the right shoulder.

* Subcostal view (long- and short-axis views) with anterior angulation. In this view, the entire sweep of the RVOT can often be visualized including the PV leaflets.

* A5C view, through clockwise angulation of transducer to bring in the RVOT.

Echo data and parameters

Qualitative evaluation of PV requires identification of valve anatomy, including bicuspid valve, prolapse, dysplasia, or

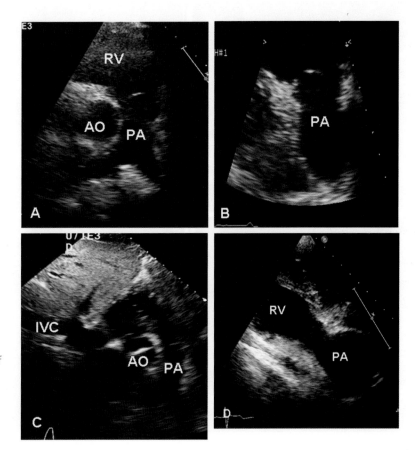

Figure 14c.13 2D TTE imaging of PV. Standard views for assessment of PV by 2D TTE on parasternal short axis (A), RV outflow (B), subcostal (C), and modified apical 5-chamber (D).

absent PV, that may help to define the mechanism of regurgitation. On the other hand, quantitative assessment of TV relies on determination of:

- Annulus and RVOT diameters, that are measured during early ejection phase from short axis or better from parasternal RV outflow view, if possible.

- M-mode pattern of the posterior pulmonary cusp movement, that helps in differentiation between PH and PS, as it is possible to recognize the presence (but not the severity) of pulmonary hypertension (➲ Fig. 14c.14). The normal pattern is formed of:

  - A wave: a small posterior movement of PV due to transmitted atrial systole.
  - B–C: systolic opening of the valve.
  - D: slight anterior movement in late systole.
  - D–E: rapid closure of the valve.
  - E–F slope: slow posterior movement in diastole before the next A wave.

- Measurement of peak systolic and diastolic pressure gradient across the valve using CW Doppler.

- Calculation of PV area using continuity equation or proximal isovelocity surface area (PISA), not routinely used

- Identification of PR at CD imaging, as diastolic jet in the RVOT, beginning at the PV, and of PS as accelerated flow beyond the stenotic PV (➲ Fig. 14c.15).

- Localization of the stenosis level (valvular, subvalvular or supravalvular) using PW Doppler. Also the shape of the velocity curve might differentiate between subpulmonic (with late systolic peak) and PS.

Technical consideration and limitations

Some technical considerations and limitations have to be known in order to improve acquisition and interpretation of PV echocardiographic images:

- Visualization of the PV leaflets in the long axis is limited especially in adults because 2D echocardiography shows only one or two posterior leaflets. During the valve opening the echo signal often disappears, to reappear as the valve closes.

- In adolescents and adults, 2D echo images are often less satisfactory.

- Visualization of PV and RVOT from long-axis projection is often problematic in large-stature adults.

- Short-axis view often is not obtainable, thus calculation of valve area by planimetry is not possible.

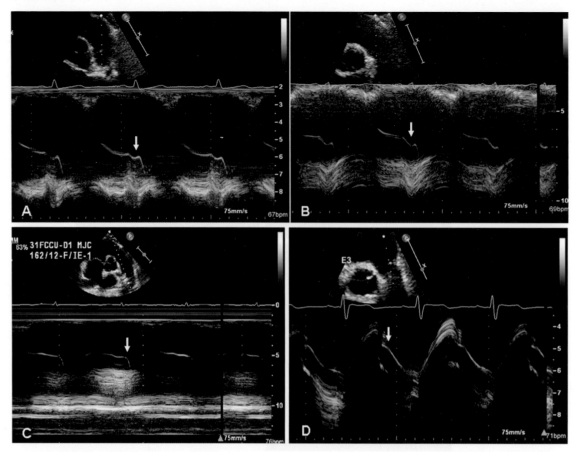

Figure 14c.14 M-mode pattern of PV. M-mode pattern of PV in normal (A), mild pulmonary hypertension (B), severe pulmonary hypertension (C), and PS (D). Arrows point to changes in a wave.

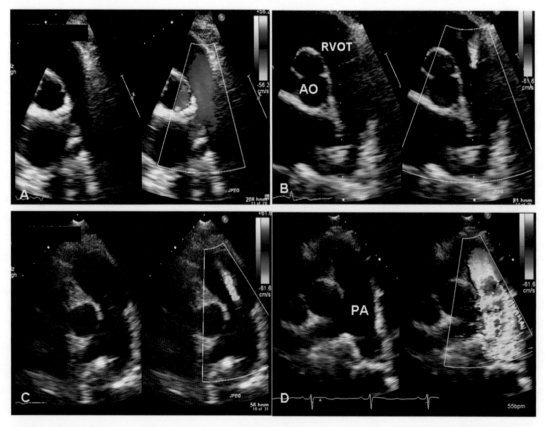

Figure 14c.15 Different colour flow patterns of PV. Parasternal short-axis view showing the colour flow pattern of normal systolic pulmonary flow (A), mild physiological PR (B), significant PR (C), and turbulent systolic flow in PS (D).

- In cases of mild PS, no abnormality is detectable either by M-mode or 2D echocardiography.

- Calculation of valve area by continuity equation or PISA method has not been validated.

- In multiple levels of stenosis (infundibular or distal branch) or in associated significant regurgitation, the peak gradient by CW Doppler may not express the actual severity. PW Doppler may be useful to detect the level of stenosis. In infundibular stenosis, the dagger- shape flow with late peaking is characteristic. The level of colour flow acceleration is also helpful.

- The extent of flow disturbance can roughly estimates the severity of PR. Planimetered colour jet areas, jet width, vena contracta, deceleration slope, and PHT by CW Doppler can be used. However, there is no method validated to standardize the grades of PR.

- In severe PR, diastolic flow reversal may be seen in the main PA that needs to be differentiated from diastolic flow due to patent ductus arteriosus.

- Colour jet area can be inaccurate in severe PR if diastolic PA and RV pressures equalized.

Assessment with two-dimensional transoesophageal echocardiography

Views

Standard and occasional views are used in TOE to image PV[7] (➔ Fig. 14c.16):

- High oesophageal position at 0-degree rotation with a long-axis view of the PA from the valve plane to its bifurcation allows imaging of RVOT.

- Horizontal (0 degrees) plane imaging from a high oesophageal position with clockwise rotation to the right, provides visualization of the bifurcation of the pulmonary artery and the PV.

- Short-axis view (RV inflow–outflow view), at mid oesophageal level 30–80 degrees with clockwise rotation to the right, allows visualization of the anterior and posterior cusps (▤ 14c.7).

- Mid and high-oesophageal view at 90 degrees, for imaging RV, PV, and the main pulmonary artery.

- Also the 90-degree long axis plane may show the PV.

- In a longitudinal or 120-degree deep gastric view, with clockwise rotation of the transducer, the entire sweep of the RV

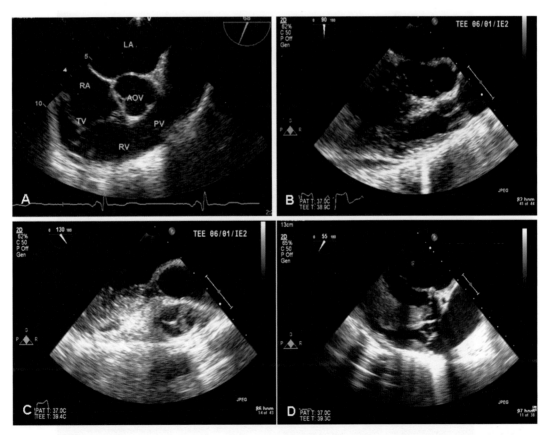

Figure 14c.16 2D TOE imaging of PV. Standard views for assessment of PV by 2D TOE; A, B) Long axis at mid-oesophageal level, C) short axis at mid-oesophageal level and D) long axis transgastric level.

inflow and outflow tracts can be obtained and simultaneous visualization of the RA, TV, RVOT, PV, and proximal pulmonary artery often accomplished.

Measurements and technical considerations

RVOT is measured in the basal view at 0 degrees. The PV is seen in its perpendicular relationship to the aortic valve in the far field of the image, so it remains virtually impossible to assess the precise morphology of valve cusps or its commissures. Moreover, calculation of maximum velocity and peak gradient by CW Doppler is not accurate due to difficulty in lining up the sample volume parallel to the flow.

Assessment with real-time three-dimensional echocardiography

Assessment of RVOT and PV annulus (shape and size) can be obtained in 95% of patients. The annulus appears as oval-shaped and the maximum diameter should be considered[8] (⊃ Fig. 14c.17). Full assessment of PV cusps and commissures could be obtained by real-time 3D TOE (🖿 14c.8). Using the x-plane (simultaneous view) of real-time 3D-TOE, the actual valve area can be visualized and measured (⊃ Fig. 14c.18).

Clinical applications

⊃ Table 14c.2 shows echo parameters regarding PV structure and function, obtained by different modalities in normal subjects, associated with possible clinical applications.

On the other hand, the assessment of PV disease is based on the following findings:

Assessment of severity of pulmonary stenosis

Direct findings of PS are domed valve on systolic opening, thickened cusps with limited mobility, exaggerated *A-dip* on M-mode (⊃ Fig. 14c.14D) and increased peak velocity across the valve (>2.0m/s). Also indirect findings of PS may be detected, such as RV hypertrophy and/or dilation (wall thickness >6mm), high RV systolic pressure estimated from TR, high RA pressure estimated from IVC size and respiratory collapse (see ⊃ Chapter 11) and evidence of post-stenotic PA dilation. A severe PS is indicated by a PV area of $1cm^2/m^2$ or less, and a peak pressure gradient greater than 60mmHg.

Selection of therapeutic modalities

Continuous follow up (every 5 to 10 years) is recommended for mild PS. Balloon or surgical intervention is indicated for severe PS, while balloon valvuloplasty is recommended for isolated PS

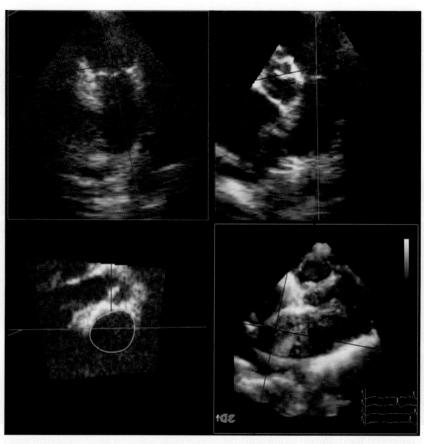

Figure 14c.17 Full volume image of real-time 3D TTE for PV and RVOT.

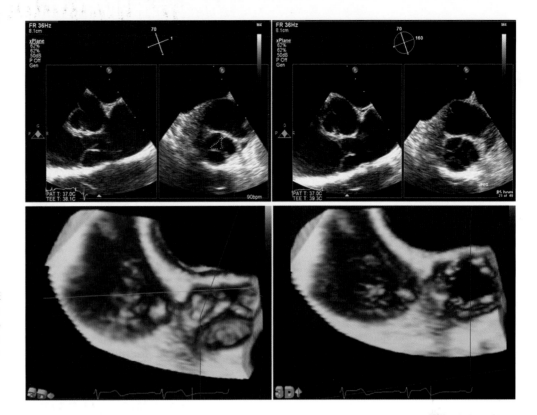

Figure 14c.18 Real-time 3DTOE x-plane. Assessment of PV area by real-time 3D TOE using X-plane to be displayed as two simultaneous views (upper panel). Zoom mode of real-time 3D TOE showing a normal PV during opening and closure (lower panel).

Table 14c.2 Normal values of PV obtained by different echo modalities and their clinical application

Parameters	Normal value	Clinical application
2D measurements		
Annulus diameter (cm)	<2.3	Determine the balloon size of valvuloplasty, Dilated annulus causes PR
Valve area (cm²)	3.5–4.5	< 1cm²/m² define severe PS
Doppler measurements		
Peak systolic velocity (m/s)	0.75 (0.6–1.1)	Increased in PS and increase pulmonary flow
Peak PR velocity (m/s)	(1.2–1.9)	Increased velocity in elevated PAP
Real-time 3DE measurements		
Annulus area	(4–6)	As in 2DE
Annulus diameter	5.2 ± 1.5	As in 2DE

if cusps are not markedly thickened or calcified. The balloon size used for valvuloplasty should be 10–20% larger than annulus. Surgical valvulotomy is the choice with calcific cusps, small and thickened annulus, and multiple levels of PS. Bioprosthetic valve replacement is indicated if PS is associated with significant PR.[9]

Personal perspective

Real-time 3D echocardiography improves the understanding of TV morphology and function which helps in decision making towards the TV disease. With good image quality, the morphological assessment of TV leaflets, commissures, and annulus can be obtained in 80–90% of patients. The oval-shaped annulus can be visualized almost in all individuals. Many studies are needed to establish the 3D echocardiographic parameters for the assessment of severity of TS and TR.

The assessment of TV annular function should be performed by real-time 3D echocardiography through cyclic changes in diameter and area and expressed as fractional shortening or fractional area change.

The use of mitral valve quantification software analysis for assessment of site and volume of the prolapsed scallop is encouraging, and the development of software for volume quantification of TV leaflets will be promising.

The use of biplane image obtained by real-time 3D TOE can help in accurate measurement of PV area because the cut plane of the short-axis view can be adjusted to pick the narrowest orifice.

References

1 Lamers WH, Viragh S, Wessels A, Moorman AFM, Anderson R. Formation of the tricuspid valve in human heart. *Circulation* 1995; **91**:111–21.

2 Anwar AM, Geleijnse ML, Soliman OI, McGhie JS, Frowijn R, Nemes A, *et al.* Assessment of normal tricuspid valve anatomy in adults by real-time three-dimensional echocardiography. *Int J Cardiovasc imaging* 2007; **23**(6):717–24.

3 Prabhu MR. Transesophageal echocardiography for tricuspid and pulmonary valves. *Ann Card Anaesth* 2009; **12**(2):167.

4 Badano LP, Agricola E, de Isla LP, Gianfagna P, Zamorano JL. Evaluation of the tricuspid valve morphology and function by trans-thoracic real-time three-dimensional echocardiography. *Eur J echocardiogr* 2009; **10**(4):477–84.

5 Anwar AM, Geleijnse ML, Soliman OI, McGhie JS, Nemes A, ten Cate FJ. Evaluation of rheumatic tricuspid valve stenosis by real-time three-dimensional echocardiography. *Heart* 2007; **93**(3):363–4.

6 Zoghbi WA, Enriquez-Sarano M, Foster E, Grayburn PA, Kraft CD, Levine RA, *et al.* Recommendations for evaluation of the severity of native valvular regurgitation with two-dimensional and Doppler echocardiography. *J Am Soc Echocardiogr* 2003; **16**(7):777–802.

7 Shanewise JS, Cheung AT, Aronson S, Stewart WJ, Weiss RL, Mark JB, *et al.* ASE/SCA Guidelines for Performing a Comprehensive Intraoperative Multiplane Transesophageal Echocardiography Examination: Recommendations of the American Society of Echocardiography Council for Intraoperative Echocardiography and the Society of Cardiovascular Anesthesiologists Task Force for Certification in Perioperative Transesophageal Echocardiography. *J Am Soc Echocardiogr* 1999; **12**:884–900.

8 Anwar AM, Soliman O, van den Bosch AE, McGhie JS, Geleijnse ML, ten Cate FJ, *et al.* Assessment of pulmonary valve and right ventricular outflow tract with real-time three-dimensional echocardiography. *Int J Cardiovasc Imaging* 2007; **23**(2):167–75.

9 Vahanian A, Baumgartner H, Bax J, Butchart E, Dion R, Filippatos G, *et al.* Guidelines on the management of valvular heart disease: The Task Force on the Management of Valvular Heart Disease of the European Society of Cardiology. *Eur Heart J* 2007; **28**:230–68.

Further reading

Galiè N, Hoeper MM, Humbert M, Torbicki A, Vachiery JL, Barbera JA, *et al.* The Task Force for the Diagnosis and Treatment of Pulmonary Hypertension of the European Society of Cardiology (ESC) and the European Respiratory Society (ERS), endorsed by the International Society of Heart and Lung Transplantation (ISHLT). *Eur Heart J* 2009; **30**:2493–537.

Lang RM, Bierig M, Devereux RB, Flachskampf FA, Foster E, Pellikka PA, *et al.* Recommendations for chamber quantification: a report from the American Society of Echocardiography's Guidelines and Standards Committee and the Chamber Quantification Writing Group, developed in conjunction with the European Association of Echocardiography, a branch of the European Society of Cardiology. *J Am Soc Echocardiography* 2005; **18**:1440–63.

Roshanali F, Saidi B, Mandegar MH, Yousefnia MA, Alaeddini F. Echocardiographic approach to the decision-making process of tricuspid valve repair. *J Thorac Cardiovasc Surg* 2010; **139**(6):1483–7.

Shemin R. Tricuspid valve disease. In: Cohn LH (ed) *Cardiac Surgery in the Adult.* New York: McGraw-Hill; 2008, pp.1111–28.

Warnes CA, Williams RG, Bashore TM, Child JS, Connolly HM, Dearani JA, *et al.* ACC/AHA 2008 Guidelines for the Management of Adults With Congenital Heart Disease: A Report of the American College of Cardiology/American Heart Association Task Force on Practice Guidelines (Writing Committee to Develop Guidelines on the Management of Adults With Congenital Heart Disease): Developed in Collaboration With the American Society of Echocardiography, Heart Rhythm Society, International Society for Adult Congenital Heart Disease, Society for Cardiovascular Angiography and Interventions, and Society of Thoracic Surgeons. *Circulation* 2008; **118**(23):e714–e833.

Additional DVD and online material

- 14c.1 Normal TV as seen by 2D TTE from parasternal RV inflow view. Colour flow showing normal systolic and diastolic flow pattern.

- 14c.2 Normal TV as seen by 2D TTE from A4C view. Colour flow showing very mild physiological TR.

- 14c.3 A4C with colour flow showing significant TR.

- 14c.4 En-face view by real-time 3D TTE showing the oval-shaped TV annulus.

- 14c.5 Real-time 3D-TTE quad-screen colour images showed severe TR. In short-axis slice, the vena contracta can be measured.

- 14c.6 PLAX view (2D TTE) showing RVOT, PV, pulmonary artery, and its main branches with normal colour flow during systole and diastole.

- 14c.7 2D TOE showing the short axis of PV in patient with PS.

- 14c.8: Quadscreen real-time 3D TOE showing the three pulmonary cusps.

- For additional multimedia materials please visit the online version of the book (http://escecho.oxfordmedicine.com).

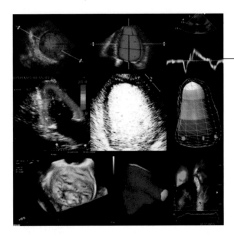

CHAPTER 15

Replacement heart valves

John B. Chambers and
Jean-Louis Vanoverschelde

Contents

Summary

Echocardiography is the gold-standard investigation for assessing replacement valve function and detecting pathology. Transthoracic echocardiography (TTE) is sufficient for assessing patients routinely with no evidence of pathology. However, in patients with suspected dysfunction, the addition of transoesophageal echocardiography is usually necessary. Stress echocardiography may also be necessary in patients with exertional symptoms unexplained by the resting TTE.

There are comprehensive International Guidelines for the echocardiographic assessment of prosthetic valves[1] and the management of clinical problems.[2,3] Stented valves placed using transcatheter techniques are rapidly becoming established.[4] The aim of this chapter is to summarize the normal appearance of replacement valves by position and also to describe the diagnosis of pathology.

Glossary

- Occluder is the mechanical part (ball, disc, leaflet) that closes the orifice.

- Patient tissue annulus is the structure formed by removing the native valve and debriding calcific deposits.

- Paraprosthetic jet means a jet of regurgitation originating outside the sewing ring and caused by a dehiscence of the valve.

- Replacement heart valve is preferred to prosthetic heart valve since replacement valves may be biological tissue.

Classification of common replacement valves

Common designs of replacement valves[5] are:

Biological

Stented xenograft

* Porcine heterograft, e.g. Hancock, Mosaic, Carpentier–Edwards (standard and supra-annular porcine), Intact, Labcor (porcine tricomposite), Biocor (porcine tri-composite).
* Pericardial (usually bovine) Baxter Perimount (pericardial), Mitroflow (bovine pericardial).

Stentless

* Autograft (Ross operation).
* Homograft, aortic or pulmonary.
* Stentless heterograft. These may be implanted as:

  · Subcoronary inclusion, e.g. Toronto (St Jude Medical), Cryolife-O'Brien, Sorin Pericarbon (pericardial), Baxter Prima, Labcor stentless, Biocor PSB tricomposite.
  · Miniroot, e.g. Cryolife-O'Brien, Baxter Prima.
  · Root, e.g. Freestyle (Medtronic), Baxter Prima, Cryolife-O'Brien root.

Mechanical

* Ball-cage, e.g. Starr–Edwards.
* Single tilting disc, e.g. Bjork–Shiley, Medtronic Hall, Monostrut, Omniscience, Ultracor.
* Bileaflet, e.g. St Jude Medical, Carbomedics, On-X, ATS, Sorin Bicarbon, Edwards Tekna, Edwards Mira.

Transcatheter valve implants

There are currently two transcatheter valve implants (TAVIs) available clinically:

* CoreValve®.
* Edwards SAPIEN®.

The preoperative echocardiogram

Echocardiography is used to assess the index valve disease, the other valves, the aorta, left ventricular (LV) function, and the right ventricle (RV) including pulmonary artery (PA) pressures. In addition it has the following roles:

Planning a Ross procedure

Ross procedure is a type of specialized aortic valve (AoV) replacement surgery, where patient's pulmonary valve (PV) is positioned at the level of diseased AoV. Then, the PV is replaced by a cryopreserved cadaveric PV. This surgical procedure is performed in children and young adults, or older particularly active patients, due to its several advantages over traditional AoV replacement: in fact, longevity of PV autograft is greater than that of biological replacement valves and does not require anticoagulation therapy.

After planning a Ross procedure, it is necessary to check that the PV is normal and that the pulmonary and aortic annuli are similar in diameter. A Ross procedure may not be advisable if the aortic annulus is large, above 27mm, since this predicts late dilation of the autograft. If the aortic root is not dilated before surgery, the Ross procedure can be performed as a mini-root rather than by implantation within the aorta.

Planning other stentless valves

A homograft almost always needs to be brought in from a tissue bank and the LV outflow tract (LVOT) diameter determines whether a large, medium, or small-sized homograft should be requested. Stentless xenografts vary in design but many need to be sized using the sinotubular junction as well as the annulus, while stented valves are sized using the patient tissue annulus alone. If the sinotubular junction is more than 10% larger than the annulus, either a stentless valve cannot be used or an associated aortoplasty must be performed. Sizing by transthoracic echocardiography (TTE), usually confirmed by intraoperative transoesophageal echocardiography (TOE), also allows the valve to be washed in advance to reduce bypass time. A stentless valve is contraindicated if there is excessive annular calcification. It is also contraindicated as an inclusion if the AoV is anatomically bicuspid.

Planning a transcatheter valve implant

It is necessary to measure the size of the aortic annulus and root to determine that a device of suitable size will be implanted. In general, TOE is superior to TTE in this regard, since it provides superior image quality. Use of three-dimensional (3D) echocardiography is also useful, since most of the examined structures are not perfectly circular in shape.

With the CoreValve®, the 26-mm prosthesis requires a native aortic annulus of 20–23mm, whereas the 29-mm prosthesis requires a native aortic annulus of 24–27mm. The 23-mm Edwards SAPIEN® prosthesis requires a native annulus diameter of 18–21mm, and the 26-mm prosthesis requires a diameter of 22–24.5mm.

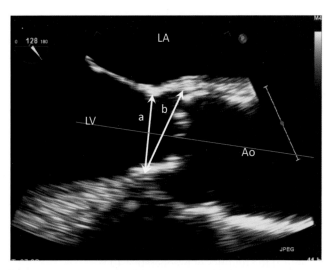

Figure 15.1 Measurement of the aortic annulus by TOE. Zoomed mid-systolic long-axis mid-oesophageal still frame of the aortic root. The aortic annulus should be measured between the hinge points of right coronary cusps and the nadir of the posterior interleaflet triangle (arrow a). Positioning the posterior caliper is sometimes difficult. It should be as close as possible to the hinge point between the anterior mitral leaflet and the nadir of the interleaflet triangle (a). One should careful avoid placing the posterior caliper in the sinus of Valsalva (b) as this leads to overestimation of annular dimensions

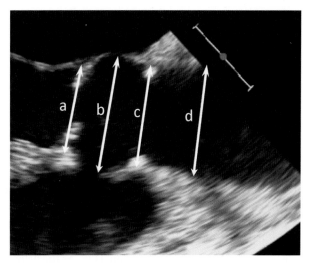

Figure 15.2 Measurements of aortic root diameters by TOE. Zoomed end-diastolic long-axis mid-oesophageal still frame of the aortic root. The dimensions of the annulus (a), the sinuses of Valsalva (b), the sinotubular junction (c), and the ascending aorta (d) should be measured as indicated.

The diameter of the aortic annulus should be carefully assessed immediately below the hinge points of the non- (or left) and the right coronary cusps of a trileaflet AoV, in a zoomed mid-systolic frame with maximal leaflet excursion, taken from a centred mid-oesophageal long-axis view at 110–150 degrees of rotation (➲ Fig. 15.1). Although the hinge point of the right coronary cusp is usually easy to identify, because the imaging plane passes through the nadir of the cusp, it is more difficult to appreciate in the posterior aspects of the valve. Indeed, in long-axis view, the imaging plane usually passes through one of the two posterior cusps (most often the non-coronary cusp) somewhere along the ascending limb of their anatomical insertion in the sinuses of Valsalva, in the posterior interleaflet triangle. This can lead to significant overestimation of annular dimensions. The posterior caliper should therefore be placed as close as possible to hinge point between the anterior mitral leaflet and the nadir of the posterior interleaflet triangle.

CoreValve® implantation also requires careful assessment of the size and dimensions of the aortic root. The aortic root is best visualized in the parasternal long-axis (PLAX) view on TTE and the mid-oesophageal long-axis view on TOE. The TOE images of the aortic root are similar to those taken for LV outflow assessment. The image needs to be frozen in a zoomed mode at end-diastole, just after the mitral valve (MV) has closed and before the AoV has opened. The aortic root walls should be parallel and the AoV orifice should be central in a trileaflet valve. All measured diameters are intraluminal from aortic wall to aortic wall, ignoring any protuberant calcium. The dimensions of both the sinuses of Valsalva and of the sinotubular junction should be obtained (➲ Fig. 15.2). The diameter of the sinuses of Valsalva is perpendicular to the long axis of the root and parallel to the aortic annular plane. It is measured as the widest intraluminal distance within the sinuses. The diameter of the sinotubular junction is usually parallel to the previous one. It is measured at the hinge point where the sinuses narrow and join the ascending aorta. Finally, the ascending aorta diameter should be measured at its widest diameter. A 26-mm CoreValve® prosthesis requires dimensions of the sinuses of Valvalva of 27mm or more, and dimensions of the sinotubular junction or ascending aorta of 40mm or less, whereas the 29-mm prosthesis requires sinuses of Valsalva of 28mm or more, and a sinotubular junction or ascending aorta of 43mm or less.

Particular attention should also be paid to the size and shape of the interventricular septum (IVS). Marked septal hypertrophy and sigmoid septa, protruding in the LVOT may cause misplacement and/or migration of the prosthesis

Perioperative echocardiography

Transcatheter valve implant

TTE is used for the transapical approach to obtain the position of the apex in order to determine the location of the intercostals' incision. The use of TOE during the procedure depends on the prosthesis implanted. During transapical implantation of an Edwards–Sapien valve, TOE should be used to verify that the apical introducer sheet and/or guidewire do not interfere with the MV apparatus, since this can cause severe transient mitral regurgitation (MR). This is best achieved using a biplane transgastric view showing at the same time a mid-ventricular section, at the level of the papillary muscle and a long-axis section at the level of the LVOT. The implanted material should always be positioned in between the two papillary muscles and chordae tendinae. Mid-oesophageal imaging is occasionally useful to ensure that the guidewire is pushed into the LVOT and not into the left atrium (LA).

TOE can sometimes help the retrograde crossing of the AoV by the delivery catheter, as it may sometimes get stuck in a calcified commissure. Echocardiography is seldom useful during the deployment of Edwards SAPIEN® valves, since it is quite often difficult to differentiate the crimped stent from its supporting balloon. By contrast, it may be helpful during the deployment of CoreValve® prostheses, which require precise placement with the ventricular end 5–10mm below the native AoV. The end of the delivery catheter is easily identified on TOE. As the delivery catheter is withdrawn, echo images are used to observe the emergence and expansion of the ventricular end of the prosthesis, as its high radial force may cause it to descend inappropriately low into the LVOT and interfere with MV function. Manual adjustment in the position is required so that the LV rim of the prosthesis covers 50% of the anterior mitral leaflet and lies above the attachment of the secondary chordae to the leaflet.

Immediately after deployment, TOE permits assessment of valve function and detection of complications, such as pericardial effusion or aortic dissection. Measurements of subvalvular and transvalvular flows are best achieved from a deep transgastric position, whereas the dimensions of the LVOT are best obtained from a mid-oesophageal long-axis position. LVOT dimensions need to be measured after deployment of the prosthesis since it usually becomes more circular and hence differs from pre-implantation measurements.

Paravalvular leaks are frequent after transcatheter valve implantation, but are rarely more than moderate in severity. The eccentric nature of the jets, as well as the combined presence of calcifications and the stent often makes it difficult to accurately grade the severity of regurgitation. Paravalvular leaks usually occur at the level of the native AoV commissures, where the stent frame is not covered by native leaflet tissue. The amount of paravalvular leak correlates with the degree of native cusp calcification, with the geometry of the deployed prosthesis and with the congruence between the prosthesis and annulus sizes (➲ Fig. 15.3). Accordingly, particular attention needs to be paid to the circularity of the deployed prosthesis in the short-axis orientation.

Conventional valve surgery

Intraoperative echocardiography is increasingly used as routine in all cardiac surgery including the implantation of replacement heart valve to:

◆ Confirm the findings of preoperative TTE.

◆ Detect new pathology, e.g. coexistent aortic dissection.

◆ Confirm annulus and sinotubular junction diameters when implanting a stentless valve.

◆ Check for an aortic root abscess or involvement of other valves in the presence of endocarditis.

◆ Detect new LV ischaemia.

◆ Assess the competency of an autograft or stentless xenograft valve after surgery.

◆ Detect significant paraprosthetic regurgitation to allow correction before closing the chest.

◆ Detect interference of cardiac structures with movement of the occluder (➲ Fig. 15.4).

◆ Detect early iatrogenic complications, e.g. a stitch placed through the non-coronary cusp after implantation of a mechanical MV.

◆ Assess an associated MV repair or tricuspid annuloplasty.

◆ Aid de-airing the heart.

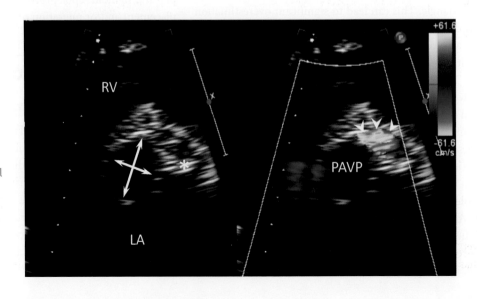

Figure 15.3 Asymmetrical deployment of an Edwards SAPIEN® prosthesis Asymmetrical deployment of an Edwards SAPIEN® prosthesis due to the presence of a large chunk of calcium in the left coronary sinus (*) and resulting in significant paraprosthetic leak at the level of the posterior commissure.

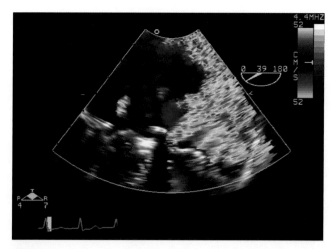

Figure 15.4 Abnormal transprosthetic mitral regurgitation on transoesophageal imaging. The patient was unstable after implantation of a bileaflet mechanical mitral valve. There was a broad jet of regurgitation originating inside the sewing ring which was intermittent as shown by the colour M-mode recording. It was caused by intermittent obstruction against the subvalvar apparatus.

Immediately after surgery

Echocardiography may be needed for assessing LV function, detecting pericardial effusions, and assessing loading conditions. Severe LV hypertrophy usually with outflow obstruction after valve replacement for severe aortic stenosis may cause LV failure and hypotension. These may be treated according to protocol with inotropic agents and diuretics which exacerbate the situation. The diagnosis is made on echocardiography and the treatment is withdrawal of inotropes, the use of drugs to slow the heart and improve LV filling, and the gradual withdrawal of diuretics.

The postoperative examination

Baseline study

A study should be performed in the early postoperative period to act as a baseline. Every valve is different and this study acts as a *fingerprint* against which to compare future studies. For example, there may be mild paraprosthetic regurgitation. If the patient presents later with fever, the finding of a paraprosthetic jet might be a sign of endocarditis if it is new, but not if it has already been documented. The timing of the baseline study depends on circumstances. Ideally it should be at the first postoperative visit usually after 4–6 weeks when the chest wound has healed, chest wall oedema has resolved, and LV function has recovered. However, if the patient is being transferred and may not return, it may be best to perform the study before hospital discharge.

Later after surgery

Routine echocardiography is not necessary if the patient is well and the examination normal. For biological valves it may be reasonable to study annually beyond about 5 years after surgery for MVs and 7 years for AoVs because of the known failure rate. The rationale is to detect failure early to allow careful follow-up and planning of elective surgery with acceptable surgical risk. Failing cusps may tear suddenly causing sudden death, shock, or pulmonary oedema.

A study is needed if malfunction is suspected from the presence of symptoms, an abnormal murmur, fever, haemolysis, or emboli despite a therapeutic international normalized ratio. Echocardiography will then be used to detect evidence of obstruction or pathological regurgitation or endocarditis as a sign of one of the possible complications of replacement heart valves:

Complications causing obstruction

Some complications can cause valve obstruction. They mainly are:

- ◆ Primary failure.
- ◆ Thrombosis.
- ◆ Pannus.
- ◆ Mechanical obstruction, e.g. by subvalvar apparatus.
- ◆ Endocarditis.

Complications causing or associated with regurgitation

Other complications may provoke or are associated with valve regurgitation. The most frequent are:

- ◆ Dehiscence.
- ◆ Endocarditis.
- ◆ Haemolysis.

Other complications

A different group of postoperative complications encompasses:

- ◆ Thromboembolism
- ◆ Anticoagulant-related bleeding

The general assessment of all patients

Clinical data required at the time of echocardiography for general assessment of the patient, must include the following:

- ◆ Type of valve and size (because these affect normal ranges).
- ◆ Date of replacement (to determine age of valve).
- ◆ Height and weight to calculate body surface area (BSA) for estimation of effective orifice area indexed (EOAi).
- ◆ Blood pressure (to help assess grade of regurgitant lesions).
- ◆ Symptoms.
- ◆ The state of the rest of the heart on echocardiography.

Sizing conventions for valves

Label size gives an approximate idea of the patient tissue annulus for which the valve is intended. However, labelling conventions vary between manufacturers and there can be 4mm or more discrepancy between the label size and the patient annulus which will accommodate that valve.[6] Furthermore, valves can be designed for either intra-annular (e.g. Carbomedics standard) or supra-annular implantation (Carbomedics 'TopHat') while some valves have both a supra-annular and intra-annular component (e.g. On-X). The surgeon may decide to place a valve designed for intra-annular use into the supra-annular position or the suture technique can force a valve into or above the annulus. These observations mean:

- That comparison of the haemodynamic function of different designs of valve cannot be made using label size.

- The label size cannot be used as surrogate for LVOT diameter in the calculation of effective orifice area (EOA) using the continuity equation.

- In avoiding patient–prosthesis mismatch (see later), the EOA needs to be known since the label size alone will not allow comparison with patient BSA.

Echocardiography of the replacement aortic valve

Imaging

On TTE, all standard views must be used with extra care taken to image the sewing ring in the parasternal short-axis (PSAX) view. This view is particularly useful to localize the origin of regurgitant jets. The movement of the cusps or occluder is imaged using PLAX and PSAX views and the apical three-chamber (A3C) view. On TOE, the reference view is at the mid-oesophageal level usually with rotation to about 30 degrees to obtain a horizontal section through the valve. As for TTE, more careful positioning of the probe is needed than for a native AoV. Rotation and flexion to insonate the plane of the sewing ring and just below this level are necessary to localize regurgitant jets. The longitudinal view rotated approximately 90 degrees further shows movement of the cusp or occluder and allows the detection of jets through the valve. Quantitative Doppler is more easily and accurately performed transthoracically since more probe and patient positions can be used.

The sutures may be visible on TOE and should not be mistaken for vegetations. Small fibrin strands are also normal (⊃ Fig. 15.5). Early after implantation, a stentless valve inserted as an inclusion will be surrounded by haematoma and oedema. This is indistinguishable from an abscess and underlines the fact that an echocardiogram cannot be interpreted outside the clinical context. Rocking of the valve suggests dehiscence which is

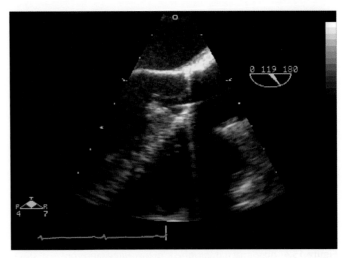

Figure 15.5 Fibrin strand attached to a bileaflet mechanical aortic valve. This is a mid-oesophageal long view on TOE

proved by overlaying colour Doppler (CD) and demonstrating a paraprosthetic regurgitant jet. Usually rocking in the aortic position implies a large dehiscence, about 40% of the sewing ring.

Quantitative Doppler

The minimum dataset is peak velocity, mean pressure gradient, and EOA[1] by the continuity equation (see ⊃ Chapter 5). It is important to derive the mean pressure gradient because it is calculated using the whole wave-form and better reflects function than the peak gradient. It is almost never appropriate to substitute the labelled size of the replacement valve for the LVOT diameter because this may differ widely from its true size.[6] For serial studies, it is reasonable to use the ratio of the velocity time intervals since this avoids measuring the LVOT.

Pressure recovery

This phenomenon is described in ⊃ Chapters 5 and 14a (for native AoV). In cases of replacement valves, it occurs in two situations: downstream from most replacement valves and between the leaflets of bileaflet mechanical valves.[8,9] Pressure recovery does not occur with valves which behave hydrodynamically as funnels in which the flow lines stay attached. Some bovine pericardial replacement valves behave as funnels. Pressure recovery is most likely to be evident if the sinotubular junction is less than 30mm in diameter. It has the effect of introducing a discrepancy between transvalvular pressure gradients measured by invasive techniques and estimated by Doppler.[9] This is not a practical problem since normal ranges are based on echocardiography rather than invasive techniques so that the interpretation of an echocardiographic study is not affected by pressure recovery.

Obstruction

Pathological obstruction is most frequently seen in biological valves and is most easily detected by the presence of thickened and immobile cusps (➲ Fig. 15.6). Thrombosis of biological valves is uncommon but may be seen after TAVI (➲ Fig. 15.7). Thickening of a biological cusp is often the earliest sign of primary failure. The mean thickness of a cusp on M-mode is 1mm,[10] and a thickness of >3mm is taken arbitrarily as a sign of thickening. This is usually a sign, not of overt thickening of the cusp, but of a small tear. This makes a small segment of the cusp turn at an angle to the ultrasound beam and look thicker. It may be associated with prolapse of the cusp and often a jet of regurgitation. About 60% of thickened cusps progress to overt failure requiring redo surgery within 2 years compared with about 1% of unthickened cusps.[10] Finding a small tear is a warning to follow the patient more carefully and, if the regurgitation progresses, to consider planning elective surgery. A proportion of biological valves develop sudden catastrophic failure as a result of an early tear or abrasion extending.

In mechanical valves, failure of the mechanical occluder may also be seen.

Normal ranges vary between valve types (see ➲ Appendix, Tables 15.1 and 15.2) but the following suggest the possibility of obstruction:[1]

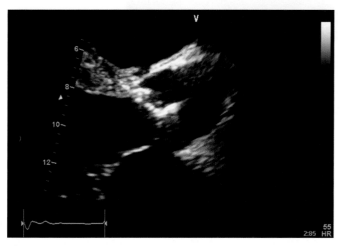

Figure 15.6 Obstructed bovine pericardial valve in the aortic position. The parasternal long-axis zoomed view on TTE showing the maximum excursion of the cusps during systole. The thickening is clear particularly of the right-coronary cusps.

- Vmax >4.0m/s.
- Mean gradient >35mmHg.
- Doppler velocity index <0.25.
- EOA <1.0cm².
- Rounded symmetrical continuous wave-form.

The interpretation of quantitative Doppler is often difficult. Overinterpretation must be avoided if the patient is well with full exercise capacity while care not to miss obstruction must be taken if the patient has symptoms. High velocities are common especially in size 19 or 21 prostheses. The challenge is to differentiate a small, but normally-functioning valve from a pathologically obstructive valve. The first step is to calculate the EOA using the continuity equation. If this is within the normal range for a valve of that size and design (see ➲ Appendix, Tables 15.1 and 15.2)[11,12] the valve is likely to be normally-functioning but small. Patient–prosthesis mismatch is diagnosed if the EOA indexed to BSA (EOAi) is less than 0.85cm2/m² (see later). If the EOAi is lower than the normal range, pathological obstruction is likely. However obstruction is most reliably detected by comparing EOA with the baseline study. Allowing for experimental error, a fall of more than 30% is likely to be significant.

Patient–prosthesis mismatch

High transvalvular velocities can occur with a normally-functioning valve if it is too small for the size of the recipient.[13] This is called patient–prosthesis mismatch[13] and is mainly a problem in the aortic position although some authors have noted an effect even for MV. Patient–prosthesis mismatch is defined by an EOAi less than 0.85cm²/m² and severe mismatch by an EOAi less than 0.65cm²/m². There is agreement that mismatch can affect mortality and LV recovery in the presence of an impaired LV.[14] A number of studies also report increased mortality and incidence of arrhythmia, reduced exercise capacity, and reduced regression of LV hypertrophy even in the presence of preserved LV systolic function.[15] However, others fail to show such an effect, sometimes because prosthetic size has been surmised from label size rather than by direct measurement of EOA.[16] It seems likely that the more severe the mismatch and the more impaired the LV systolic function, the more likely that the patient will be affected clinically. Ideally the incidence of patient–prosthetic mismatch should be minimized by the surgeon selecting a valve design with the optimum EOA for the measured patient tissue annulus. A chart of the EOAs of all valves kept in the department should be available in the operating theatre.

Regurgitation

Minor regurgitation is normal in virtually all mechanical valves. Early valves had a closing volume as the leaflet closed followed by true regurgitation around the occluder. For the Starr–Edwards, there is a small closing volume and usually little or no true regurgitation. The single tilting disc valves have both types of regurgitation, but the pattern may vary. The Bjork–Shiley valve has a minor and major jet from the two orifices while the Medtronic Hall valve has a single large jet through a central hole in the disk.

The bileaflet valves have continuous leakage through the pivotal points where the lugs of the leaflets are held in the housing (➲ Fig. 15.8). These are thought to prevent the formation of thrombus at sites of stasis and are called *washing jets*. They are usually found in formation, two from each pivotal point giving a

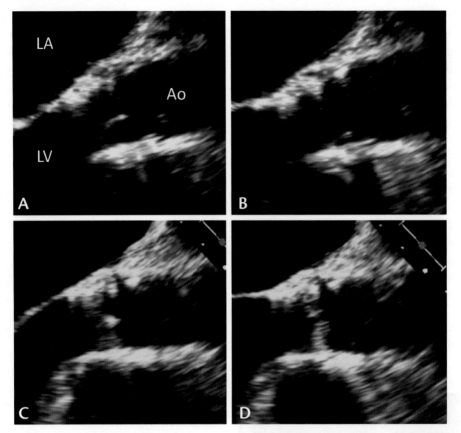

Figure 15.7 Acute thrombosis of a Edwards SAPIEN® aortic prosthesis. End-diastolic (A and C) and end-systolic (B and D) still frames showing an Edwards SAPIEN® aortic prosthesis immediately post implantation (upper rows) and during an episode of acute thrombosis (lower row). Note the abnormal thickening and reduced systolic excursion of the thrombosed cusps.

characteristic appearance on imaging in a plane just below the valve. Sometimes these single pivotal washing jets divide into two or three separate *plumes* and in some valve designs such as the St Jude Medical there may be a jet around the edge of one or other leaflet. The jets are invariably low in momentum so that they are homogenous in colour with aliasing confined to the base of the jet.

Regurgitation through the valve is also increasingly reported in normal biological valves. This is mainly because echocardiography machines are increasingly sensitive. Stentless valves including homografts and autografts are more likely than the stented valves to have minor regurgitant jets, usually at the point of apposition of all three cusps or at one or more commissure. In stented valves, the regurgitation is usually at the point of apposition of the cusps.

The same methods of quantifying regurgitation can be used as for native regurgitation.[17] However, assessing the height of an aortic jet relative to the LVOT diameter may be difficult if it is eccentric and care must be taken to measure the diameter of dilation to its axis. Multiple small normal transprosthetic jets cannot be quantified accurately, but this is not necessary in clinical practice. For paraprosthetic jets, the proportion of the circumference of the sewing ring occupied by the jet gives an approximate guide to severity: mild (<10%), moderate (10–25%), severe (>25%).

Echocardiography of the replacement mitral valve

Imaging

On TTE, PLAX and PSAX views, and all apical views with multiple angulation and off-axis cuts are needed to insonate the whole sewing ring. The subcostal view is helpful to show paraprosthetic jets since the effect of shielding is minimized. For TOE, the low oesophageal four-chamber view is the reference view and from here rotation of the probe to two- and three- chamber planes together with anteflexion and retroflexion allows interrogation of the whole of the sewing ring. The transverse short-axis transgastric view is useful for imaging the whole sewing ring.

The occluder in mechanical valves should open quickly and fully and reduced opening is a reliable sign of obstruction provided that LV function is good. Severe impairment of LV function may also cause reduced valve opening, but this will be associated with a thin, low-velocity inflow signal on colour mapping. In normal bileaflet valves there may be slight oscillation of the leaflets during diastole and slight temporal asymmetry of closure. Off-axis insonation in these valves can show one leaflet

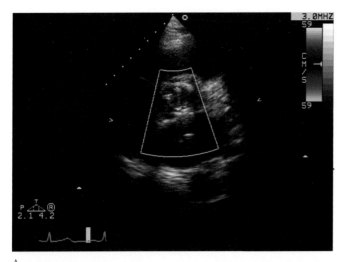

A

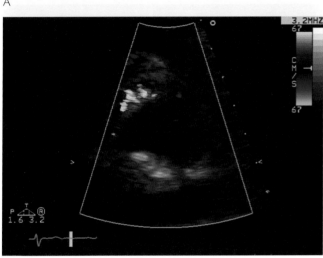

B

Figure 15.8 Bileaflet mechanical valve in the aortic position. A) A parasternal short-axis view on TTE view. There are two thin washing jets from each pivotal point. In (B) there is a paraprosthetic jet beginning clearly beyond the sewing ring

better than the other and give the spurious suggestion of obstruction. In biological valves, the cusps should be thin (1–2mm) and fully mobile with no prolapse behind the plane of the annulus. The colour map should entirely fill the orifice in all views. In an obstructed biological valve, it is possible for the colour map to be restricted at the orifice but to expand before the tips of the stents and it is possible to miss this sign. Unlike in the aortic position, rocking of the sewing ring may occur as a result of retention of the native posterior leaflet, but a true dehiscence is obvious from the gap opening between annulus and sewing ring and by the presence of a jet on colour mapping.

As for the aortic position, it is normal to see stitches and fibrin strands. It is also normal to see echoes resembling bubbles in the LV (◗ Fig. 15.9). These occur with all designs but are most frequent with bileaflet mechanical valves. Their origin is not firmly established. They are probably benign although occasional reports link them to abnormalities of higher cognitive function.

Obstruction

Heavily calcified cusps and reduced occluder motion are the most reliable signs of obstruction since the cusps, disc, or leaflets are usually imaged easily from the mitral position even on TTE. In a bileaflet mechanical valve, partial obstruction may be obvious when one leaflet clearly moves less than the other (◗ Fig. 15.10). Even if image quality is suboptimal, colour mapping can identify obstruction by showing a narrowed, high-velocity inflow jet with *wrap-around* aliasing (◗ Fig. 15.11) although TOE may sometimes be necessary to confirm this. In a stenotic stented biological valve, the jet can be narrow at the level of the immobile cusps, but can expand rapidly to fill the orifice towards the tips of the stents. It is therefore easy to miss the abnormality. Severe impairment of LV function may also cause reduced valve opening, but this will be associated with a thin, low-velocity inflow signal on colour mapping.

In the diagnosis of obstruction, quantitative Doppler is relatively less important in the mitral position than imaging and colour mapping. The minimum dataset is peak velocity, mean pressure gradient and pressure half-time (PHT) (see ◗ Chapter 5). The PHT is dependent on LV and left atrial function as well as MV function. In moderate or severe native or prosthetic stenosis, the mitral orifice dominates the PHT, but in a normal prosthetic valve or mild native stenosis, the PHT mainly reflects LV diastolic function. Thus small changes in PHT reflect loading conditions, heart rate, or drugs rather than a change in MV function. The Hatle formula (220/PHT) is not valid in normally-functioning mitral prostheses. The mean pressure gradient provides a reasonable description of valve function. Obstruction can be suspected:[1]

- Greatly prolonged PHT usually in excess of 200ms.
- Peak transmitral velocity >2.0m/s.
- Mean gradient >7mmHg.

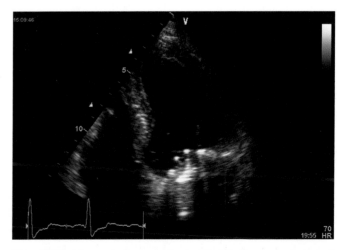

Figure 15.9 Microcavitations associated with a bileaflet mechanical mitral valve. Transthoracic study from the apical 4-chamber view.

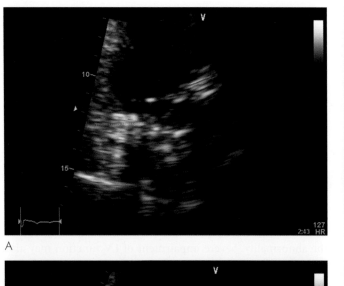

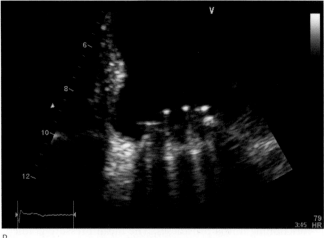

Figure 15.10 Obstructed bileaflet mechanical mitral valve. In this TTE four-chamber view failure of the lateral leaflet to open is shown in (A) in comparison to a normal valve in (B).

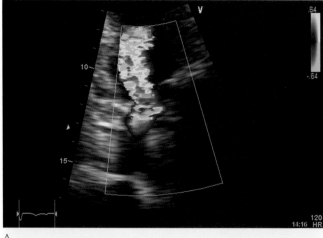

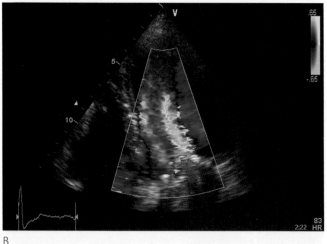

Figure 15.11 Colour imaging in an obstructed bileaflet mechanical mitral valve. These are the same patients as shown in ➲ Fig. 15.10. In the TTE four-chamber view (A) there is a narrowed, high velocity inflow map while the lateral part of the orifice lacks flow. By comparison flow fills the whole orifice in a normal valve (B).

In less severe obstruction, particularly with restriction of only one leaflet in a bileaflet mechanical valve, the PHT may be only mildly prolonged, to around 150ms. A change from immediate postoperative values may be obvious. Normal ranges are less variable than for the aortic position (see ➲ Appendix, Table 15.3).[11]

TOE is essential for determining the cause of obstruction in mechanical valves: thrombosis, pannus, mechanical obstruction by septal hypertrophy or retained chordae, or vegetations as a result of endocarditis. Thrombus (➲ Fig. 15.12) and also vegetations are associated with low density echoes, while pannus is typically highly echogenic (➲ Fig. 15.13). A thrombus is usually larger than pannus and more likely to extend into the left atrium and the appendage. However minor pannus may be overlain by thrombus so conclusive differentiation may not be possible. The clinical history may also be useful. A shorter duration of symptoms and inadequate anticoagulation suggests thrombus rather than pannus. Onset of symptoms less than a month from surgery predicts thrombus as a period of 6 months or more is usually necessary for pannus formation.

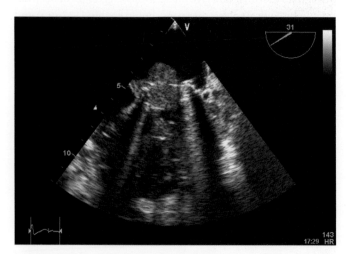

Figure 15.12 Thrombus. Transoesophageal four-chamber view showing a bileaflet mechanical mitral valve obstructed by a large thrombus.

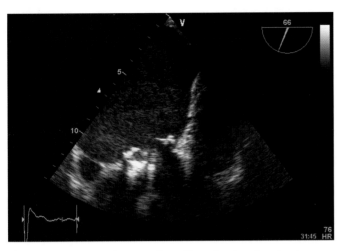

Figure 15.13 Pannus. Transoesophageal four-chamber view showing obstruction of one leaflet of a bileaflet mechanical mitral valve by a layer of highly echogenic pannus.

Regurgitation

Normal transprosthetic jets are particularly well seen in the mitral position (➲ Fig. 15.14) and may easily be misdiagnosed as pathological. Although the regurgitant fraction (RF%) is usually no larger than 10–15%, the associated colour jet can look large, up to 5cm long and 1cm wide. The RF% is directly related to the size of the valve and is also larger at low cardiac output (CO). A recognized clinical catch is the patient with a low CO as a result of a non-prosthetic cause such as LV failure who is found to have apparently large transprosthetic jets on TOE. It is important not to *treat the echocardiogram* and reoperate in this situation. Abnormal regurgitation through the valve occurs if the leaflet is prevented from closing as a result of thrombus, septal hypertrophy, or a chord (➲ Fig. 15.4).

Paraprosthetic regurgitation is differentiated from transprosthetic regurgitation by the jet having its origin outside the sewing ring. However, it may sometimes be difficult to locate the *neck* of

the jet and the distal parts of jets detected within the left atrium need to be followed carefully back to their origin. The neck and flow acceleration region within the LV can be imaged on TTE in all patients with moderate or severe paraprosthetic regurgitation (➲ Fig. 15.15). However, the location and size of the neck is also better seen on TOE (➲ Fig. 15.16) particularly 3D TOE (➲ Fig. 15.17). Important clues that TOE is necessary are:

♦ The patient is breathless.

♦ The LV is hyperdynamic.

Although paraprosthetic leaks are pathological by definition, they may be small and of no clinical significance. They are particularly frequent immediately after surgery and may resolve as endothelium covers the edge of the sewing ring. However small paraprosthetic jets, while of no haemodynamic significance, may still cause haemolysis so that haemolytic anaemia is an indication for TOE.

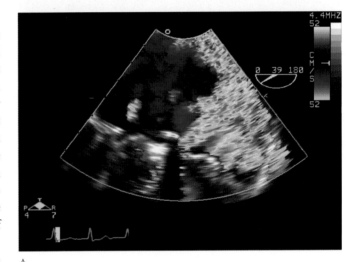

A

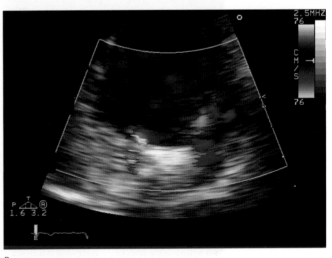

B

Figure 15.15 Paraprosthetic mitral regurgitation. The neck and intra-LV flow acceleration of a moderate of large paraprosthetic jet can usually be seen on TTE by careful angulation of the probe. The position can be described using a 'clock-face' and the grade of regurgitation is approximately given by the proportion of the sewing ring occupied.

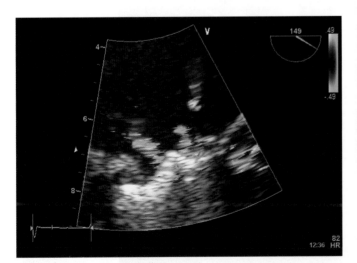

Figure 15.14 Normal transprosthetic mitral regurgitation. The bileaflet mechanical valve fully open and there are two plumes of regurgitation from the pivotal point and one around the leaflet.

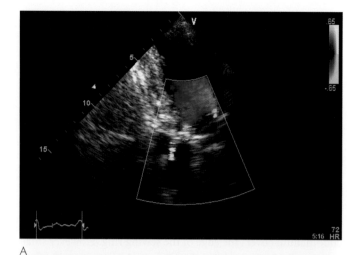

A

B

Figure 15.16 Paraprosthetic mitral regurgitation on TTE and TOE. On TTE this apical two-chamber view shows an apparently small intra-atrial jet (A), while on TOE (B) there is a broad jet.

Quantifying regurgitation uses the same methods as for native regurgitation[17] although as in the aortic position, the proportion of the circumference of the sewing ring occupied by a paraprosthetic jet gives an additional guide to severity.

Echocardiography of the replacement pulmonary valve

Imaging

The pulmonary valve (PV) is imaged on TTE from the PLAX view tilted to the right, from the PSAX view at the level of the AoV, and from the subcostal approach. On TOE it is imaged from the low oesophageal view by rotating clockwise from the long-axis view of the aorta. It can also be imaged from a deep transgastric view in a 120-degree imaging plane.

Obstruction

The minimum dataset is peak velocity and mean pressure gradient. Obstruction is suggested by cusp thickening or immobility with narrowing of the colour flow signal or by the following:[1,18]

- A single peak velocity >2m/s in a homograft or >3.0m/s in any other type of valve.

- A progressive rise in serial estimates is more reliable.

- New impairment of RV function.

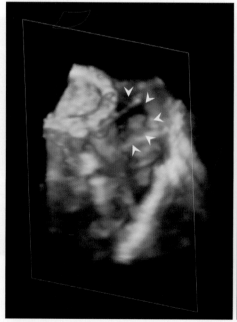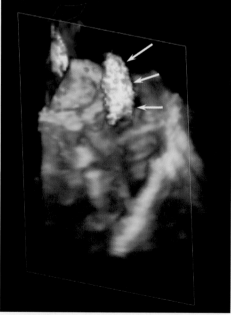

Figure 15.17 Paraprosthetic mitral regurgitation. 3D view of a partial dehiscence of a mitral mechanical prosthesis. The area of dehiscence is indicated by the arrow heads (left). The paravalvular leak is indicated by the arrows (right).

Regurgitation

Pulmonary regurgitation can be quantified by comparing the jet width to the annulus diameter as mild (<25%), moderate (26–50%), and severe (>50%). In severe pulmonary regurgitation, the PHT is short, often less than 100ms,[19] the jet is dense, and the RV is dilated and hyperdynamic.

Echocardiography of the replacement tricuspid valve

Imaging

The tricuspid valve (TV) is imaged on TTE from the PLAX view rotated medially, from the PSAX view, from the A4C view, and from the subcostal approach. All views, particularly from the apex will need multiple tilting to obtain optimal views of the RV and TV. On TOE the valve is imaged from the bicaval view obtained in the low oesophageal four-chamber view, with further 90 degrees of rotation and anticlockwise rotation of the probe. It is also shown from a transgastric view with 90-degree rotation.

Obstruction

The minimum dataset is peak velocity, mean pressure gradient, and PHT.[1] Obstruction is shown by reduced cusp or occluder motion with a narrowed colour signal. On transthoracic imaging, an engorged, unreactive inferior vena cava with a dilated right atrium and small RV are useful indirect signs. The following should also suggest obstruction:[20,21]

◆ A transtricuspid peak velocity >1.5m/s.

◆ Mean pressure gradient >5mmHg.

◆ PHT >240ms.

As for the mitral position, TOE is essential for determining the cause of obstruction in mechanical valves: thrombosis, pannus, or vegetations as a result of endocarditis.

Regurgitation

As for the mitral position, minor transprosthetic tricuspid regurgitation is normal. A paraprosthetic jet should be assessed by its width, which is most easily measured using 3D. Other methods of quantification are as for native tricuspid regurgitation:[17] jet shape and density, RV volume load, hepatic vein systolic flow reversal.

Stress echocardiography

This is not performed routinely but should be considered in any patient with exertional symptoms where the diagnosis is

not clear. The aim is to test for valve dysfunction, coexistent coronary disease, and on occasion new or worsening mitral regurgitation. Dobutamine and supine bicycle exercise are most commonly used. Treadmill exercise gives additional information about exercise capacity but is less frequently used because it makes recording information about the LV as well as the AoV relatively hard.

Comprehensive normal ranges and precise cut-points are not available. It is likely that a similar level as for native valves is a guide to significant obstruction, for example, a mean gradient increase greater than 15mmHg. In clinical practice, a combination of exact reproduction of symptoms with no wall motion abnormality and a large rise in pressure difference is highly suggestive of abnormal valve dynamics. For valves other than caged-ball valves, a peak instantaneous velocity above 5.0m/s on exercise is likely to be abnormal.

For the mitral position no normal ranges or cut-points exist, but data from native valves suggests that obstruction is likely if the mean pressure gradient is normal at rest (usually <7mmHg) and rises above 18mmHg after exercise[22] or if the estimated pulmonary artery pressure rises above 60mmHg.

Endocarditis

Suspected endocarditis is one of the most frequent indications for echocardiography in patients with replacement heart valves. Endocarditis affecting biological replacement valves result in vegetation similar to those occurring in native heart valve, while infective process at the level of mechanical replacement valves often cause paravalvular abscess (*ring abscess*) and discrete vegetations may be not seen.

Vegetations and local complications (dehiscence, abscess, perforation, fistula) may be obvious even on TTE especially if the valve is biological. However, if the valve is mechanical, vegetations are often difficult to detect transthoracically and TOE is then necessary (➲ Fig. 15.18). The reasons for failure of TTE in detecting mechanical replacement valve vegetations usually reside on reverberations and acoustic shadowing. Echocardiographic findings that may increase clinical suspicious of endocarditis of mechanical replacement valves on TTE are Doppler evidence of valve dysfunction or instability, a raise of pulmonary artery pressure that cannot be justified by other causes and a change in chamber dimensions. In general the sensitivity for vegetations is 15% on TTE and 90% on TOE.[23]

For the detection of complications both approaches are complementary. TTE is more sensitive for the detection of anterior aortic root abscess (➲ Fig. 15.19) while TOE is more sensitive for posterior root abscesses. Similar to abscess of native heart valves, paravalvular abscess of replacement valves may appear echodense or echo-free. When infective process persists, an aneurysm may develop at the site of valve abscess.

However echocardiography should not be part of the initial investigation of fever since the yield both of TTE and TOE is then exceptionally low.[24,25] Furthermore there is the risk of making a spurious diagnosis of endocarditis. It is never possible to differentiate vegetations from a segment of disrupted cusp. Nor it is possible to differentiate generalized valve thickening as a result of infection from primary failure even on TOE. Similarly, normal swelling and haematoma around a recently-implanted stentless valve cannot be differentiated from an abscess.

When transoesophageal echocardiography is necessary

TOE is necessary more frequently than with native valves especially for replacement valves in the mitral position because of the problem of shielding:

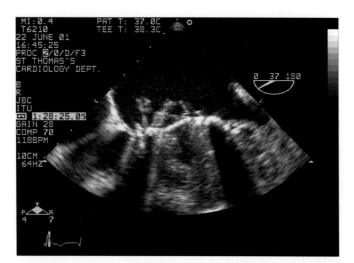

Figure 15.18 Vegetations on TOE. This patient with a bileaflet mechanical mitral valve had a fever and grew meticillin-resistant *Staphylococcus aureus* in multiple blood culture. This is a TOE four-chamber view

◆ When endocarditis is suspected particularly for mechanical valves. However, vegetations and complications may be obvious transthoracically and anterior aortic root abscesses are better seen transthoracically than transoesophageally. If the transthoracic study is diagnostic, it is only necessary to have a transoesophageal study if surgery is being discussed in order to check the other valves and to look for an abscess. This can be performed perioperatively.

◆ Despite a normal transthoracic study, if valve dysfunction is suspected from the presence of an abnormal murmur,

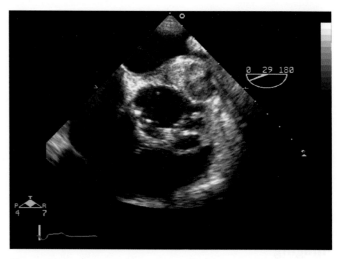

Figure 15.19 Aortic root abscess. This patient had a stentless aortic valve replacement with fever and MSSA on multiple blood cultures. There was an extensive abscess well seen on TTE

breathlessness, or haemolysis.

◆ The grade of mitral regurgitation is uncertain on transthoracic examination

◆ Thromboembolism recurs despite adequate anticoagulation since this suggests the presence of vegetation or alternatively of pannus acting as a nidus for thrombus formation.

◆ Obstruction of a mechanical valve to differentiate thrombosis from the other causes and to decide whether surgery or thrombolysis should be considered.

Conclusions

There are some key points:

◆ Quantitative Doppler should always be interpreted in the clinical context; normal ranges vary with design, position, and size.

◆ Velocities are flow dependent; always calculate EOA for valves in the aortic position.

◆ Do not use valve size in place of LVOT diameter in calculating the EOA.

◆ The PHT method for calculating EOA is not valid in normal replacement mitral valves.

◆ Transvalvular regurgitation is normal in almost all mechanical valves and many biological valves.

◆ TTE and TOE are complementary and should not be considered in isolation.

Personal perspective

If we had a replacement heart valve we would ensure that we had a postoperative study and would keep a copy of the report against which to compare future studies. Assuming this was normal and there were no other abnormalities we would not want further studies unless clinically indicated. If we had a biological valve we would elect to have a routine study beyond 7 rather than the 5 years recommended in European Society of Cardiology and American Heart Association guidelines since third-generation valves have good expected durability. If we had a fever we would not want TOE unless there was a reasonable clinical suspicion of endocarditis, for example, a blood culture growing an organism capable of causing endocarditis. We would want to have echocardiography and clinical follow-up in a specialist valve clinic and would want to be referred to an expert centre if there were a suspicion of malfunction.

Appendix

Normal values for prosthetic function. Mean (standard deviation).[26]

Table 15.1 Aortic position: biological

	Vmax m/s	Peak ΔP mmHg	Mean ΔP mmHg	EOA cm^2
Stented porcine: Carpentier–Edwards standard as example (values similar for Carpentier–Edwards supra-annular, Intact, Hancock I and II and Mosaic, Biocor, Epic)				
19mm		43.5 (12.7)	25.6 (8.)	0.9 (0.2)
21mm	2.8 (0.5)	27.2 (7.6)	17.3 (6.2)	1.5 (0.3)
23mm	2.8 (0.7)	28.9 (7.5)	16.1 (6.2)	1.7 (0.5)
25mm	2.6 (0.6)	24.0 (7.1)	12.9 (4.6)	1.9 (0.5)
27mm	2.5 (0.5)	22.1 (8.2)	12.1 (5.5)	2.3 (0.6)
29mm	2.4 (0.4)		9.9 (2.9)	2.8 (0.5)
Stented Bovine Pericardial: Baxter Perimount as example (similar Mitroflow, Edwards Pericardial, Labcor-Santiago, Mitroflow)				
19mm	2.8 (0.1)	32.5 (8.5)	19.5 (5.5)	1.3 (0.2)
21mm	2.6 (0.4)	24.9 97.70	13.8 (4.0)	1.3 (0.3)
23mm	2.3 (0.5)	19.9 (7.4)	11.5 (3.9)	1.6 (0.3)
25mm	2.0 (0.3)	16.5 (7.8)	10.7 (3.8)	1.6 (0.4)
27mm		12.8 (5.4)	4.8 (2.2)	2.0 (0.4)
Homograft				
22mm	1.7 (0.3)		5.8 (3.2)	2.0 (0.6)
26mm	1.4 (0.6)		6.8 (2.9)	2.4 (0.7)
Stentless				
Whole root as inclusion: St Jude Toronto (similar to Prima)				
21mm		22.6 (14.5)	10.7 (7.2)	1.3 (0.6)
23mm		16.2 (9.0)	8.2 (4.7)	1.6 (0.6)
25mm		12.7 (8.2)	6.3 (4.1)	1.8 (0.5)
27mm		10.1 (5.8)	5.0 (2.9)	2.0 (0.3)
29mm		7.7 (4.4)	4.1 (2.4)	2.4 (0.6)
Cryolife–O'Brien (similar to Freestyle)				
19mm			9.0 (2.0)	1.5 (0.3)
21mm			6.6 (2.9)	1.7 (0.4)
23mm			6.0 (2.3)	2.3 (0.2)
25mm			6.1 (2.6)	2.6 (0.2)
27mm			4.0 (2.4)	2.8 (0.3)

Table 15.2 Aortic position: mechanical

Single tilting disc

Medtronic-Hall (similar values Bjork–Shiley monostrut and CC, Omnicarbon and Omnisceince)

	Vmax m/s	Peak ΔP mmHg	Mean ΔP mmHg	EOA cm²
20mm	2.9 (0.4)	34.4 (13.1)	17.1 (5.3)	1.2 (0.5)
21mm	2.4 (0.4)	26.9 (10.5)	14.1 (5.9)	1.1 (0.2)
23mm	2.4 (0.6)	26.9 (8.9)	13.5 (4.8)	1.4 (0.4)
25mm	2.3 (0.5)	17.1 (7.0)	9.5 (4.3)	1.5 (0.5)
27mm	2.1 (0.5)	18.9 (9.7)	8.7 (5.6)	1.9 (0.2)

Bileaflet mechanical

Intra-annular: St Jude standard (similar Carbomedics standard, Edwards Mira, ATS, Sorin Bicarbon)

	Vmax m/s	Peak ΔP mmHg	Mean ΔP mmHg	EOA cm²
19mm	2.9 (0.5)	35.2 (11.2)	19.0 (6.3)	1.0 (0.2)
21mm	2.6 (0.5)	28.3 (10.0)	15.8 (5.7)	1.3 (0.3)
23mm	2.6 (0.4)	25.3 (7.9)	13.8 (5.3)	1.6 (0.4)
25mm	2.4 (0.5)	22.6 (7.7)	12.7 (5.1)	1.9 (0.5)
27mm	2.2 (0.4)	19.9 (7.6)	11.2 (4.8)	2.4 (0.6)
29mm	2.0 (0.1)	17.7 (6.4)	9.9 (2.9)	2.8 (0.6)

Intra-annular modified cuff or partially supra-annular: MCRI On-X (similar St Jude Regent, St Jude HP, Carbomedics Reduced cuff, Medtronic Advantage)

	Vmax m/s	Peak ΔP mmHg	Mean ΔP mmHg	EOA cm²
19mm	21.3 (10.8)	11.8 (3.4)	1.5 (0.2)	
21mm	16.4 (5.9)	9.9 (3.6)	1.7 (0.4)	
23mm	15.9 (6.4)	8.6 (3.4)	1.9 (0.6)	
25mm	16.5 (10.2)	6.9 (4.3)	2.4 (0.6)	

Supra-annular: Carbomedics TopHat

	Vmax m/s	Peak ΔP mmHg	Mean ΔP mmHg	EOA cm²
21mm	2.6 (0.4)	30.2 (10.9)	14.9 (5.4)	1.2 (0.3)
23mm	2.4 (0.6)	24.2 (7.6)	12.5 (4.4)	1.4 (0.4)
25mm		1.6 (0.3)	1.6 (0.3)	9.5 (2.9)

Ball and cage: Starr–Edwards

	Vmax m/s	Peak ΔP mmHg	Mean ΔP mmHg	EOA cm²
23mm	3.4 (0.6)	32.6 (12.8)	22.0 (9.0)	1.1 (0.2)
24mm	3.6 (0.5)	34.1 (10.3)	22.1 (7.5)	1.1 (0.3)
26mm	3.0 (0.2)	31.8 (9.0)	19.7 (6.1)	
27mm		30.8 (6.3)	18.5 (3.7)	
29mm		29.3 (9.3)	16.3 (5.5)	

Table 15.3 Mitral position

	Vmax m/s	Peak ΔP mmHg
Stented porcine: Carpentier–Edwards (similar Intact, Hancock)		
27mm	6.0 (2.0)	
29mm	1.5 (0.3)	4.7 (2.0)
31mm	1.5 (0.3)	4.5 (2.0)
33mm	1.4 (0.2)	5.4 (4.0)
Pericardial: Ionescu–Shiley (similar Labcor-Santiago, Hancock pericardial, Carpentier–Edwards pericardial		
25mm	1.4 (0.2)	4.9 (1.1)
27mm	1.3 (0.2)	3.2 (0.8)
29mm	1.4 (0.2)	3.2 (0.6)
31mm	1.3 (0.1)	2.7 (0.4)
Single tilting disc: Bjork–Shiley monostrut (similar Omnicarbon)		
25mm	1.8 (0.3)	5.6 (2.3)
27mm	1.7 (0.4)	4.5 (2.2)
29mm	1.6 (0.3)	4.3 (1.6)
31mm	1.7 (0.3)	4.9 (1.6)
33mm	1.3 (0.3)	
Bileaflet: Carbomedics (similar St Jude)		
25mm	1.6 (0.2)	4.3 (0.7)
27mm	1.6 (0.3)	3.7 (1.5)
29mm	1.8 (0.3)	3.7 (1.3)
31mm	1.6 (0.4)	3.3 (1.1)
33mm	1.4 (0.3)	3.4 (1.5)
Caged ball: Starr–Edwards		
28mm	1.8 (0.2)	7.0 (2.8)
30mm	1.8 (0.2)	7.0 (2.5)
32mm	1.9 (0.4)	5.1 (2.5)

References

1 Zoghbi WA, Chambers JB, Dumesnil JG, Foster E, Gottdiener JS, Grayburn PA, et al. American Society of Echocardiography recommendations for evaluation of prosthetic valves with two-dimensional and Doppler echocardiography. J Am Soc Echo 2009; 22:975–1014.

2 Bonow RO, Carabello BA, Kanu C, de Leon AC Jr, Faxon DP, Freed MD, et al. ACC/AHA 2006 guidelines for the management of patients with valvular heart disease: a report of the American College of Cardiology/American Heart Association Task Force on Practice Guidelines (writing committee to revise the 1998 Guidelines for the Management of Patients With Valvular Heart Disease). Circulation 2006; 114:e84–231.

3 Vahanian A, Baumgartner H, Bax J, Butchart E, Dion R, Filippatos G, et al. Guidelines on the management of valvular heart disease. Eur Heart J 2007; 28:230–68.

4 Descoutures F, Himbert D, Lepage L, Iung B, Detaint D, Tchetche D, et al. Contemporary surgical or percutaneous management of severe aortic stenosis in the elderly. Eur Heart J 2008; 29:1410–7.

5 Jamieson WR. Current and advanced prostheses for cardiac valvular replacement and reconstruction surgery. Surg Technol Int 2002; 10:121–49.

6 Chambers J, Oo L, Naracott A, Lawford P, Blauth C. Nominal size in six bileaflet mechanical aortic valves: a comparison with orifice size and a biological equivalent. J Thorac Cardiovasc Surg 2003; 125:1388–93.

7 Chambers JB, Spiropoulos G. Estimation of the aortic orifice area: comparison of the classical and modified forms of the continuity equation. Am J Noninvasive Cardiol 1993; 7:259–62.

8 Levine RA, Cape EG, Yoganathan AP. Pressure recovery distal to stenoses: expanding clinical applications of engineering principles. J Am Coll Cardiol 1993; 21:1026–8.

9 Baumgartner H, Khan S, DeRobertis M, Czer L, Maurer G. Discrepancies between Doppler and catheter gradients in aortic prosthetic valves in vitro. A manifestation of localized gradients and pressure recovery. Circulation 1990; 82:1467–75.

10 Alam M, Goldstein S, Lakier JB. Echocardiographic changes in the thickness of porcine valves with time. Chest 1981; 79:663–8.

11 Rosenhek R, Binder T, Maurer G, Baumgartner H. Normal values for Doppler echocardiographic assessment of heart valve prostheses. J Am Soc Echo 2003; 16: 1116–27.

12 Rajani R, Mukherjee D, Chambers J. Doppler echocardiography in normally functioning replacement aortic valves: a review of 129 studies. J Heart Valve Dis 2007; 16:519–35.

13 Pibarot P, Dumesnil JG. Prosthesis-patient mismatch: definition, clinical impact, and prevention. Heart 2006; 92:1022–9.

14 Ruel M, Al-Faleh H, Kulik A, Chan KL, Mesana TG, Burwash IG. Prosthesis-patient mismatch after aortic valve replacement predominantly affects patients with preexisting left ventricular dysfunction: effect on survival, freedom from heart failure, and left ventricular mass regression. J Thorac Cardiovasc Surg 2006; 131:1036–44.

15 Blais C, Dumesnil JG, Baillot R, Simard S, Doyle D, Pibarot P. Impact of prosthesis-patient mismatch on short-term mortality after aortic valve replacement. Circulation 2003; 108:983–8.

16 Blackstone EH, Cosgrove DM, Jamieson WR, et al. Prosthesis size and long-term survival after aortic valve replacement. J Thorac Cardiovasc Surg 2003; 126:783–96.

17 Zoghbi WA, Enriquez-Sarano M, Foster E, et al. ASE recommendations for evaluation of the severity of native valvular regurgitation with two-dimensional and Doppler echocardiography. J Am Soc Echocardiogr 2003; 16:777–802.

18 Novaro GM, Connolly HM, Miller FA. Doppler hemodynamics of 51 clinically and echocardiographically normal pulmonary valve prostheses. Mayo Clin Proc 2001; 76:155–60.

19 Rodriguez RJ, Riggs TW. Physiologic peripheral pulmonary stenosis in infancy. Am J Cardiol 1990; 66:1478–81.

20 Connolly HM, Miller FA, Taylor CL, et al. Doppler hemodynamic profiles of 82 clinically and echocardiographically normal tricuspid valve prostheses. Circulation 1993; 88:2722–7.

21 Koyobashi Y, Nagata S, Ohmori F, et al. Serial Doppler echocardiographic evaluation of bioprosthetic valves in the tricuspid position. J Am Coll Cardiol 1996; 27:1693–7.

22 Reis G, Motta MS, Barbosa MM, Esteves WA, Souza SF, Bocchi EA. Dobutamine stress echocardiography for noninvasive assessment and risk stratification of patients with rheumatic mitral stenosis. J Am Coll Cardiol 2004; 43:393–401.

23 Schulz R, Werner GS, Fuchs JB, Andreas S, Prange H, Ruschowski W, Krenzer H. Clinical outcome and echocardiographic findings

of native and prosthetic valve endocarditis in the 1990s. *Eur Heart J* 1996; **17**:281–8.

24 Greaves K, Mou D, Patel A, Celermajer DS. Clinical criteria and appropriate use of transthoracic echocardiography for the exclusion of endocarditis. *Heart* 2003; **89**:273–5.

25 Thangaroopan A, Choy B. Is transesophageal echocardiography overused in the diagnosis of infective endocarditis? *Am J Cardiol* 2005; **95**:295–7.

26 Rimington H, Chambers J. Echocardiography: Guidelines for Reporting, 2nd edition. New York: Informa Healthcare; 2007.

Further reading

Bonow RO, Carabello BA, Kanu C, de Leon AC Jr, Faxon DP, Freed MD, et al. ACC/AHA 2006 guidelines for the management of patients with valvular heart disease: a report of the American College of Cardiology/American Heart Association Task Force on Practice Guidelines (writing committee to revise the 1998 Guidelines for the Management of Patients With Valvular Heart Disease). *Circulation* 2006; **114**:e84–231.

Grunkemeier GL, Li H-H, Naftel DC, Starr A, Rahimtoola SH. Long-term performance of heart valve prostheses. *Curr Probl Cardiol* 2000; **25**:73–156.

Vahanian A, Baumgartner H, Bax J, Butchart E, Dion R, Filippatos G, *et al.* Guidelines on the management of valvular heart disease. *Eur Heart J* 2007; **28**:230–68.

Zoghbi WA, Chambers JB, Dumesnil JG, Foster E, Gottdiener JS, Grayburn PA, *et al.* American Society of Echocardiography recommendations for evaluation of prosthetic valves with two-dimensional and Doppler echocardiography. *J Am Soc Echo* 2009; **22**:975–1014.

➲ For additional multimedia materials please visit the online version of the book (🕮 http://escecho.oxfordmedicine.com).

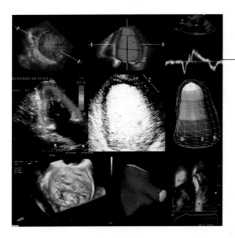

CHAPTER 16

Infective endocarditis

Gilbert Habib and Franck Thuny

Contents

Summary

Echocardiography plays a key role in the assessment of infective endocarditis. It is useful for the diagnosis of endocarditis, the assessment of severity of the disease, the prediction of short-term and long-term prognosis, the prediction of embolic risk, the management of the complications of endocarditis, and the follow-up of patients under specific antibiotic therapy.

The 'Guidelines on the prevention, diagnosis, and treatment of infective endocarditis' of the European Society of Cardiology and the 'Recommendations for the practice of echocardiography in infective endocarditis' of the European Association for Echocardiography recently underlined the value and limitations of echocardiography in infective endocarditis, and gave clear recommendations for the optimal use of both transthoracic echocardiography and transoesophageal echocardiography in infective endocarditis.

Introduction

The role of echocardiography in the assessment of infective endocarditis is fundamental.[1] This imaging tool is useful for diagnosis and the prediction of embolic risk of infective endocarditis, for the prediction of short-term and long-term prognosis, and the follow-up of patients under antibiotic therapy. Echocardiography is also useful for the diagnosis and management of the complications of infective endocarditis, helping the physician in decision making, particularly when a surgical therapy is considered. Recent guidelines underlined the great value of echocardiography in infective endocarditis and gave useful information concerning its correct use in clinical practice.[2,3]

Diagnostic value of echocardiography

The major echocardiographic criteria for infective endocarditis are vegetation and abscess.[4] Other echocardiographic findings are only suggestive.

Vegetations

Anatomical features

Anatomically, infective endocarditis is characterized by a combination of vegetations and destructive lesions. Vegetation is defined as an infected mass attached to an endocardial structure, or on implanted intracardiac material (➲ Table 16.1). Vegetations are typically attached on the low pressure side of the valve structure, but may be located anywhere on the components of the valvular and subvalvular apparatus, as well as on the mural endocardium of the cardiac chambers or the ascending aorta.[3] When large and mobile, vegetations are prone to embolism and less frequently to valve or prosthetic obstruction.

Echographic features

Vegetations present as oscillating or non-oscillating intracardiac masses on valve or other endocardial structures, or on implanted intracardiac material[2] (🎞 16.13 and 16.14). Echocardiography is the reference method for the diagnosis of vegetation. When typical, vegetation presents as an oscillating mass attached on a valvular structure (➲ Figs. 16.1 and 16.2; 🎞 16.1 and 16.2), with a motion independent to that of this valve. However, vegetation may also present as a non-oscillating mass and with an atypical location (➲ Fig. 16.3).

Vegetations are usually localized on the atrial side of the atrioventricular valves, and on the ventricular side of the aortic and pulmonary valves. The reported sensitivity for the diagnosis of vegetation is about 75% for transthoracic echocardiography (TTE) and 85–90% for transoesophageal echocardiography (TOE). In addition, both TTE and TOE are useful to assess the size and mobility of the vegetation, as well as its evolution under antibiotic therapy.[5]

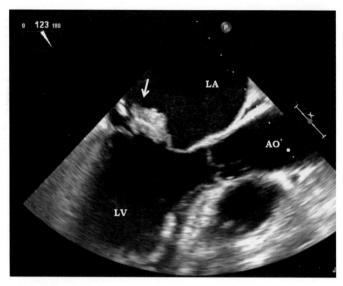

Figure 16.1 Vegetation on mitral valve. Large vegetation on the anterior mitral leaflet with chordae rupture (arrow) (TOE). Ao, aorta; LA, left atrium; LV, left ventricle.

Difficult situations

The correct identification of vegetations is sometimes difficult. A negative echocardiography may be observed in about 15% of infective endocarditis.[3] The main situations in which the identification of vegetations may be difficult include very small or absent vegetations and presence of pre-existent severe lesions (mitral valve [MV] prolapse, degenerative lesions, and prosthetic valves). The diagnosis may be difficult at the early stage of the disease, when vegetations are not yet present or too small to be identified. In one series,[6] vegetation was observed by TOE in

Table 16.1 Anatomical and echocardiographic definitions*

	Surgery/necropsy	Echocardiography
Vegetation	Infected mass attached to an endocardial structure, or on implanted intracardiac material	Oscillating or non-oscillating intracardiac mass on valve or other endocardial structures, or on implanted intracardiac material
Abscess	Perivalvular cavity with necrosis and purulent material not communicating with the cardiovascular lumen	Thickened, non-homogeneous perivalvular area with echodense or echolucent appearance
Pseudoaneurysm	Perivalvular cavity communicating with the cardiovascular lumen	Pulsatile perivalvular echo-free space, with colour-Doppler flow detected
Perforation	Interruption of endocardial tissue continuity	Interruption of endocardial tissue continuity traversed by colour-Doppler flow
Fistula	Communication between 2 neighbouring cavities through a perforation	Colour-Doppler communication between 2 neighboring cavities through a perforation
Valve aneurysm	Saccular outpouching of valvular tissue	Saccular bulging of valvular tissue
Dehiscence of a prosthetic valve	Dehiscence of the prosthesis	Paravalvular regurgitation identified by TTE/TOE, with or without rocking motion of the prosthesis

*Reproduced with permission from Habib G, Hoen B, Tornos P, Thuny F, Prendergast B, Vilacosta I, *et al*. Guidelines on the prevention, diagnosis, and treatment of infective endocarditis (new version 2009): The Task Force on the Prevention, Diagnosis, and Treatment of Infective Endocarditis of the European Society of Cardiology (ESC). *Eur Heart J* 2009; **30**:2369–413.

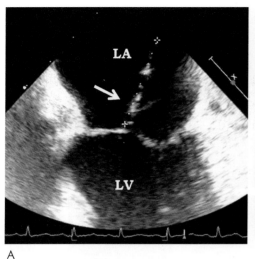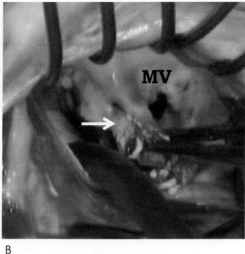

Figure 16.2 Echocardiographic and anatomical correlations. A) TOE: long vegetation on the anterior mitral leaflet (arrow). B) Anatomical correlation: large vegetation (black arrow). LA, left atrium; LV, left ventricle; MV, mitral valve.

only 81%, among 93 patients with anatomically confirmed infective endocarditis. In another series, among 105 patients with suspected infective endocarditis, 65 had an initial negative TOE; in 3 cases, vegetation appeared on a repeat TOE.[7] For this reason, repeat TTE or TOE examination must be performed 7–10 days after the first examination when the clinical level of suspicion is still high (➲ Fig. 16.4; 🔳 16.10 and 16.11).

Sensitivity and specificity of echocardiography are lower in specific subgroups including cardiac device-related[8–10] and prosthetic valve[11–15] infective endocarditis (➲ Fig. 16.5; 🔳 16.16.). In both situations, TOE has a better sensitivity than TTE, but both examinations are finally necessary and recommended in all patients.[2–3] Because of the lower diagnostic value of echocardiography, Duke criteria also present with a lower

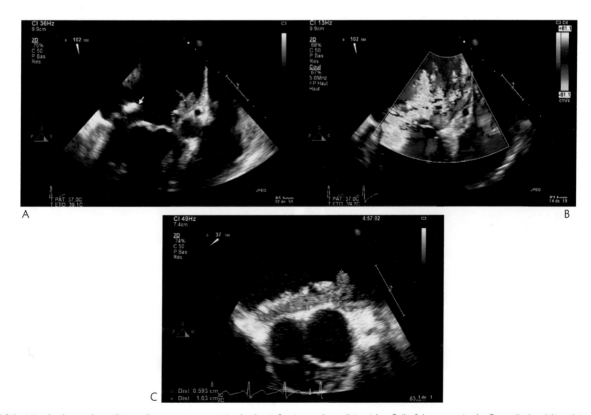

Figure 16.3 Mitral valve endocarditis and consequences. Mitral valve infective endocarditis with a flail of the posterior leaflet at P1 level (A, white arrow). This lesion leads to a severe mitral insufficiency with an excentric regurgitant jet (B). Vegetations in the left atrium represent contamination by this 'infected' mitral regurgitation (C).

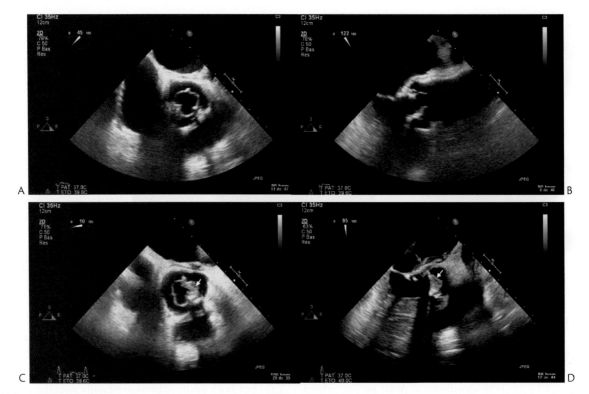

Figure 16.4 Detection of infective endocarditis over time. Evolution of TOE performed in a patient with an aortic bioprosthetic valve and a clinical suspicion of endocarditis. The first TOE was normal with no vegetation and no abscess (A and B). A second TOE was performed 5 days later and showed a new large vegetations on the bioprosthetic cusps (white arrow) and a periannular abscess (red arrow).

sensitivity in these specific subgroups.[6] It is of utmost importance to keep in mind that, in both cardiac device-related and prosthetic infective endocarditis, a negative echocardiography does not rule out the clinical suspicion.

Conversely, false diagnosis of infective endocarditis may occur in other situations: for example, it may be difficult to differentiate between vegetations and thrombi, cusp prolapse, cardiac tumours, myxomatous changes, Lambl's excrescences, strands, or non-infective vegetations (marantic endocarditis).[16] Non-infective vegetations are impossible to differentiate from infective vegetations. They can be suspected in the presence of small and multiple vegetations, changing from one examination to another, and without associated abscess or valve destruction.

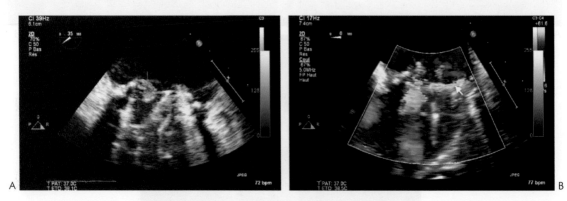

Figure 16.5 Vegetation on prosthetic valves. TOE showing a large vegetation (red arrow) on the annulus of a mitral mechanical prosthetic valve hampering the leaflets closure (A) and leading to an intraprosthetic regurgitation (B, white arrow).

Abscess

Anatomical features

Abscesses represent the second most typical findings suggesting infective endocarditis. They are more frequent in aortic and prosthetic valve. Anatomically, they are defined as perivalvular cavity with necrosis and purulent material not communicating with the cardiovascular lumen[2] (▣ 16.3). Abscess may be complicated by a communication with the cardiovascular lumen (*pseudoaneurysm*) (▣ 16.12) and by fistulization into an adjacent cavity[17] (➲ Table 16.1).

Echographic features

Abscess typically presents as a perivalvular zone of reduced echo density, without colour flow detected inside[3] (➲ Figs. 16.6 and 16.7). The sensitivity of TTE is about 50%, that of TOE 90%. The additional value of TOE is much higher for the diagnosis of abscess than for the diagnosis of vegetation. For this reason, TOE must be systematically performed in aortic valve (AoV) infective endocarditis, and as soon as an abscess is suspected.

Abscess may be complicated by a pseudoaneurysm, which presents as a pulsatile perivalvular echo free-space with colour Doppler flow inside (➲ Fig.16.8), and by fistulization displayed at echocardiography as a colour Doppler communication between two adjacent cavities.

All these perivalvular lesions are more frequently observed in aortic endocarditis and then involve the mitral-aortic intervalvular fibrosa[18] (▣ 16.4–16.6).

Difficult situations

Despite use of TOE, diagnosis of a perivalvular abscess may be difficult in cases of small abscess or when echocardiography is performed very early in the course of the disease or in the immediate postoperative period after aortic root replacement and Bentall procedure. In this last situation, a thickening of the aortic wall may be observed in the absence of infective endocarditis, mimicking abscess formation. Reduced diagnostic value of TOE has recently been reported in patients with abscess localized around calcification in the posterior mitral annulus.[19] ➲ Figure 16.9 shows an example of mitral annulus abscess with anatomical correlation. Finally, a normal echocardiogram does not completely rule out infective endocarditis, even if TOE is performed and even in expert hands. A repeat examination has to be performed in case of high level of clinical suspicion.

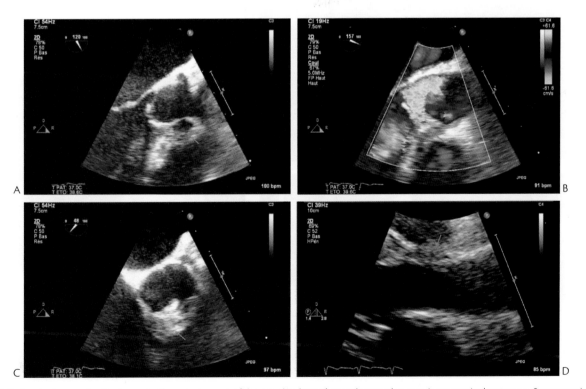

Figure 16.6 Aortic abscess. Aortic abscess in the anterior part of the annulus (arrow) near the membranous interventricular septum. Severe aortic regurgitation through this periannular complication.

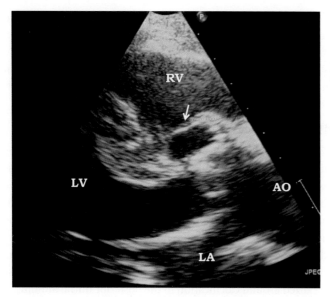

Figure 16.7 Aortic bioprosthetic abscess (TTE). Presence of an anterior free space corresponding to an abscess (arrow). AO, aorta; LA, left atrium; LV, left ventricle; RV, right ventricle.

Other echocardiographic findings

Other echocardiographic features have less sensitivity and specificity but may be suggestive of the diagnosis of infective endocarditis. They include new dehiscence of a prosthetic valve, valve destruction and prolapse, aneurysm, and/or perforation of a valve.

Perforation of the anterior leaflet of MV is a relatively frequent complication of AoV infective endocarditis (🔳 16.7–16.9). It is best visualized by TOE and may be observed either isolated or as a complication of a MV aneurysm[20] (➲ Fig. 16.10).

New dehiscence of a prosthetic valve represents the third main diagnostic criterion for infective endocarditis in the Duke classification,[4] and may be the only echocardiographic sign of infective endocarditis in some patients (🔳 16.15). TOE has a better sensitivity than TTE for this diagnosis, especially in mitral prosthetic valve endocarditis.

In addition, both TTE and TOE are useful for the assessment of the underlying valve disease, and for the assessment of

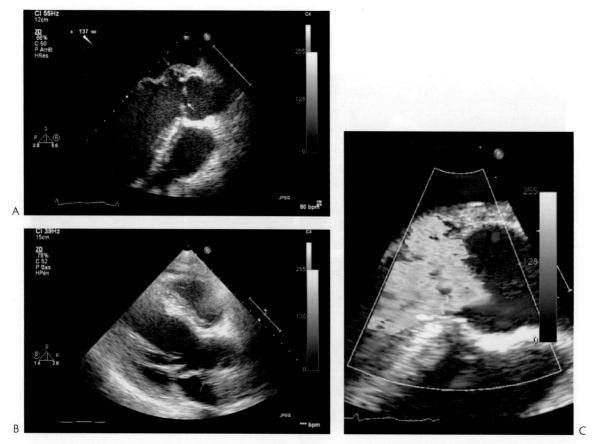

Figure 16.8 Pseudoaneurysm of the mitral-aortic fibrosa. Pseudoaneurysm of the mitral-aortic fibrosa (A) (red arrow) due to an eccentric severe aortic regurgitation (C) in a patient with a *Staphylococcus aureus* endocarditis. This lesion can be evidenced by TTE (B).

APPOINTMENT CARD

Name:

Date of appointment: 4/12/2015

Time of appointment: 12:20pm

ASDA OPTICIANS

If you would like to rearrange your appointment please contact us:

Asda Stores Ltd, Gillingham Pier 4794,
Dynamo Way, Gillingham, Kent, ME7 1RZ

Tel: 01732 753131

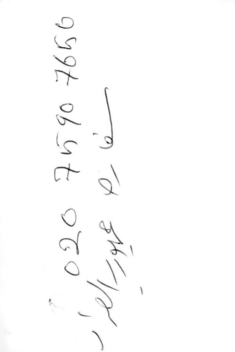

0920 7590 7656

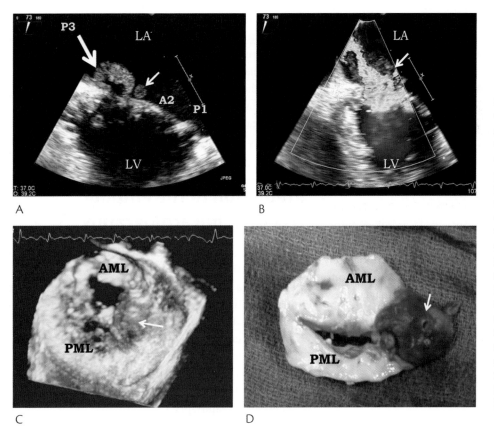

Figure 16.9 Infective endocarditis with commissural abscess and perforation. Severe native valve infective endocarditis with commissural abscess and perforation. A) Vegetation and pseudoaneurysm (thick arrow) of the posterointernal commissure of the mitral valve, associated with a small vegetation (thin arrow). B) Fistulization of the pseudoaneurysm into the left atrium causing massive mitral regurgitation (arrow). C) 3D echocardiography showing the commissural abscess (arrow). D) Anatomical correlation: surgical specimen showing the commissural abscess (arrow). AML, anterior mitral leaflet; LA, left atrium; LV, left ventricle; PML, posterior mitral leaflet.

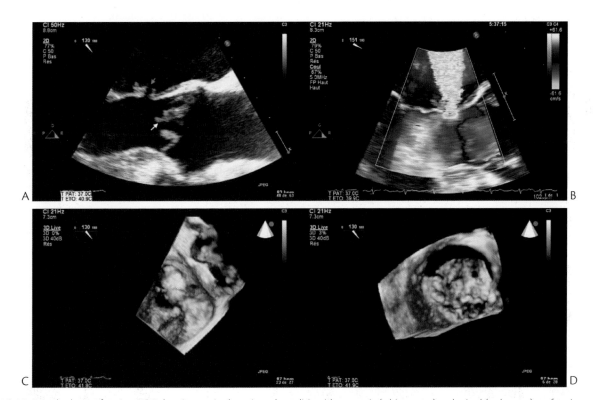

Figure 16.10 Mitral valve perforation. TOE showing a mitral-aortic endocarditis with an aortic (white arrow) and mitral (red arrow) perforation (A and B). Part (C) shows the mitral perforation by real-time 3D TOE from an atrial view. Part (D) shows the mitral perforation by real-time 3D TOE from a ventricular view.

consequences of infective endocarditis, the evaluation of left and right ventricular function, the quantification of valve regurgitation/obstruction, and the estimation of pulmonary pressures.[3]

Indications of different echocardiographic modalities in infective endocarditis

The respective indications of TTE and TOE have been recently summarized in the 2009 European Society of Cardiology guidelines[2] and in the EAE 'Recommendations for the practice of echocardiography in infective endocarditis'.[3] Echocardiography must be performed in several very different clinical situations, including heart failure, cerebral embolism, pacemaker infection, or isolated fever. Infective endocarditis must be suspected in the presence of fever associated with regurgitant heart murmur, known cardiac disease, bacteraemia, new conduction disturbance, and embolic events of unknown origin.[2]

TTE must be performed first in all cases, because it is a non-invasive technique giving useful information both for the diagnosis and the assessment of severity of infective endocarditis. TOE must also be performed in the majority of patients with suspected infective endocarditis, because of its better image quality and better sensitivity, except in case of good quality negative TTE associated with a weak clinical suspicion (➲ Fig. 16.11).

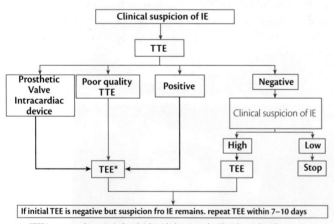

If initial TEE is negative but suspicion fro IE remains. repeat TEE within 7–10 days

*TEE is not mandatory in isolated right-sided native valve IE with good quality TEE examination and unequivocal echocardiographic findings.

Figure 16.11 Diagnosis of infective endocarditis. Algorithm showing the role of echocardiography in the diagnosis and assessment of infective endocarditis. IE, infective endocarditis; TOE, transoesophageal echocardiography; TTE, transthoracic echocardiography. Adapted with permission from Habib G, Hoen B, Tornos P, Thuny F, Prendergast B, Vilacosta I, et al. Guidelines on the prevention, diagnosis, and treatment of infective endocarditis (new version 2009): The Task Force on the Prevention, Diagnosis, and Treatment of Infective Endocarditis of the European Society of Cardiology (ESC). Eur Heart J 2009; **30**:2369–413.

Intracardiac echocardiography has been occasionally reported in case reports or short series, but adds little information to conventional echocardiography. The use of three-dimensional (3D) echocardiography is not better than TTE or TOE for the diagnosis of vegetation, but may be useful for the diagnosis and assessment of abscesses, false aneurysms, MV anterior leaflet perforation, and other destructive consequences of infective endocarditis.[2]

Prediction of the embolic risk by echocardiography

Embolic events are a frequent and life-threatening complication of infective endocarditis, with a total risk of embolism of 20–50%, and a risk of new embolic event (i.e. occurring after initiation of antibiotic therapy) of 6–21%.[1] Cerebral embolism is the most frequent and severe localization of embolism. Conversely, embolic events may be totally silent in about 20% of patients with infective endocarditis, especially in case of splenic or cerebral embolisms, and must be diagnosed by systematic non-invasive imaging.

Echocardiography plays a major role in the assessment of embolic risk, although this prediction remains difficult in the individual patient.[21–24] Several factors have been associated with an increased risk of embolism:

- Size and mobility of vegetations.
- Localization of the vegetation on the MV.
- Increasing or decreasing size of the vegetation under antibiotic therapy.
- Type of microorganism.
- Previous embolism.
- Multivalvular endocarditis.
- Biological markers.

Among them, the size and mobility of vegetations are the most potent independent predictors of new embolic event in patients with infective endocarditis. A significant relationship has been shown between presence of vegetation and occurrence of embolism, as well as between vegetation size and mobility and the incidence of embolism. Consequently, measurement of vegetation size by echocardiography (particularly TOE) is of crucial importance. Patients with left-sided infective endocarditis and very large (>15mm) and mobile vegetations must be considered as at high risk of embolism and need specific management.[2]

In addition, the risk of embolism is particularly high during the first days following the initiation of antibiotic therapy and decreases after 2 weeks.[23] For this reason, the benefit of surgery to prevent embolization will be greatest during the first week of antibiotic therapy, when the embolic rate is highest.

Prognostic value of echocardiography

Echocardiography also plays an important role both in the short-term and long-term prognostic assessment of patients with infective endocarditis.

Prognostic assessment at admission

The in-hospital mortality rate of patients with infective endocarditis is still high, ranging from 9.6–26%. Thus, accurate prediction of the risk of in-hospital death is desirable, allowing aggressive strategy to be performed in order to reduce the risk of death. Several echocardiographic features have been associated with a worse prognosis, including perivalvular complications, severe native or prosthetic valve regurgitation or obstruction, low left ventricular ejection fraction, pulmonary hypertension, large vegetations, and premature MV closure or other signs of elevated diastolic pressures. Consequently, prognostic assessment at admission can be performed using simple clinical, microbiological, and echocardiographic parameters, and should be used to choose the best therapeutic option.[25]

Long-term prognosis

After hospital discharge, the main complications include recurrence of infection, heart failure, need for valve surgery, and death. The 6-month mortality remains high in infective endocarditis, ranging from 22–27%.[26–29] The presence of a vegetation, its size, and its multivalvular location are echocardiographic features associated with a worse prognosis. In a recent series, large vegetations (>15mm length) were associated with a worse prognosis.[21]

To prevent late complications and death, both clinical and echocardiographic follow-up are recommended after discharge. The recent European Society of Cardiology guidelines[2] recommend performing an initial baseline TTE at the completion of antimicrobial therapy, and serial examinations at 1, 3, 6, and 12 months during the first year following completion of therapy. Repeat TOE is usually not necessary after discharge, except in selected patients with incomplete surgical treatment or persistent valve or prosthetic dysfunction.

Echocardiography and decision making

Echocardiography plays a crucial role both for the decision to operate or not and for the choice of the optimal timing of surgery.[30] Indications for surgery in infective endocarditis may be subdivided in three categories: haemodynamic, infectious, and embolic indications.[2]

Haemodynamic indications

Heart failure represents the main indication for surgery in infective endocarditis. Urgent echocardiography is required as soon as symptoms or signs of heart failure are detected.[3] Recent European guidelines recommend early surgery to be performed in patients with acute regurgitation and heart failure, as well as in patients with obstructive vegetations.[2] Echocardiography is useful in both situations. In acute regurgitation, it allows a detailed assessment of valve lesions, a quantification of valve regurgitation, and the evaluation of the haemodynamic tolerance of the regurgitation (cardiac output, pulmonary artery pressures, left and right ventricular function). Some echocardiographic features suggest the need for urgent surgery including premature MV closure (in aortic infective endocarditis), massive regurgitation, and extensive destructive valvular lesions[1–3] (➲ Fig. 16.12). The second haemodynamic indication is obstructive vegetation. In this latter situation, echocardiography provides both the mechanism of obstruction and its

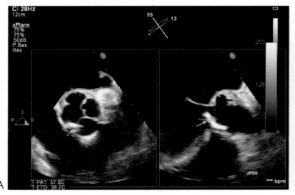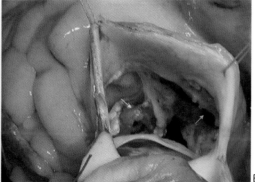

Figure 16.12 Destructive aortic infective endocarditis. Patient with a destructive aortic infective endocarditis: TOE (A) and surgical view (B) showing large pseudoaneurysm (purple arrow) and aortic vegetations (yellow arrow).

quantification. Elevated transvalvular gradients and reduced orifice area can be measured with Doppler echocardiography (see ➲ Chapter 5).

Infectious indications

The infectious complications needing surgery include persisting fever, poor response to antibiotic therapy, and locally uncontrolled infection.[2] Locally uncontrolled infection includes abscess, false aneurysm, fistula, and enlarging vegetation. Echocardiography plays a key role in the assessment of perivalvular lesions, including abscess, false aneurysm, fistula, and aneurysm/perforation (➲ Fig. 16.13). Unless severe comorbidities are present, surgery must be performed when a perivalvular complication is diagnosed by echocardiography. Surgery is urgent in such patients, except in cases of extensive perivalvular lesions associated with severe heart failure, which may need emergency surgery. Rarely, medical therapy alone may be attempted in patients with small non-staphylococcal abscesses (surface area $<1cm^2$) without severe valve regurgitation and without heart failure, in case of rapid and favourable response to antibiotic therapy. Finally, enlarging vegetations under therapy indicates urgent surgery, justifying repeat TTE/TOE in the follow-up of patients with infective endocarditis.

Embolic indications

Since echocardiography plays a major role in the measurement of the vegetation size and thus prediction of the risk embolism, careful measurement of the maximal vegetation size at time of diagnosis and during follow-up is strongly recommended as part of the risk stratification, using both TTE and TOE.[3]

The Task Force on the Prevention, Diagnosis, and Treatment of Infective Endocarditis of the European Society of Cardiology[2] recommends surgical therapy in case of large (>10mm) vegetation following one or more embolic episodes, and when the large vegetation is associated with other predictors of complicated course (heart failure, persistent infection under therapy,

abscess, and prosthetic endocarditis), indicating an earlier surgical decision. The decision to operate early in isolated very large vegetation (>15mm) is more difficult. Surgery may be preferred when a valve repair seems possible, particularly in MV infective endocarditis. Anyhow, the most important point is that the surgery, if needed, must be performed on an urgent basis.

Intraoperative echocardiography

Intraoperative TOE is recommended in all patients with infective endocarditis undergoing cardiac surgery.[2] It is of utmost importance for the final assessment of valvular and perivalvular lesion, just before surgery, and is particularly useful to assess the immediate result of conservative surgery and in cases of complex perivalvular repair. Intraoperative TOE is particularly useful in homograft surgery, which is relatively frequently used in infective endocarditis. Finally, post-pump intraoperative TOE also serves as a reference document of the surgical result for subsequent postoperative echocardiography. In addition, a post-pump intraoperative TOE also helps in the assessment and treatment of difficult weaning from the cardiopulmonary bypass pump and can guide difficult de-airing.[31]

Conclusion

Echocardiography plays a key role in infective endocarditis, both concerning its diagnosis, the diagnosis of its complications, its follow-up under therapy, and its prognostic assessment. Echocardiography is particularly useful for the initial assessment of embolic risk. TOE plays a major role both before surgery and during surgery. Echocardiographic results must be taken into consideration for both the surgical decision and the choice of the optimal timing for surgery. Recent advances in 3D imaging are promising in the better assessment of patients with infective endocarditis.

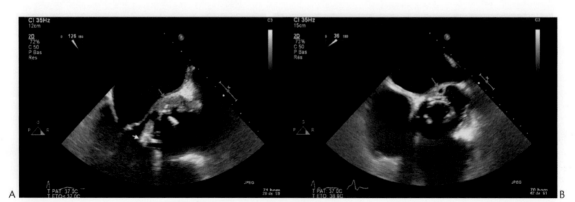

Figure 16.13 Assessment of perivalvular lesion. TOE showing a large abscess (red arrows) around an aortic bioprosthetic valve and a large vegetation (white arrow).

Personal perspective

Although a very old disease, infective endocarditis is also a changing disease, with a new epidemiology, an increasing number of elderly patients, of cases affecting prosthetic valves or intracardiac devices, and of nosocomial cases, which represent up to 30% of all cases of infective endocarditis. In all these situations, echocardiography will play an essential role, both for the diagnosis, the evaluation, and, more importantly, the management of patients with infective endocarditis.

Echocardiographic results must be taken into consideration for both the decision to operate on patients or not and the choice of the optimal timing for surgery. Recent advances in 3D imaging offer additional importance to the echographic evaluation of patients with infective endocarditis. In all cases, however, the results of echocardiographic studies may be interpreted taking into account the clinical features of the patient.

References

1 Habib G. Embolic risk in subacute bacterial endocarditis. Role of transesophageal echocardiography. *Curr Cardiol Rep* 2003; **5**: 129–36.

2 Habib G, Hoen B, Tornos P, Thuny F, Prendergast B, Vilacosta I, *et al.* Guidelines on the prevention, diagnosis, and treatment of infective endocarditis (new version 2009): The Task Force on the Prevention, Diagnosis, and Treatment of Infective Endocarditis of the European Society of Cardiology (ESC). *Eur Heart J* 2009; 30:2369–413.

3 Habib G, Badano L, Tribouilloy C, Vilacosta I, Zamorano JL, Galderisi M, *et al.* Recommendations for the practice of echocardiography in infective endocarditis. *Eur J Echocardiogr* 2010; **11**(2):202–19.

4 Durack DT, Lukes AS, Bright DK. New criteria for diagnosis of infective endocarditis: utilization of specific echocardiographic indings. Duke Endocarditis Service. *Am J Med* 1994; **96**:200–9.

5 Rohmann S, Erbel R, Darius H, Gorge G, Makowski T, Zotz R, *et al.* Prediction of rapid versus prolonged healing of infective endocarditis by monitoring vegetation size. *J Am Soc Echocardiogr* 1991; 4:465–74.

6 Habib G, Derumeaux G, Avierinos JF, Casalta JP, Jamal F, Volot F, *et al.* Value and limitations of the Duke criteria for the diagnosis of infective endocarditis. *J Am Coll Cardiol* 1999; 33:2023–9.

7 Sochowski RA, Chan KL. Implication of negative results on a monoplane transesophageal echocardiographic study in patients with suspected infective endocarditis. *J Am Coll Cardiol* 1993; **21**:216–21.

8 Klug D, Lacroix D, Savoye C, Goullard L, Grandmougin D, Hennequin JL, *et al.* Systemic infection related to endocarditis on pacemaker leads: clinical presentation and management. *Circulation* 1997; **95**:2098–107.

9 Vilacosta I, Sarriá C, San Román JA, Jiménez J, Castillo JA, Iturralde E, *et al.* Usefulness of transesophageal echocardiography for diagnosis of infected transvenous permanent pacemakers. *Circulation* 1994; **89**:2684–7.

10 Victor F, De Place C, Camus C, Le Breton H, Leclerq C, Pavin D, *et al.* Pacemaker lead infection : echocardiographic features, management, and outcome. *Heart* 1999; **81**:82–7.

11 Piper C, Korfer R, Horstkotte D. Prosthetic valve endocarditis. *Heart* 2001; **85**:590–3.

12 Habib G, Thuny F, Avierinos JF. Prosthetic valve endocarditis: current approach and therapeutic options. *Prog Cardiovasc Dis* 2008; **50**:274–81.

13 Lamas CC, Eykyn SJ. Suggested modifications to the Duke criteria for the clinical diagnosis of native valve and prosthetic valve endocarditis: analysis of 118 pathologically proven cases. *Clin Infect Dis* 1997; **25**:713–19.

14 Pedersen WR, Walker M, Olson JD, Gobel F, Lange HW, Daniel JA, *et al.* Value of transesophageal echocardiography as an adjunct to transthoracic echocardiography in evaluation of native and prosthetic valve endocarditis. *Chest* 1991; **100**: 351–6.

15 Perez-Vazquez A, Farinas MC, Garcia-Palomo JD, Bernal JM, Revuelta JM, Gonzalez-Macias J. Evaluation of the Duke criteria in 93 episodes of prosthetic valve endocarditis: could sensitivity be improved? *Arch Intern Med* 2000; **160**:1185–91.

16 Habib G. Management of infective endocarditis. *Heart* 2006; **92**:124–30.

17 Anguera I, Miro JM, Vilacosta I, Almirante B, Anguita M, Munoz P, *et al.* Aorto-cavitary fistulous tract formation in infective endocarditis: clinical and echocardiographic features of 76 cases and risk factors for mortality. *Eur Heart J* 2005; **26**:288–97.

18 Karalis DG, Bansal RC, Hauck AJ, Ross JJ, Jr., Applegate PM, Jutzy KR, *et al.* Transesophageal echocardiographic recognition of subaortic complications in aortic valve endocarditis. Clinical and surgical implications. *Circulation* 1992; **86**:353–62.

19 Hill EE, Herijgers P, Claus P, Vanderschueren S, Peetermans WE, Herregods MC. Abscess in infective endocarditis: the value of transesophageal echocardiography and outcome: a 5-year study. *Am Heart J* 2007; **154**:923–8.

20 Vilacosta I, San Román JA, Sarria C, Iturralde E, Graupner C, Batlle E, *et al.* Clinical, anatomic, and echocardiographic characteristics of aneurysms of the mitral valve. *Am J Cardiol* 1999; **84**:110–13, A119.

21 Thuny F, Di Salvo G, Belliard O, Avierinos JF, Pergola V, Rosenberg V, *et al.* Risk of embolism and death in infective endocarditis: prognostic value of echocardiography: a prospective multicenter study. *Circulation* 2005; **112**:69–75.

22 Di Salvo G, Habib G, Pergola V, Avierinos JF, Philip E, Casalta JP, *et al.* Echocardiography predicts embolic events in infective endocarditis. *J Am Coll Cardiol* 2001; **37**:1069–76.

23 Steckelberg JM, Murphy JG, Ballard D, Bailey K, Tajik AJ, Taliercio CP, *et al.* Emboli in infective endocarditis: the prognostic value of echocardiography. *Ann Intern Med* 1991; **114**:635–40.

24 Vilacosta I, Graupner C, San Román JA, Sarria C, Ronderos R, Fernandez C, *et al.* Risk of embolization after institution of antibiotic therapy for infective endocarditis. *J Am Coll Cardiol* 2002; **39**:1489–95.

25 San Román JA, López J, Vilacosta I, Luaces M, Sarria C, Revilla A, Ronderos R, Stoermann W, Gomez I, Fernandez-Aviles F. Prognostic stratification of patients with left-sided endocarditis determined at admission. *Am J Med* 2007; **120**:369. e1–7.

26 Hasbun R, Vikram HR, Barakat LA, Buenconsejo J, Quagliarello VJ. Complicated left-sided native valve endocarditis in adults: risk classification for mortality. *JAMA* 2003; **289**(15):1933–40.

27 Wallace SM, Walton BI, Kharbanda RK, Hardy R, Wilson AP, Swanton RH. Mortality from infective endocarditis: clinical predictors of outcome. *Heart* 2002; **88**:53–60.

28 Vikram HR, Buenconsejo J, Hasbun R, Quagliarello VJ. Impact of valve surgery on 6-month mortality in adults with complicated, left-sided native valve endocarditis. A propensity analysis. *JAMA* 2003; **290**:3207–14.

29 Hill EE, Herijgers P, Claus P, Vanderschueren S, Herregods MC, Peetermans WE. Infective endocarditis: changing epidemiology and predictors of 6-month mortality: a prospective cohort study. *Eur Heart J* 2007; **28**:196–203.

30 Habib G, Avierinos JF, Thuny F. Aortic valve endocarditis; is there an optimal surgical timing? *Curr Op Cardiol* 2007; **22**:77–83.

31 Shapira Y, Weisenberg DE, Vaturi M, Sharoni E, Raanani E, Sahar G, Vidne BA, Battler A, Sagie A. The impact of intraoperative transesophageal echocardiography in infective endocarditis. *Isr Med Assoc J* 2007; **9**:299–302.

Further reading

Durack DT, Lukes AS, Bright DK. New criteria for diagnosis of infective endocarditis: utilization of specific echocardiographic findings. Duke Endocarditis Service. *Am J Med* 1994; **96**:200–9.

Habib G, Hoen B, Tornos P, Thuny F, Prendergast B, Vilacosta I, *et al.* Guidelines on the prevention, diagnosis, and treatment of infective endocarditis (new version 2009): The Task Force on the Prevention, Diagnosis, and Treatment of Infective Endocarditis of the European Society of Cardiology (ESC). *Eur Heart J* 2009; **30**:2369–413.

Habib G, Badano L, Tribouilloy C, Vilacosta I, Zamorano JL, Galderisi M, *et al.* Recommendations for the practice of echocardiography in infective endocarditis. *Eur J Echocardiogr* 2010; **11**(2):202–19.

Habib G, Derumeaux G, Avierinos JF, Casalta JP, Jamal F, Volot F, *et al.* Value and limitations of the Duke criteria for the diagnosis of infective endocarditis. *J Am Coll Cardiol* 1999; **33**:2023–9.

Hasbun R, Vikram HR, Barakat LA, Buenconsejo J, Quagliarello VJ. Complicated left-sided native valve endocarditis in adults: risk classification for mortality. *JAMA* 2003; **289**(15):1933–40.

Karalis DG, Bansal RC, Hauck AJ, Ross JJ, Jr., Applegate PM, Jutzy KR, *et al.* Transesophageal echocardiographic recognition of subaortic complications in aortic valve endocarditis. Clinical and surgical implications. *Circulation* 1992; **86**:353–62.

San Román JA, López J, Vilacosta I, Luaces M, Sarria C, Revilla A, *et al.* Prognostic stratification of patients with left-sided endocarditis determined at admission. *Am J Med* 2007; **120**:369.e1–7.

Sochowski RA, Chan KL. Implication of negative results on a monoplane transesophageal echocardiographic study in patients with suspected infective endocarditis. *J Am Coll Cardiol* 1993; **21**:216–21.

Steckelberg JM, Murphy JG, Ballard D, Bailey K, Tajik AJ, Taliercio CP, *et al.* Emboli in infective endocarditis: the prognostic value of echocardiography. *Ann Intern Med* 1991; **114**:635–40.

Thuny F, Di Salvo G, Belliard O, Avierinos JF, Pergola V, Rosenberg V, *et al.* Risk of embolism and death in infective endocarditis: prognostic value of echocardiography: a prospective multicenter study. *Circulation* 2005; **112**:69–75.

Additional DVD and online material

■ 16.1 TOE in '90-degree bi-atrial view' showing two thin mobile vegetations on one of pacemaker leads in the right atrium.

■ 16.2 TOE showing a very large and highly mobile vegetation implanted on the pacemaker right ventricular lead and going through the tricuspid valve.

■ 16.3 TTE showing a large and mobile tricuspid vegetation in an intravenous drug user.

■ 16.4 TOE showing a very large and mobile tricuspid vegetation in an intravenous drug user.

■ 16.5 First TOE (45-degree view) performed in a patient with an aortic bioprosthetic valve and a clinical suspicion of endocarditis. This exam does not show any vegetation or abscess.

■ 16.6 TOE (45-degree view) performed 5 days later showing two vegetations on the bioprosthetic cusps.

■ 16.7 TOE showing a large vegetation on the annulus of a mitral mechanical prosthetic valve hampering the leaflets closure.

■ 16.8 TOE showing a large abscess of the anterior mitral leaflet with a very large and mobile vegetation associated with a possible chordae rupture.

■ 16.9 Patient with a destructive aortic infective endocarditis. TOE showing a large pseudo-aneurysm of posterior aortic annulus and aortic vegetations.

■ 16.10 TTE showing an aneurysm of the mitral-aortic fibrosa.

■ 16.11 TOE (120-degree view) showing an aneurysm of the mitral-aortic fibrosa and a prolapse of the right coronary aortic cusp.

■ 16.12 TOE showing a severe aortic regurgitation with an eccentric jet toward the mitral-aortic fibrosa.

▣ 16.13 TOE (120-degree view) showing a mitral-aortic endocarditis with an aortic and mitral perforation.

▣ 16.14 TOE (120-degree view and colour Doppler) showing a mitral-aortic endocarditis with an aortic and mitral perforation.

▣ 16.15 Real-time 3D TOE in an atrial view showing the mitral perforation.

▣ 16.16 TOE (120-degree view) showing a large abscess around the annulus of an aortic bioprosthetic valve and a large vegetation. The bioprosthetic valve moves during all the cardiac cycle because of a large dehiscence

⮑ For additional multimedia materials please visit the online version of the book (🕮 http://escecho.oxfordmedicine.com).

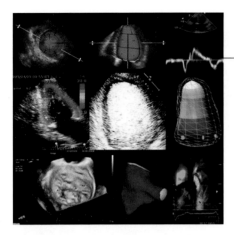

CHAPTER 17

Cardiomyopathies

G. Karatasakis and G.D. Athanassopoulos

Contents

Summary

Echocardiography is a key diagnostic method in the management of patients with cardiomyopathies.

The main echocardiographic findings of hypertrophic cardiomyopathy are asymmetric hypertrophy of the septum, increased echogenicity of the myocardium, systolic anterior motion, turbulent left ventricular (LV) outflow tract blood flow, intracavitary gradient of dynamic nature, mid-systolic closure of the aortic valve and mitral regurgitation. The degree of hypertrophy and the magnitude of the obstruction have prognostic meaning. Echocardiography plays a fundamental role not only in diagnostic process, but also in management of patients, prognostic stratification, and evaluation of therapeutic intervention effects.

In idiopathic dilated cardiomyopathy, echocardiography reveals dilation and impaired contraction of the LV or both ventricles. The biplane Simpson's method incorporates much of the shape of the LV in calculation of volume; currently, three-dimensional echocardiography accurately evaluates LV volumes. Deformation parameters might be used for detection of early ventricular involvement. Stress echocardiography using dobutamine or dipyridamole may contribute to risk stratification, evaluating contractile reserve and left anterior descending flow reserve. LV dyssynchrony assessment is challenging and in patients with biventricular pacing already applied, optimization of atrio-interventricular delays should be done. Specific characteristics of right ventricular dysplasia and isolated LV non-compaction can be recognized, resulting in an increasing frequency of their prevalence. Rare forms of cardiomyopathy related with neuromuscular disorders can be studied at an earlier stage of ventricular involvement.

Restrictive and infiltrative cardiomyopathies are characterized by an increase in ventricular stiffness with ensuing diastolic dysfunction and heart failure. A variety of entities may produce this pathological disturbance with amyloidosis being the most prevalent. Storage diseases (Fabry, Gaucher, Hurler) are currently treatable and early detection of ventricular involvement is of paramount importance for successful treatment. Traditional differentiation between constrictive pericarditis (surgically manageable) and the rare cases of restrictive cardiomyopathy should be properly performed.

Hypertrophic cardiomyopathy

Introduction

Hypertrophic cardiomyopathy (HCM) is an autosomal dominant genetic heart disease. The morphological characteristics consist of a hypertrophic, non-dilated left ventricle (LV) in the absence of an apparent cause of hypertrophy. Patients with HCM may develop hypertension or aortic stenosis (AS). The diagnosis in these cases should not rely solely on morphological characteristics. However, in most cases, the degree of hypertrophy is unexpectedly high when the severity of the AS or the duration and the severity of hypertension are taken into account. HCM is probably the most frequent cardiomyopathy, and is considered as the first cause of sudden cardiac death in young age. Its prevalence can be as high as 1/500 in the general population. The annual mortality rate varies from 1–6% and most of the deaths occur suddenly in children and young adults of whom 22% are previously asymptomatic.

Physiopathology

Hypertrophy, myocardial disarray interstitial fibrosis, and small coronary arteries abnormalities are the pathological characteristics of HCM. Disarray is often extensive and may involve significant portions of the LV and right ventricle (RV). Interstitial fibrosis is more pronounced in the interventricular septum (IVS) as well as abnormalities of the intramural coronary arteries wall.

Sudden cardiac death in young age is the most dramatic symptom of HCM. Systolic dysfunction occurs late in the course of the disease, in up to 10% of patients with HCM and is characterized by wall thinning and LV dilation. Heart failure (HF) with *preserved* systolic function is very common, with the disease being used as a paradigm of diastolic dysfunction. Myocardial ischaemia is due to intramural coronary arteries wall changes and demand–supply imbalance. The genetic substrate of HCM is missense mutations that involve an amino acid substitution. Numerous mutant genes have been identified, the most common being β-myosin heavy chain and myosin binding protein C. The pleomorphic nature of the disease phenotype parallels the heterogeneity of its genetic substrate.[1]

Echocardiography morphological characteristics

The main morphological criterion for the diagnosis of HCM is the presence of asymmetric septal hypertrophy.

Patterns of hypertrophy

Four main types of hypertrophy distribution have been proposed. Type I involves the anterior segment of the IVS, type II involves the anterior and the inferior septum, type III involves the anterolateral wall of the IVS (⮞ Fig 17.1) and type IV

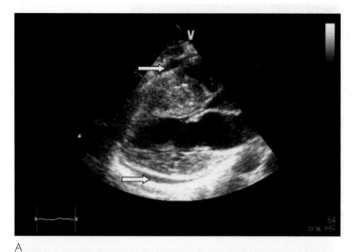

A

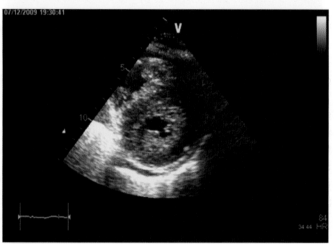

B

Figure 17.1 Hypertrophic cardiomyopathy: type III. A) Parasternal long-axis view of a patient with hypertrophic cardiomyopathy, diffuse hypertrophy (type III), and small pericardial effusion (arrows). B) Parasternal short-axis view of the same patient with hypertrophic cardiomyopathy, type III.

involves the apex (⮞ Fig 17.2). The majority of patients (52%) exhibit type III pattern of hypertrophy while type II and IV (apical) is observed in 20% and 18%. It is interesting that the degree of hypertrophy is recently considered a major determinant of the disease course in patients with wall thickness greater than 30mm, having a 40% risk of sudden death.[3] However, no clear distinction of subtypes of the disease according to the wall thickness can be made.

The presence of *angled* ventricular septum can be erroneously interpreted as asymmetric septal hypertrophy. This can become a diagnostic dilemma especially in elderly patients with an uncertain history of hypertension. The term hypertrophic cardiomyopathy of the elderly is controversial. The condition seems to be more common in women, the hypertrophy is localized and the hypertrophy is mild. It is unclear whether elderly patients with localized hypertrophy of the septum or septal bulge should be diagnosed as HCM. Left ventricular diastolic diameter is normal

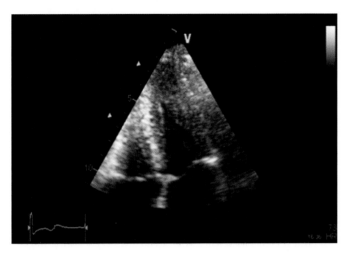

Figure 17.2 Hypertrophic cardiomyopathy: type IV. Apical four-chamber view of a patient with hypertrophy of the distal septum and the distal lateral wall.

or even dilated in these patients. Right ventricular involvement is also very rare in this subgroup. Patients with more diffuse patterns of hypertrophy and lack of 'accompanying' findings such as systolic anterior motion are more difficult to diagnose. Conversely patients with a localized form of hypertrophy as well as patients with intracavitary obstruction at rest are easier to diagnose. On the other hand, the presence of LV outflow tract obstruction (LVOTO) is not synonymous with HCM.

Several reports are dealing with the possibility of a linkage among the genetic disorder, the phenotypic expression in terms of hypertrophy pattern and the clinical outcome. In one study[4] it has been suggested that patients with mutations of the cardiac myosin binding protein C do not exhibit hypertrophy until middle age and beyond. Delayed expression of hypertrophy and a benign clinical course may hinder the recognition of the heritable nature of mutations in the cardiac myosin binding protein C gene. Furthermore, in another study[5] troponin T mutations were found in 15% of families with the disease and are related with mild or subclinical hypertrophy but increased probability of sudden cardiac death in young age.

Cavity size

LV dimensions are usually small. The size of the LV can be used to differentiate HCM from other causes of hypertrophy. LV hypertrophy caused by hypertension is usually accompanied by ventricular dilation. Athlete's heart and aortic stenosis can also be differentiated on the basis of LV size from HCM. Left atrium (LA) is dilated in most patients with HCM. This is due to the increased diastolic pressure of the ventricle and to the coexistence of mitral regurgitation (MR). Right heart chambers are usually of normal dimensions.

Echocardiographic appearance of the myocardium

Myocardial thickness and appearance are important for the echocardiographic diagnosis of HCM. The ratio of IVS to posterior wall thickness has been extensively used as a basic diagnostic criterion for a definite diagnosis. A cut-off point for this ratio with high sensitivity but relatively low specificity is 1.3,[6] while a value of 1.5 seems to be more specific.[7] However, the lack of specific measurement sites limits the value of this diagnostic criterion. The myocardial appearance on the echocardiogram is another characteristic of HCM. The myocardium is of increased echogenicity with *sparkling* or *ground glass* appearance which was considered the echocardiographic equivalent of myocardial disarray and fibrosis (➲ Fig 17.3). However, similar myocardial appearance can be seen in cardiac amyloidosis. The differential diagnosis between HCM and cardiac amyloidosis will be based on the concentric character of hypertrophy and the systolic dysfunction of amyloidosis. Involvement of the RV myocardium can also be seen in patients with HCM.

Endocardial thickening at the site of systolic anterior motion–septal contact point

In patients with systolic anterior motion (SAM), the repeated contact of the mitral apparatus with the IVS may result to a characteristic *notch* of the septal endocardium at the point of SAM-septal contact. This contact lesion is not specific for HCM (➲ Fig 17.4).

Geometric changes of the mitral apparatus

The mitral apparatus exhibits anterior displacement in patients with HCM. This displacement is due to the translocation of the papillary muscles tips, caused by the septal hypertrophy.[8] Because of this reduction of the distance between the tips of the papillary muscles, an apparent excess of leaflet tissue is formed and low tension is applied to the leaflets through the chordae tendineae. The mitral leaflets appear elongated, oversized for the cavity size, and provide the substrate for the functional characteristic of LVOTO.

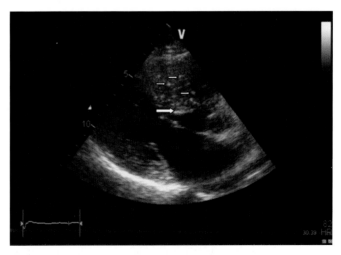

Figure 17.3 Parasternal long-axis view of a patient with hypertrophic cardiomyopathy. Diastolic frame. Note the increased echogenicity of the endocardium at the point of contact with the anterior mitral leaflet (large arrow) and the 'ground glass' appearance of the myocardium (small arrows).

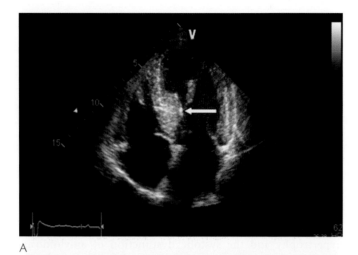

A

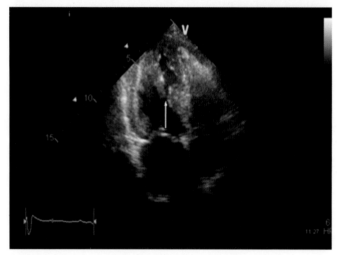

B

Figure 17.4 Asymmetric hypertrophy of the basal septum. A) Apical four-chamber view of a patient with hypertrophic cardiomyopathy. Diastolic frame. Asymmetric hypertrophy of the basal septum and endocardial thickening at the SAM septal contact point (arrow). B) Apical long-axis view of the same patient. Note the close vicinity of the asymmetrically hypertrophied septum with the posteromedial papillary muscle (arrow).

Functional features

Systolic function of the ventricles

HCM was considered for years a paradigm of *pure* diastolic dysfunction with normal or *super normal* contractility. This was before the possibility to evaluate longitudinal function and myocardial strain and strain rate (SR) by tissue Doppler (TD) imaging. Systolic function of both ventricles remains apparently normal throughout the natural history of the disease in the majority of cases. However, longitudinal thickening, strain and SR may result impaired even in the early stages of disease. At end stage, significant impairment of contractility may occur resulting from myocardial fibrosis. Coexisting coronary artery disease (CAD) or repeated surgical procedures may contribute to this loss of contractility.

Mechanisms of generation of intracavitary gradients

LVOTO and SAM of mitral valve (MV) leaflet were initially recognized by M-mode echocardiography. Geometric changes of the mitral apparatus and asymmetric hypertrophy of the septum provide the anatomic substrate for the development of intraventricular pressure gradient.

Systolic anterior motion of mitral valve

Several mechanisms have been proposed for the initiation and maintenance of the SAM. Venturi phenomenon is involved: the initial flow acceleration because of the anatomical narrowing of LV outflow tract (LVOT) produces high blood velocity and low pressure in the LVOT which *sacks* the mitral apparatus towards the septum.[9,10] The part of the mitral apparatus which plays a predominant role in the generation of SAM is usually the tip of the anterior mitral leaflet. When the mitral apparatus touches the IVS, the SAM is *complete*. Complete SAM lasting for more than 30% of systole is associated with significant LVOTO.[11] The SAM can be visualized by M-mode and two-dimensional (2D) echocardiography from the parasternal long-axis (PLAX) and short-axis (PSAX) views and the apical four- (A4C) and three-chamber (A3C) views by 2D echocardiography (➲ Figs. 17.5 and 17.6).

Premature closure of the aortic valve

This systolic reduction of the normal initial opening of the aortic cusps occurs abruptly at late systole. It is a secondary phenomenon due to the SAM and the intracavitary gradient. It can be documented by M-mode echocardiography and is often accompanied by systolic fluttering of the valve cusps. It occurs simultaneously with SAM–septal contact and the delayed peaking of the systolic flow gradient.

Types of obstruction: dynamic versus fixed

Dynamic outflow gradient is identified by Doppler echocardiography. The exact location of the obstruction can be

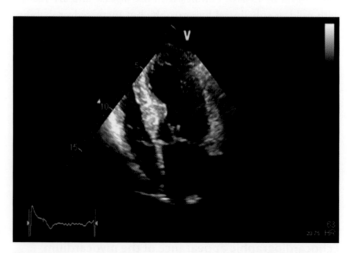

Figure 17.5 Complete SAM in apical four-chamber view. Systolic frame, apical four-chamber view of a patient with hypertrophic cardiomyopathy and complete SAM.

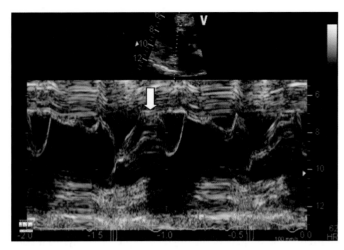

Figure 17.6 M-mode recording of complete SAM. Complete SAM (arrow) in a patient with hypertrophic cardiomyopathy. M-mode tracing.

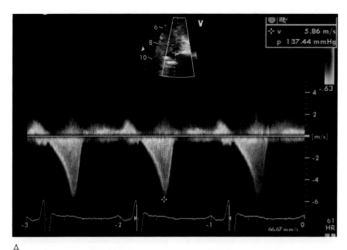

A

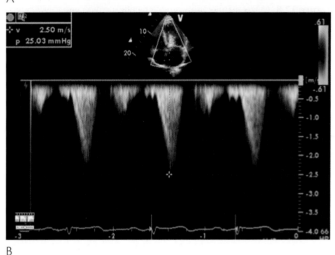

B

Figure 17.7 Late peaking of the flow. A) Continuous Doppler recording of a patient with significant intracavitary obstruction. The flow velocity is peaking in late systole and the pattern indicates dynamic obstruction. B) Continuous wave Doppler recording of a patient with hypertrophic cardiomyopathy, moderate intracavitary gradient, and late peaking characteristic of dynamic obstruction.

documented by colour Doppler (CD) and pulsed wave (PW) Doppler echocardiography. By continuous wave (CW) Doppler recording from the apical windows, the flow gradient pattern exhibits late peaking of the flow velocity curve. The recognition of the late peaking of the Doppler flow signal is important to distinguish the dynamic obstruction of HCM from the fixed subaortic aortic stenosis. In the latter no evidence of late peaking exists and the flow pattern is similar to the valvular aortic stenosis.

Apical flow acceleration

Using PW Doppler relatively high systolic velocity with late peaking is evident at the apical region in patients with HCM. This can be used as a diagnostic criterion of the disease.[12]

Doppler characteristics of dynamic obstruction

The characteristic flow pattern of dynamic flow obstruction is the late peaking of the flow. The other important feature is the variability of the LVOT velocity (➲ Fig 17.7).

Mechanisms of generation of MR and Doppler echocardiographic features of MR

MR in HCM is related to the geometric changes of the mitral apparatus and the generation of the SAM. MR due to secondary changes of the valve is not uncommon. Typically the MR jet due to geometric changes of the mitral apparatus is directed posteriorly. This is due to the fact that the anterior leaflet is elongated and contacts the septum to a greater degree than the posterior leaflet. Conversely when the MR is due to the combination of the geometric changes of the mitral apparatus and secondary morphologic changes, the direction of the jet is variable. The development of mitral annular calcification may also interfere with the mechanism of the regurgitation and the direction of the jet. The severity of MR is related to the distance of the leaflets during systole, and the severity of the obstruction.[13] Patients with HCM have very small end-systolic volume. Consequently an

amount of regurgitant volume (RVol) that is well tolerated in patients with chronic MR of other aetiology can be difficult to cope with in patients with HCM (➲ Fig 17.8).

Provoking manoeuvres of intracavitary gradient

The inhalation of amyl nitrate was used during the echocardiographic study to increase the degree of intracavitary obstruction or to provoke intracavitary gradients in patients with the *non-obstructive* form of the disease. Amyl nitrate produces simultaneous venous and arterial dilation and increases obstruction by reducing both preload and afterload. This approach based on provoking manoeuvres to the physiological features of HCM is no longer in use because it was proven that its clinical value and prognostic yield was limited despite the fact that recently clinical importance of the severity of intracavitary obstruction has been reemphasized. Conversely the combination of echocardiography with treadmill exercise test may reveal significant increase of intracavitary gradient. The relation with patients'

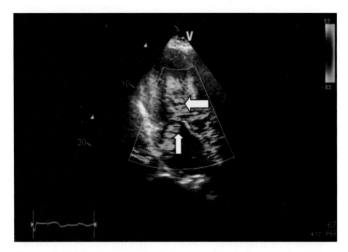

Figure 17.8 Mitral regurgitation in hypertrophic cardiomyopathy. Apical long-axis view with colour Doppler display. Turbulent flow in the left ventricular outflow tract (horizontal arrow). Moderate mitral regurgitation with the jet directed posteriorly (vertical arrow).

symptoms is the great advantage of physiological exercise over amyl nitrate and other pharmacological interventions

Diastolic function

Diastolic dysfunction is considered the most significant mechanism producing symptoms in HCM.[14] Impaired LV diastolic filling was extensively studied with the clinical application of spectral Doppler. Filling impairment reflects the impairment of the other two components of diastole—the chamber stiffness and the relaxation. All diastolic components are affected by the hypertrophy, inactivation of myofibrils, ischaemia because of decreased coronary flow delayed relaxation.

The mitral inflow diastolic pattern (◉ Fig 17.9) demonstrates increased isovolumic relaxation time (IVRT), decreased flow velocity during rapid filling of the ventricle (E wave), prolonged deceleration time (DT), of the E wave and increased velocity during atrial contraction (A wave). These abnormalities may remain throughout the clinical course of the disease. In the few patients who demonstrate progression from the *hyper-contractile* small LV to the dilated hypocontractile fibrotic ventricle of end-stage disease the inflow pattern changes dramatically. Very high

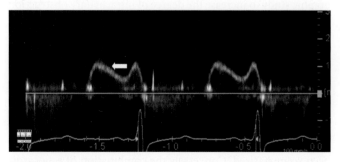

Figure 17.9 Mitral inflow in hypertrophic cardiomyopathy. Mitral inflow of a patient with hypertrophic cardiomyopathy. Prolonged deceleration of the E wave (arrow).

and ill sustained E wave with shortened DT and a small A wave are the characteristics of the stage.

Longitudinal function

TD velocity and strain imaging is a developing imaging method offering further insights to the analysis of ventricular function in patients with HCM (◉ Fig. 17.10).

The E/E′ ratio, with E′ representing the diastolic velocity of the mitral annulus during rapid filling of the LV, correlates with relaxation parameters and filling pressure.[15] The regional myocardial fibre disarray which is the pathological hallmark of the disease and results in locally dysfunctioning myocardium can be depicted by the lack of systolic deformation.[16] The decrease of the systolic velocity of the mitral annulus below 4cm/s is considered a bad prognostic sign.[17] Diastolic abnormality detectable by TD imaging can be evident prior to the appearance of classical 2D echocardiographic finding.[18–21]

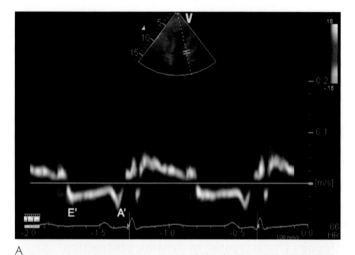

A

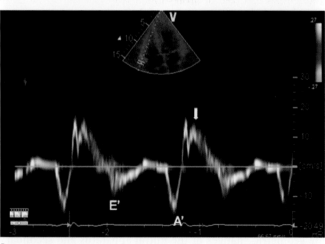

B

Figure 17.10 Tissue Doppler velocity tracing in hypertrophic cardiomyopathy. A) Tissue Doppler velocity tracing of the lateral mitral annulus with prominent A′ wave. The systolic velocity of the lateral mitral annulus is >4cm/s. B) Tissue Doppler velocity tracing of a patient with hypertrophic cardiomyopathy exhibiting normal systolic velocity of the tricuspid annulus (arrow). The E′ is also normal. The A′ is prominent.

Limitations and pitfalls
Erroneous measurement of wall thickness

The precise measurement of the wall thickness is very important for the correct diagnosis of HCM. The complete distinction of the endocardium on both sides of the IVS is sometimes difficult especially in obese patients with large chest. Structures of the RV such as false tendons, trabeculae, and moderator band represent significant sources of overdiagnosis in HCM. The presence of angled IVS especially in elderly patients can also be misinterpreted. The display of several echocardiographic views and the performance of a complete echocardiographic examination is the way to overcome these diagnostic pitfalls. The PSAX view is particularly useful in distinguishing the RV trabeculae from the septum. Conversely the apical views cannot be used for the distinction of RV trabeculae or the moderator band from the septum.

Differential diagnosis from secondary hypertrophy

Differential diagnosis from other forms of hypertrophy will be based on the presence of a stenotic aortic valve, the LV size, which is usually enlarged in patients with hypertrophy due to hypertension, and in the presence of systolic dysfunction in patients with amyloidosis. Phaeochromocytoma and Friedreich's ataxia are more rare causes of hypertrophy. Fabry disease can easily be misdiagnosed as HCM. Given the possibility for enzyme replacement therapy, the differential diagnosis is important and will be based on the measurement of enzyme levels in patients with Fabry disease.

Athlete's heart

Individuals involved in professional, semiprofessional, or competitive sport activities raise a significant amount of medicolegal issues. Sudden unexpected death during an athletic activity of a young individual is usually a dramatic event. The real clinical and prognostic yield of the discovery of a hypertrophied LV in a young athlete is not totally understood. Body surface area (BSA), type and intensity of athletic activity, as well as duration of the athletic season determine the degree of LV hypertrophy that may reach 16mm in elite athletes. Therefore the recommendation to perform echocardiograms as screening tests in children ready to start their involvement in sports is not justified and would be a disaster in economic terms. A solution for differential diagnosis could be the screening of athletes off season with the *physiological* hypertrophy expected to regress without intense training.

Assessment of therapy
Evaluation of gradient reduction by medical therapy

The measurement of the intracavitary gradient by CW Doppler in a patient with HCM at baseline and after therapy with negative inotropic agents emphasizes the possibility of echo to be used as a clinical tool. Beta-blockers without vasodilation effect and disopyramide with a significant negative inotropic effect combined with suppression of ventricular arrhythmias seem to have less contraindication than verapamil and diltiazem. Although no clear benefit on survival has been proven, there is some benefit on symptomatic status as well as on the degree of obstruction.

Selection of atrioventricular delay after DDD pacing

The induction of asynchronous contraction of the basal IVS may decrease the LVOTO and reduce intracavitary gradient. After the initial enthusiasm with the method, it was clarified that placebo effect was interfering, so that the indication for dual chamber pacing in HCM is currently restricted to patients with significant gradient, symptoms refractory to medical therapy, and contraindications for alcohol septal ablation or myectomy. However patients who have a dual chamber pacemaker implanted may improve LV filling by prolonging atrioventricular (AV) delay, so that the improvement of filling will not produce more vigorous contraction. Measuring cardiac output by echocardiography in different levels of AV delay permits optimization of timing of cardiac events to produce the highest output.

Alcohol ablation: patient selection, monitoring, assessment of outcome

The infusion of ethanol into the septal perforator and the consequent necrosis of the basal septum mimics the effect of surgical myectomy without the need for operation. The location of the proper branch is done by injecting intracoronary contrast agents (see ➲ Chapter 7). The myocardial region to be selected is the site of endocardial thickening at the place of SAM–septal contact. Use of contrast echocardiography determines occurrence of smaller infarcts with lower levels of creatine kinase-MB (CKMB), less need for pacemaker implantation[22] and reduction of intracavitary gradient at rest and during follow-up.

Intraoperative guidance of surgical septal myectomy and mitral valve surgery

Surgical myectomy of the septum in HCM can be performed with a mortality rate of less than 2%. The operation is technically demanding and requires a lengthy learning curve which is difficult to achieve given the relatively low frequency of this operation. The operation is associated with long-lasting symptomatic improvement in patients with significant intracavitary gradient. There is also some evidence from non-randomized studies for survival benefit and reduction of rate of sudden cardiac death. The identification of a significant resting gradient in a symptomatic patient who does not respond to medical therapy and is unsuitable for alcohol ablation is the initial indication for surgical myectomy. Echocardiography may investigate the exact mechanism of SAM and MR defining the anatomic parts involved and setting the need for MV surgery. Echocardiography will also assess the aortic valve prior to surgical myectomy to evaluate the degree of concomitant aortic regurgitation. The intraoperative use of transoesophageal echocardiography is important because the surgical field is not clearly visible through the aortic valve and the aortic annulus. The removal of the hypertrophied muscle is done almost blindly and the surgeons tend to remove less muscle to avoid iatrogenic ventricular septal defects and damage of the conduction system. The use of intraoperative echocardiography enables immediate assessment of the residual gradient before the patient leaves the operating theatre.[23]

Screening of relatives

Screening methods of first-degree relatives of patients with HCM may range from physical examination with 12-lead electrocardiogram (ECG) to genetic analysis. Echocardiography is the most widely used screening test for relatives of patients with HCM. The diagnostic criteria used in relatives of patients with HCM are wider than in individuals that are screened for other reasons. Mild echocardiographic hypertrophy should be interpreted differently in a relative of a patient with HCM, especially if in young age. Young children first-degree relatives of patients with HCM should be regularly screened at 5-year intervals because the complete phenotypic expression of HCM may delay for several years.[24]

Dilated cardiomyopathy

Introduction

Idiopathic dilated cardiomyopathy (DCM) is characterized by dilation and impaired contraction of the LV or both ventricles. DCM can lead to progressive refractory HF and represents the majority of heart transplantation referrals. It is also associated with a high rate of sudden death and a mortality rate of 15–50% at 5 years.[25] Early diagnosis of DCM is of prognostic importance because an effective treatment started at the beginning of the disease may delay the development of symptomatic HF.

Aetiology

The aetiology and the pathogenetic mechanisms are unknown in half of the patients. The most prevalent toxic cause of DCM is alcohol.[26] Genetic transmission of the disease is detectable in at least 25% of DCM patients.[26] However, the true frequency is still probably underestimated as no clinical or histopathological characteristic allows a distinction between familial and non-familial cases. As many as 30% of index cases of DCM will have other family members with evidence of LV dysfunction or enlargement on echocardiography. Familial DCM is heterogeneous,[27] with autosomal trait prevailing and variable

clinical features. Based on clinical and molecular genetic data, different forms are distinguished. Familial DCM is clinically and diagnostically the same as other forms of DCM, so family history is essential. The autosomal dominant forms are the most common inheritance accounting for about 85–90% of cases.

Hereditary DCM as an autosomal dominant includes the following mutations of protein-coding genes:

◆ Cytoskeleton: desmin, tafazin, b-sarcoglycan, d-sarcoglycan, dystrophin, metavinculin.
◆ Intercellular connections: vinculin.
◆ Nuclear envelope: laminin A/C, emerin.
◆ Sarcomer: troponin T, heavy chain in beta-myosin, actin, telotonin.
◆ Ionic channels: phospholamban (calcium pump), a subunit of the heart potassium channel sensitive to triphosphate.
◆ Mitochondrion DNA.

Sarcomere gene mutations responsible for causing HCM are also associated with DCM (MYBPC3; MYH7; TNNT2; cardiac troponin I, TNNI3; tropomyosin, TPM1; cardiac actin, ACTC) and they account for 10–15% of familial DCM. Lamin A/C (LMNA) is the most frequent disease-associated gene for familial DCM with conduction system disease. LMNA gene is involved in up to 30–50% of patients with cardiac conduction disorders and DCM.[28–31] Dilated cardiomyopathy caused by LMNA gene defects are highly penetrant, adult onset, malignant diseases characterized by a high rate of heart failure and life-threatening arrhythmias, predicted by New York Heart Association (NYHA) functional class, competitive sport activity and type of mutation.[32]

The majority of the skeletal muscle dystrophies, including the Duchenne and Becker types, may have cardiac involvement. In some families, cardiac involvement may be dominant and present first.[33] Some forms of cardiomyopathies, which are difficult to classify, may also belong in the DCM group. Patients may present with very mild symptoms and a dilated LV. These cases may be early forms of DCM and their frequency is increased in asymptomatic family members of index DCM cases.[34]

Myocardial fibrosis may occur without any clear cause and be associated with ventricular arrhythmias rather than LV dilation and HF. Such cases have been equated in the past with healed myocarditis but are increasingly being recognized as familial, although the genes are not identified.

DCM can be split into groups according to the evidence of chronic myocarditis/viral persistence. Modifications of therapy based on immunosuppression have been proposed accordingly.[35]

Diagnostic criteria

An ECG is essential for DCM. In poor echo windows, cardiac magnetic resonance (CMR) may be useful and contrast echocardiography should be performed. Diagnostic criteria for DCM are represented by depressed contractile function indices and increased LV dimensions: in particular, diagnosis of DCM is formulated in presence of an ejection fraction (EF) less than 0.45 and/or a fractional shortening of less than 25%, and a LV end-diastolic dimension (LVEDD) higher than 112% of predicted value corrected for age and body surface area (BSA). A value greater than 112% of the predicted one represents two standard deviations from the mean corrected for age and BSA, and is given by the following formula:[36]

$$[45.3 \times (\text{body surface area})1/3 - (0.03 \times \text{age}) - 7.2] \pm 12\%$$

A more conservative cut-off of higher than 117% (two standard deviations + 5%) has been proposed in order to increase specificity for family studies.[37] However, a value of 112% is probably just as predictive of disease if systolic function is also abnormal.[37]

Moreover, anatomical changes, which occur throughout the natural history of the disease, may be easily detected by 2D echocardiography. They include:

♦ Dilation of the LV.

♦ Changes in the shape of the LV (from ellipsoidal to spherical).

♦ Changes in spatial configuration of the MV and subvalvular apparatus.

♦ Enlargement of the LA, the RV and the right atrium (RA).

2D and Doppler echocardiography provide information on LV size, systolic and diastolic function. They may be considered as indicators of an unfavourable prognosis in DCM.[38] Such indicators are summarized as follows (➲ Figs. 17.11 and 17.12):

♦ LV end-systolic diameter (LVESD) >55mm and LV end-diastolic diameter (LVEDD) >64mm.

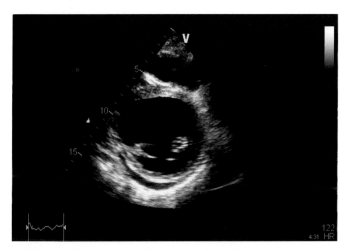

Figure 17.11 Large end-diastolic diameter. LV short-axis: endiastolic diameter >70mm with small pericardial effusion.

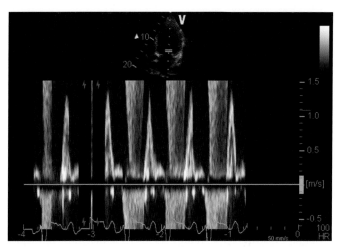

Figure 17.12 Restrictive filling pattern. Mitral inflow with restrictive pattern of LV filling.

♦ LVEF <40%.

♦ Sphericity index <1.5.

♦ dP/dt <600mmHg/s.

♦ Tei index (myocardial performance index) >0.4.

♦ Restrictive mitral inflow pattern.

♦ Pseudonormalization of mitral inflow.

Familial dilated cardiomyopathy

The clinical status of members of families with familial DCM should be evaluated.[39] Major and minor criteria have been established in order to achieve the diagnosis in the first-degree relative of patients with DCM. Major criteria are represented by defined criteria for DCM:

♦ Presence of two or more affected individuals in a single family.

♦ Presence of a first-degree relative of a DCM patient, with well documented unexplained sudden death[25] at less than 35 years of age.

Minor criteria consist in:

♦ Unexplained supraventricular (atrial fibrillation or sustained arrhythmias) or ventricular arrhythmias, frequent (>1000/24h) or repetitive (three or more beats with >120 beats/min) before the age of 50.

♦ LV dilation >112% of the predicted value.

♦ LV dysfunction: EF <50% or fractional shortening <28%.

♦ Unexplained conduction disease: II or III atrioventricular conduction defects, complete LV bundle branch block, sinus nodal dysfunction.

♦ Unexplained sudden death or stroke before 50 years of age.

- Segmental wall motion abnormalities in the absence of intra-ventricular conduction defect or ischaemic heart disease.

European guidelines for the study of familial DCM[37] propose that the diagnosis of familial DCM would be fulfilled in a first-degree relative in the presence of:

- Both LV dilation and systolic dysfunction.
- LV dilation (>117%) + one minor criterion.
- Three minor criteria.

Diagnostic process also requires that exclusion criteria[39] are considered:

- Systemic arterial hypertension (AH), defined as systemic blood pressure >160/100mmHg documented and confirmed at repeated measurements and/or evidence of target-organ disease.
- Coronary heart disease, represented by obstruction >50% of the luminal diameter in a major branch.
- History of chronic excess of alcohol consumption, defined as consumption >40g/day for female and >80g/day for males for more than 5 years, according to the World health Organization criteria, with remission of DCM after 6 months of abstinence.
- Clinical, sustained, and rapid supraventricular arrhythmias.
- Systemic diseases.
- Pericardial diseases.
- Congenital heart disease.
- Cor pulmonale.

Clinically there are a lot of important causes of secondary DCM that include alcohol and cocaine abuse, HIV infection, metabolic abnormalities, as well as the cardiotoxicity of anti-cancer drugs—most notably doxorubicin and newly introduced drugs that inhibit tyrosine kinases. The following four specific disorders are particularly important to recognize in that correct diagnosis has a major impact on patient management and chance for recovery.

- Stress cardiomyopathy or *takotsubo cardiomyopathy* or *broken heart syndrome*: this is an acute cardiomyopathy that can be provoked by a stressful or emotional situation. This cardiomyopathy is most common among middle-aged women, appears to be related to catecholamine release, and in most cases is fully reversible with supportive care.
- Peripartum cardiomyopathy: this is defined as a cardiomyopathy manifesting between the last month of pregnancy and 6 months postpartum. Inflammatory factors are highly implicated and some studies reveal a high incidence of lymphocytic inflammation. It is important to differentiate peripartum cardiomyopathy from a chronic cardiomyopathy exacerbated by the volume load occurring during pregnancy (see ➲ Chapter 18).

- Tachyarrhythmia induced cardiomyopathy: patients may develop a DCM with congestive HF in the face of recurrent or persistent tachycardias. There is a high rate of full recovery with control of the arrhythmia. This cardiomyopathy is notable for the degree to which it phenotypically resembles idiopathic DCM, yet is characterized by a remarkable degree of recovery in LV function once the arrhythmia is controlled. Patients should be carefully monitored by echocardiography in order to identify signs of recovery in the weeks to months following presentation.
- Alcoholic Cardiomyopathy: it is the most common secondary cardiomyopathy. Phenotypically and clinically, it closely resembles idiopathic DCM.

Echocardiographic analysis of dilated cardiomyopathy

Systolic function

The presence of diffuse wall motion abnormalities (WMAs) suggests DCM. However, the sign is not specific since there are often cases of non-uniform distribution of wall motion/thickening abnormalities in DCM.[40] Parameters commonly assessed by echocardiography are load dependent, i.e. LVEF, dP/dt, and stroke volume. There are several less load dependent measures of global systolic function that may allow a more comprehensive assessment of ventricular function. These include:

- Elastance (emax), which can be derived from the end systolic pressure–volume or pressure–dimension relationships.
- Cyclic variation of integrated backscatter.
- LV strain/strain rate.[43,44]

Strain and strain rate appear to be less affected by cardiac motion and segmental myocardial tethering. Despite recognized limitations, the most common measure of systolic function derived from echocardiography is the LVEF. The biplane Simpson's method using two apical views incorporates much of the shape of the LV in its calculation of volume; this is particularly important in the myopathic heart with its alterations in shape. Currently 3D echocardiography provides a unique tool to evaluate accurately LV volumes.[43]

Diastolic function

The transmitral and pulmonary venous Doppler recordings combined with the mitral annular TD velocity is used to identify patterns of impaired ventricular relaxation and restriction to filling. The propagation of blood flow in the LV cavity can be quantified by colour M-mode. The flow propagation velocity is inversely proportional to *Tau* (time constant of isovolumic relaxation). The ratio of transmitral E velocity to mitral annular E′ velocity (E/E′) is related linearly to LA pressure. As LA pressure increases, LV diastolic dysfunction in patients with DCM progressively evolves from impaired ventricular relaxation to restrictive filling pattern throughout pseudonormal stage (see ⮕ Chapter 9). Delayed relaxation is characterized by a decreased transmitral Doppler E/A ratio, a prolonged transmitral Doppler E wave deceleration time (>240ms), and a pulmonary venous Doppler systolic/diastolic velocity ratio greater than 1. A progressive increase in the LV end-diastolic pressure can alter this pattern of delayed relaxation, resulting in pseudonormal transmitral Doppler pattern, which will have a normal E/A ratio, a pulmonary venous Doppler systolic/diastolic wave velocity ratio less than 1 and a reduced TD annular E′ wave velocity (<10cm/s). With further increases in LA pressure, the transmitral E wave DT decreases and the E/A ratio increases resulting in a restrictive pattern, with E wave DT less than 150ms, E/A ratio greater than 2, and mitral annular TD E′ velocity less than 10cm/s.

Functional valve regurgitation

In DCM, the atrioventricular valve incompetence is typically *functional* and reflects geometric distortions of the chambers. The closure of the valve leaflets tends to be displaced towards the ventricle and is known as incomplete valve closure (⮕ Fig 17.13). Mitral RV (regurgitant volume) is determined by parameters including mitral annulus diameter, dyssynchrony, tenting height (area) and contractility of the LV mid-lateral wall.[44] In the presence of aortic and mitral regurgitant Doppler velocity profiles, and since in DCM there is no obstruction to left heart inflow or outflow, LA and LV end-diastolic pressures can be estimated using the simplified Bernoulli's equation (⮕ Equation 5.3). LA systolic pressure and LV diastolic pressure may be calculated, as described in ⮕ Chapter 5 (see ⮕ Fig 5.19).

Risk stratification

LVEF has long been the primary index used as a marker of risk in HF and its strength has been demonstrated even in the elderly.[45] During exercise ergometry in DCM, maximum oxygen consumption is related to LV and RV dimensions and

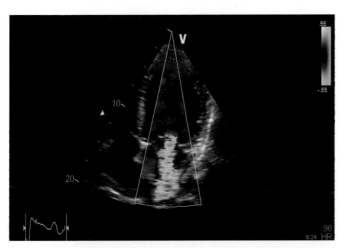

Figure 17.13 Functional mitral regurgitation. Significant mitral regurgitation (central jet with an estimated PISA orifice 0.30mm²).

filling pattern, and to LVEF. Both systolic and diastolic dysfunction influence functional capacity. The transmitral PW Doppler DT correlates with maximum oxygen consumption.[46] Restrictive LV filling pattern is frequent in DCM, is associated with more severe disease and it is a powerful indicator of increased mortality risk and need for heart transplantation.[47]

The amino-terminal propeptide of type III procollagen is associated with restrictive filling pattern in DCM.[48] In symptomatic DCM restrictive filling pattern of transmitral Doppler, especially a DT less than 140ms, may be the single best predictor of cardiac death, being related with a threefold mortality rate.[48] In DCM, persistence of restrictive filling at 3 months is associated with a high mortality and transplantation rate. The patients with reversible restrictive filling have a high probability of improvement and better survival.[49]

In DCM with LVEF less than 25% and DT greater than 130ms, the intermediate 2-year survival is almost 70%, whereas patients with a LVEF of 25% or more had a 2-year survival of 95% or higher, regardless of DT. Markers of diastolic dysfunction correlated strongly with congestive symptoms, whereas variables of systolic function were the strongest predictors of survival. Consideration of both LVEF and DT allows identification of subgroups with divergent long-term prognoses.[50]

Blunted pulmonary vein flow (decreased systolic phase), reduced EF, older age, and increased heart rate (HR) are independent predictors of ominous outcome in descending order of power.[51] MR is marker of a large subgroup of patients with DCM *protected* from LV thrombus formation, but it is also a sensitive marker of decreased survival. Presence of LV apical thrombus is related with an increased incidence of stroke/transient ischaemic attacks (± 2% per year), without any implication on survival.[51]

Non-invasive assessment of pulmonary hypertension using CW Doppler of tricuspid regurgitation (TR) can predict morbidity and mortality in DCM.[52] In DCM and mild-to-moderate symptoms of HF, echocardiography is sufficiently reproducible to be used for determination of treatment effects in longitudinal studies.[53]

The Doppler index (Tei index) reflects disease severity and has incremental prognostic value in DCM. Ease of use, no geometric dependency, excellent separation of clinical groups, and a strong relation to outcome enhance its appeal.[54]

RV function is an important predictor of prognosis in DCM. Not only do individuals with biventricular dysfunction have a worse NYHA functional class, but they also have more severe LV dysfunction and worse long-term prognosis.[55] RV enlargement is a strong marker for adverse prognosis in DCM, as well as that RV long axis excursion[56] and longitudinal velocity.[57]

In both ischaemic and DCM, the prognostic value of TR is important.[57] In addition to the presence of impaired LV systolic function, increasing degrees of MR have a direct impact on survival.[58]

LV synchrony is a marker of prognosis and it has been shown that those with widened QRS duration have a poorer long-term survival than those with coordinated wall motion.[59]

Dyssynchrony in dilated cardiomyopathy

Left bundle branch block is common in DCM and subsequent intraventricular dyssynchrony (see ➲ Chapter 6) results in ineffective cardiac contraction and HF. The presence of LV dyssynchrony[60,61] is most important for response to cardiac resynchronization therapy (CRT).

Intraventricular mechanical dyssynchrony best predicts who will have a good response to CRT (➲ Fig 17.14) (see ➲ Chapter 6). Echocardiographic measures of dyssynchrony, aimed at improving patient selection criteria or CRT, do not appear to have a clinically relevant impact on improving response rates when studied in a multi-centre setting such as PROSPECT.[62] Dyssynchrony measured by strain imaging does provide better predictive value for identifying responders than dyssynchrony by tissue velocity (➲ Fig 17.15).

In cases of DCM patients with biventricular pacing already applied, adequate programming of the CRT device is needed. Programming of the device has to be tailored for each patient and is obtained by the optimization of AV and interventricular delays (see ➲ Chapter 6).

Strain imaging analysis is a sensitive means to delineate the presence of dyssynchrony in early phase of cardiomyopathy. Reversed apical rotation and loss of LV torsion in DCM is associated with significant LV remodelling, increased electrical dyssynchrony, reduced systolic function, and increased filling pressures, indicating a more advanced disease stage.[63] Strain-based LV radial dyssynchrony and E/E′ as well as LV torsion are related to diastolic untwisting performance in DCM. In DCM, all torsional, systolic and diastolic deformational parameters are

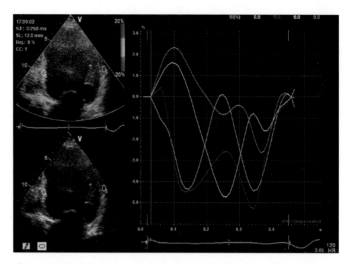

Figure 17.15 Colour tissue Doppler longitudinal strain profiles. Colour tissue Doppler-derived longitudinal strain profiles from the septum and lateral wall with obvious discordance.

decreased. Corresponding 3D components of systolic and diastolic deformations were closely coupled. Considerable variation in the direction of basal and apical rotation exists in a subset of DCM.[64] HF patients who are candidates for CRT frequently display longitudinal rotation—a swinging motion of the heart when imaged in a horizontal long-axis plane. Clockwise longitudinal rotation is linked to presence of DCM, with small impact of QRS duration. Longitudinal rotation is an important predictor of end-systolic volume decrease during CRT in DCM.[65]

Role of stress echocardiography in dilated cardiomyopathy

There is no consensus about the protocol to be used in patients with LV systolic dysfunction. EF is the most frequently used

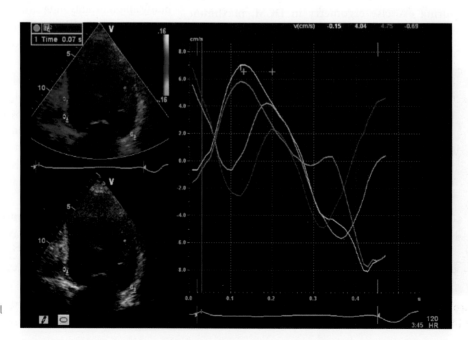

Figure 17.14 Colour tissue Doppler velocity profiles. Colour tissue Doppler-derived velocity profiles from the septum and lateral wall with obvious discordance.

index of LV performance. An increase in EF by more than 5% or change from baseline EF by more than 20% during stress echocardiography identifies patients with preserved LV contractile reserve and better prognosis.

Dobutamine

Since β-receptor downregulation and desensitization is a marker of progressive deterioration of LV systolic function,[66] it is expected that improvement in contractility during low-dose dobutamine infusion is greater in patients with preserved β-receptor function who will subsequently improve. LV end-systolic volume of more than 150mL after low-dose dobutamine echocardiography (LDDE) and no decrease of LV end-diastolic volume after dobutamine are significant predictors of combined end-point (of cardiac death or need for cardiac transplantation).[67] Contractile reserve is correlated well with peak oxygen consumption.[68] Percentage change in end-systolic volume index post-LDDE was associated with ominous prognosis. LDDE may further refine prognosis in DCM with maximal oxygen consumption between 10–14mL/kg/ min (grey zone for risk stratification).[69] This finding may be used for prioritization of patients for cardiac transplantation.

In patients with suspected tachycardiomyopathy, improvement of contractile function induced by low-dose dobutamine has a prognostic significance. In fact, when performed in patients with chronic atrial fibrillation and DCM, LDDE can predict recovery of LV function after cardioversion to sinus rhythm.[70] Changes in LV wall motion score index and ejection fraction during LDDE are predictive of improvement of LV systolic performance during medium-term follow-up.[71]

Use of high-dose dobutamine echocardiography (HDDE) is not associated with serious complications in DCM, having a feasibility of almost 90%. The most common adverse event, requiring discontinuation of dobutamine, are complex ventricular arrhythmias, noted in 8% of patients (frequent multifocal ventricular extra systoles in 6.4% and no sustained ventricular tachycardia in 1.6%).[72]

Early in the course of DCM, dobutamine-induced change in LV contractile response and geometry is able to predict late spontaneous recovery of LV systolic performance.[73] Increased LV mass is associated with better outcome in DCM[74] and the presence of LV hypertrophy implies the presence of myocardial contractile reserve. Dobutamine-induced change in wall motion score index (WMSI) is able to identify patients at greater risk for cardiac death and carries superior prognostic information than change in LV ejection fraction.[72]

Contractile reserve indices assessed by HDDE correlate with myocardial histomorphometric features, suggesting that contractile reserve is related to the degree of histological rearrangement in DCM. Myocyte diameter and interstitial fibrosis showed strongest correlation with change in WMSI followed by change in LVEF.[75]

Dipyridamole

Dipyridamole may be used instead of dobutamine to evoke contractile response, since it is less arrythmogenic[76] and better tolerated.[77] Ability of dipyridamole to recruit contractile reserve is mediated through increase in coronary blood flow and accumulation of endogenous adenosine.[78] Decrease in WMSI with a variation versus baseline (Δ) >0.15 during dipyridamole identifies patients who are more likely to survive more than 3 years.[79] Reported overall feasibility of dipyridamole stress echo was almost 100%.

Dobutamine and dipyridamole stress echocardiography have similar feasibility and prognostic accuracy in DCM risk stratification.[80] The worst prognostic combination was the presence of restrictive filling pattern at rest in the absence of contractile reserve post dipyridamole (Δ WMSI <0.15).[81]

Coronary flow reserve in dilated cardiomyopathy

In DCM patients, coronary flow reserve (CFR) is often impaired. CFR is reduced but with a substantial individual variability, only partially related with the level of systolic and diastolic dysfunction. The clinical functional class is the strongest predictor of CFR reduction in these patients, with lowest flow reserve found in more advanced NYHA class.[82] A reduced CFR (CFR <2) is an independent prognostic marker of bad prognosis.[83] Reduced CFR combined with absence of inotropic reserve (identified as a Δ WMSI post dipyridamole >0.25) have additive value in predicting a worse prognosis.[84] Combined evaluation of contractile reserve and CFR in DCM is currently recommended.[85]

Dynamic performance of right ventricle

Increase in RV ejection fraction (RVEF) to more than 35% during exercise is the only independent predictor of event-free survival in advanced HF.[86] Preserved RV contractile reserve (measured by pressure–area relations) induced by LDDE was associated with a good 30-day outcome in patients with NYHA class IV HF.[87]

Fractional area change greater than 9% identifies patients with more favourable outcome. Tissue velocities of the RV free wall have clinical relevance and should be measured, especially when decision for LV assist device has to be made (➲ Fig 17.16). More importantly, these data suggest that patients in whom contractile reserve of both ventricles is preserved will most likely have good prognosis.

Arrhythmogenic right ventricular dysplasia

First recognized in young subjects with normal exercise tolerance who died suddenly, arrhythmogenic right ventricular

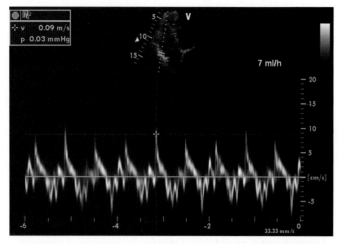

Figure 17.16 Right ventricular tissue Doppler imaging. Pulsed Doppler tissue velocity of the right ventricular free wall in a patient candidate for left ventricular assist device. Following dobutamine infusion the peak velocity remains low, implying incompetent right ventricle to support the circulation, necessitating a biventricular support as bridge to heart transplantation.

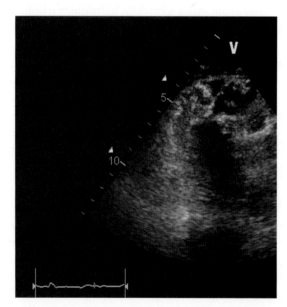

Figure 17.17 Right ventricular apex aneurysm. Right ventricular apex with thinning of the wall and aneurysm combined with a mesh of trabeculations.

dysplasia (ARVD) is characterized by areas in the RV where there is transmural replacement of the myocytes largely by adipose tissue, but with some fibrosis leading to focal areas of aneurismal dilation of the *triangle of dysplasia*: diaphragmatic, infundibular and apical RV regions (➲ Figs. 17.17 and 17.18). While RV involvement is universal, the LV is involved less frequently and the degree of involvement is less severe.

About a third of cases have concomitant LV involvement with fibro-fatty replacement of myocytes, often subpericardial and maximal on the posterior wall. In most but not all cases the myocardial involvement, while acting as a substrate for arrhythmias, does not significantly reduce RV or LV contractile function.[88] Actually, the frequency of ARVD is impossible to

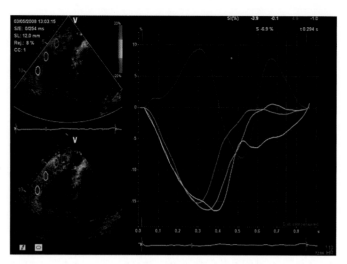

Figure 17.18 Doppler tissue imaging in ARVD. Right ventricular free wall with distortion of strain curves (derived by colour Doppler tissue imaging) near to the apex.

establish accurately, because the less striking cases are underdiagnosed both during life and after death. It appears to be a major cause of sudden death in young people in northern Italy.

TD imaging and 2D strain-derived parameters[89] are superior to conventional echocardiographic parameters in identifying RV dysplasia and may have additional value in the diagnostic workup of patients with suspected disease.

Isolated left ventricular non-compaction

While isolated left ventricular non-compaction (IVNC) remains an *unclassified* form of cardiomyopathy, its echocardiographic and clinical features have recently been characterized and IVNC is now being recognized with increasing frequency. In the largest published series of isolated IVNC, such disease was diagnosed in 17 of 37 555 adult ECGs, with a prevalence of 0.05%.

IVNC, which results from an interruption of the normal process of embryological myocardial compaction, is associated with a risk of systolic dysfunction, systemic embolization, and ventricular arrhythmias.[90] Accurate recognition requires knowledge of the echo features, which include the presence of a thin (compacted) epicardium and a thick, spongy endocardial (non-compacted) surface with extensive trabeculation and sinusoid formation. Extent of trabeculation is defined by more than three trabeculae apically to the papillary muscles, visible in one echocardiographic image plane.[91] Communication between the deep intertrabecular spaces and the ventricular cavity can be demonstrated by CD imaging and/or contrast echo (see ➲ Chapter 7). In the majority of cases the non-compacted myocardium involves the mid lateral, apical, or inferior walls.

A ratio of non-compacted to compacted myocardium higher than 2:1 is diagnostic of this entity. Additionally, both regional and generalized LV hypokinesis has been observed in this condition. Right ventricular involvement has been described in some patients with this condition. The hypokinetic segments can occur in both the affected area and the surrounding normally compacted myocardial segments. Although some authors postulate IVNC to be a distinct cardiomyopathy, there are several indications that it has a heterogeneous aetiology. Often believed to be a congenital cardiac abnormality, IVNC may occur as an acquired disease. IVNC is commonly associated with neuromuscular disorders[92,93] such as myoadenylate deaminase deficiency, mitochondriopathy, myotonic dystrophy, Becker's muscular dystrophy, Barth syndrome, Friedreich's ataxia, and Pompe disease. Because of its rarity, IVNC has been often overlooked. As a consequence of the increasing awareness of IVNC, however, IVNC is also falsely diagnosed. Increased trabeculations might occur during the evolution of LV dysfunction and remodelling in the idiopathic DCM (➲ Fig 17.19) *LV solid body rotation*, with near absent LV twist, may be a new sensitive and specific, objective and quantitative, functional diagnostic criterion for IVNC.[94]

Friedreich's ataxia

Friedreich's ataxia (FRDA) is an inherited neurodegenerative disorder associated with cardiomyopathy and impaired glucose tolerance. The genetic basis for FRDA is a GAA trinucleotide repeat expansion in the first intron of gene X25, which encodes for the protein Frataxin. The most common echocardiographic abnormality is asymmetrical LV hypertrophy and thickening of

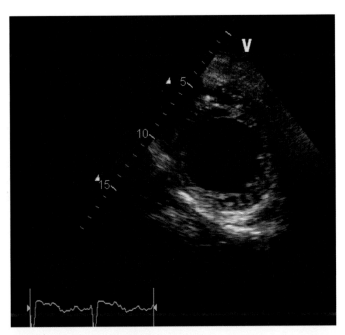

Figure 17.19 Left ventricular non-compaction. Increased trabeculations in the inferolateral wall at the apical cross-section (parasternal short axis) in a patient with idiopathic DCM with decompensated heart failure (NYHA IV).

the papillary muscles, although the range of abnormalities appears to be wide. Myocardial velocity gradients (MVG) by TD imaging in systole and during rapid ventricular filling phase of early diastole are reduced in patients with FRDA who are without cardiac symptoms.[95]

Age-corrected MVGs were inversely related to the size of the GAA triple repeat expansion in all phases of the cardiac cycle. They hypothesize that the abnormal MVG reflects the decreased myocardial contractility and relaxation secondary to abnormal mitochondrial function resulting from reduced levels of Frataxin in FRDA.

Myotonic dystrophy (Steinert disease)

Myotonic dystrophy is a multisystem disorder that affects skeletal muscle and smooth muscle, as well as the eye, heart, endocrine system, and central nervous system. Its prevalence is estimated at 1/20 000.[96] Myotonic dystrophy is inherited in an autosomal dominant manner. Diagnosis is confirmed by detection of an expansion of the CTG trinucleotide repeat in the DMPK gene (chromosomal locus 19q13.2–q13.3).

Cardiac conduction defects of varying degrees of severity are common, up to 90% in one series. Less commonly, cardiomyopathy may occur.[97]

Subclinical impairment of LV contractility may be detected using conventional 2D echocardiography and TD Imaging. Systolic motion at the basal lateral and basal septal segments as well as lateral velocities were significantly lower in subjects with myotonic dystrophy when compared to controls. Furthermore, peak systolic velocities correlated inversely with neurological severity.[98]

Duchenne/Becker muscular dystrophy

Becker muscular dystrophy (BMD) is an X-linked recessive muscular disease characterized by progressive muscular weakness and cardiac involvement caused by dystrophin abnormalities in all striated muscles as well as in the myocardium. The prevalence is estimated at 2.38/100 000.[99]

Eventually patients as well as female carriers will develop a DCM. Both in BMD patients and in female carriers myocardial damage can be detected in a preclinical stage through minor electrocardiographic and echocardiographic signs.

Most of the regional pulsed TD diastolic indices were decreased in BMD patients and carriers.[100] Besides confirming systolic alterations of BMD patients with reduced LVEF, pulsed TD has detected early segmental systolic abnormalities in BMD patients with normal LVEF and in female carriers. TD imaging alteration may represent an independent marker of early systolic dysfunction compared to standard echocardiographic parameters.

In Duchenne patients, significant decreases in radial and longitudinal peak systolic strain, and peak systolic and early diastolic myocardial velocities were found in the LV inferolateral and anterolateral walls. The prognostic significance of this early ventricular involvement warrants further longitudinal follow-up.[101]

Becker muscular dystrophy has a high heart transplantation rate in the 5 years after diagnosis of cardiomyopathy. Serial echocardiography demonstrates a different disease course for Duchenne and Becker patients compared with idiopathic DCM patients.

Restrictive and infiltrative cardiomyopathy

Introduction

Relative to the dilated and hypertrophic cardiomyopathies, restrictive cardiomyopathy occurs with lower frequency in the developed world. The pathophysiological identity of restrictive cardiomyopathy is the increase in stiffness of the ventricular walls, which causes HF because of impaired diastolic filling. In early stages, systolic function may be normal.

Restrictive cardiomyopathy must be distinguished from constrictive pericarditis, which is also characterized by normal or nearly normal systolic function but abnormal ventricular filling. Differentiation of these two conditions is of clinical importance because pericardial constriction may be treated with pericardiectomy.

Approximately 50% of cases of restrictive cardiomyopathy result from specific clinical disorders, whereas the remainder represents an idiopathic process. The most common specific cause of restrictive cardiomyopathy is infiltration caused by amyloidosis.

Classification of restrictive cardiomyopathy

Aetiological classification of types of restrictive cardiomyopathy[102] encompasses:

- Myocardial forms, which are distinguished in:

  - Non-infiltrative, such as idiopathic cardiomyopathy, scleroderma pseudoxanthoma elasticum, diabetic cardiomyopathy

  - Infiltrative, such as amyloidosis, sarcoidosis, Gaucher disease, Hurler disease, fatty infiltration

  - Storage disease, such as haemochromatosis, Fabry disease, glycogen storage disease

- Endomyocardial forms, such as endomyocardial fibrosis, Hypereosinophilic syndrome, carcinoid heart disease,

metastatic cancers, radiation, toxic effects of anthracycline, drugs causing fibrous endocarditis (serotonin, methysergide ergotamine, mercurial agents, busulfan).

Amyloidosis

Amyloidosis is a disease process that results from tissue deposition of proteins that have a unique secondary structure (twisted β-pleated sheet fibrils). Primary amyloidosis results from the deposition of portions of immunoglobulin light chain (designated as AL). Secondary amyloidosis (also known as reactive systemic amyloidosis) results from excessive production of a non-immunoglobulin protein known as AA.

Echocardiography reveals increased ventricular wall thickness with small intracavitary chambers, enlarged atria, and a thickened interatrial septum. Systolic function is normal early in the course of the disease but progressive LV dysfunction ensues with advancing amyloid deposition.[103] The walls of the ventricles often reveal a distinctive appearance with a sparkling and granular texture, most likely resulting from the amyloid deposition itself. The cardiac valves may have a thickened appearance but typically have normal excursion. Mild-to-moderate pericardial effusions may be present but do not advance to tamponade (→ Fig 17.20–17.22). Patterns of chamber hypertrophy are, on occasion, regional, mimicking HCM.[104] The echocardiographic appearance of thickened LV walls associated with low voltage on ECG is valuable for differentiation from pericardial disease.

Inherited and acquired infiltrative disorders

The heritable metabolic disorders include Fabry disease, Gaucher disease, the glycogenoses, and the mucopolysaccharidoses (Hurler). Early diagnosis is increasingly important because of the availability, in some cases, of effective enzyme replacement therapy.

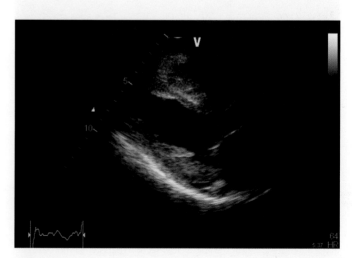

Figure 17.20 Diffuse increase of wall thickness in amyloidosis. Long axis of left ventricle with diffuse increase of wall thickness.

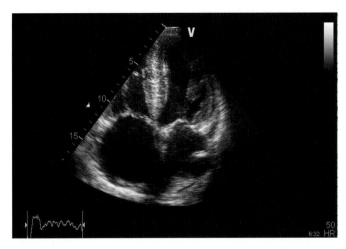

Figure 17.21 Septal thickening and granular texture in amyolidosis. Apical four-chamber view with intense septal thickening and granular texture. There is also thickening of mitral and tricuspid valve and gross atrial dilation.

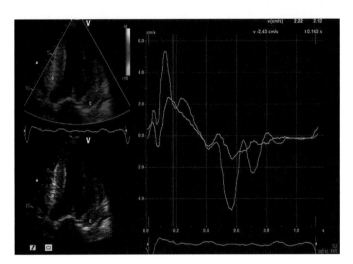

Figure 17.22 Tissue Doppler imaging in amyloidosis. Tissue Doppler imaging of septum and lateral wall with decrease of systolic and diastolic velocity (more in the septum).

Fabry disease

Fabry disease (angiokeratoma corporis diffusum universale) is an X-linked recessive disorder that results in deficiency of alpha-galactosidase A, a lysosomal enzyme, and the resultant accumulation of glycosphingolipids in lysosomes in the endothelium. Patients with absent alpha-galactosidase activity exhibit widespread systemic manifestations with prominent kidney and cutaneous manifestations, whereas those with an attenuated level of enzyme activity have atypical variants of Fabry disease that may cause isolated myocardial disease. Patients often experience angina pectoris and myocardial infarction caused by the accumulation of lipid species in the coronary endothelium, although epicardial coronary arteries are angiographically normal. The ventricular walls are thickened and have mildly diminished diastolic compliance with normal systolic function. Mild MR may be present due to the thickening

of the leaflet and occasionally aortic valve is involved. Diastolic abnormalities detected by Doppler echocardiography may be one of the earlier manifestations preceding cardiac hypertrophy. Males almost always present with symptomatic cardiovascular involvement, whereas female carriers may be completely asymptomatic or have only minimal symptoms (➲ Figs. 17.23 and 17.24). Echocardiography demonstrates increased ventricular wall thickness, which may mimic HCM. Low plasma alpha-galactosidase A activity offer a definitive diagnosis, which has therapeutic implications because enzyme replacement therapy for Fabry disease is safe and effective. TD imaging can provide early detection of cardiac involvement in Fabry disease and represents the most accurate and sensitive non-invasive tool for the diagnosis of myocardial dysfunction and for the assessment

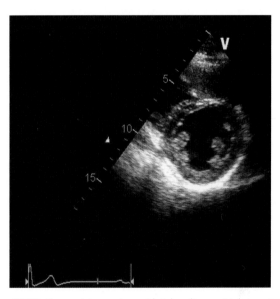

Figure 17.23 Short axis in a patient with Fabry disease. LV short axis with mild wall thickening (obvious papillary muscles).

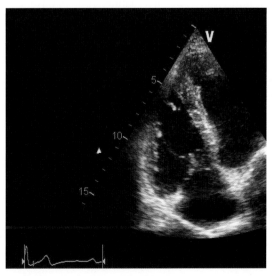

Figure 17.24 RV in a patient with Fabry disease. Apical view of the RV with thickened free wall.

of cardiac improvement during enzyme replacement therapy.[105] The detection of TD abnormalities in female carriers may represent a hint for an invasive assessment of cardiac involvement. Treatment of Fabry cardiomyopathy with recombinant alpha-galactosidase A should best be started before myocardial fibrosis has developed to achieve long-term improvement in myocardial morphology and function and exercise capacity. The *double peak sign* in strain-rate imaging tracings seems to be a reliable tool to diagnose regional fibrosis.

Gaucher disease

Gaucher disease results from a heritable deficiency of β-glucosidase, which leads to an accumulation of cerebrosides in diffuse organs. Cardiac disease manifests as a stiffened ventricle caused by reduced chamber compliance, leading to impaired cardiac performance. Other manifestations include LV failure and enlargement, haemorrhagic pericardial effusion, and sclerotic, calcified left-sided valves. Gaucher disease is responsive to enzyme replacement therapy, or in more extreme cases, hepatic transplantation; both therapies contribute to reducing tissue infiltration by cerebrosides and can lead to varying degrees of clinical improvement.

Haemochromatosis

Haemochromatosis results from excessive deposition of iron in a variety of parenchymal tissues. The most frequent form of haemochromatosis is inherited as an autosomal recessive disorder that arises from a mutation in the HFE gene, which codes for a transmembrane protein that is responsible for regulating iron uptake in the bowel and liver. Haemochromatosis may also arise from ineffective erythropoiesis secondary to a defect in haemoglobin synthesis or may be acquired as a result of chronic and excessive oral or parenteral intake of iron (or blood transfusions as in thalassaemias). Cardiac toxicity results directly from the free iron moiety in addition to adverse effects of tissue infiltration. The early manifestation of cardiac involvement is the restrictive type diastolic dysfunction detected by conventional Doppler echocardiography in the advanced stage of iron load[106] or earlier in a patient's life by new biochemical markers (as NT-proBNP). Iron overload is also the main reason for LV dysfunction and cardiomyopathy. Chelation therapy is the most important way of prediction of cardiomyopathy presentation and LV dysfunction reversal, while its additional therapy is the common one of dilated cardiomyopathy.

Glycogen storage disease

Patients with type II, III, IV, and V glycogen storage diseases may have cardiac involvement. However, survival to adulthood is rare with the exception of patients with type III disease (glycogen debranching enzyme deficiency). The most typical cardiac involvement is LV hypertrophy, with electrocardiographic and echocardiographic findings, often with the absence of symptoms. A subset of patients may present with overt cardiac dysfunction, arrhythmias, and presentation of a dilated cardiomyopathy.

Sarcoidosis

Sarcoidosis is a systemic inflammatory condition characterized by the formation of non-caseating granulomas, (lungs, reticuloendothelial system, skin). Cardiac involvement is recognized in 20–30% of autopsies of affected patients. The clinical manifestations of sarcoid heart disease result from infiltration of the conduction system and myocardium with a restrictive cardiomyopathy caused by increased ventricular chamber stiffness. Echocardiography may demonstrate either global or regional LV dysfunction and rarely may reveal aneurysm formation (basal septum).

Endomyocardial disease

A common form of restrictive cardiomyopathy found in a geographical location close to the equator is known as endomyocardial disease (EMD). Variants are described that, despite similar phenotypes, are likely unique processes, both manifesting as aggressive endocardial scarring obliterating the ventricular apices and subvalvular regions. Endomyocardial fibrosis or Davies disease occurs primarily in tropical regions, in contrast to the other disease (Löffler endocarditis parietalis fibroplastica, or the hypereosinophilic syndrome).

Primary restrictive cardiomyopathy

Primary restrictive cardiomyopathy is characterized by restricted ventricular filling resulting from an idiopathic non-hypertrophied myocardial abnormality (i.e. stiffening fibrosis or decreased compliance or both). Idiopathic restrictive cardiomyopathy is a rare entity distinguished from the other forms of restrictive cardiomyopathy by the presence of normal ventricular wall thickness. This disease is seen in individuals where other aetiologies for cardiomyopathy have been excluded such as connective tissue disease, carcinoid syndrome, amyloidosis, haemochromatosis, eosinophilic syndrome, malignancy, radiation exposure, cardiotoxic drug exposure, or a history of alcohol abuse. In addition, these individuals do not have a history of ischaemic heart disease, treated hypertension for more than 5 years, or organic valvular, pericardial, or congenital diseases.[107]

Ventricular systolic function usually is preserved in the initial stage, but diastolic pressure is elevated, which in turn results in increased atrial pressures and marked biatrial enlargement. Therefore, the characteristic morphological features of primary restrictive cardiomyopathy include ventricular cavities of normal size; normal wall thicknesses, with relatively preserved global systolic function and biatrial enlargement. Restrictive cardiomyopathy has restrictive diastolic filling pattern. The typical haemodynamic feature of restrictive cardiomyopathy is the *dip-and-plateau* configuration in the ventricular diastolic pressure tracing. This haemodynamic feature produces shortened DT of E wave in the mitral inflow pattern. With the increase in LA pressure, the MV opens at a higher pressure, resulting in a decrease in IVRT. High atrial pressure also results in an increased transmitral pressure gradient, increased E mitral velocity, and decreased systolic pulmonary venous flow velocity. Because of high ventricular pressure at end-diastole, atrial contraction does not contribute significantly to ventricular filling, and A velocity is usually decreased. As a result, the E/A ratio is markedly increased (>2.0). Because of the increase in atrial pressure, venous flow velocity decreases during systole and increases with diastole. In contrast to constrictive pericarditis, hepatic vein diastolic flow reversal is greater during inspiration. Myocardial relaxation is impaired so that mitral annulus E' velocity is usually less than 7cm/s (when obtained from the septal annulus).[108]

Typical Doppler features in restrictive cardiomyopathy are as follows:

- Mitral and tricuspid inflow:
  - Increased E velocity: mitral >1m/s, tricuspid >0.7m/s.
  - Decreased A velocity: mitral <0.5m/s, tricuspid <0.3m/s.
  - Increased E/A ratio: >2.0.
  - Shortened DT: <160 ms.
  - Decreased IVRT: <70 ms.
- Pulmonary and hepatic vein flow:
  - Systolic velocity less than diastolic velocity.
- Increased diastolic flow reversal in the hepatic vein during inspiration.
- Increased atrial flow reversal velocity and duration in pulmonary vein.
- Tissue Doppler imaging from the septal mitral annulus:
  - Decreased systolic velocity: S <5cm/s.
  - Decreased early diastolic velocity: E<7cm/s.

Restrictive cardiomyopathy should be distinguished from restrictive haemodynamics or physiology. Male sex, LA dimension larger than 60mm, age older than 70 years, and each increment of the NYHA functional class doubled the risk of death.

Post-transplant echocardiographic evaluation

Echocardiographic evaluation of patients after a cardiac transplant usually is performed in order to assess cardiac anatomy and function and to detect potential RV or LV dysfunction, secondary to lack of myocardial preservation during surgery, or to coronary artery disease development or to occurrence of transplant reject. Pericardial effusion is a common finding in these patients, while mitral or tricuspid regurgitation can be due to ventricular dysfunction and dilation.

Normal findings

LV and RV size and wall thickness usually are normal, as well as valvular function. A biatrial enlargement can be detected, with a prominent ridge between the donor and recipient portions of both atria: when visible, atrial suture line to be differentiated by abnormal atrial mass. Pericardial effusion often is seen during the first days after the transplant and tends to disappear in a few weeks. Interventricular septum shows an altered motion with anterior displacement in systole and a slight decrease in thickness. Pulmonary artery pressure may be persistently elevated and can be measured by tricuspid regurgitant flow.

Abnormal findings

Echocardiographic examination of patients with suspected cardiac dysfunction after transplant is similar to that of any other patients, but requires recognition of typical findings characterizing post-transplant heart. Pericardial effusion usually is loculated due to inflammatory adhesions, so that its detection should be performed by a careful research from multiple echocardiographic views.

Transplant rejection

Transplant rejection is characterized by increased LV mass and myocardial echogenicity and decreased systolic function. Because early stages of transplant rejection are subtle, echocardiographic evaluation of diastolic function can be obtained in order to allow a prompted adjustment of immunosuppressive therapy. In fact, early acute rejection cause an increased early diastolic deceleration slope with a decreased pressure half-time (PHT), a decreased isovolumic relaxation time (IVRT), and an increased E wave velocity. A change greater than 20% in E wave velocity or greater than 15% in PHT and IVRT compared to baseline is considered diagnostic for early rejection. However, in many clinical centres such echocardiographic features are not taken into account, and transvenous endomyocardial biopsy continues to be largely performed for diagnosis of transplant rejection. Usually echocardiography is used as guide for such procedure: subcostal approach mostly is performed due to better visualization of RV and IVS, but also apical view may be useful.

Transplant coronary artery disease

Increased survival of patients after cardiac transplant causes development of CAD also in transplanted heart. Atherosclerotic process affects both epicardial coronary artery and microvasculature due to relevant intimal hyperplasia. In these patients, exercise stress echocardiography may provide false-negative results due to diffuse involvement of coronary arteries masking regional WMAs, while dobutamine stress echocardiography seems to be more accurate. Coronary angiography always is fundamental to confirm diagnosis and often requires intravascular ultrasound imaging of coronary arteries.

Personal perspective

HCM is not as rare as it was thought to be. The attention of the medical community focuses on this disease because of the high incidence of sudden death in young age. Echocardiography is very important for the diagnosis although in patients with borderline hypertrophy or *other apparent causes of hypertrophy* further testing, mainly genetic, is definitely needed. Prognostically, echocardiography has some additive value over the classical markers of sudden death as family history of sudden death, sustained ventricular arrhythmias, and previous cardiac arrest.

The prevalence of familial DCM is expected to increase with the expansion of genetic studies. Patients may present with very mild symptoms and a dilated LV. Diagnostic algorithms for triage of subclinical forms of myopathy are evolving and echocardiography is going to be involved. 3D analysis will provide better volumetric analysis of myopathic ventricles and will provide robust deformation analysis in the early phase of cardiomyopathy. Resynchronization therapy is going to expand. Use of stress echocardiography should be a standard procedure, for better risk stratification in the era of expanding use of ventricular supportive implantable devices.

Evolving drug treatment of storage diseases calls for more intensive screening for cardiac involvement. Deformation imaging using strain and twist/torsion analysis may provide insight in earlier forms of myopathic involvement. Familial cases with milder phenotypes may become candidates for specific therapy as in the case of Fabry disease.

References

1 Bos JM, Towbin JA, Ackerman MJ. Diagnostic, prognostic and thepareutic implications of genetic testing for hypertrophic cardiomyopathy. *J Am Coll Cardiol* 2009; **54**:201–11.

2 Seidman JG, Seidman CE. The genetic basis for cardiomuyopathy. From mutation identification to mechanistic paradigms. *Cell* 2001; **104**:557–67.

3 Spirito P, Belone P, Harris KM, Bernabò P, Bruzzi P, Maron BJ. Magnitude of left ventricular hypertrophy and risk of sudden death in hypertrophic caridomyopathy. *N Engl J Med* 2000; **324**:1778–85.

4 Nimura H, Bachinski LL, Sangwatanaraj S, Watkins H, Chudley AE, McKenna W, *et al*. Mutations in the gene for cardiac myosin-binding protein C and late-onset familial hypertrophic cardiomyopathy. *N Engl J Med* 1998; **338**:1248–57.

5 Watkins H, McKenna WJ, Thierfelder L, Suk HJ, Anan R, O Donoghue A, *et al*. Mutations in the genes for cardiac troponin T and alpha-tropomyosin in hypertrophic cardiomyopathy. *N Engl J Med* 1995; **332**:1058–64.

6 Henry WL, Clark CE, Epstein SE. Asymmetric septal hypertrophy. Echocardiographic identification of the pathognomonic anatomic abnormality of IHSS. *Circulation* 1973; **47**:225–233.

7 Rakowski H, Sasson Z, Wigle ED. Echocardiographic and Doppler assessment of hypertrophic cardiomyopathy. *J Am Soc Echocardiogr* 1988; **1**:31–47.

8 Martin RP, Rakowski H, French J, Popp RL. Idiopathic hypertrophic subaortic Stenosis viewed by wide-angle, phased-array echocardiography. *Circulation* 1979; **59**:1206–17.

9 Sherrid MV, Gunsburg DZ, Moldenhauer S, Pearle G. Systolic anterior motion begins at low left ventricular outflow track velocity in obstructive hypertrophic cardiomyopathy. *J Am Coll Cardiol* 2000; **36**:1344–54.

10 Maron BJ, Nishimura RA, Danielson GK. Pitfalls in clinical recognition and a novel operative approach for hypertrophic cardiomyopathy with severe outflow obstruction due to anomalous papillary muscle. *Circulation* 1998; **98**:2505–8.

11 Pollick C, Rakowski H, Wigle ED. Muscular subaortic stenosis. The quantitative relationship between systolic anterior motion and the pressure gradient. *Circulation* 1984; **69**:43–9.

12 Nihoyannopoulos P, Karatasakis G, Joshi J, Gilligan D, Oakley C. intraventricular systolic flow mapping in hypertrophic cardiomyopathy. *Echocardiography J Cardiov Ultr and Allied Tech* 1993; **10**:121–32.

13 Yu E, Omran AS, Wigle ED, Williams WG, Siu SC, Rakowski H. Mitral regurgitation in hypertrophic obstructive cardiomyopahty. Relationship to obstruction and relief with myectomy. *J Am Coll Cardiol* 2000; **36**:2219–25.

14 Nihoyannopoulos P, Karatasakis G, Frenneaux M, McKenna WJ, Oakley CM. Diastolic function in hypertrophic cardiomyopahty. Relation to exercise capacity. *J Am Coll Cardiol* 1992; **19**:536–40.

15 Bijnens BH, Cikes M, Claus P, Sutherland GR. Velocity and deformation imaging for the assessment of myocardial dysfunction. *Eur J Echocardiogr* 2009; **10**:216–26.

16 De Backer J, Matthys D, Gillebert TC, De Paepe A, De Sutter J. The use of tissue doppler imaging for the assessment of changes in myocardial structure and function in inherited cardiomyopathies. *Eur J Ecocardiogr* 2005; **6**:243–50.

17 Bayrak F, Kahveci G, Mutlu B, Sonmez K, Degertekin M. Tissue Doppler imaging to predict clinical course of patients with hypertrophic cardiomyopathy. *Eur J Echocardiogr* 2008; **9**:278–83.

18 Panza JA, Maron BJ. Relation of electrocardiographic abnormalities to evolving left ventricular hypertrophy in hypertrophic cardiomyopathy during childhood. *Am J Cardiol* 1989; **63**:1258–65.

19 Ho CY, Sweitzer NK, McDonough B, Maron BJ, Casey SA, Sedman JG, *et al*. Assessment of diastolic function with Doppler

tissue imaging to predict genotype in preclinical hypertrophic cardiomyopathy. *Circulation* 2002; **105**:2997.

20 Hagège AA, Dubourg O, Desnos M, Mirochnik R, Isnard G, Bonne G, et al. Familial hypertrophic cardiomyopathy. Cardiac ultrasonic abnormalities in genetically affected subjects without echocardiographic evidence of left ventricular hypertrophy. *Eur Heart J* 1998; **19**:490–9.

21 Nagueh SF, Bachinski LL, Meyer D, Hill R, Zoghbi WA, Tam JW, et al. Tissue Doppler imaging consistently detects myocardial abnormalities in patients with hypertrophic cardiomyopathy and provides a novel means for an early diagnosis before and independently of hypertrophy. *Circulation* 2001; **104**:128–30.

22 Lakkis NM, Nagueh SF, Kleiman NS, Killip D, He ZX, Verani MS, et al. Echocardiography-guided ethanol septal reduction for hypertrophic obstructive cardiomyopathy. *Circulation* 1998; **98**:1750–1755.

23 Marwick TH, Stewart WJ, Lever HM, Lytle BW, Rosenkranz ER, Duffy CI, et al. Benefits of intraoperative echocardiography in the surgical management of hypertrophic cardiomyopathy. *J Am Coll Cardiol* 1992; **20**:1066–72.

24 Nimura H, Bachinski LL, Sangwatanaroj S, Watkins H, Chudley AE, McKenna W, et al. Mutations in the gene for cardiac myosin-binding protein C and late-onset familial hypertrophic cardiomyopathy. *N Engl J Med* 1998; **338**:1248–57.

25 Graham RM, Owens WA. Pathogenesis of inherited forms of dilated cardiomyopathy. *N Engl J Med* 1999; **341**:1759–62.

26 Michels W, Mills P, Miller F, Tajik A J, Chu J S, Driscoll D J, et al. The frequency of familial dilated cardiomyopathy in a series of patients with idiopathic dilated cardiomyopathy. *N Engl J Med* 1992; **326**:77–82.

27 Grunig E, Tasman JA, Kuherer H, Franz W, Kubler W, Katus HA. Frequency and phenotypes of familial dilated cardiomyopathy. *J Am Coll Cardiol* 1998; **31**: 186–94.

28 Fatkin D, MacRae C, Sasaki T, Wolff MR, Porcu M, Frenneaux M, et al. Missense mutations in the rod domain of the lamin A/C gene as causes of dilated cardiomyopathy and conduction-system disease. *N Engl J Med* 1999; **341**:1715–24.

29 Brodsky G, Muntoni F, Miocic S, Sinagra G, Sewry C, Mestroni L. Lamin A/C gene mutation associated with dilated cardiomyopathy with variable skeletal muscle involvement. *Circulation* 2000, **101**:473–6.

30 Hershberger RE, Hanson E, Jakobs PM, Keegan H, Coates K, Bousman S, et al. A novel lamin A/C mutation in a family with dilated cardiomyopathy, prominent conduction system disease, and need for permanent pacemaker implantation. *Am Heart J* 2002, **144**:1081–6.

31 Arbustini E, Pilotto A, Repetto A, Repetto A, Grasso M, Negri A, et al. Autosomal dominant dilated cardiomyopathy with atrioventricular block: a lamin A/C defect-related diseas. *J Am Coll Cardiol* 2002, **39**:981–90.

32 Pasotti M, Klersy C, Pilotto A, Marziliano N, Rapezzi C, Serio A, et al. Long-term outcome and risk stratification in dilated cardiolaminopathies. *J Am Coll Cardiol* 2008, **52**:1250–60.

33 Politano L, Nigro V, Nigro G, et al. Development of cardiomyopathy in female carriers of Duchenne and Becker muscular dystrophies. *JAMA* 1996; **275**:1335–8.

34 Manolio TA, Baughman KL, Rodeheffer R, Pearson TA, Bristow JD. Prevalence and etiology of idiopathic dilated cardiomyopathy (summary of a National Heart, Lung and Blood Institute Workshop). *Am J Cardiol* 1992; **69**:1459–66.

35 Kuhl U, Noutsias M, Seeberg B, Schultheiss HP. Immunological evidence for a chronic intramyocardial inflammatory process in dilated cardiomyopathy. *Heart* 1996; **75**:295–300.

36 Henry WL, Gardin JM, Ware JH. Echocardiographic measurements in normal subjects from infancy to old age. *Circulation* 1980; **62**:1054–61.

37 Mestroni L, Maisch B, McKenna WJ, Schwartz K, Charron P, Rocco C, et al. on behalf of the Collaborative Research Group of the European Human and Capital Mobility Project on Familial Dilated Cardiomyopathy, Guidelines for the study of familial dilated cardiomyopathies. *Eur Heart J* 1999; **20**:93–102.

38 Feigenbaum H, Armstrong WF, Ryan T. *Faigenbaum's Echocardiography*. 6th ed. Philadelphia, PA: Lippincott Williams and Wilkins, 2006, pp.537–546.

39 Richardson P. Report of the WHO/ISFC task force on the definition and classification of cardiomyopathy. *Circulation* 1996; **93**:341–2.

40 Diaz RA, Nihoyannopoulos P, Athanassopoulos G, Oakley CM. Usefulness of echocardiography to differentiate dilated cardiomyopathy from coronary-induced congestive heart failure. *Am J Cardiol* 1991; **68**(11):1224–7.

41 Denault AY, Gorcsan J 3rd, Mandarin WA, et al. LV performance assessed by echocardiographic automated border detection and arterial pressure. *Am J Physiol* 1997; **272**(1 Pt 2):H138–47.

42 Heimdal A, Stoylen A, Torp H, et al. Real-time strain rate imaging of the left ventricle by ultrasound. *J Am Soc Echocardiogr* 1998; **11**:1013–19.

43 De Castro S, Caselli S, Maron M, Pelliccia A, Cavarretta E, Maddukuri P, et al. Left ventricular remodelling index (LVRI) in various pathophysiological conditions: a real-time three-dimensional echocardiographic study. *Heart* 2007; **93**(2):205–9.

44 Donal E, De Place C, Kervio G, Bauer F, Gervais R, Leclercq C, et al. Mitral regurgitation in dilated cardiomyopathy: value of both regional LV contractility and dyssynchrony. *Eur J Echocardiogr* 2009; **10**(1):133–8.

45 Gottdiener JS, McClelland RL, Marshall R, Shemanski L; Furberg CD, Kitzman DW, et al. Outcome of congestive heart failure in elderly persons: influence of LV systolic function: the cardiovascular health study. *Ann Intern Med* 2002; **147**:631–9.

46 Pepi M, Agostoni P, Marenzi G, Dorai E, Guazzi M, Lauri G, et al. The influence of diastolic and systolic function on exercise performance in heart failure due to dilated cardiomyopathy or ischemic heart disease. *Eur J Heart Fail* 1999; **1**(2):161–7.

47 Pinamonti B, Di Lenarda A, Sinagra G, Camerini F. Restrictive LV filling pattern in dilated cardiomyopathy assessed by Doppler echocardiography: clinical, echocardiographic and hemodynamic correlations and prognostic implications. Heart Muscle Disease Study Group. *J Am Coll Cardiol* 1993; **22**(3):808–15.

48 Rossi A, Cicoira M, Golia G, Zanolla L, Franceschini L, Marino P, et al. Amino-terminal propeptide of type III procollagen is associated with restrictive mitral filling pattern in patients with dilated cardiomyopathy: a possible link between diastolic dysfunction and prognosis. *Heart* 2004; **90**(6):650–4.

49 Lapu-Bula R, Robert A, De Kock M, D'Hondt AM, Detry JM, Melin JA, et al. Risk stratification in patients with dilated cardiomyopathy: contribution of Doppler-derived LV filling. *Am J Cardiol* 1998; **82**(6):779–85.

50 Pinamonti B, Zecchin M, Di Lenarda A, Gregori D, Sinagra G, Camerini F. Persistence of restrictive LV filling pattern in dilated

cardiomyopathy: an ominous prognostic sign. *J Am Coll Cardiol* 1997; **29**(3):604–12.

51 Rihal CS, Nishimura RA, Hatle LK, Bailey KR, Tajik AJ. Systolic and diastolic dysfunction in patients with clinical diagnosis of dilated cardiomyopathy. Relation to symptoms and prognosis. *Circulation* 1994; **90**(6):2772–9.

52 Dini FL, Dell'Anna R, Micheli A, Michelassi C, Rovai D. Impact of blunted pulmonary venous flow on the outcome of patients with LV systolic dysfunction secondary to either ischemic or idiopathic dilated cardiomyopathy. *Am J Cardiol* 2000; **85**(12):1455–60.

53 Blondheim DS, Jacobs LE, Kotler MN, Costacurta GA, Parry WR. Dilated cardiomyopathy with mitral regurgitation: decreased survival despite a low frequency of LV thrombus. *Am Heart J* 1991; **122**(3 Pt 1):763–71.

54 Abramson SV, Burke JF, Kelly JJ Jr, Kitchen JG 3rd, Dougherty MJ, Yih DF, *et al.* Pulmonary hypertension predicts mortality and morbidity in patients with dilated cardiomyopathy. *Ann Intern Med* 1992; **116**(11):888–95.

55 Jansson K, Dahlström U, Karlberg KE, Karlsson E, Nyquist O, Nylander E. The value of repeated echocardiographic evaluation in patients with idiopathic dilated cardiomyopathy during treatment with metoprolol or captopril. *Scand Cardiovasc J* 2000; **34**(3): 293–300.

56 Dujardin KS, Tei C, Yeo TC, Hodge DO, Rossi A, Seward JB. Prognostic value of a Doppler index combining systolic and diastolic performance in idiopathic-dilated cardiomyopathy. *Am J Cardiol* 1998; **82**(9):1071–6.

57 Juillière Y, Barbier G, Feldmann L, Grentzinger A, Danchin N, Cherrier F. Additional predictive value of both left and right ventricular ejection fractions on long-term survival in idiopathic dilated cardiomyopathy. *Eur Heart J* 1997; **18**(2):276–80

58 Karatasakis GT, Karagounis LA, Kalyvas PA, Manginas A, Athanassopoulos GD, Aggelakas SA, *et al.* Prognostic significance of echocardiographically estimated right ventricular shortening in advanced heart failure. *Am J Cardiol* 1998; **82**(3):329–34.

59 Meluzín J, Spinarová L, Dusek L, Toman J, Hude P, Krejcí J. Prognostic importance of the right ventricular function assessed by Doppler tissue imaging. *Eur J Echocardiogr* 2003; **4**(4):262–71.

60 Hung J, Koelling T, Semigran MJ, Dec GW, Levine RA, Di Salvo TG. Usefulness of echocardiographically determined tricuspid regurgitation in predicting event-free survival in severe heart failure secondary to idiopathic-dilated cardiomyopathy or to ischemic cardiomyopathy. *Am J Cardiol* 1998; **82**:1201–3, A10.

61 Koelling TM, Aaronson KD, Cody RJ, Bach DS, Armstrong WF. Prognostic significance of mitral regurgitation and tricuspid regurgitation in patients with LV systolic dysfunction. *Am Heart J* 2002; **144**:524–9.

62 Fauchier L, Marie O, Casset-Senon D, Babuty D, Cosnay P, Fauchier JP. Interventricular and intraventricular dyssynchrony in idiopathic dilated cardiomyopathy: a prognostic study with Fourier phase analysis of radionuclide angioscintigraphy. *J Am Coll Cardiol* 2002; **40**:2022–30.

63 Popescu BA, Beladan CC, Calin A, Muraru D, Deleanu D, Rosca M, *et al.* LV remodelling and torsional dynamics in dilated cardiomyopathy: reversed apical rotation as a marker of disease severity. *Eur J Heart Fail* 2009; **11**(10):945–51.

64 Saito M, Okayama H, Nishimura K, Ogimoto A, Ohtsuka T, Inoue K, *et al.* Determinants of LV untwisting behaviour in patients with dilated cardiomyopathy: analysis by two-dimensional speckle tracking. *Heart* 2009; **95**(4):290–6.

65 Popovi ZB, Grimm RA, Ahmad A, Agler D, Favia M, Dan G, *et al.* Longitudinal rotation: an unrecognised motion pattern in patients with dilated cardiomyopathy. *Heart* 2008; **94**(3):e11.

66 Fowler MB, Laser JA, Hopkins GL, Minobe W, Bristow MR. Assessment of beta-adrenergic receptor pathway in the intact failing human heart: progressive receptor down-regulation and subsensitivity to agonist response. *Circulation* 1986, **74**: 1290–302.

67 Drozd J, Krzeminska-Pakula M, Plewka M, Ciesielczyk M, Kasprzak JD. Prognostic value of low dose dobutamine echocardiography in patients with dilated cardiomyopathy. *Chest* 2002; **121**:1216–22.

68 Scrutinio D, Napoli V, Passantino A, Ricci A, Lagioia R, Rizzon P. Low-dose dobutamine responsiveness in idiopathic dilated cardiomyopathy: relation to exercise capacity and clinical outcome. *Eur Heart J* 2000; **21**(11):927–34.

69 Paraskevaidis IA, Adamopoulos S, Kremastinos Th: Dobutamine echocardiographic study in patients with nonischemic dilated catdiomyopathy and prognosticall borderline values of peak exercise oxygen consumption: 18-month follow-up study. *J Am Coll Cardiol* 2001, **37**:1685–91.

70 Paelinck B, Vermeersch P, Stockman D, Convens C, Vaerenbeg M: Usefulness of low-dose dobutamine stress echocardiography in predicting recovery of poor LV function in atrial fibrillation dilated cardiomyopathy. *Am J Cardiol* 1999; **83**:1668–70.

71 Kitaoka H, Takata T, Yabe N, Hitomi N, Furuno T, Doi YL. Low dose dobutamine stress echocardiography predicts the improvement of LV systolic function in dilated cardiomyopathy. *Heart* 1999, **81**:523–27.

72 Pratali L, Picano E, Otaševi! P, Vigna C, Palinkas A, Cortigiani L, *et al.* Prognostic significante of the dobutamine echocardiography test in idiopathic dilated cardiomyopathy. *Am J Cardiol* 2001, **88**(12):1374–8.

73 Naqvi TS, Goel RK, Forrester JS, Siegel RJ. Myocardial contractile reserve on dobutamine echocardiography predicts late spontaneous improvement in cardiac function in patients with recent onset idiopathic dilated cardiomyopathy. *J Am Coll Cardiol* 1999, **34**:1537–44.

74 Ida K, Sersu MF, Fujieda K. Pathologic significance of LV hypertrophy in dilated cardiomyopathy. *Clin Cardiol* 1996, **19**:704–8.

75 Otaševic P, Popovic ZB, Vasiljevic JD, Vidakovic R, Pratali L, Vlahovic A, *et al.* Relation of myocardial histomorphometric features and LV contractile reserve assessed by high-dose dobutamine stress echocardiography in patients with idiopathic dilated cardiomyopathy. *Eur J Heart Fail* 2005, **7**:49–56.

76 Perper EJ, Segall GM. Safety of dipyridamole-thallium imaging in high risk patients with known or suspected coronary artery disease. *J Nucl Med* 1991; **32**(11):2107–14.

77 Pingitore A, Picano E, Varga A, Gigli G, Cortigiani L, Previtali M, *et al.* Prognostic value of pharmacological stress echocardiography in patients with known or suspected coronary artery disease: a prospective, large-scale, multicenter, head-to-head comparison between dipyridamole and dobutamine test. Echo-Persantine International Cooperative (EPIC) and Echo- Dobutamine International Cooperative (EDIC) Study Groups. *J Am Coll Cardiol* 1999, **34**:1769–77.

78 Biaggioni I, Olafsson B, Robertson RM, Hollister AS, Robertson D: Cardiovascular and respiratory effects of adenosine in conscious man. Evidence for chemoreceptor activation. *Circ Res* 1987, **61**:779–86.

79 Pratali L: Prognostic value of contractile reserve during dipyridamole stress-echocardiography in idiopathic dilated cardiomyopathy. *Eur J Heart Fail* 2005

80 Pratali L, Otasevic P, Neskovic A, Molinaro S, Picano E. Prognostic value of pharmacologic stress echocardiography in patients with idiopathic dilated cardiomyopathy: a prospective, head-to-head comparison between dipyridamole and dobutamine test. *J Card Fail* 2007; **13**(10):836–42.

81 Pratali L, Otasevic P, Rigo F, Gherardi S, Neskovic A, Picano E. The additive prognostic value of restrictive pattern and dipyridamole-induced contractile reserve in idiopathic dilated cardiomyopathy. *Eur J Heart Fail* 2005; **7**(5):844–51.

82 Santagata P, Rigo F, Gherardi S, Pratali L, Drozdz J, Varga A, Picano E. Clinical and functional determinants of coronary flow reserve in non-ischemic dilated cardiomyopathy: an echocardiographic study. *Int J Cardiol* 2005; **105**(1):46–52.

83 Rigo F, Gherardi S, Galderisi M, Pratali L, Cortigiani L, Sicari R, Picano E. The prognostic impact of coronary flow-reserve assessed by Doppler echocardiography in non-ischaemic dilated cardiomyopathy. *Eur Heart J* 2006; **27**(11):1319–23.

84 Rigo F, Gherardi S, Galderisi M, Sicari R, Picano E. The independent prognostic value of contractile and coronary flow reserve determined by dipyridamole stress echocardiography in patients with idiopathic dilated cardiomyopathy. *Am J Cardiol* 2007; **99**(8):1154–8.

85 Sicari R, Nihoyannopoulos P, Evangelista A, Kasprzak J, Lancellotti P, Poldermans D, *et al.* Stress Echocardiography Expert Consensus Statement—Executive Summary. *Eur Heart J* 2009; **30**:278–89.

86 DiSalvo TG, Mathier M, Semigran MJ, Dec GW. Preserved right ventricular ejection fraction predicts exercise capacity and survival in advanced heart failure. *J Am Coll Cardiol* 1995, **25**:1143–53.

87 Gorcsan J, Murali S, Counihan PJ, Mandarino WA, Kormos RL. Right ventricular performance and contractile reserve in patients with severe heart failure: assessment by pressure-area relations and association with outcome. *Circulation* 1996, **94**:3190–7.

88 Corrado D, Basso C, Thiene G, McKenna WJ, Davies MJ, Fontaliran F, *et al.* Spectrum of clinicopathologic manifestations of arrhythmogenic right ventricular cardiomyopathy/dysplasia: a multicenter study. *J Am Coll Cardiol* 1997; **30**:1512–20.

89 Teske AJ, Cox MG, De Boeck BW, Doevendans PA, Hauer RN, Cramer MJ. Echocardiographic tissue deformation imaging quantifies abnormal regional right ventricular function in arrhythmogenic right ventricular dysplasia/cardiomyopathy. *J Am Soc Echocardiogr* 2009; **22**(8):920–7.

90 Jenni R, Oechslin E, Schneider J, Attenhofer Jost C, Kaufmann PA, *et al.* Echocardiographic and pathoanatomical characteristics of isolated LV non-compaction: a step towards classification as a distinct cardiomyopathy. *Heart* 2001; **86**:666–71.

91 Stöllberger C, Blazek G, Wegner C, Winkler-Dworak M, Finsterer J. Neuromuscular and cardiac comorbidity determines survival in 140 patients with left ventricular hypertrabeculation/noncompaction. *Int J Cardiol* 2010; Mar 10 [Epub ahead of print].

92 Hughes, William J McKenna. New insights into pathology of inherited cardiomyopathies: *Heart* 2005; **91**:257–264.

93 Stollberger C, Finsterer J. Cardiologic and neurologic findings in LV hypertrabeculation/non-compaction related to wall thickness, size and systolic function. *Eur J Heart Fail* 2005; **7**:95–7.

94 van Dalen BM, Caliskan K, Soliman OI, Nemes A, Vletter WB, Ten Cate FJ, *et al.* LV solid body rotation in non-compaction cardiomyopathy: a potential new objective and quantitative functional diagnostic criterion? *Eur J Heart Fail* 2008; **10**(11): 1088–93.

95 Dutka DP, Donnelly JE, Palka P, Lange A, Nunez DJ, Nihoyannopoulos P. Echocardiographic characterization of cardiomyopathy in Friedreich's ataxia with tissue Doppler echocardiographically derived myocardial velocity gradients. *Circulation* 2000; **102**(11):1276e82.

96 Hawley RJ, Milner MR, Gottdiener JS, Cohen A. Myotonic heart disease: a clinical follow-up. *Neurology* 1991; **41**(2 Pt1):259e62.

97 Fung KC, Corbett A, Kritharides L. Myocardial tissue velocity reduction is correlated with clinical neurologic severity in myotonic dystrophy. *Am J Cardiol* 2003; **92**(2):177e81.

98 Bushby KMTM, Gardner-Medwin D. Prevalence and incidence of Becker muscular dystrophy. *Lancet* 1991; **337**(8748):1022e4.

99 Agretto A, Politano L, Bossone E, Petretta VR, D'Isa S, Passamano L, *et al.* Pulsed Doppler tissue imaging in dystrophinopathic cardiomyopathy. *J Am Soc Echocardiogr* 2002; **15**(9):891e9.

100 Mertens L, Ganame J, Claus P, Goemans N, Thijs D, Eyskens B, *et al.* Early regional myocardial dysfunction in young patients with Duchenne muscular dystrophy. *J Am Soc Echocardiogr* 2008; **21**(9):1049–54.

101 Connuck DM, Sleeper LA, Colan SD, Cox GF, Towbin JA, Lowe AM, *et al.* Pediatric Cardiomyopathy Registry Study Group. Characteristics and outcomes of cardiomyopathy in children with Duchenne or Becker muscular dystrophy: a comparative study from the Pediatric Cardiomyopathy Registry. *Am Heart J* 2008; **155**(6):998–1005.

102 Richardson P. Report of the WHO/ISFC task force on the definition and classification of cardiomyopathy. *Circulation* 1996; **93**:341–2.

103 Moyssakis I, Triposkiadis F, Rallidis L, Hawkins P, Kyriakidis M, Nihoyannopoulos P. Echocardiographic features of primary, secondary and familial amyloidosis. *Eur J Clin Invest* 1999; **29**: 484–9.

104 Palka P, Lange A, Donnelly JE, Scalia G, Burstow DJ, Nihoyannopoulos P. Doppler tissue echocardiographic features of cardiac amyloidosis. *J Am Soc Echocardiogr* 2002; **15**:1353–60.

105 Weidemann F, Niemann M, Breunig F, Herrmann S, Beer M, Störk S, Voelker W, Ertl G, Wanner C, Strotmann J. Long-term effects of enzyme replacement therapy on Fabry cardiomyopathy: evidence for a better outcome with early treatment. *Circulation* 2009; **119**(4):524–9.

106 Kremastinos DT, Tsiapras DP, Tsetsos GA, Rentoukas EI, Vretou HP, Toutouzas PK. Left ventricular diastolic Doppler characteristics in beta-thalassemia major. *Circulation* 1993; **88**:1127–1135.

107 Malissa J Wood, Michael H Picard. Utility of echocardiography in the evaluation of cardiomyopathies. *Heart* 2004; **90**:707–712.

108 Hatle LK, Appleton CP, Popp RL. Differential of constrictive pericarditis and restrictive cardiomyopathy by Doppler echocardiography. *Circulation* 1989; **79**:357–70.

Further reading

Elliott P. Diagnosis and management of dilated cardiomyopathy. *Heart* 2000; **84**:106–12.

Gorcsan J 3rd, Abraham T, Agler DA, Bax JJ, Derumeaux G, Grimm RA, *et al.* Echocardiography for cardiac resynchronization therapy: recommendations for performance and reporting—a report from the American Society of Echocardiography Dyssynchrony Writing Group endorsed by the Heart Rhythm Society. American Society of Echocardiography Dyssynchrony Writing Group. *J Am Soc Echocardiogr* 2008; **21**:191–213.

Graham RM, Owens WA. Pathogenesis of inherited forms of dilated cardiomyopathy. *N Engl J Med* 1999; **341**:1759–62.

Hughes S, McKenna WJ. New insights into pathology of inherited cardiomyopathies: *Heart* 2005; **91**:257–64.

Mestroni L, Maisch B, McKenna WJ, Schwartz K, Charron P, Rocco C, *et al.* on behalf of the Collaborative Research Group of the European Human and Capital Mobility Project on Familial Dilated Cardiomyopathy. Guidelines for the study of familial dilated cardiomyopathies. *Eur Heart J* 1999; **20**:93–102.

Pasotti M, Klersy C, Pilotto A, Marziliano N, Rapezzi C, Serio A, *et al.* Long-term outcome and risk stratification in dilated cardiolaminopathies. *J Am Coll Cardiol* 2008, **52**:1250–60.

➲   For additional multimedia materials please visit the online version of the book (http://escecho.oxfordmedicine.com).

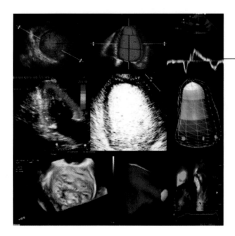

CHAPTER 18

Cardiac involvement in systemic diseases

Andreas Hagendorff

Contents

Summary

Systemic diseases are generally an interdisciplinary challenge in clinical practice. Systemic diseases are able to induce tissue damage in different organs with ongoing duration of the illness. The heart and the circulation are important targets in systemic diseases. The cardiac involvement in systemic diseases normally introduces a chronic process of alterations in cardiac tissue, which causes cardiac failure in the end stage of the diseases or causes dangerous and life-threatening problems by induced acute cardiac events, such as myocardial infarction due to coronary thrombosis. Thus, diagnostic methods—especially imaging techniques—are required, which can be used for screening as well as for the detection of early stages of the diseases. Two-dimensional echocardiography is the predominant diagnostic technique in cardiology for the detection of injuries in cardiac tissue—e.g. the myocardium, endocardium, and the pericardium—due to the overall availability of the non-invasive procedure.

The quality of the echocardiography and the success rate of detecting cardiac pathologies in patients with primary non-cardiac problems depend on the competence and expertise of the investigator. Especially in this scenario clinical knowledge about the influence of the systemic disease on cardiac anatomy and physiology is essential for central diagnostic problem. Therefore the primary echocardiography in these patients should be performed by an experienced clinician or investigator. It is possible to detect changes of cardiac morphology and function at different stages of systemic diseases as well as complications of the systemic diseases by echocardiography.

The different parts of this chapter will show proposals for qualified transthoracic echocardiography focusing on cardiac structures which are mainly involved in different systemic diseases.

Physiological conditions influencing Cardiovascular system

Athlete's heart

The cardiac adaptation to physical activity, especially long-term training, is a complex mechanism. Left ventricular (LV) hypertrophy is generally a cardiovascular risk factor. Thus, an increase of LV mass in athletes can be assumed to be linked to an unfavourable prognosis.

In the literature, however, the term physiological cardiac hypertrophy in athletes is used. This implies that intermittent pressure and volume overload during sustained exercise training induces LV hypertrophy with preserved myocardial structure which is characterized by normal pattern of gene expression and collagen metabolism. This hypertrophy will not cause progression into LV dysfunction and has to be completely reversible.

In athlete's heart, two types of physiological hypertrophy can be distinguished. During endurance training and dynamic exercise (e.g. running, skiing, soccer), volume overload occurs inducing eccentric LV hypertrophy. During strength training and static exercise (e.g. weight-lifting, gymnastics, wrestling) pressure overload occurs inducing concentric LV hypertrophy.

The echocardiographic findings to document volume overload are increased LV end-diastolic volume (LVEDV), increased LV wall thickness, increased right ventricular (RV) diastolic dimensions, and increased inferior vena cava (IVC) dimension. The echocardiographic findings to document pressure overload are normal heart cavity size in the presence of an increasing wall thickness.

To detect LV hypertrophy conventional M-mode is commonly used. Three-dimensional (3D) echocardiography should be performed for accurate LV mass determination. Echocardiography is certainly able to detect and monitor cardiac changes due to sustained exercise training. The discussion, however, whether or not LV hypertrophy in athletes can be accepted as normal or healthy, is still ongoing. It is important to detect pathological hypertrophy like hypertrophic cardiomyopathy which is the most common cause of sudden cardiac death in athletes. Hypertrophy per se will enlarge diffusion layers. The longer the distance for oxygen diffusion, the earlier endocardial hypoxia will occur during a stress induced mismatch between energy supply and energy consumption. Endocardial hypoxia at maximum stress will serve per se as an arrhythmogenic substrate which predisposes to malignant arrhythmias. Therefore, LV hypertrophy in athletes should be interpreted with caution.

The detection of pathological hypertrophy will be aggravated by the misuse of amphetamines and other drugs in high performance sport. The detection of fibrosis in LV wall thickening by tissue Doppler (TD) imaging as well as by delayed enhancement using cardiac magnetic resonance (CMR) should be integrated into the diagnostic procedure to differentiate between the so-called physiological and pathophysiological LV hypertrophy.

Heart during pregnancy

Pregnancy induces physiological changes of the cardiovascular system in order to enable adequate delivery of oxygenated blood to peripheral tissue and fetus. Due to the increased circulating blood volume and the decreased systemic vascular resistance the general echocardiographic findings in pregnancy are a left and right atrial and ventricular dilation, an increased stroke volume (SV) and cardiac output (CO), and changes in mitral and tricuspid valve coaptation—often combined with a mild mitral and tricuspid valve regurgitation. Regurgitation velocities of the atrioventricular valves are slightly increased. Small pericardial effusions are frequently found. The adaptation of the cardiovascular system to chronic volume overload peaks during the third trimester.

Echocardiography is important before pregnancy to detect risk patients. Women with cardiac diseases like dilated cardiomyopathy, obstructive valve lesions, moderate to severe regurgitations, and pulmonary hypertension are not able to adapt to the increase of blood volume. The decision to continue pregnancy or to induce abortion in women with structural heart disease is difficult, has to be performed individually due to the desire to have children, and requires accurate evaluation by echocardiography.

The normal increase of CO in pregnancy is about 30–50% during the third trimester. In the peripartum period a further increase of about 15% occurs. Thus, women at high risk during labour, who are not able to accommodate to the increases in preload, have to undergo section Caesarean. The high-risk group of women includes patients with dilated cardiomyopathy, obstructive valvular stenosis including pulmonary stenosis, moderate to severe valvular insufficiencies, and severe systemic and pulmonary hypertension. If women of this patient cohort become pregnant and an indicated abortion is refused due to individual reasons, they have to be monitored by echocardiography to estimate the risk of acute cardiac failure. Thus echocardiography in these patients has to be periodically performed—especially during the last trimester in short-term follow-ups. During in vitro fertilization, myocardial oedema, pericardial and pleural effusion, and thrombotic complications can be observed and should be detected and monitored by echocardiography.

A further disorder with unknown aetiology is the peripartum cardiomyopathy which occurs during the last month of pregnancy or within the first few months after delivery. It is supposed to be related to a pre-existing cardiomyopathy. The echocardiographic findings are the enlargement of all cardiac cavities—primarily the LV, pericardial and pleural effusion, and often mural thrombi in the cardiac cavities. Pulmonary hypertension due to pulmonary embolism can be detected. The course of peripartum cardiomyopathy differs between complete recovery and persisting cardiomegaly with LV dysfunction.

Diseases with a main influence on coronary arteries and thoracic arteries

Hypertension

Echocardiography in patients with suspected hypertension is very important as a screening tool for LV hypertrophy. LV hypertrophy reflects end-organ damage of arterial hypertension (AH) and should be treated according to the guidelines. Therefore the measurements of wall thickness should be performed with accuracy.[1] The M-mode using the parasternal approach is still the most common way for the detection of LV wall thickness (see ⊃ Chapter 2). The main problem of M-mode-measurements using a monoplane probe is still the standardization (⊃ Fig. 18.1; ◼ 18.1–18.4). Every wrong transducer position will produce increased wall thickness.

With ongoing hypertensive heart disease a mismatch of energy supply and consumption occurs mainly in the end territories of the coronary arteries due to severe myocardial hypertrophy. Thus severe hypertension normally causes stunning phenomena in the apical inferior/inferoseptal region, which reflects the end territory of the left anterior descending artery.

However, coronary sclerosis can produce narrowing of coronary arteries in every part of the coronary tree which can also produce hypokinesia as well as post-systolic shortening in every other region of the LV. In suspected coronary artery disease (CAD) in patients with hypertensive heart disease, stress echocardiography should be additionally performed.

In severe hypertensive heart disease, congestive heart failure (HF) with severe reduced global LV function can be found. Important complications of AH are, for example, aneurysm of the ascending aorta, severe aortic valve regurgitation (AR), dissection of the thoracic aorta, acute myocardial infarction, and moderate to severe mitral valve regurgitation (MR) in hypertensive heart failure[2] (⊃ Fig. 18.2; ◼ 18.5–18.8).

In patients with AH, assessment by echocardiography of the following items is required:

♦ LV wall thickness.

♦ Global systolic LV function (Teichholz, Simpson).

♦ Regional LV wall motion abnormalities (WMAs).

♦ Diastolic function.

♦ Valvular morphology and function.

♦ Right ventricular (RV) function.

♦ Pulmonary hypertension.

Diabetes

In patients with diabetes mellitus there is an increased incidence of large vessel atherosclerosis as well as of intimal thickening

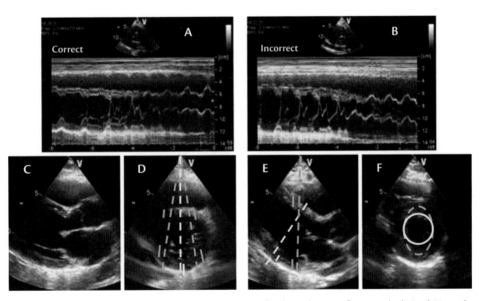

Figure 18.1 Standardized transthoracic examination in echocardiography: reason for the technique of a correctly derived M-mode sweep (A) and an incorrectly derived M-mode-sweep (transducer position derived too far in the caudal and lateral direction) (B). Correct parasternal long-axis view (C) and parasternal short-axis view (D). Incorrect parasternal long-axis view (E) and parasternal short-axis view (F). Possible incorrect scan lines in the short axis (secant slices) in the case of M-mode derivations from the long axis are shown in part (D). Incorrect scanning results in measurements with LV diameters that are too small and LV walls that are too thick (see outlined paths—correct in yellow, incorrect in orange). Incorrect transducer positions derived too far in the caudal and lateral direction result in measurements with LV diameters that are too large and LV walls that are too thick (see outlined paths—correct in yellow, incorrect in orange) (E and F).

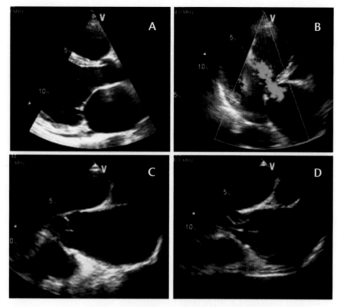

Figure 18.2 Example of complications of arterial hypertension.
Congestive heart failure in hypertensive heart disease (A); severe aortic regurgitation due to aortic annular dilation (B); aneurysm of the ascending aorta (C); and Stanford A dissection (D).

and inflammatory changes within the small arteries. Because it is reported that these patients have an abnormal or absent pain response to myocardial ischaemia mainly due to an autonomic nervous system dysfunction, echocardiography should focus on detection of regional wall motion disturbances.

Regional WMA evaluation should be performed not only by visual analysis, but also by modern techniques, able to detect minor changes in the regional kinetics: these techniques encompass the assessment of regional post-systolic contraction by M-mode, TD, and speckle tracking.

With ongoing disease, diastolic dysfunction can occur without significant regional systolic dysfunction. Due to the increased amount of collagen and other particles in the myocardial interstitium, the ventricular compliance is markedly impaired and pseudonormal as well as restrictive filling patterns can be observed. For estimation of LVEDP, the E/E' ratio should be always performed in patients with diabetes.

Furthermore, due to the high coincidence of CAD and diabetes, stress echocardiography is recommended in some guidelines at least every 2 years.[3]

In patients with diabetes, assessment by echocardiography of the following items is required:

◆ Global systolic LV function (Teichholz, Simpson).

◆ Regional LV WMAs.

◆ Diastolic function.

◆ Valvular morphology and function.

◆ RV function.

◆ Pulmonary hypertension.

Rheumatoid arthritis and other collagen vascular diseases

Rheumatoid arthritis and other collagen vascular diseases[4] can cause inflammatory processes in all parts of the heart. An important proportion of patients with rheumatoid arthritis (>20%) has intimal inflammation and oedema which can cause coronary artery stenosis with consecutive regional wall motion defects due to repetitive myocardial ischaemia. An interesting issue is the determination of coronary flow reserve (CFR) in these patients by vasodilator stress echocardiography (see also ➲ Chapter 13). In normal patients the CFR during adenosine administration is more than 2.5. In patients with rheumatoid arthritis and other collagen vascular diseases, dysfunction of coronary reactivity can be detected by this test. A pathological CFR can be explained in these patients either by significant epicardial stenosis due to inflammatory processes and/or concomitant coronary sclerosis or by microvessel disease (➲ Fig. 18.3; 🎞 18.9 and 18.10).

Heart valves are also involved by inflammation and formation of granuloma, in patients with rheumatoid arthritis and other collagen vascular diseases. Often regurgitations of the mitral and aortic valve can be observed.

The most common finding in patients with collagen vascular diseases is pericardial fluid. The appearance of *granular sparkling echos* causes an unspecific enhanced myocardial texture which may be due to the inflammatory myocardial processes or the nodula formation in the myocardium.

In patients with rheumatoid arthritis and other collagen vascular diseases, assessment by echocardiography of the following items is required:

◆ Myocardial texture.

◆ Global systolic LV function (Teichholz, Simpson).

◆ Regional left ventricular wall motion abnormalities.

◆ Diastolic function.

◆ Valvular morphology and function.

◆ RV function.

◆ Pulmonary hypertension.

◆ Coronary flow reserve by vasodilator stress echocardiography (optional).

Takayasu arteritis

Takayasu arteritis is an inflammatory disease of the medium- and large-sized arteries mostly observed in the aortic arch and the thoracic arterial branches. Due to the intimal proliferation, scarring and vascularization of the media, and disruption and/or degeneration of the elastic lamina vessel narrowing and/or occlusion and sometimes local thrombosis occur. The echocardiographic findings depend on the main effect of the systemic disease. Due to induced hypertension left and right ventricular

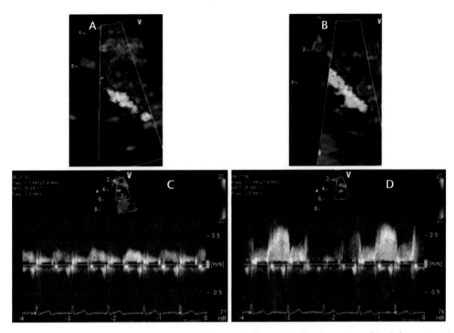

Figure 18.3 Coronary flow reserve. Example for non-invasive analysis of coronary flow in the distal portions of the left anterior descending artery. Color-coded illustration of the distal portion of the left anterior descending artery at rest (A), and during adenosine infusion (B). Coronary flow profile at rest (C) and during adenosine infusion (D) documenting a normal coronary flow reserve.

hypertrophy as well as aortic regurgitation (AR) can be observed. Pulmonary hypertension is often induced. In acute stages of the disease severe LV dysfunction and cardiac failure can be observed. Regional WMAs are rarely detected because coronaries are seldom affected. The experienced sonographer will often find abnormalities like stenosis, aneurysm due to poststenotic dilations, and occlusion of the aortic branches.

Kawasaki disease

Kawasaki disease is a mucocutaneous lymph node syndrome characterized by an acute, febrile systemic disease in children. The acute course of the disease is normally benign; however, in almost all severe cases vasculitis of the vasa vasorum of the coronary arteries occur. In acute fatal cases arteritic complications like myocardial infarction due to formation of aneurysm and subsequent thrombosis, and left ventricular dysfunction due to perimyocarditis can be observed.

The main common manifestation in adolescents after Kawasaki disease is the occurrence of acute myocardial ischaemia and myocardial infarction due to occlusion induced by severe aneurysm formation of the coronary arteries. Thus, the experienced sonographer will be able to detect enlargement of the proximal portions of the coronary arteries, because the aneurysm formation mostly affects the proximal parts of the coronary arteries, which can be analysed from the parasternal view. Due to myocardial ischaemia and consecutive inferior wall motion defects disturbances of the suspension of the mitral valve (MV) with concomitant mitral regurgitation (MR) can be found.

Syphilitic aortitis

The cardiovascular effects of a systemic infection with *Treponema pallidum* are due to the slowly progressive inflammatory course of the disease leading to a so-called tertiary stage or to the late syphilis. The cardiovascular manifestations of the syphilis are generally limited to the large thoracic vessels. The pathomechanism of aortitis is a medial necrosis due to endarteritis obliterans of the vasa vasorum, which destructs the elastic tissue of the vessel wall. With time, saccular aneurysms mostly in the ascending and transverse segments of the aorta will be formed. Syphilitic aneurysms do not normally lead to dissection. As concomitant effects, aortic valve regurgitation due to aortic annular dilation and ostium stenosis of the coronary arteries can be observed. Thus, the echocardiographic investigation in patients with a history of syphilis should focus on analysis of the thoracic aorta including suprasternal and transoesophageal views.

Marfan syndrome and Ehlers–Danlos syndrome

Marfan syndrome is defined by characteristic changes of the connective tissue system affecting the skeleton, the eyes, and the cardiovascular system. Ehlers–Danlos syndrome is another heritable disorder of the connective tissue. The weakness of the connective tissue mainly causes an aortic root dilation with a high risk of dissection. The echocardiographic findings are the dilation of the aortic annulus, of the sinuses of Valsalva, and of the ascending aorta. This entity is known as annuloaortic ectasia. Concomitant with this finding an AR can be observed.

Mitral annular dilation and chordae elongation of the MV often cause MV prolapse and concomitant MV regurgitation. The acute cardiovascular complication of Marfan syndrome is aortic dissection. The echocardiographic investigation in patients with Marfan or Ehlers–Danlos syndrome should focus on exact evaluation of aortic dimensions, especially in repetitive follow-up investigation to detect the optimal time point for necessary surgical intervention.

Temporal or giant cell arteritis

Giant cell arteritis is a systemic vasculitis involving the large- and medium-sized arteries, mostly the carotid arteries. The echocardiographic findings show aortic aneurism formation and in some acute cases aortic dissection. Aortic regurgitation due to aortic annular dilation and thickening of the aortic cusps due to inflammatory processes will be observed. A concomitant myocarditis can induce LV systolic and diastolic dysfunction. Pericardial effusion is often seen in the presence of concomitant pericarditis.

Hereditary haemorrhagic telangiectasia (Osler–Weber–Rendu)

Osler–Weber–Rendu disease is an autosomal dominant disease with systemic telangiectasia which primary affects the skin. It is characterized by primary arteriovenous malformations within the dermal microcirculation. The mucosal arteriovenous malformations can explain the tendency of bleeding complications in these patients. The formation of arteriovenous fistulas—especially in the pulmonary circulation—can cause hypoxemia and paradoxical embolism. The echocardiographic investigation should focus on the detection of high CO, the determination of shunt volume by measurement of Qp/Qs (see ➲ Chapter 5), and the evaluation of shunts by contrast echocardiography performed with right heart contrast agents (see ➲ Chapter 7). In contrast to interatrial communication defects the wash-in of microbubbles into the left atrium (LA) is some heart cycles later (3–4 RR intervals) than the wash-in into the right atrium (RA). In the presence of interatrial communication defects the wash in of microbubbles normally occurs simultaneously.

In patients with suspected arteritis and vascular problems, assessment by echocardiography of the following items is required:

◆ Assessment of LV size.

◆ Assessment of aortic dimension in different views, including suprasternal views.

◆ Assessment of the coronary ostia determined by the parasternal views.

◆ Assessment of morphology and function of the aortic valve (AoV).

◆ Analysis of RV function.

◆ Assessment of pulmonary hypertension.

◆ Optional: determination of arteriovenous shunts by contrast echocardiography.

Diseases with a main influence on heart valves

Rheumatic fever

Rheumatic fever is an inflammatory disease due to group A streptococci infection. The involvement of the heart occurs in the acute stage of the disease (which is actually rare in industrial countries due to the common use of antibiotic treatment) as well as during chronic conditions—mainly due to deformation processes of the heart valves.

Acute disease

In the acute inflammatory stage nearly all patients develop cardiac manifestation of the disease. The most characteristic involvement of rheumatic fever is verrucous valvulitis due to rheumatic endocarditis. Fibrous thickening and adhesion of the valvular commissures and chordae cause valvular deformation which is clearly detectable by echocardiography. The functional alterations lead to variable degrees of valvular stenosis and/or regurgitation which have to be quantified by Doppler echocardiography.

The less known consequence of acute rheumatic fever is the effect on myocardial tissue, in which inflammatory reactions occur. The local swelling and fragmentation of collagen fibres is histologically described by the myocardial Aschoff body, which can be seen in echocardiography as an enhanced myocardial texture. Large focal myocardial inflammation is sometimes combined with bride reflections within the myocardium. In some cases myocardial inflammation will induce acute myocardial HF. In addition, as a sign of a pancardiac disease acute rheumatic fever can produce pericardial effusions which are characterized by fibrinous structures at the visceral side of the pericardium.

Chronic disease

All acute cardiac alterations of rheumatic fever normally result in chronic manifestations of the disease. Valvular lesions depend on the amount of scarring of the valves as well as of the myocardium which determine the location, lesion, and severity of the valvular heart disease. The most common valvular lesion in post-rheumatic disease is the mitral valve stenosis (MS). Echocardiographic evaluation of MS is performed as described in ➲ Chapter 14b (➲ Fig. 18.4).

The AoV is less frequently affected than the MV. Morphologically the doming of the aortic cusps can be observed in case of adhesion. Post-rheumatic aortic regurgitation is more frequent than post-rheumatic aortic stenosis. In rare cases

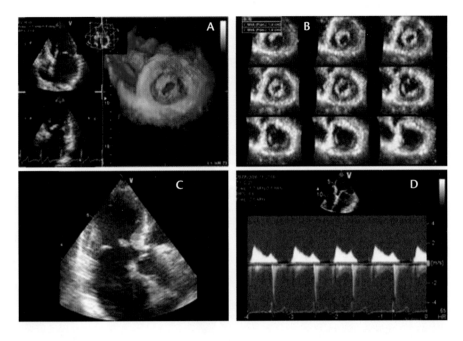

Figure 18.4 Multidimensional imaging of a post-rheumatic mitral valve stenosis.
Conventional multidimensional view from the apex to the mitral valve (A); 12-slice view for analysis of mitral valve orifice (B); conventional two-dimensional view in the apical long axis (C); and the continuous wave Doppler spectrum of mitral flow (D).

mitral, aortic, and tricuspid valve are affected. The non-invasive haemodynamic assessment of all valvular stenosis and insufficiencies has to be performed in these patients by echocardiography.

The progression of valvular calcification and sclerosis, the risk of endocarditis, and the risk of thrombus formation determine the further requirements of echocardiography in these patients.

The variability of the duration and severity of myocardial inflammation determines the degree of myocardial damage. The chronic rheumatic myocarditis or post-rheumatic myocarditis is characterized by severe systolic dysfunction. The differentiation between rheumatic and other causes of myocarditis can only be performed by the detection of other typical post-rheumatic cardiac as well as extracardiac manifestations. An isolated rheumatic myocarditis is not common due to the pancardiac nature of the rheumatic fever.

The pericardial effusion which is observed in the early stage of rheumatic fever often becomes calcified, but only in rare cases can significant pericardial constriction be observed.

In patients with rheumatic fever, assessment by echocardiography of the following items is required:

◆ Global systolic LV function (Teichholz, Simpson).

◆ Regional LV WMAs.

◆ Valvular morphology.

◆ Severity of stenosis and/or regurgitation of all valves involved.

◆ RV function.

◆ Pulmonary hypertension.

Systemic lupus erythematosus and antiphospholipid syndrome

The characteristic findings in echocardiography are endocardial lesions described by Libman and Sacks. The locations of the warty lesions are mostly described at the angles of the atrioventricular valves and at the ventricular surface of the mitral valve. However, the abacterial verrucous conglomerates can also be observed at the AoV. The valvular alterations are usually not haemodynamically relevant. However, in rare cases significant valvular stenosis and/or regurgitation can be observed (➲ Fig. 18.5).

In patients with lupus erythematosus, coronary arteritis may induce coronary stenosis with consecutive myocardial ischaemia. Acute myocardial infarction due to acute coronary inflammation is described. On the other hand, coronary sclerosis is often induced by hypertension and/or glucocorticoid therapy. Thus, regional wall motion of the LV has to be accurately analysed.

Pericardial effusion can be detected in most of the patients with systemic lupus erythematosus. In later stages of the disease pericardial constriction has to be verified or excluded.

A further important issue is the analysis of the RV and its function. Recurrent interstitial lupus pneumonitis with episodes of fever, dyspnoea, and cough causes pulmonary fibrosis. Therefore, the patients often develop pulmonary hypertension with RV hypertrophy. Early stages of RV affection can be determined by measuring a prolonged pulmonary pre-ejection interval in comparison to the aortic pre-ejection interval. RV function should be documented by TAPSE and TD spectra of the basal ventricular wall during follow-up investigations.

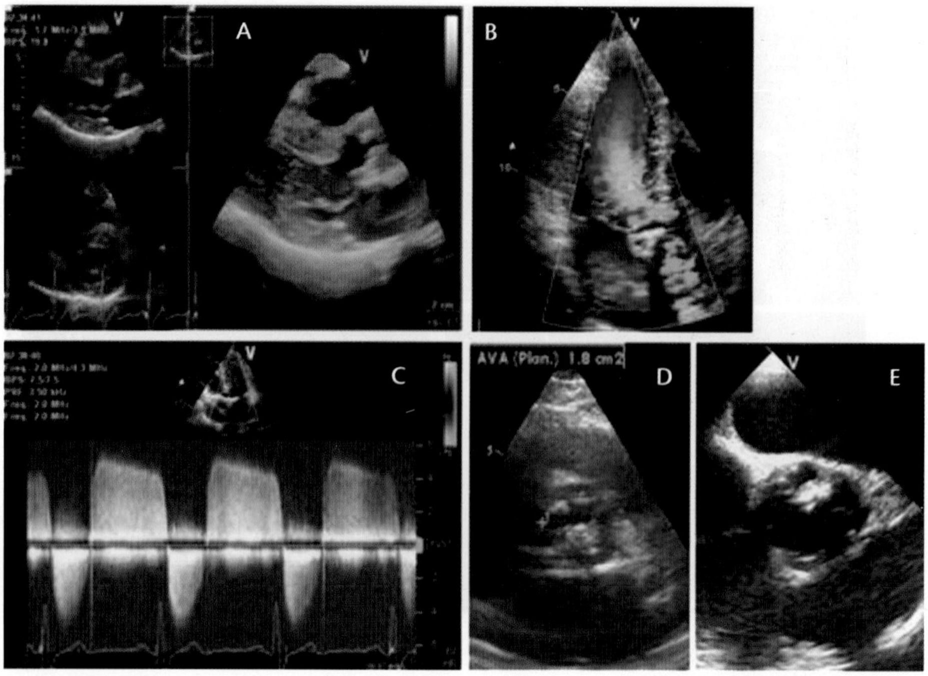

Figure 18.5 Example of Libman–Sacks endocarditis of the aortic valve. Multidimensional illustration (A); colour-coded illustration of systolic flow in the apical long-axis view (B); continuous wave Doppler spectrum documenting stenotic as well as regurgitant flow (C); and planimetry of the valvular orifice by transthoracic (D) and transoesophageal echocardiography (E).

In patients with antiphospholipid syndrome, valvular affections are also common, causing primarily valvular regurgitations. The echocardiographic analysis should additionally focus on LV dysfunction. Dilated cardiomyopathy and regional WMAs can be found due to vascular affections with consecutive myocardial ischaemia. Due to coronary thrombosis myocardial infarction can occur. Thrombus formation in the cardiac cavities and the aorta can be observed due to thrombophilia in patients with antiphospholipid syndrome. Thromboembolic complications originating from the venous system often induce chronic pulmonary hypertension due to chronic pulmonary embolism. In severe stages of the disease notching of the pulmonary flow signal can be detected.

In patients with systemic lupus erythematosus and/or antiphospholipid syndrome, assessment by echocardiography of the following items is required:

◆ Global systolic LV function (Teichholz, Simpson).
◆ Regional LV WMAs.
◆ Valvular morphology.
◆ Severity of stenosis and/or regurgitation of all valves involved.
◆ RV function.
◆ Pulmonary hypertension.

Carcinoid

The carcinoid tumours are mostly located in the gastrointestinal tract. The enterochromaffin cells secrete a variety of hormones which can induce valvular heart disease by destruction of the heart valves. Due to the gastrointestinal location of the tumour the lesions are almost exclusively on the right side of the heart. The characteristic lesion is usually a significant tricuspid valve regurgitation in combination with a relative pulmonary stenosis due to RV enlargement. In the end stage of the disease, RV failure due to severe tricuspid and pulmonary insufficiency will be detected. TTE focuses on the analysis of RV size and function as well as of the RV valves (➲ Fig. 18.6).

The distinct documentation of RV morphology and function—using modern techniques a triplane or multidimensional evaluation of the RV should be performed—is mandatory. Pulsed wave (PW) and continuous wave (CW) Doppler spectra through the tricuspid and pulmonary valve should be acquired for estimation of systolic, mean, and end-diastolic pulmonary pressure. RV preload has to be characterized by volume status of the inferior caval vein. Therapeutical options depend on RV function and on the individual prognosis of the patients. Thus, patients can only be treated in the presence of severe tricuspid and/or pulmonary regurgitations if RV function is preserved. Right heart failure in the end stage of the disease can be documented by diastolic flow through the pulmonary valve during inspiration (Fontan breathing) using PW Doppler.

In patients with carcinoid tumours, assessment by echocardiography of the following items is required:

◆ Global systolic LV function (Teichholz, Simpson).
◆ Regional LV WMAs.
◆ Valvular morphology, especially the tricuspid and pulmonary valve.
◆ Severity of stenosis and/or regurgitation of all valves involved.

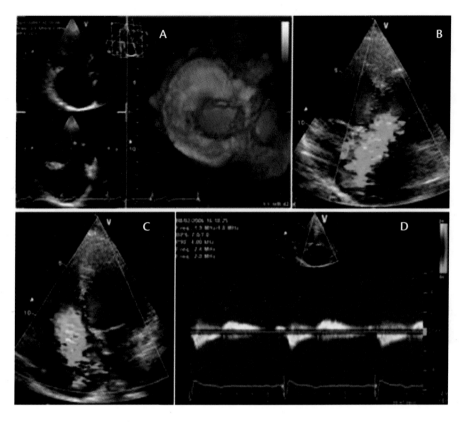

Figure 18.6 Example of tricuspid valve destruction in a patient with carcinoid. Multidimensional illustration (A); colour-coded illustration of systolic tricuspid flow in the apical two-chamber view of the right ventricle (B); and the apical four-chamber view (C); continuous wave Doppler spectrum through the tricuspid valve (D).

♦ RV function.

♦ Pulmonary hypertension.

Diseases with a main influence on myocardial tissue damage

Amyloidosis

Amyloidosis is defined by extracellular depositions of the fibrous protein amyloid. The clinical manifestation depends mainly on the involved organ system. Amyloidosis is associated with different diseases, e.g. multiple myeloma and other haemato-oncological disorders, chronic infective diseases like osteomyelitis and tuberculosis, or chronic inflammatory diseases like rheumatoid arthritis. Furthermore, amyloidosis is observed with aging and with long-term dialysis.

Cardiac manifestation is indicated by a significant wall thickening of the LV and the RV. Echocardiography cannot distinguish between hypertrophy, myocardial oedema, or myocardial thickening due to pathological depositions. The thickening of the LV wall is normally symmetric. At the beginning of myocardial deposition of amyloid the size of the LV cavity is normal. With ongoing disease diffuse hypokinesia occurs which is often pronounced in septal regions. The myocardium shows typically a hyper-reflective *granular sparkling*. With increasing wall thickening the size of the LV and RV cavities is reduced mocking

hypercontractility instead of reduced myocardial function. At the end stage of amyloidosis a severe restrictive filling pattern of the cavities can typically be observed which is combined with an individual poor prognosis of the patient. In these patients the atrial cavities are significantly enlarged in comparison to the ventricles (◑ Fig. 18.7).

Pericarditis with effusion is observed very rarely in patients with amyloidosis.

In patients with amyloidosis, assessment by echocardiography of the following items is required:

♦ Myocardial texture

♦ Global systolic LV function (Teichholz, Simpson)

♦ Regional LV WMAs

♦ Diastolic function

♦ Pericardial effusion

Haemochromatosis and other storage diseases (Fabry disease)

Haemochromatosis is an iron-storage disorder with potential tissue damage and functional impairment of the organ systems involved. Cardiac manifestation occurs in 25–20% of the disease. The most common cardiac manifestation is congestive HF. Echocardiography usually documents an enlargement of all cardiac cavities. The morphological entity is comparable to dilated or idiopathic cardiomyopathy.

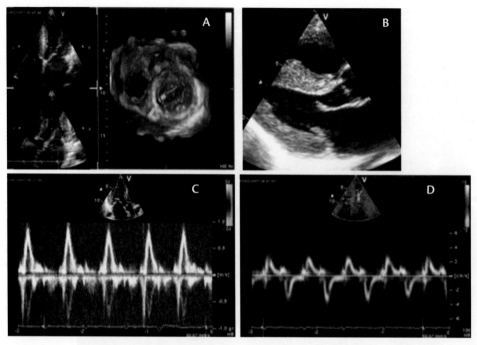

Figure 18.7 Example of amyloidosis in a patient with multiple myeloma. Multidimensional illustration (A); illustration of myocardial texture with 'granular sparkling' (B); pulsed wave Doppler spectrum of the mitral flow documenting restrictive filling pattern (C); and pulsed wave tissue Doppler spectrum of the basal septal myocardium (D).

Among several storage diseases Fabry disease shows the most important cardiac manifestations. Fabry disease is induced by an accumulation of galactosylgalactosylglucosylceramide due to a deficiency of the enzyme α-galactosidase A. The disorder is X-linked. In men symptoms develop within the third and fourth decade, in women usually one decade later. Echocardiography documents LV wall thickening in early stages due to the lipid deposition. With ongoing disease increasing lipid deposition can cause myocardial damage with alterations of the valvular function and/or myocardial infarction. Thus, during follow-up echocardiography distinct analysis of regional wall motion has to be performed.

Other storage diseases like leucodystrophies, Niemann–Pick disease or Gaucher disease very rarely have cardiac manifestations. Due to recurrent pulmonary infections and infiltrates pulmonary hypertension can be detected by echocardiography.

In patients with haemochromatosis and other storage diseases, assessment by echocardiography of the following items is required:

◆ Myocardial texture.

◆ LV wall thickness.

◆ Global systolic LV function (Teichholz, Simpson).

◆ Regional LV WMAs.

◆ Diastolic function.

◆ Valvular function.

◆ RV function.

Systemic sclerosis (scleroderma) and other tissue diseases (mixed connective tissue disease, ankylosing spondylitis, Reiter syndrome)

Systemic sclerosis is characterized by an overproduction of collagen presumably due to an aberrant regulation of fibroblast cell growth or to an increased synthesis of connective tissue. Because immunologic abnormalities and perivascular damage is observed in systemic sclerosis, immunological and vascular mechanisms are discussed in the pathogenesis of this disease. Scleroderma produces fibrosis of the skin, vessels, and visceral organs like gastrointestinal tract, lungs, kidneys, and heart.

The most often observed clinical cardiac problem in patients with systemic sclerosis is a pericarditis without effusion, which cannot be detected by echocardiography.

Two entities of myocardial damage can be observed by echocardiography in patients with scleroderma. Firstly, cardiomyopathy is directly caused by myocardial fibrosis; granular sparkling, wall thickening due to oedema and/or fibrosis, WMAs, and mostly regurgitations of the atrioventricular valves will be observed due to retraction of the leaflets induced by scarring and/or dilation of the ventricles. Secondly, LV as well as RV dysfunction may be induced by systemic or pulmonary AH. In end-stage disease congestive left HF as well as cor pulmonale are described.

A further cardiac problem is caused by intermittent vasospasm. Episodes of Prinzmetal's angina may induce regional wall motion disturbances. With ongoing duration of a hyper-reactive α-adrenergic coronary vasoconstriction myocardial infarction may occur in this patient cohort.

In other connective tissue diseases such as mixed connective tissue disease, ankylosing spondylitis, and Reiter syndrome, different echocardiographic findings depending on the leading characteristic may be found. In most patients with mixed connective tissue disease, signs of pericarditis can be found. In ankylosing spondylitis and Reiter syndrome alterations of the AoV, dilation of the aortic root, and LV dysfunction are common. Nevertheless, the sonographer has to perform an accurate documentation of the echocardiographic findings, because all possible findings due to the affection of the myocardium, the coronaries, and the valves can be found in patients with connective tissue diseases.

In patients with systemic sclerosis and other connective tissue diseases, assessment by echocardiography of the following items is required:

◆ Myocardial texture.

◆ Global systolic LV function (Teichholz, Simpson).

◆ Regional LV WMAs.

◆ Diastolic function.

◆ Valvular function.

◆ Pericardial effusion.

Sarcoidosis

In sarcoidosis accumulation of lymphocytes and phagocytes causes epitheloid granulomas interacting with the tissue of the organ involved. A small proportion of patients with sarcoidosis will have cardiac manifestation. LV wall is most common affected by granuloma formation. The tissue damage is normally in the mid-myocardial layers and causes regional WMAs. Furthermore due to papillary muscle dysfunction restriction of the chordae tendineae will be induced causing insufficiencies of the atrioventricular valves. Right heart affection is potentially induced by pulmonary manifestation of the disease causing pulmonary AH.

In patients with severe cardiac manifestation of sarcoidosis congestive HF can occur documented by severe LV dysfunction in echocardiography.

In patients with sarcoidosis, assessment by echocardiography of the following items is required:

◆ Myocardial texture.

◆ Global systolic LV function (Teichholz, Simpson).

◆ Regional LV WMAs.

◆ Diastolic function.

◆ Valvular function.

◆ Pericardial effusion.

Eosinophilic endomyocardial disease and hypereosinophilic syndrome

The eosinophilic endomyocardial disease is also known as Loeffler's endocarditis or fibroplastic endocarditis. In some patients with hypereosinophilia the heart is predominantly involved. Presumably due to a local inflammatory process the endocardium and the underlying myocardium in both ventricles are thickened. The local inflammatory reaction—mostly in the apical regions of the ventricles—induces a local thrombogenic milieu which predisposes to thrombus formation. Thus, large mural thrombi can be observed within the LV and RV which are able to compromise the cardiac cavities and to serve as source of systemic and pulmonary embolism. In echocardiography it has to be emphasized that in patients with Loeffler's endocarditis thrombus formation can be observed in the presence of complete normal regional wall motion.

Sometimes a local cardiac tissue hypereosinophilia can produce thrombus formation. Then, normal global and regional wall motion with apical thrombus formation is present without peripheral hypereosinophilia (➲ Fig. 18.8).

Loeffler's endocarditis has to be separated from the endomyocardial fibrosis which can be found in tropical and subtropical regions. This disease is mainly characterized by fibrous endocardial lesions mainly in the inflow tract of the left and right ventricle. Thus, the atrioventricular valves are often involved with the sequelae of regurgitation. However, in some patients thrombotic masses are also found in the apical regions.

In patients with eosinophilic endomyocardial disease, assessment by echocardiography of the following items is required:

◆ Myocardial texture.

◆ LV wall thickness.

◆ Global systolic LV function (Teichholz, Simpson).

◆ Regional LV WMAs.

◆ Diastolic function.

◆ Thrombus formations.

◆ Valvular function.

◆ Pericardial effusion.

Endocrine diseases

Hyperthyroidism

In patients with hyperthyroidism, increased CO has to be determined by echocardiographic investigation. It can be quantitatively measured by Doppler techniques and semiquantitatively estimated by turbulences within the LV using colour Doppler (CD) imaging. The tachycardia-induced diastolic dysfunction can be observed at early stages of the disease. With ongoing disease compensatory mechanisms can be detected, such as increase in LV mass as well as tachycardia-induced cardiomyopathy.

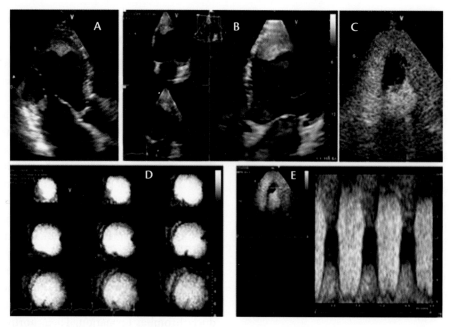

Figure 18.8 Loeffler's endocarditis. Example of Loeffler's endocarditis with apical thrombus formation in the left ventricular cavity. Conventional illustration in the apical long-axis view (A) and multidimensional illustration of the thrombus formation (B); thrombus illustration by contrast imaging using perfusion imaging technique (C); illustration by nine slices using contrast echocardiography (D); illustration of missing perfusion in the thrombus formation by anatomical M-Mode during contrast infusion documenting normal regional apical contraction and normal myocardial replenishment in the tissue near the thrombus formation (E).

A secondary pulmonary hypertension is a not common finding in patients with hyperthyroidism.

Hypothyroidism

In patients with hypothyroidism two pathological entities have to be considered. Firstly, due to significant elevations of cholesterol and triglycerides, severe coronary arteriosclerosis is common. Thus, echocardiography should detect regional WMAs with the same attention as in the other risk groups of hypertension and diabetes. Secondly, due to the increased capillary permeability, pericardial effusion can often be observed. In the presence of a circular pericardial effusion the end-diastolic distance between the pericardial layers should be determined behind the LV using M-mode. In the presence of localized pericardial effusion different reproducible views should be acquired to document possible changes during follow-up investigations. Because of its chronic genesis pericardial tamponade is very rare. Patients with severe hypothyroidism are often sent for echocardiography because of suspected congestive heart failure due to the clinical signs of peripheral oedema, dyspnoea, hypotension, and pleural effusion.

In patients with hyper- and hypothyroidism, assessment by echocardiography of the following items is required:

- Assessment of global systolic LV function (Teichholz, Simpson).
- Assessment of regional LV WMAs.
- Assessment of diastolic function.
- Assessment valvular morphology and function.
- Assessment of RV function.
- Assessment of pulmonary hypertension.
- Assessment of pericardial effusion.

Phaeochromocytoma

In patients with phaeochromocytoma, the effects of catecholamine-induced hypertension on the cardiovascular system can be detected. In echocardiography LV hypertrophy and hypertrophic cardiomyopathy with and without dynamic LV outflow tract obstruction (LVOTO) as well as diastolic dysfunction can be observed at early stages. With ongoing disease, LV dilation and LV remodelling has to be analysed by echocardiography.

Acromegaly

Acromegaly or gigantism is normally due to pituitary adenomas with growth hormone production. The disease produces myocardial wall thickening mostly due to hypertrophy induced by AH, but also due to myocardial fibrosis. Most of the patients with acromegaly develop a specific cardiomyopathy and congestive HF in the absence of other underlying heart diseases, if the patients remain untreated.

Drug-induced cardiomyopathy due to ergot alkaloids and appetite suppressants

Ergot alkaloids can induce fibrotic and serosal inflammatory disorders causing pulmonary and pleural fibrosis with pleural effusion and consecutive pulmonary hypertension, myocardial fibrosis with consecutive LV dysfunction, and endocardial fibrosis with consecutive valvular dysfunction. During treatment with ergot alkaloid HF can be induced directly due to the sequelae of peripheral vasoconstriction or indirectly by concomitant drugs which inhibit the CYP2C9 or CYP3A4 pathway. Beside myocardial insufficiency, pericardial fibrosis can also be observed. Thus, echocardiographic investigation to detect signs of constrictive pericarditis has to be performed. Another reason for HF is valvular heart diseases due to valvular fibrosis mostly induced by regurgitations. Echocardiographic monitoring is recommended every 6–12 months during treatment with ergot alkaloid.

In patients receiving treatment for appetite suppression (amphetamines, fluramines), acute HF and an association with myocardial infarction have been observed. Furthermore, appetite suppressants can induce severe systemic and pulmonary hypertension as well as valvular destruction due to serotonergic effect. Thus, echocardiographic monitoring due to cardiac complications should be performed in patients undergoing treatment with appetite suppressants.

Chagas disease

Chagas disease is a tropical parasite disease induced by the flagellate protozoan *Trypanosoma cruzi* transmitted by the blood-sucking assassin bugs. The typical acute symptoms are normally local swelling and acute HF. The typical echocardiographic findings are LV posterior wall hypokinesis with minimal involvement of the interventricular septum (IVS) as well as LV apical aneurysms. The disease becomes more and more important in Europe because transmission can occur by blood and organ donation, vertically from the mother to the child, and by food contaminated with faeces of the assassin bug. In this context trypanosomes may enter blood circulation via oropharyngeal microlesions.

Cardiac effects of systemic infections and sepsis

Systemic infections induce symptomatic tachycardia due to temperatures or chronic anaemia which physiologically causes diastolic dysfunction. Furthermore, they can directly cause myocardial depression by specific toxins. Thus, LV systolic dysfunction and HF can frequently be observed in patients with severe infections and sepsis. Myocarditis and pericarditis are often accompanying diseases in systemic infection.

Bacterial and fungal endocarditis can be the cause of septicaemia as well as the sequelae of a bacteriaemia due to an infective focus. In all cases with suspected and documented systemic infection TTE and transoesophageal echocardiography (TOE) should be performed in short-term intervals to detect lesions of endocarditis (vegetations, abscess formation).

Cardiotoxic effects of cancer therapy

Myocardium can be directly damaged by pharmacological agents (adriamycin, daunorubicine, emetine, lithium, phenothiazine). Acute and chronic myocardial damage can be induced during chemotherapy in patients with cancer,. Thus, it is recommended to evaluate cardiac function before and during cancer treatment. Antracycline derivatives may produce acute HF due to a toxic effect with an inflammatory pattern such as in patients with myocarditis. Further well-known cardiotoxic drugs are cyclophosphamide and 5-fluorouracil.

The main problem for monitoring of this patient cohort is a reduced LV function due to other reasons before starting the cardiotoxic chemotherapy. In these cases an individual decision for starting and continuation of chemotherapy can be made by repetitive control investigations with echocardiography to document objectively a further deterioration of myocardial function due to the treatment. Thus, analysis of myocardial function should be quantitatively be performed—especially using modern features like TD and speckle tracking as well as multidimensional echocardiography.

In all patients with cancer treatment the risk of bacteraemia due to leucopenia exists. Thus, echocardiography should additionally focus on the detection of lesions due to endocarditis during every follow-up investigation.

In patients undergoing chemotherapy, assessment by echocardiography of the following items is required:

- Global systolic LV function (Teichholz, Simpson).
- Regional LV WMAs.
- Pericardial effusion.
- Lesions due to endocarditis.

Diseases with a main influence on pericardium

Uraemia

In patients with chronic renal failure, uraemia is one of the main symptoms of fluid retention. Especially in the pre-end stage of renal failure, haemodynamically non-relevant pericardial effusion is a common echocardiographic finding. In patients after initiation of dialysis, pericarditis can occur as a complication of viral infections. Echocardiography is suitable for monitoring the effects of fluid retention in uraemic patients by the detection of cardiovascular abnormalities due to circulatory volume overload. The detection of an increased RV preload (volume status of the inferior caval vein) and an increased LVEDP (E/E′ ratio) by echocardiography is mandatory in follow-up investigations to prevent acute congestive HF and pulmonary oedema.

In patients with uraemia, assessment by echocardiography of the following items is required:

- Global systolic LV function (Teichholz, Simpson).
- Regional LV WMAs.
- Diastolic function.
- Pericardial effusion.
- Pulmonary hypertension.

Polyserositis

Viral infections

In patients with general viral infections the detection of pericardial fluid (Horowitz classification type B, C, and D) without any haemodynamic relevance can be observed if peri-myocardial affection is present.

In patients with acquired immunodeficiency syndrome cardiac affections can often be observed. Most of the patients have haemodynamically non-relevant pericardial effusions. Due to the most common clinical manifestation of the human immunodeficiency virus infection—opportunistic infections—the patients develop pulmonary hypertension and RV hypertrophy. In the end stage of the disease multinodular vascular nodules of Karposi's sarcoma can cause focal myocarditis with concomitant pericardial effusion.

In viral myocarditis, pericardial effusion is mostly an accompanying finding. Myocarditis is normally characterized by different stages of LV dysfunction and thrombus formation within the cardiac cavities.

In patients with viral infections, assessment by echocardiography of the following items is required:

- Global systolic LV function (Teichholz, Simpson).
- Pericardial effusion and analysis of its haemodynamic relevance.

Neoplastic syndrome

Analysis of pericardial effusion should be carefully performed in patients with suspected or known cancer disease. Especially in patients with breast, lung, and prostate cancer or melanoma pericardial effusion can be the first finding of metastatic dispersal.

In end-stage diseases all kinds of pericardial effusion can be observed. In cases of pericardial haemorrhage (e.g. lung cancer, melanoma) severe pericardial fluid can cause swinging hearts; in cases of metastatic infiltration (e.g. lung and breast cancer) large masses can be detected within the pericardial space; in cases of penetration (e.g. oesophageal cancer) purulent pericarditis can be observed (➲ Fig. 18.9).

In patients with neoplastic syndrome, assessment by echocardiography of the following items is required:

- Global systolic LV function (Teichholz, Simpson).
- Pericardial effusion and analysis of its haemodynamic relevance.

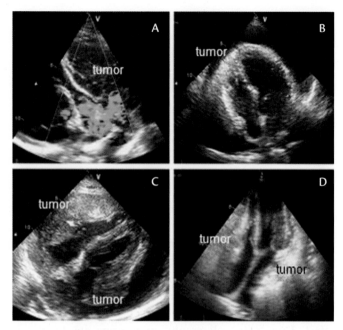

Figure 18.9 Different pericardial affections in neoplastic syndrome. Examples of different pericardial affections in neoplastic syndrome. Small pericardial effusion in a patient with mediastinal lymphoma (A); swinging heart in patient (B); tumour masses in a patient with lung cancer (C); and purulent pericardial space after pericardial-oesophageal fistula in a patient with oesophageal cancer (D).

Effects of cancer therapy on pericardium

In patients with radiation therapy chronic pericardial effusion can be observed. Some new agents in cancer therapy induce severe serositis. Therefore, recurrent echocardiography should be performed in patients receiving tyrosine kinase inhibitors. Continuation or alterations of the treatment regimen often depend on severe fluid formation in the pericardial and/or pleural space.

In patients with suspected diseased pericardium due to chemotherapy, assessment by echocardiography of the following items is required:

- Global systolic LV function (Teichholz, Simpson).
- Pericardial effusion and analysis of its haemodynamic relevance.

Graft-versus-host reaction

The graft-versus-host reaction is one of the major complications of marrow transplantation. Usually skin and intestinal involvement is predominant in these patients. However, serositis is a common phenomenon in these patients. Beside the haemodynamical relevance of the pericardial fluid, echocardiography should focus on the detection of endocarditis due to the risk of cardiac infection in the presence of skin and intestinal lesions.

In patients with graft-versus-host reaction, assessment by echocardiography of the following items is required:

- Global systolic LV function (Teichholz, Simpson).

◆ Pericardial effusion and analysis of its haemodynamic relevance.

Diseases with a main influence on right ventricular function

Obesity

In obese patients there is a general affect on the heart due to the chronic volume and pressure overload. Thus, two main cardiac manifestations will occur due to the predominant stress.

Primary pulmonary congestion is observed if pulmonary vessel resistance is increased due to an obesity-induced hypoventilation syndrome.[5] Then, impairment of right heart function in relation to the increase of pulmonary arterial pressure (PAP) can be documented. In echocardiography a distinct analysis of RV wall thickening and regional RV contraction should be performed. Normally RV hypertrophy can be well evaluated in parasternal views because scan lines are perpendicular to the free anterior RV wall. RV function can be described by the contraction amplitude of the right ventricular outflow tract as well as by the TAPSE (see ➲ Chapter 11). The longitudinal RV velocities can be additionally analysed by TD. The more isovolumetric relaxation peaks are present in the RV, the worse the effect on RV. The deviation of the IVS has to be described by different short-axis views. Doppler echocardiography enables the analysis of the severity of pulmonary hypertension (see ➲ Chapter 5 and 11) (➲ Fig. 18.10).

If systemic hypertension in obese patients is the predominant problem, eccentric hypertrophy normally can be observed due to the severe volume overload. Ventricular enlargement is therefore not primarily due to fatty infiltrations of the myocardium, but is due to haemodynamic compensation of the increase in total and central blood volume. With duration of obesity, combination of systemic hypertension and diabetes is obligate. Thus, echocardiography should document severity of LV hypertrophy as well as global and regional LV wall motion.

In obese patients, assessment by echocardiography of the following items is required:

◆ Global systolic LV function (Teichholz, Simpson).

◆ Regional LV WMAs.

◆ RV morphology and function.

◆ Valvular morphology and function, especially of the tricuspid valve.

◆ RV preload.

Chronic obstructive lung disease

In patients with chronic obstructive lung disease mild-to-moderate pulmonary hypertension is common due to severe

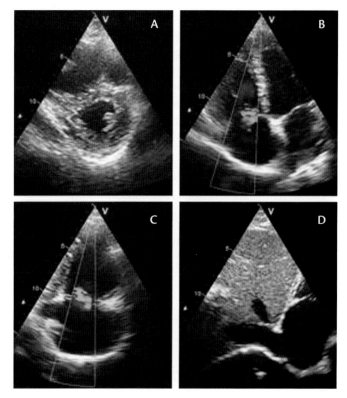

Figure 18.10 Cor pulmonale. Example of cor pulmonale in an obese patient using two dimensional imaging (A); colour-coded illustration of systolic tricuspid flow in the apical two-chamber view of the right ventricle (B) and the apical four-chamber view (C); subcostal view showing dilated inferior venacava (D).

obstructive bronchitis, emphysema, and/or asthma bronchiale. Pulmonary hypertension is due to vasoconstriction induced by alveolar hypoxia and hypercarbia. RV enlargement and hypertrophy have to be detected in early stages of the disease by echocardiography. With ongoing disease a complete analysis of RV morphology and function has to be performed. End stage of the disease is characterized by RV failure presenting with interventricular systolic and diastolic deviation, *normal* velocities of the tricuspid regurgitation due to the loss of RV contraction, and dilated central veins without any modulation by breathing.

In patients with chronic obstructive lung disease, assessment by echocardiography of the following items is required:

◆ Global systolic LV function (Teichholz, Simpson).

◆ Regional LV WMAs.

◆ RV morphology and function.

◆ Valvular morphology and function, especially of the tricuspid valve.

◆ RV preload.

Lung fibrosis

In patients with lung fibrosis the increase of pulmonary pressure is often fully compensated. Thus, in echocardiography only a RV hypertrophy is recognized in the presence of normal

RV volume. Because tricuspid regurgitation is often minimal or not present, and normal dimensions with normal behaviour of the central veins are documented, pulmonary hypertension will be not detected. In these patients estimation of pulmonary pressure has to be performed by analysis of the pulmonary regurgitation signal. In further stages of the disease decompensation of the RV with tricuspid annular dilation and severe tricuspid regurgitation occurs.

In patients with lung fibrosis, assessment by echocardiography of the following items is required:

◆ Global systolic LV function (Teichholz, Simpson).

◆ Regional LV WMAs.

◆ RV morphology and function.

◆ Valvular morphology and function, especially of the tricuspid valve.

◆ RV preload.

Liver cirrhosis

In patients with ascites refractory to drug treatment, cardiac cirrhosis due to RV failure or to constrictive pericarditis has to be considered. Echocardiographic investigation should intensively focus on right heart morphology and function. In the presence of severe TV regurgitation and right heart failure, evaluation of RV function is mandatory to clarify therapeutical options for further treatment (drug treatment, surgical intervention, heart transplantation). In patients with bad acoustic windows and dilated central venous system, echocardiography should detect possible constrictive pericarditis. Due to pericardial calcification the 2D visualization of the heart by echocardiography is mostly limited. Thus, diagnosis should be found by Doppler echocardiography using MV flow pattern, PW TD of the MV annulus, and the detection of breathing dependency between MV and TV inflow.

Personal perspective

Cardiac involvement in systemic diseases is common. The diagnostic challenge of echocardiography in these patients consists of the responsibility of the investigator to detect the respective pathological findings at an early stage of the disease in order to be able to introduce the correct therapy. Examples of the importance of the correct diagnosis are the detection of distinct regional WMAs due to different coronary processes, of diastolic dysfunction due to inflammation or storage diseases, of right heart dysfunction due to constrictive pericarditis or lung diseases, of high CO due to arteriovenous malformations, and of valvular dysfunction due to carcinoid or specific drug treatment. The efficacy of echocardiographic diagnosis, however, depends on the practical skill, the experience, and competence of the investigator. The diagnostic yield can only be enhanced with the clinical knowledge of the investigator regarding the specific systemic diseases. With other words, the physician or sonographer, who performs echocardiography, has to know what he/she is looking for to have a high success rate of pathological findings.

References

1 Hagendorff A, Transthoracic echocardiography in adult patients–a proposal for documenting a standardized investigation. *Ultraschall Med* 2008; 29(4):344–65.

2 Mancia G, De Backer G, Dominiczak A, Cifkova R, Fagard R, Germano G, *et al.* 2007 Guidelines for the management of arterial hypertension: The Task Force for the Management of Arterial Hypertension of the European Society of Hypertension (ESH) and of the European Society of Cardiology (ESC). *Eur Heart J* 2007; 28(12):1462–536.

3 Rydén L, Standl E, Bartnik M, Van den Berghe G, Betteridge J, de Boer MJ, *et al.* Guidelines on diabetes, pre-diabetes, and cardiovascular diseases: executive summary. The Task Force on Diabetes and Cardiovascular Diseases of the European Society of Cardiology (ESC) and of the European Association for the Study of Diabetes (EASD). *Eur Heart J* 2007; 28(1):88–136.

4 Hagendorff A, Pfeiffer D, Echocardiographic functional analysis of patients with rheumatoid arthritis and collagen diseases. *Z Rheumatol* 2005; 64(4):239–48.

5 Galiè N, Hoeper MM, Humbert M, Torbicki A, Vachiery JL, Barbera JA, *et al.* Guidelines for the diagnosis and treatment of pulmonary hypertension: The Task Force for the Diagnosis and Treatment of Pulmonary Hypertension of the European Society of Cardiology (ESC) and the European Respiratory Society (ERS), endorsed by the International Society of Heart and Lung Transplantation (ISHLT). *Eur Heart J* 2009; 30(20):2493–537.

Further reading

Mancia G *et al.* 2007 Guidelines for the management of arterial Hypertension. *European Heart Journal.* (2007); 28:1462–1536.

Vahanian A *et al.* Guidelines on the management of valvular heart disease. *European Heart Journal.* (2007); 28: 230–268.

Galie N *et al.* Guidelines for the diagnosis and treatment of pulmonary hypertension. *European Heart Journal.* (2009); 30: 2493–2537.

Nagueh FN *et al.* Recommendations for the Evaluation of Left Ventricular Diastolic Function by Echocardiography. *J Am Soc Echocardiography.* (2009); 22: 107–133.

Additional DVD and online material

- 18.1 A correctly set parasternal long-axis view for M-mode measurements.
- 18.2 A correctly set parasternal short-axis view for M-mode measurements.
- 18.3 An incorrectly set parasternal long-axis view may provide too large LV diameters and too thick LV walls.
- 18.4 Possible incorrect settings in the short axis derived from an incorrect long-axis view.
- 18.5 PLAX view in a hypertensive patient with congestive heart failure.
- 18.6 A3C view showing a severe aortic regurgitation due to aortic annular dilation.
- 18.7 PLAX view showing an aneurysm of the ascending aorta.
- 18.8 PLAX view in a patient with Stanford A dissection.
- 18.9 Colour Doppler imaging of anterior descending artery with coronary flow at rest.
- 18.10 Colour Doppler imaging of anterior descending artery with coronary flow during adenosine infusion.

- For additional multimedia materials please visit the online version of the book (http://escecho.oxfordmedicine.com).

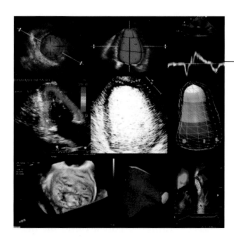

CHAPTER 19

Pericardial disease

Bernard Cosyns and Bernard Paelinck

Contents

Summary

The ability of ultrasound to elucidate the functional and structural abnormalities of pericardial disease is powerful. Due to multimodality imaging possibilities and to its portability, echocardiography is the technique of choice for the diagnosis of pericardial disease. Although other non-invasive technologies have been developed to provide information about the pericardium, echocardiography remains the first and often only diagnostic method needed to make a definitive diagnosis and guide appropriate treatment in patients with pericardial effusion, cardiac tamponade, or constrictive pericarditis. It allows differential diagnosis with restrictive cardiomyopathy and can easily be performed for guiding pericardiocentesis.

Normal pericardial anatomy

The pericardium is a sac enveloping the heart. It consists of two layers: the visceral one (contiguous to the epicardium) and the parietal or fibrous one, thicker with an element of protection and fixity. The pericardium reflects around the right border of the aorta and than crosses the anterior part of pulmonary artery (PA) trunk, the origin of the left PA, posterior part of the PA bifurcation, and finally the posterior part of the aorta to go back to the right border of the aorta (➲ Fig. 19.1).

In clinical practice, the pericardium can be evaluated by M-mode and two-dimensional (2D) and three-dimensional (3D) echocardiography. Echocardiography is an important tool in the diagnosis and management of pericardial disease and is usually one of the first diagnostic procedures used to evaluate patient with suspected pericardial abnormality.

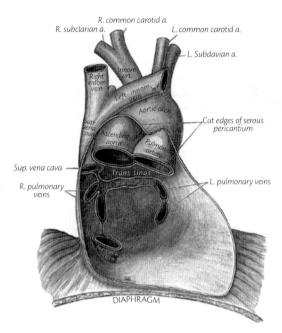

Figure 19.1 Pericardium. Anatomical representation of lines of pericardial reflection.

Pericardial effusion

Detection of pericardial effusion

Pericardial effusion is the filling of pericardial space with an amount of fluid or blood as a result of a wide variety of pathological conditions affecting the pericardium:

♦ Inflammatory disease: pericarditis with infective aetiology (most commonly viral, less frequently bacterial), pericarditis due to autoimmune disorders, myocarditis, myocardial infarction, cardiac surgery, chemotherapy, and radiation therapy.

♦ Traumatic disease: chest trauma, aortic dissection, rupture of ventricular free wall.

♦ Miscellaneous: tumours, uraemic state, hypothyroidism, other metabolic disorders.

The physiological consequences of pericardial effusion depend on both the amount of effusion and the rate of its accumulation. In chronic pathological conditions and in the absence of adequate therapy, pericardial effusion slowly accumulates and persists over time, without haemodynamic consequences. Conversely, the acute and rapid filling of pericardial space, as occurs during myocardial rupture or aortic dissection, causes a raise of intrapericardial pressure with subsequent compression of cardiac chambers and clinical instability. This results in a life-threatening condition, named *cardiac tamponade* (see later). In the setting of acute myocardial infarction, free wall rupture in the pericardium is responsible for 15–20% of early death. In this particular case, pericardiocentesis is not helpful to improve haemodynamics and urgent surgery is indicated.

Aortic dissection should be suspected in every patient with chest pain and pericardial effusion. In this setting, pericardial effusion is a criterion of severity and pericardiocentesis is contraindicated.

The first choice echocardiographic modality for detection and quantification of a pericardial effusion is 2D echocardiography. Pericardial effusion is visualized as an echo-free space, external to myocardial wall. Small amount of fluid (5–10mL) can be detected in normal conditions in parasternal long-axis (PLAX) view as a small echo-free space in the posterior atrioventricular junction, increasing in size during systole (◑ Fig. 19.2). When the amount of effusion is more than 25mL, the echo-free space extends circumferentially around the heart and persists throughout the cardiac cycle; in extreme cases, in which effusion is massive, the heart may have a *swinging* motion within the pericardial sac. Haemorrhagic effusion with intra-pericardial haematoma shows a density similar to that of myocardium (◑ Fig. 19.3), whereas the presence of intrapericardial structures conveys a poor specificity and only masses suggesting tumour with intramyocardial extension are diagnostic (◑ Figs. 19.4 and 19.5). The presence of air within the pericardial sac (pneumopericardium), as occurs due to oesophageal perforation, impairs visualization of cardiac chambers.

2D echo detection of pericardial effusion must be completed by additional views including parasternal short-axis (PSAX), apical, and subcostal views, since pericardial effusion may be localized and may be seen only in certain tomographic views (see later). In every case, M-mode measurement of echo-free space size provides a semiquantitative assessment of fluid amount (see later). The sensitivity of 2D and colour Doppler (CD) modalities may be low in cases of subacute free wall rupture: the performance of contrast echocardiography may be

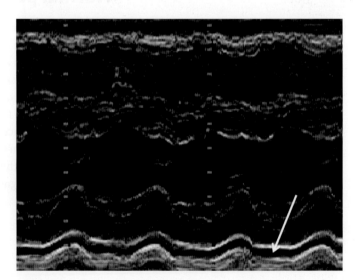

Figure 19.2 Small amount of pericardial fluid. M-mode from parasternal long-axis view: a small amount of fluid can be detected in normal conditions and can be identified as a small echo-free space (arrow) in the posterior atrioventricular junction, increasing in size during systole (arrow).

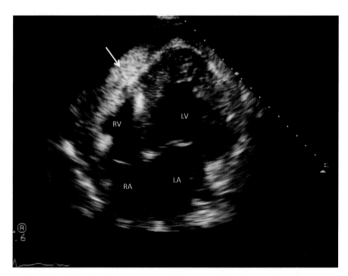

Figure 19.3 Intrapericardial haematoma. Illustration in apical four-chamber view of intrapericardial haematoma (arrow). The density of the haematoma is similar to myocardium and may produce loculated effusion with tamponade. LA, left atrium; LV, left ventricle; RA, right atrium; RV, right ventricle.

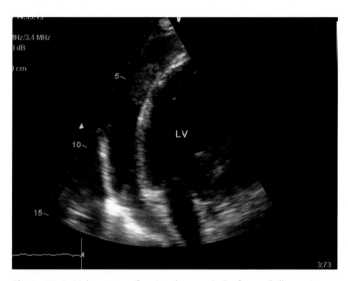

Figure 19.4 Melanoma perforating the ventricular free wall. Illustration in apical three-chamber view of a metastasis from a malignant melanoma perforating the ventricular free wall and producing a pericardial effusion. LV, left ventricle.

helpful to unmask the rupture tear responsible for haemorrhagic effusion.

After cardiac surgery or during some inflammatory processes, pericardial effusion may be localized or *loculated*, due to the presence of fibrin which creates adhesions between pericardial layers. Localized pericardial effusion may cause an isolated compression of cardiac chambers, pulmonary veins, or even vena cava inflow: detection of such effusions is challenging and should be performed by standard and non-standard echocardiographic views. Conversely, the assessment of pericardial effusion may be affected by poor quality images, particularly in postoperative conditions or after invasive procedures;

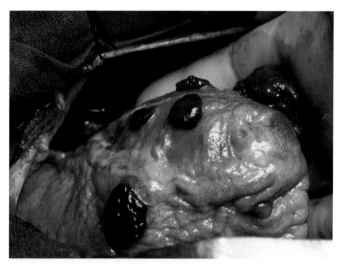

Figure 19.5 Melanoma metastasis with intramyocardial extension. Macroscopic view of the melanoma metastasis with intramyocardial extension as illustrated in ➲ Fig. 19.4.

transoesophageal echocardiography (TOE) may be required in evaluating these patients.

Quantitation of pericardial fluid

The evaluation of the amount of pericardial fluid is of modest interest and can only be semiquantitative although 3D echo may determine pericardial volume. Many severity scales have been proposed without wide clinical acceptance (from physiological to large effusion). A circumferential echo-free space less than 0.5cm is considered as *small* (<100mL). A free space less or equal to 1cm, is considered as *moderate* (100–500mL), and more than 1cm as *large* (500mL).

Differentiation between pericardial and pleural effusion

The reflection of the pericardium around the pulmonary veins limits the size of a pericardial effusion behind the left atrium (LA). Therefore, a fluid collection behind the LA is more likely pleural than pericardial (➲ Fig. 19.6). The position of echo-free space relatively to adjacent structures, as visualized in PLAX view, is a useful marker for distinguishing pericardial from pleural effusion: in fact, fluid appearing in PLAX view anterior to the descending aorta is typically pericardial, whereas pleural effusion usually is localized posterior to the aorta. However, there are exceptions and the distinction between pleural and pericardial may be more difficult. In any case, the presence of a pleural effusion on the left side allows imaging of the heart from the back.

Differentiation between pericardial effusion and pericardial fat

Pericardial fat increases with age and obesity. Fat is usually observed at the level of the anterior part of the heart without any pathological significance (➲ Fig. 19.7). It can be differentiated from effusion by a higher density (white echoes) with

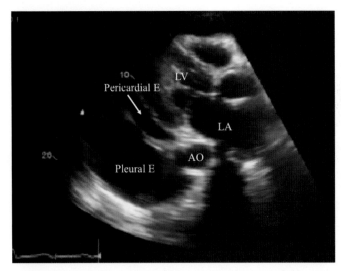

Figure 19.6 Pericardial and pleural effusion. Long-axis view of pericardial and simultaneous pleural effusion. Typically, the fluid appearing anterior to the descending aorta is pericardial. Ao, descending aorta; E, effusion; LA, left atrium; LV, left ventricle.

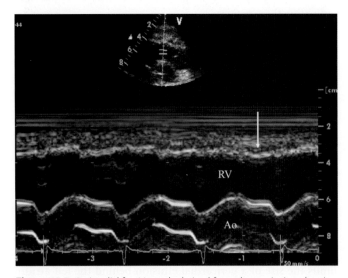

Figure 19.7 Pericardial fat. M-mode derived from short-axis view showing fat (arrow), usually observed at the level of the anterior part of the heart without any pathological significance. It can be differentiated from effusion by a higher density (white echoes). Ao, ascending aorta, RV, right ventricle.

ultrasound compared to fluid but this distinction may be difficult and computed tomography may be required to make the distinction between fat and effusion.

Diagnosis of cardiac tamponade

Cardiac tamponade is a life-threatening condition, in which the elevation of intrapericardial pressure above normal filling pressure of the heart, due to accumulation of pericardial effusion, results in decreased left ventricular (LV) preload and subsequent fall of cardiac output with severe haemodynamic alterations. The limit of pericardial stretch is dependent not only on amount of effusion but also on the rate at which effusion accumulates. The lower pressure cardiac chambers (atria) are

affected before the higher pressure cardiac chambers (ventricles). Compressive effect is more likely to be seen in the phase of cardial cycle when filling pressure within a cavity is lower, as occurs during systole for the atria and during diastole for the ventricles. Thus, such pericardial effusion produces an elevation of intracardiac filling pressures, a decrease of ventricular filling, and subsequently in stroke volume. Echocardiography is required to confirm the presence of effusion, to assess its haemodynamic impact, and to establish the cause of tamponade.

In normal conditions, inspiration decreases intrathoracic pressure resulting in increase in venous return, right cavities filling, and right ventricular (RV) stroke volume. As a consequence, pulmonary venous return, LV filling, and stroke volume will decrease slightly (⮁ Fig. 19.8). However, these variations do not exceed 30%. All clinical situations that increase intrathoracic or intrapericardial pressures will induce an exaggerated increase of these reciprocal variations of ventricular filling, stroke volume, and decrease arterial blood pressure by more than 10mmHg. This will lead to *pulsus paradoxus*. Note that pulsus paradoxus may be absent in the presence of severe LV dysfunction, regional right atrial (RA) effusion, positive pressure breathing, atrial septal defect (ASD), pulmonary arterial (PA) obstruction, and severe aortic regurgitation (AR). Conversely, pulsus paradoxus may be present in patients with chronic obstructive lung disease without any pericardial effusion.

The echocardiographic signs of tamponade are:

◆ A RA collapse (⮁ Fig. 19.9) or inversion during systole (time of collapse/time of cardiac cycle with a ratio >0.34 improves specificity).

◆ The RV diastolic collapse, best viewed in PLAX and PSAX views (⮁ Fig. 19.10) in early diastole: it reflects rise of intrapericardial pressure above the intracardiac pressure and, for this reason, may be delayed in case of pulmonary hypertension or RV hypertrophy.

◆ Swinging heart, which means that the four cardiac chambers are free floating within the pericardial effusion in a phasic manner (⮁ Fig. 19.11).

◆ Occasionally compression of the LA or the LV.

◆ Reciprocal changes in ventricular volumes can be observed with a septum moving toward the LV with inspiration and toward the RV during expiration.

◆ A plethora of inferior vena cava (IVC) and blunted respiratory changes can also occur (⮁ Fig. 19.12).

◆ Doppler findings in tamponade consist of exaggeration of the respiratory variations in filling, outflow tract, and hepatic veins velocities. Respiratory variation of the tricuspid inflow is the earliest feature of tamponade. It is therefore recommended to decrease the sweep velocity around 25m/s to demonstrate these respiratory variations and to use a respirometer.

Expiration   Inspiration

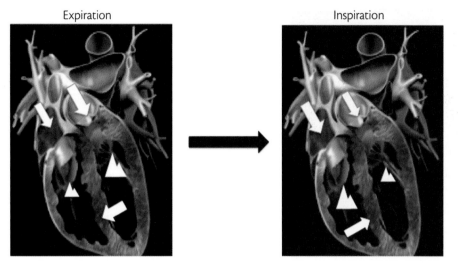

Figure 19.8 Respiratory variations of ventricular filling. In normal conditions, inspiration decreases intrathoracic pressure resulting in increase in venous return, right cavities filling, and right ventricular stroke volume. As a consequence, pulmonary venous return, left ventricular filling, and stroke volume will decrease slightly.

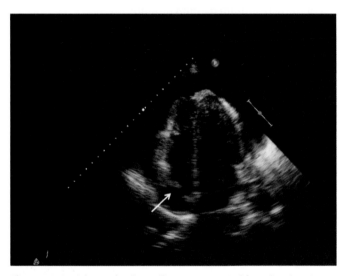

Figure 19.9 Right atrial collapse. Illustration in apical four-chamber view of right atrial collapse (arrow). LA, left atrium; LV, left ventricle; RA, right atrium; RV, right ventricle.

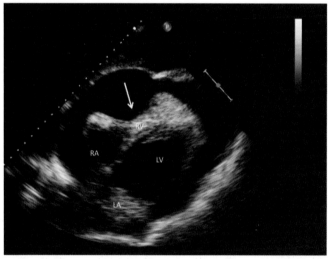

Figure 19.10 Right ventricular collapse. Illustration in subcostal view of right ventricular collapse (arrow). LA, left atrium; LV, left ventricle; RA, right atrium; RV, right ventricle.

Reciprocal changes in ventricular volumes occur as result of *ventricular interdependence* due to the relatively fixed combined cardiac volume. As LV filling decreases with inspiration, mitral valve (MV) opening is delayed and isovolumic relaxation time is prolonged, so that E wave velocity is low. In right-side cardiac chambers ventricular filling is increased during inspiration and decreased during expiration. Such ventricular interdependence transmit to pulmonary and hepatic venous flow, causing alternate increase of forward and reversal flows: an inspiratory increase and expiratory decrease of forward flow with increase of reversal flow at the hepatic vein level, opposed to inspiratory decrease and expiratory increase of pulmonary venous forward flow. Doppler findings should be recorded in urgent conditions to demonstrate haemodynamic impairment during cardiac tamponade, also in the absence of simultaneous respirometer recordings.

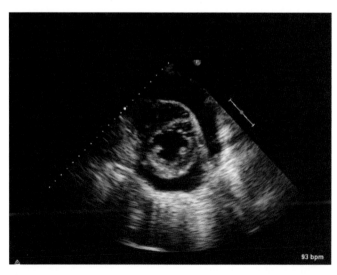

Figure 19.11 Swinging heart. Illustration in short-axis view of swinging heart due to large circumferential effusion.

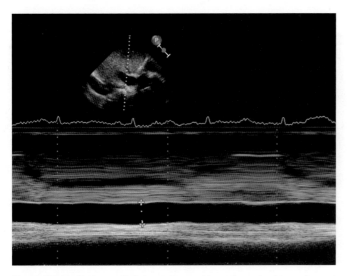

Figure 19.12 Plethora of inferior vena cava. M-mode tracing from subcostal view with plethora of inferior vena cava and blunted respiratory changes.

Echo-guided pericardiocentesis

Pericardiocentesis is the most effective and life-saving procedure in cases of cardiac tamponade. A blind percutaneous access to pericardium may cause severe complications, such as pneumothorax, puncture of the cardiac wall, and death. Echocardiography plays a major role in pericardiocentesis to determine the distribution and the depth of the effusion and to guide direction of the needle. During the procedure, continuous echocardiography has been proposed, usually by subcostal view and eventually combined with the injection of air gas microbubbles (see ⇨ Chapter 7) in the pericardial space, to generate contrast and define the tip of the needle. Echocardiography is also required after the procedure to assess the completeness of fluid removal.

Constrictive pericarditis

Constrictive pericarditis is a pathological condition characterized by impaired cardiac diastolic function due to a thickened, inflamed or adherent, frequently calcified pericardium. Commonly it occurs as consequence of previous cardiac surgery and radiotherapy or as evolution of effusive pericarditis, when a great amount of fibrin replaces pericardial effusion. Frequently, constrictive pericarditis is misdiagnosed, but should be suspected in most patients with heart failure, particularly in the presence of normal left ventricular systolic function and predisposing factors. Pericardial calcifications seen on chest radiography may facilitate diagnosis, but they are lacking in most patients.

2D, Doppler, and tissue Doppler (TD) imaging provide useful information to formulate a correct diagnosis. Characteristic findings on M-mode and 2D echocardiography are:

◆ Thickened pericardium.

◆ Abnormal interventricular septal motion.

◆ Respiratory variations in ventricular filling.

◆ Diastolic flattening of LV posterior wall.

◆ Dilated IVC.

Pericardial thickening appears as increased echogenicity of the pericardium on 2D echocardiography and as multiples parallel reflections posterior to LV on M-mode recordings. However, since pericardium is usually more echogenic than other cardiac structures, it can be difficult to distinguish thickened from normal pericardium. Sometimes pericardial thickness appears normal on 2D transoesophageal echocardiography (TOE), despite haemodynamic features of pericardial constriction: in these cases, the correlation of echocardiographic thickening with histopathological specimen is poor. Other imaging techniques, such as computed tomography (CT) and cardiac magnetic resonance (CMR) may be more sensitive for this diagnosis. The sensitivity of TOE is higher when showing a thickening of the pericardium of 3mm or more.

Usually, the contractility and the size of the LV appear normal with 2D echo and the atria may be of normal size. A *flattened* motion of posterior wall can be observed in diastole as an abrupt posterior motion of ventricular septum (septal *bounce*) in early diastole (⇨ Fig. 19.13). Dilated IVC and hepatic veins are common. A premature diastolic opening of the pulmonary valve (PV) can be present.

Although the physiopathology is different from tamponade, the haemodynamics characteristics of constriction in regard to respiratory variation in left and right filling are similar. In tamponade, the resistance to ventricular filling is present during the complete duration of diastole. In constrictive pericarditis, the early filling is preserved. Constrictive pericarditis is characterized by the isolation of the cardiac chambers from intrathoracic respiratory pressure changes and by a fixed end-diastolic

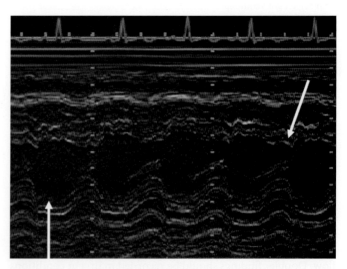

Figure 19.13 M-mode assessment of constrictive pericarditis. M-mode from parasternal long axis view: 'flattened' motion of posterior wall in diastole and abrupt posterior motion of ventricular septum (septal 'bounce') in early diastole (arrows).

ventricular volume. Inspiration reduces pressure within the thorax as well as into pulmonary vein. Due to rigid pericardium, such decreased pressure is not fully transmitted to pericardial and intracardiac spaces. Thus, the pressure gradient guides diastolic LV filling only in early diastole, when the atrial pressures are elevated. In this phase, ventricular filling is very rapid. However, when relaxing ventricle meets the non-compliant pericardium, LV diastolic pressure raises rapidly and filling declines by mid-diastole. At the end of diastole, RA, RV, wedge pulmonary pressure, arterial, and LV pressures are equally elevated. The increase in atrial afterload impairs atrial contraction. The rigid pericardium increases the ventricular interdependence through the septum (Fig. 19.14). Decrease of LV filling during inspiration allows filling of the RV, by leftward motion of interventricular septum (IVS); conversely, increase of LV filling during expiration reduces simultaneous RV filling, by shifting of IVS to the right.

Doppler diagnosis of pericardial constriction

Mitral and tricuspid forward flow patterns reflect respiratory changes in ventricular filling. Doppler features of constriction show a prominent *Y* descent on hepatic vein or superior vena cava flow pattern, a LV inflow with a prominent E wave with rapid early diastolic deceleration slope, and a small A wave (Fig. 19.15). An increase in LV isovolumic relaxation time by greater than 20% on first beat after inspiration and respiratory variations with increase in RV filling of more than 40% and decrease in LV filling by 25% can be observed (Fig. 19.16). At the level of pulmonary veins, systolic flow varies as often or more than diastolic flow with respiration and hepatic vein diastolic filling flow decreases or is absent with marked expiratory reversal (Fig. 19.17). Note that classic Doppler patterns of constrictive pericarditis may require preload reduction

Expiration   Inspiration

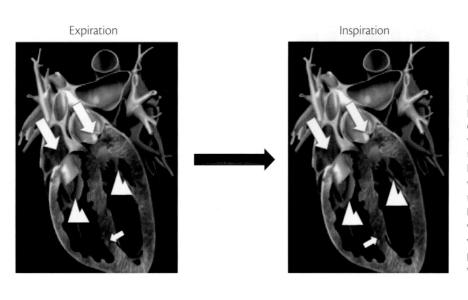

Figure 19.14 Constrictive pericarditis. Constrictive pericarditis: exaggerated increase of the reciprocal variations of ventricular filling with respiration, the rigid pericardium is coupling both ventricles, increasing the ventricular interdependence through the septum (arrows). Inspiration increases right ventricular return, right ventricular filling, and decreases pulmonary venous return and left ventricular filling.

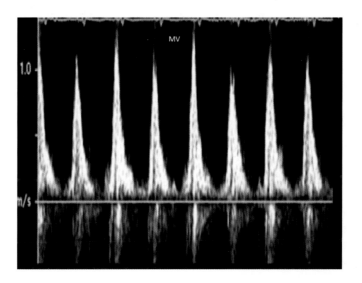

Figure 19.15 Left ventricular inflow pattern in constrictive pericarditis. Illustration of Doppler tracing in a patient with constrictive pericarditis: left ventricular inflow with a prominent E wave with rapid early diastolic deceleration slope and a small A wave.

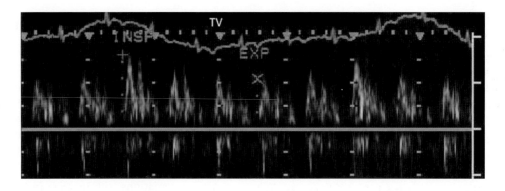

Figure 19.16 Respiratory variations in right ventricular filling. Illustration of Doppler tracing in a patient with constrictive pericarditis: respiratory variations with increase in right ventricular filling greater than 40%.

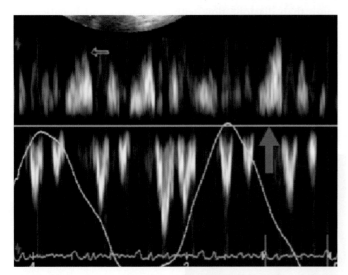

Figure 19.17 Respiratory variations in hepatic vein flow. Doppler tracing from hepatic veins showing diastolic filling flow decrease and with marked expiratory reversal (arrow).

e.g. head-up tilting to be unmasked. In some clinical conditions (i.e. malignancy or radiotherapy), a combination of constriction and tamponade may be present. In this case, haemodynamic impairment will persist and Doppler findings appear more similar to constriction after pericardiocentesis.

Usually, echocardiographic diagnosis of constrictive pericarditis is based on the following criteria:

◆ Respiratory variation greater than 25% in E wave velocity at the level of mitral valve.

◆ Increased reversal flow during expiration at the hepatic vein level.

However, the lack of respiratory variation in mitral valve inflow pattern should not rule out the diagnosis of constrictive pericarditis, but any other complementary signs should be carefully searched. TD imaging provides additional information by assessment of mitral septal annulus velocity. In fact, in myocardial disease, the mitral septal annulus velocity is decreased (<7cm/s), because LV relaxation is impaired. Conversely, in constrictive pericarditis, such velocity is normal or increased: this occurs because, while lateral diastolic expansion of LV

cavity is limited by rigid pericardium, the longitudinal motion of the heart is preserved or even exaggerated. As pericardial constriction worsens, longitudinal motion and mitral septal annulus velocity increase: such phenomenon has been named annulus paradoxus. Moreover, contrary to what happens in myocardial disease, E/E′ appears inversely proportional to pulmonary capillary wedge pressure and E′ usually is higher with expiration than with inspiration.

Differential diagnosis versus restrictive cardiomyopathy

The distinction between constrictive pericarditis and restrictive cardiomyopathy often is challenging, because these pathological conditions show similar clinical and haemodynamic profiles and are based on abnormal diastolic function associated with preserved systolic function (for details regarding restrictive cardiomyopathy, see ➔ Chapter 17). However, while in restrictive cardiomyopathy the myocardium becomes non-compliant due to fibrosis and infiltrative diseases, in constrictive pericarditis diastolic function is altered by non-compliant and thickened pericardium.

The great majority of the M-mode or 2D echo signs previously described can be observed in both conditions. The main differences that can be found in constriction compared to restriction are summarized as follows:

◆ Thickening of the pericardium.

◆ Wall motion abnormalities (WMAs) of the septum are found more often, such as reciprocal respiratory variation in septal motion.

◆ Less often, dilation of the atria.

◆ Usually no LV hypertrophy.

Doppler flow analysis may be more useful. Typically, respiratory changes may not be observed in restrictive cardiomyopathy because MV opening occurs when respiration has little effect on transmitral pressure gradient. Patients with restrictive cardiomyopathy show a blunting of the systolic wave velocity and a decrease in the ratio of systolic to early diastolic wave

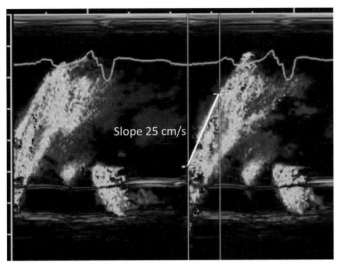

Figure 19.18 Velocity of propagation of mitral inflow. The velocity of propagation of mitral inflow determined from M-mode colour Doppler is usually reduced in restriction (<55cm/s).

velocity throughout the respiratory cycle, with a large atrial reversal wave and without any significant respiratory variation.

The velocity of propagation of mitral inflow determined from M-mode CD is usually reduced in restriction whereas it is normal or increased in constriction (>55cm/s) (⊃ Fig. 19.18).

An echocardiographic study of LV mechanics may be helpful for the distinction of these two clinical entities. Patients with constrictive pericarditis have high-velocity early diastolic biphasic IVS motion (>7cm/s) by TD imaging. Patients with restrictive cardiomyopathy and intrinsic myocardial abnormalities have reduced longitudinal deformation of the LV base and reduced early diastolic longitudinal velocities. A lateral or septal early diastolic mitral annular velocity of more than 8cm/s on pulsed TD has been proposed as a cut-off value to differentiate between constrictive pericarditis and restrictive cardiomyopathy. However, age, gender, focal zone of endomyocardial fibrosis (heterogeneity of the disease), regional LV dysfunction, and mitral annulus calcification have to be taken into account and may limit the ability for differentiating with restrictive cardiomyopathy. By speckle-tracking imaging, patients with constrictive pericarditis have significantly reduced net LV twist and torsion compared with normal subjects and patients with restrictive cardiomyopathy.

Pitfalls in differentiating restrictive cardiomyopathy versus cor pulmonale

Respiratory variations of the mitral inflow can be observed in other clinical entities as pulmonary embolism, RV infarction, global heart failure secondary to cardiomyopathy, pleural effusion, and chronic obstructive lung disease. In the last condition, hepatic veins or superior vena cava flow increases with inspiration, because of significant fall in intrathoracic pressure, which transmits to cardiac chambers and raises RV filling. In case of pericardial constriction, such systemic venous flow remains relatively unchanged with respiration. On the other hand, mitral inflow velocities rarely show a restrictive pattern in chronic obstructive lung disease.

Pericardial cysts

These are usually asymptomatic, benign developmental abnormalities with a portion of the parietal pericardium disconnected from pericardial sac (no communication). A pericardial cyst may be located in the right or left costophrenic angle, in superior mediastinum, and hilum. Frequently, it is a rare incidental finding but needs to be differentiated from other masses, particularly malignant tumours, cardiac chamber enlargement, and diaphragmatic hernia. At echocardiography, they appear as a round or elliptical echo-free space adjacent to a cardiac chamber, often filled with clear fluid.

Congenital absence of the pericardium

This is an uncommon and benign congenital abnormality mainly affecting men and defined as the total (or, less commonly, partial) absence of pericardium. The echo findings may be variable. The heart may appear shifting to left chest, hypermobile (exaggerated cardiac motion), with an apparent RV enlargement in parasternal windows due to malposition of the RV, abnormal ventricular septal motion (mimicking RV overload). Multiple imaging modalities are recommended to confirm the diagnosis. Congenital absence of the left pericardium may result in reduced LV torsion. The partial absence of pericardium may lead to herniation and/or strangulation of a portion of the heart. Moreover, congenital absence of the pericardium is usually associated with other congenital abnormalities, such as ASD, bicuspid aortic valve and bronchogenic cysts. The echo features are dependent on which portion of the heart is involved and often diagnosis requires to be confirmed by CT or CMR.

Personal perspective

Pericardial disease diagnosis has been one of the first main applications of echocardiography. Today, in clinical practice, the pericardium can be evaluated by M-mode, 2D, Doppler, and 3D echocardiography. New modalities based on TD imaging, speckle tracking imaging, and contrast echocardiography have recently increased the power of ultrasound to help in the diagnosis of this disease. TOE may also be indicated in selected cases. All these modalities used in combination have been of great help in the understanding of the physiopathology of pericardial disease. A cluster of specific echocardiographic signs makes the diagnosis more confident even in the absence of suggestive clinical signs. Finally, echocardiography remains the modality of choice for the treatment and the follow-up of patients with pericardial disease.

Further reading

Oh JK, Seward JB, Tajik AS. *The Echo Manual*, 3rd ed. Philadelphia, PA: Lippincott Williams and Wilkins; 2007

Otto C. *Textbook of Clinical Echocardiography*, 4th ed. Philadelphia, PA: Saunders; 2009

European guidelines of clinical practice in cardiology.

Papers of interest on echocardiography from the European Association of Echocardiography.

➲ For additional multimedia materials please visit the online version of the book (🔗 http://escecho.oxfordmedicine.com).

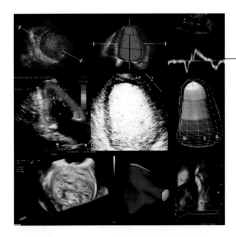

CHAPTER 20

Tumours and masses

M.J. Andrade

Contents

Summary

Transthoracic and transoesophageal echocardiography is the first-line diagnostic tool for imaging space-occupying lesions of the heart. Cardiac masses can be classified as tumours, thrombi, vegetations, iatrogenic material, or normal variants. Occasionally, extracardiac masses may compress the heart and create a mass effect. Cardiac masses may be suspected from the clinical presentation. This is the case in patients with an embolic event presumed of cardiac origin or in patients with infective endocarditis. Otherwise, a cardiac mass can be identified during the routine investigation of common, non-specific cardiac manifestations or as an incidental finding.

In general, an integrated approach which correlates the patient's clinical picture with the echocardiographic findings may reasonably predict the specific nature of encountered cardiac masses and, in the case of tumours, discriminate between primary versus secondary, and benign versus malignant. Furthermore, echocardiography alone or with complementary imaging modalities, can provide information to help decide on the resectability of cardiac tumours, enhance effective diagnosis and management of infective endocarditis, and assist in planning therapy and follow-up. Because several normal structures and variants may mimic pathological lesions, a thorough knowledge of potential sources of misinterpretation is crucial for a correct diagnosis. After surgical resection, histological investigation is mandatory to confirm the diagnosis.

Cardiac tumours

The rarity and heterogeneous clinical presentation of cardiac tumours make the diagnosis difficult. Until they produce a mass effect by obstructing cardiac chambers and great vessels or until they cause pulmonary or systemic embolization, complete heart block, or cardiac tamponade, tumours in the heart remain asymptomatic. Secondary malignancies of the heart are far more common than primary ones (20–40 times). Ninety per cent of all primary cardiac tumours are benign. The frequency and type of cardiac tumours in adults differ from those in children.[1,2]

Primary benign tumours

Myxoma

Myxoma is the most common benign primary cardiac tumour (70%). It occurs most commonly in the left atrium (LA, 75%), but can arise in the right atrium (RA) or in the ventricles. Although familial cases associated with multiple endocrine syndromes do occur, sporadic myxoma represents the large majority. It tends to occur in middle-age women as isolated lesions, attached through a fibrovascular stalk to the region of the fossa ovalis in the interatrial septum.

Cardiac myxomas have variable echocardiographic features, sometimes atypical. Most cardiac myxomas are globular in appearance, have a regular and smooth surface, and sizes ranging from 4–8cm in diameter. Less frequently they may be multilobular or with very irregular and friable surfaces (◑ Fig. 20.1). Their echogenicity is usually not homogeneous, frequently with areas of echolucency, and occasionally with areas of calcification—a useful finding to differentiate them from large thrombus. Mobility depends on the size of the myxomas and the characteristics of the stalk, but prolapsing into ventricles through the mitral or tricuspid valves during diastole is a very common finding for atrial located tumours (◑ Fig 20.2; ◙ 20.1–20.4). Besides the evaluation of location, size, contours, mobility, and echogenicity of the tumour, it is very important during the echo examination to identify the site of tumour attachment, to ensure that the tumour does not involve the

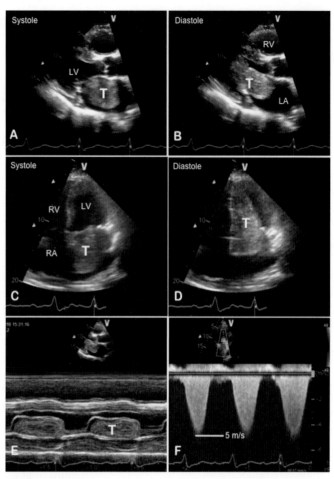

Figure 20.2 Mobility of left atrial myxoma. Large left atrial myxoma (T) recorded from the parasternal long-axis (A, B) and from the apical four-chamber views (C, D) in systole (A, C) and diastole (B, D). During diastole, the tumour prolapses into the left ventricle (LV), completely obstructing the mitral valve orifice (B, D). E) M-mode recording at the level of the mitral valve of a prolapsing LA myxoma. A dense array of wavy tumour echos is seen behind the anterior leaflet of the mitral valve. F) Continuous wave Doppler recording of tricuspid regurgitation velocity of the same patient. Peak velocity is 5m/s, corresponding to a 100mmHg transtricuspid gradient.

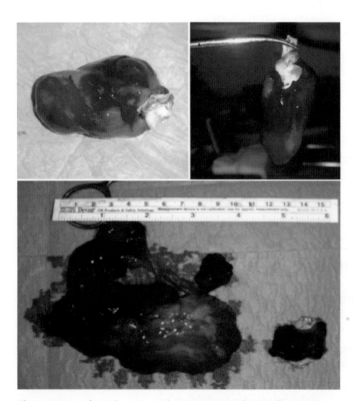

Figure 20.1 Left atrial myxomas that were removed surgically. Note the difference in appearance: the top myxoma has a smooth surface while the bottom one is villous, more friable, and prone to tissue fragmentation and embolism. (Courtesy of Rute Couto MD, and Rui Rodrigues MD.)

valve leaflets, and to exclude the possibility of multiple masses. For cardiac myxomas, two-dimensional (2D) echocardiography from multiple views was found to be highly accurate in providing all the relevant information for surgery.[3] However, in cases of very large myxomas that nearly fill the LA chamber in intimal contact with large portions of the LA endocardium throughout the cardiac cycle, the stalk may be not clearly seen. In these cases transoesophageal echocardiography (TOE) may be needed in planning the surgical approach (◑ Fig. 20.3; ◙ 20.5–20.7). Particularly, all four pulmonary veins, and superior and inferior vena cavae must be carefully looked at for any local extension of the tumour. The degree to which the tumour causes functional obstruction to ventricular diastolic filling can be evaluated qualitatively by colour flow imaging and, quantitatively, by evaluation of the Doppler trace of the ventricular inflow, showing the typical signs of mitral stenosis in cases of LA myxomas, or tricuspid stenosis in RA myxomas.[4]

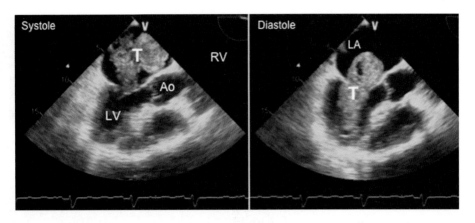

Figure 20.3 Longitudinal transoesophageal view of a large left atrial myxoma (T). In systole (left) it remains inside the left atrium, while in diastole (right) it enters the mitral valve orifice, virtually occluding forward flow.

A variable degree of atrioventricular valves regurgitation is common, as well as increased right ventricular (RV) systolic pressure (➲ Fig. 20.1F). Postoperatively, complete excision should be documented by echocardiography. Sequential long-term follow-up is indicated because recurrent myxomas have been reported, particularly with a familial form of this disease.

Papillary fibroelastoma

Papillary fibroelastoma (PFE) is the most common heart valve tumour, representing 10% of the encountered cardiac tumours in autopsy series. Papillary fibroelastomas are usually small, the majority less than 1cm in diameter, mostly pedicled by a short stalk. They are typically found on aortic and mitral valves, less frequently on tricuspid and pulmonary valves, or even in the mural non-valvular endocardium (➲ Figs. 20.4 and 20.5; ▣ 20.8–20.10). Regardless of their size, these highly mobile tumours with a frond-like appearance have the potential for systemic or pulmonary embolization. Despite its typical shape, imaging techniques may fail to differentiate PFE from other cardiac masses so the differential diagnosis has to be made with other heart tumours, thrombi, vegetations, valvular calcification, and Lambl's excrescences. Because of their small size, TOE is superior to TTE in diagnosing these tumours.[5] Although there is a debate for resection of the asymptomatic PFE, surgical

excision should be considered for left-sided lesions regardless of their size, in order to hinder future embolic and haemodynamic complications.

Rhabdomyoma

Rhabdomyoma is the most common cardiac tumour during fetal life and childhood. These tumours are usually located within the ventricles but they may also originate in the atrium or in the atrioventricular junction. Fetal diagnosis of cardiac rhabdomyoma is most commonly made after incidental detection of multiple intracardiac masses. A strong association of multiple cardiac rhabdomyomas with tuberous sclerosis has long been recognized.[6,7]

Macroscopically, rhabdomyomas appear uniform, round, and solid, and are brighter than the neighbouring healthy myocardium. Rhabdomyomas are most commonly multiple and intramural, but intracavitary extensions are found in up to 50% of patients. Echocardiography is diagnostic and shows multiple homogeneous bright intramural masses with luminal extensions (➲ Fig. 20.6; ▣ 20.11 and 20.12).

The outcome of antenatally detected cardiac rhabdomyomas is favourable. After birth, regression of the tumour in infancy is an expected outcome, and complete resolution of more than 80% of the tumours may occur during early childhood.

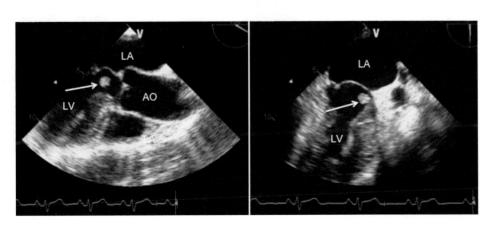

Figure 20.4 Papillary fibroelastoma of the mitral valve. Transoesophageal echocardiography views from a young man who had an embolic event. Transducer position at 134 (left) and 90 degrees (right) shows a small (8mm) mass on the ventricular surface of the anterior mitral leaflet, which corresponded to a papillary fibroelastoma of the mitral valve.

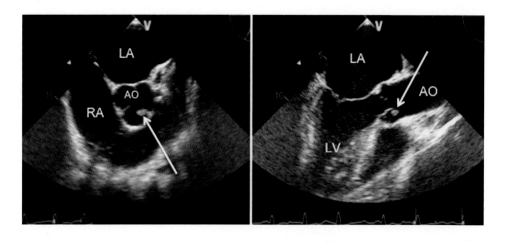

Figure 20.5 Papillary fibroelastoma of the aortic valve. Transverse (left) and longitudinal (right) transoesophageal views of a small mass attached to the arterial surface of the aortic valve in a patient after an embolic myocardial infarction. These rather small tumours can be missed by transthoracic echocardiography.

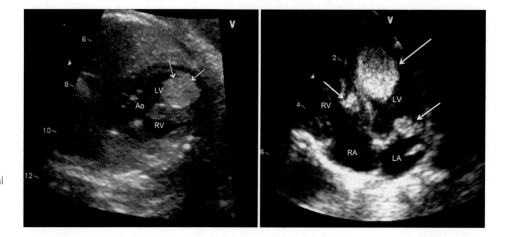

Figure 20.6 Rhabdomyoma. Fetal echocardiography (left) and transthoracic apical four-chamber view (right) from a baby showing multiple cardiac tumours (arrows) in both ventricles and on the mitral valve. This is a typical example of rhabdomyoma. (Courtesy of Ana Teixeira, MD.)

Echocardiography is the tool of choice to monitor the haemodynamic significance of the tumour and its evolution. Surgical intervention should be preserved only for sick patients with symptoms of severe obstruction or intractable arrhythmias.

Fibroma

Cardiac fibroma is the second most common primary cardiac neoplasm in infants and children after rhabdomyoma. On echocardiography, cardiac fibroma usually appears as a solitary intramural homogeneous echogenic lesion, rounded, with a fibrous whorled cut surface (➲ Fig. 20.7). The usual location of the tumour is in the ventricular septum (IVS) or the left ventricular (LV) free wall, and the size of the tumour may vary from 1–10cm. Calcification of the central portion of the tumour is pathognomonic for fibroma reflecting poor blood supply to the mass. Because of the potential for cardiac fibromas to cause heart failure (HF) or arrhythmias, complete surgical resection is recommended in symptomatic cases. Echocardiography is helpful in following the growth of the tumour. After surgery, periodic echocardiography may be necessary to monitor for recurrence.

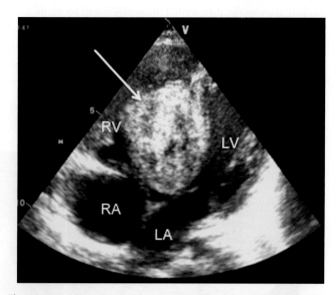

Figure 20.7 Fibroma. Apical four-chamber view from a young child showing a voluminous fibroma (arrow) located in the interventricular septum, causing left ventricular outflow tract obstruction. (Courtesy of Rui Anjos, MD.)

Lipomas

Cardiac lipomas are rare lesions and occur exclusively in adults. They are encapsulated subepicardial masses. They are commonly silent but rarely may cause symptoms including arrhythmias and atrioventricular block.

Pericardial cysts

Pericardial cysts, the most common pericardial tumour, are usually small, and most often discovered as incidental findings. Patients have an excellent prognosis.

Primary malignant tumours

Ninety-five per cent of primary cardiac malignancies are sarcomas (➲ Fig. 20.8). They can arise in any part of the heart but angiosarcoma, the more common type, arises preferentially in the RA and has a predilection for male sex. Multiple attachment sites and infiltration of contiguous structures (chamber walls, valves, and vessels), and irregular pericardial thickening are indicative of malignancy. Invasion of adjacent structures is common and metastases to the lungs, brain, bone, and colon develop in the majority of cases of angiosarcoma.[8] Rhabdomyosarcomas are most common in adult males, children, and adolescents. They can occur in any heart chamber, are often multicentric, and frequently invade cardiac valves and interfere with valve function. As compared to angiosarcoma, the tumour rarely invades beyond the parietal pericardium. Fibrosarcomas can be seen within the left or right heart chambers and they may spread to surrounding structures.[9]

Primary cardiac lymphomas (PCLs) represent 5% of primary cardiac malignancies but it is thought that their incidence is rising in relation with the increase in prevalence of AIDS and transplanted population.

The prognosis for malignant primary cardiac tumours is generally extremely poor. The therapy depends on the tumour type, size, histology, location, and evidence of metastatic spread.

Surgery, chemotherapy, and radiotherapy may prolong survival. Because some tumours such as PCL respond to chemotherapy, aggressive diagnostic procedures should be applied early after diagnosis. In cases where a malignant type of cardiac tumour is suspected from echocardiographic imaging features, additional imaging modalities such as computed tomography (CT) or cardiac magnetic resonance (CMR) and positron emission tomography (PET) are useful in providing information about extracardiac involvement as well as to measure tumour metabolism and proliferation.[8,9]

Metastatic cardiac tumours

Malignant tumours spread to the heart by direct extension, lymphatic spread, haematogenous spread, and by intracavitary extension from inferior vena cava (IVC) or throughout the pulmonary veins. Metastatic tumours are mostly located in the epicardial surface of the heart. Although an higher rate of metastization to the heart occur in rare tumours such as melanoma, malignant germ cell neoplasm, and malignant thymoma, the greatest number of malignant cardiac lesions originate from lung tumours in men, breast tumours in women, and from common types of cancer such as stomach, liver, ovary, and colon. Because 90% of cases with secondary cardiac involvement by malignant disease are clinically silent, echocardiography should be performed to rule out intracardiac or pericardial involvement after a patient's history of known malignancy elsewhere who presents with cardiac symptoms (➲ Fig. 20.9; ◪20.13–20.15). The differential diagnosis of pericardial effusion in a patient with known malignancy includes malignant pericardial effusion, radiation-induced pericarditis, drug-induced pericarditis, and idiopathic pericarditis. The diagnosis is often confirmed by cytological analysis of pericardial fluid removed for diagnostic or therapeutic pericardiocentesis.

In the presence of a floating mass extending through the IVC within the right cardiac chambers, suspicion for intracardiac

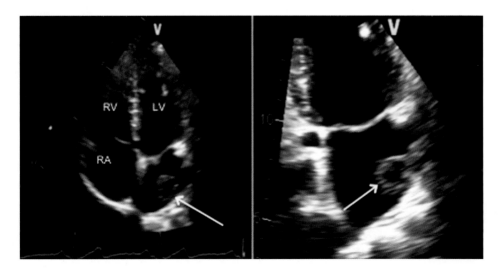

Figure 20.8 Sarcoma. Apical four-chamber (left) and two-chamber (right) views of a left atrial mass (arrows) that corresponded to a primary sarcoma removed completely with surgery.

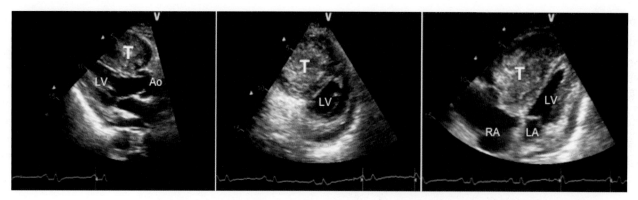

Figure 20.9 Metastases from a primary germ cell tumour. Bulky right-sided metastases causing right ventricular outflow obstruction in a patient with a primary germ cell tumour, which presented with syncope. A small pericardial effusion also is present.

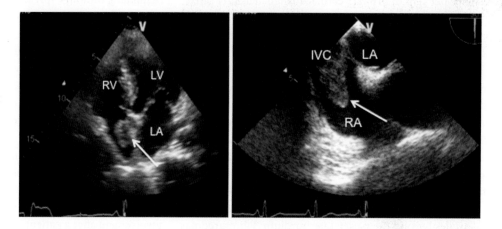

Figure 20.10 Metastases from a pelvic tumour. Apical four-chamber (left) view showing a right atrial mass close to the interatrial septum (arrow). Transverse transoesophageal (right) view disclosed the mass attached to the junction of the inferior vena cava and right atrium. This was a pelvic tumour that reached the heart through the venous system.

extension of renal cell tumour, pelvic leiomyoma, or hepatocellular carcinoma should be retained, and such a finding should prompt radiographic evaluation of the abdomen and the pelvis (⬦ Fig. 20.10; ◼ 20.16).

The delineation of a therapeutic strategy for secondary cardiac tumours should be conducted with oncology specialists, and before cardiac surgery is considered, a detailed anatomical definition of the extension of involvement usually requires the combination of echocardiography with CT and/or CMR. For right-sided tumours where histological analysis is needed, TOE-guided transvenous biopsy is recommended, as it allows direct visualization of both the tumour and the bioptome positioning.[8] Intracardiac echocardiographic (ICE) guidance for trans-jugular biopsy of right-sided cardiac masses has also been described as useful and safe.[10]

Non-neoplastic masses

Thrombi

Intracardiac thrombi tend to form when there is stasis of blood flow. They are usually associated with cardiac disease, homogeneous, and are associated with cardiac diseases and dilated cardiac chambers.

Atrial thrombi

LA thrombi classically reside in the atrial appendage, but can also form in the body of the LA. The presence of an enlarged chamber, atrial fibrillation, a stenotic mitral valve (MV), low cardiac output (CO) state, and spontaneous contrast echoes, all favour blood stasis and thrombus formation.

While TTE may provide visualization of larger thrombi located in the body of the LA (⬦ Fig. 20.11), a transoesophageal window is usually required to detect thrombus in the LA appendage (⬦ Fig. 20.12), small atrial thrombi, or to evaluate patients with technically difficult studies. Size, echogenicity, and mobility of LA thrombi are widely variable, and occasionally, differentiation from other masses myxoma in particular, may not be easy (⬦ Fig. 20.13; ◼ 20.17).

Left ventricular thrombi

LV thrombus is a frequent and potentially dangerous complication of ischaemic heart disease (IHD). Ventricular thrombi formation usually occurs in the early phase of anterior myocardial infarction or in poorly contracting ventricles (⬦ Fig. 20.14).[11] They are most often located in the LV apex in association with anterior and larger infarcts, with a reported incidence of 10–40%. The diagnosis of ventricular thrombus has important

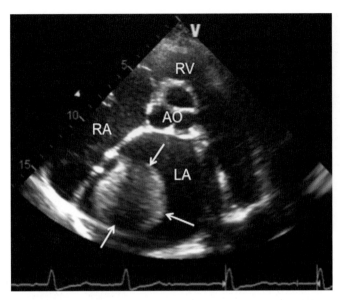

Figure 20.11 TTE view of left atrial thrombus. Transthoracic short-axis view showing a large thrombus (arrows) in the left atrium.

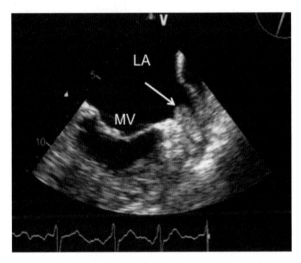

Figure 20.12 TOE view of left atrial thrombus. TOE imaging showing a thrombus (arrow) in the left atrial appendage in a patient with atrial fibrillation.

clinical and therapeutical implications because of the increased risk of systemic embolization, and of the rationale for antico-agulation. The timing of the LV assessment is crucial, as throm-bus formation that develop over the next few days after a myocardial infarction will be missed if echocardiography is applied just at the time of admission. Although TTE is the rou-tine diagnostic procedure in assessing patients with LV thrombi, its sensitivity is limited by the quality of the acoustic window and poor contrast between thrombus and adjacent myocar-dium. Great caution should be taken in making such a diagno-sis if the systolic function is normal, or if the mass has a band or thread-like appearance, since apical trabeculae may be misin-terpreted as thrombi. Moreover, apical abnormalities can be difficult to visualize. This is because native tissue harmonic echocardiography is weak at the near field. Contrast opacifica-tion facilitates the identification of apical abnormalities (see ◐ Chapter 7). Hence, contrast echocardiography is now recog-nized as the technique of choice for establishing or excluding the presence of LV apical thrombus (◐ Fig. 20.15), and assist in the differential diagnosis with other apical abnormalities (apical hypertrophic cardiomyopathy, LV non-compaction, and ven-tricular pseudoaneurysm). Newer technologies such as CMR and CT are likely superior in this regard.[12,13]

Right-side thrombi

Thrombi in the right side of the heart usually originate from lower extremity peripheral veins or grow on pacing wires or indwelling catheters. They are mobile, have a characteristic popcorn or snake-like appearance, and almost always are asso-ciated with pulmonary embolism. These pleomorphic thrombi are mainly localized in the RA, frequently move back and forth through the tricuspid orifice, and may cause cardiovascular col-lapse when entrapment occurs. In patients with acute pulmo-nary embolism, TTE finds the presence of right-sided heart thrombi in 4–18%. While direct visualization of a thrombus in the pulmonary artery is attained with echocardiography in only few cases, indirect signs of acute pulmonary hypertension and RV overload may be accepted to establish the diagnosis

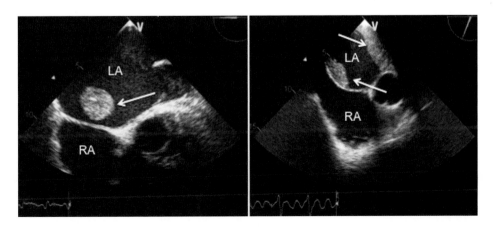

Figure 20.13 Multiple left atrial thrombi. TOE imaging of left atrial thrombi. Transverse transoesophageal views showing a free-floating thrombus (left) and multiple mural thrombi (right).

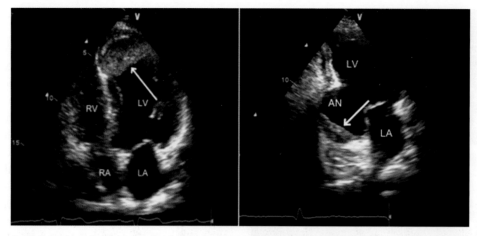

Figure 20.14 Left ventricular thrombi. Apical four-chamber (left) view showing a large apical thrombus (arrow) in a patient after a large anterior myocardial infarction. Apical two-chamber (right) view from a patient with inferoposterior myocardial infarction that developed a large aneurysm. A mural thrombus is seen (arrow).

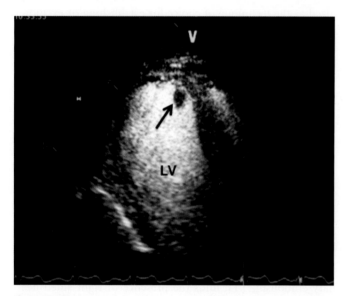

Figure 20.15 LV apical thrombus at contrast echocardiography. Contrast echocardiography showing a left ventricular apical thrombus (arrow) in a patient with a history of myocardial infarction.

(➲ Fig. 20.16). In this clinical scenario, echocardiography is a significant tool in risk stratification and decision making regarding the choice of therapeutic interventions.

Thrombus straddling the patent foramen ovale (PFO) is a rare event. There is a strong association of thrombus straddling the PFO with thromboembolic disease, frequently with severe pulmonary embolism but also with paradoxical embolism. Increased pulmonary and RV pressure could support clot migration across the PFO by interauricular pressure gradient reversal. Because thrombus straddling the PFO is usually not visualized by TTE, TOE has an essential role in cases where an intracardiac mass is diagnosed, or thromboembolic disease or pulmonary embolism is associated with systemic embolism suspected of paradoxical embolism.[14]

Vegetations

Echocardiography is an essential tool for the evaluation of patients with infective endocarditis (IE), which should be performed as soon as IE is suspected. Echocardiographic findings that provide evidence of IE includes vegetations, periannular abscesses, aneurysms, leaflets perforation, fistulas, or valvular dehiscence (see ➲ Chapter 16). Haemodynamic consequences of the infection and prognostic information concerning risk of embolization and/or need for cardiac surgery are provided by TTE and TOE, especially in cases of suspected prosthetic valve or intracardiac device infective endocarditis (see ➲ Chapter 16).

On 2D echocardiography, a valvular vegetation appears as a linear or round, irregular echogenic mass of few millimetres to several centimetres size, on a valve or supporting structure, frequently showing oscillations or fluttering, in the path of a regurgitant jet, or on an iatrogenic device (➲ Figs. 20.17 and 20.18; 🖪 20.18–20.20). Their echodensity is relatively low (similar to myocardium) in the early stages, and increases over time.

Right-sided IE is most frequently observed in intravenous drug abusers, mainly those HIV seropositives with advanced immunosuppression (🖪 20.21). Whilst the tricuspid valve is the usual site of infection in intravenous drug abusers, pulmonary and Eustachian valve infection may also be observed. Right-sided vegetations are usual large in size and easy to identify with TTE.

As indications for pacemakers and implantable cardioverter defibrillators expand, there is a rising incidence of device-related complications. Cardiac device-related infective endocarditis involves most commonly the leads or the tricuspid valve. Both TTE and TOE are recommended as soon as the diagnosis is suspected (➲ Fig 20.17; 🖪 20.18–20.21). Recently some case reports highlighted the potential role of high-resolution ICE for the demonstration of lead's vegetations when TOE is non-diagnostic. The size of the vegetations may influence the decision about whether to perform lead extraction percutaneously or surgically.[15]

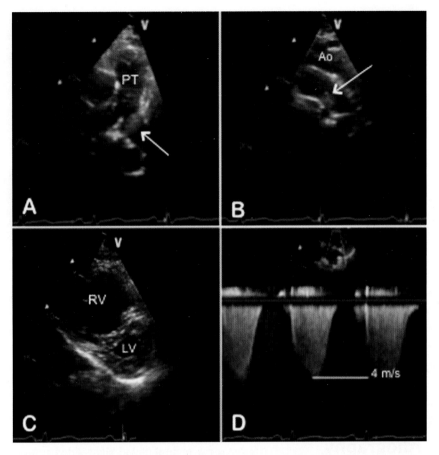

Figure 20.16 Pulmonary embolism. A) Parasternal transthoracic echocardiographic view of pulmonary trunk (PT) and its bifurcation into right and left pulmonary arteries, showing a large thrombus (arrow) almost occluding the left artery. B) Visualization of the thrombus in the left pulmonary artery from the suprasternal view. C) Parasternal short-axis view demonstrating the D-shaped left ventricle (LV) cavity and enlarged right ventricular (RV) cavity in pulmonary hypertension. D) Tricuspid regurgitation velocity recording by continuous wave Doppler. Transtricuspid gradient derived from the peak Doppler velocity corresponds to 64mmHg.

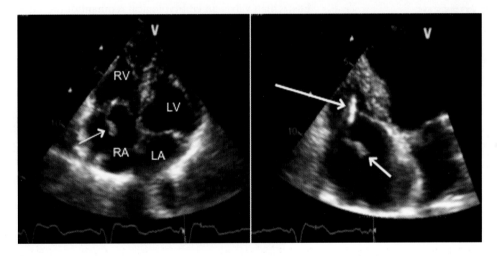

Figure 20.17 Vegetation on a pacemaker wire. TTE views of a patient with a vegetation (short arrows) associated with a pacemaker wire (long arrow).

Usefulness of contrast echocardiography for assessment of intracardiac masses

As stated earlier, 2D contrast enhancement is an accurate method for the identification of intracardiac thrombi (➲ Fig. 20.15). Moreover, contrast echocardiography has been shown to aid in the differentiation of cardiac masses, since standard echocardiography is not a reliable method for their tissue characterization.

Three different echocardiographic patterns regarding pixel intensity in intracardiac masses may occur:

◆ Complete lack of enhancement by contrast agent suggesting thrombi, as they are generally avascular.

◆ Partial enhancement with decreased pixel intensity in comparison with the myocardium, suggesting a poor blood supply mass such as myxomas.

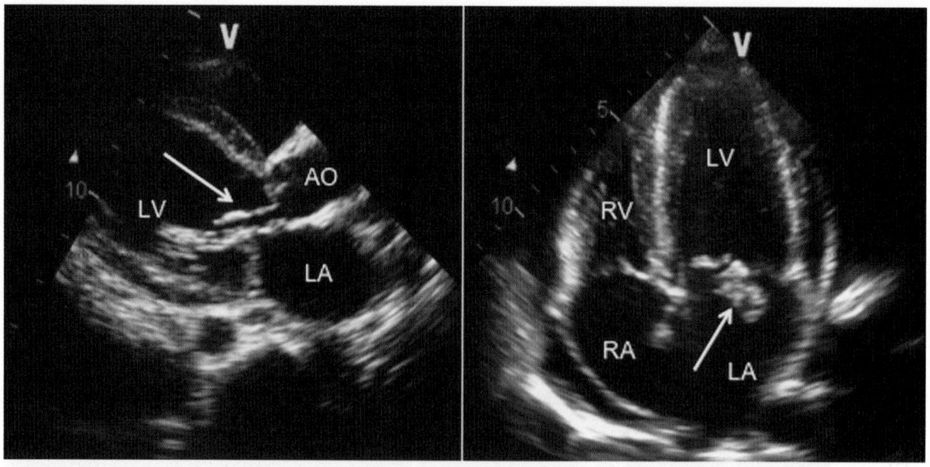

Figure 20.18 Aortic and mitral valves vegetations. TTEs of aortic (left) and mitral (right) valves vegetations illustrating the usual initial site of attachment: in the ventricular surface for the aortic valve and in the atrial surface for the mitral valve (arrows).

◆ Greater enhancement than the adjacent myocardium, suggesting a highly vascular tumour. Most malignant rapidly growing tumours have neovascularization, which explains the intense contrast enhancement after contrast echo injection.[16–21]

Added value of real-time three-dimensional echocardiography in assessing cardiac masses

Real-time three-dimensional echocardiography (RT3DE) allows a detailed anatomy of a region of interest to be obtained. Regarding the evaluation of cardiac masses, it can provide accurate information not only of the size and shape but also of the volume, surface characteristics, and composition of the mass, as well as its relationship to adjacent structures (➲ Fig 20.19). Additional advantages of RT3D include the improved visualization of the true apex (better visualization of thrombi), and LA appendage with 3DMTOE (differentiating pectinate muscles from thrombi). Finally, through expansion of the diagnostic capabilities of 2D imaging in assessing cardiac structure and function, RT3D may represent an added value for surgical planning, and accurate and reproducible evaluation of LV function in patients with cardiac tumours treated with cardiotoxic agents.[22–24]

Normal anatomical variants

Variations within normality and less frequently encountered morphologies do not necessarily denote disease or pathology. Several anatomical variants of normal structures throughout the heart may mimic pathological lesions, and be misdiagnosed as tumours, thrombi, or vegetations. A thorough knowledge of these normal anatomical variants is important for reaching a correct diagnosis, as it may have implications on further investigation and the patient's management.[25]

Most of these anatomical variants are located in the RA. The Chiari network is characterized by elongated and fenestrated highly mobile curvilinear echos interconnecting the crista terminalis, interatrial septum, IVC, and coronary sinus valves. Its prevalence is 2% in normal hearts and it is seldom clinically important. When doubts arise with TTE, TOE is helpful to differentiate it from vegetations, ruptured chordae of the tricuspid valve, or a pedunculated right-sided tumour. A prominent Eustachian valve, an embryological remnant of the valve of the inferior vena cava best identified in subcostal views, may also be mistaken for a pathological atrial mass. The Thebesian valve represents the valve of the sinus venosus and can be seen as a semilunar endocardial flap visualized best in the right heart

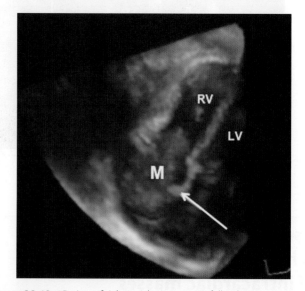

Figure 20.19 3D view of right atrial myxoma. 3D full-volume reconstruction echocardiography of a large right atrial myxoma. Detailed information of the mass volume and contour is provided as well as confirmation of the site of attachment in the interatrial septum (arrow). (Courtesy of Jorge Almeida, MD, Cardio-Thoracic Surgery Centre, Hospital São João, Porto, Portugal.)

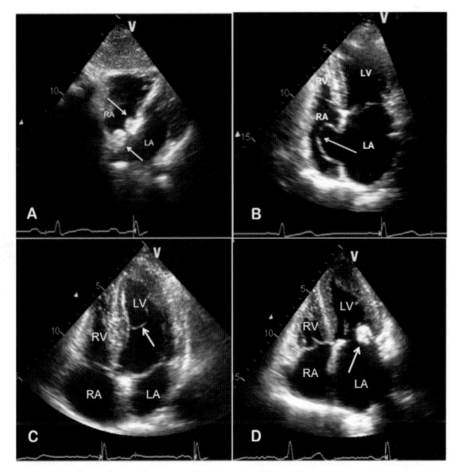

inflow view. The crista terminalis runs along the lateral atrial wall, between the right sides of the two-venacaval orifices.

Lipomatous hypertrophy of the interatrial septum (LHIS) is a benign cardiac mass characterized by massive fatty deposits in the interatrial septum that appears unusually thick. The mass has a typical dumbbell shape sparing the membrane of the fossa ovalis (➲ Fig 20.20A). LHIS should be considered in the differential diagnosis of any cardiac mass involving the IAS. Recognition of this lesion is of paramount importance because it can be mistaken with a malignant tumour leading to unwarranted surgical removal. Surgical management of LHIS should be limited to patients with intractable severe rhythm disorders, haemodynamic instability, and symptoms of SVC syndrome or RA obstruction.[26,27]

Aneurysms bulging from the interatrial septum are usually incidental findings (➲ Fig 20.20B). They have been associated with septal defects, atrial arrhythmias, and systemic and pulmonary embolisms. In rare instances, interatrial septal aneurysms mimic atrial masses.

In the LA the normal ridge between the LA appendage and left superior pulmonary vein, when thick and prominent, may be mistaken for an abnormal mass. On evaluation of LA appendage with TOE, caution has to be used to differentiate prominent pectinate muscles from thrombi.[28] TOE is largely superior to TTE in characterizing atrial masses.

In the ventricles, RV moderator band, LV bands or false tendons, normal or aberrant trabeculae or chordae, and prominent papillary muscles are further examples of normal cardiac structures that can be mistaken for pathological entities (➲ Fig 20.20C).

In the valves, Lambl's excrescences are thin, mobile, filiform structures, also known as valvular strands. Most often they occur on the ventricular side of the aortic valve. The differential diagnosis for Lambl's excrescences includes fibroelastoma, thrombi, and vegetations. The clinical importance of these valvular strands remains unclear. For asymptomatic patients, conservative follow-up is recommended.[29] Finally, caseous calcification of the mitral annulus is a rare form of periannular calcification that generally appears as a calcified mass with a central echolucent area that may lead to diagnostic errors (➲ Fig 20.20D).

Spontaneous echo contrast may be seen in the LA when there is stasis of blood flow, or in the LV, especially in the region of an apical aneurysm. Spontaneous echo contrast can also be

Figure 20.20 Anatomical variants. A) Subcostal view of lipomatous hypertrophy of the atrial septum (arrows). Note the characteristic dumbbell shape appearance. B) Atrial septal aneurysm (arrow) seen on TTE in a four-chamber view. C) Left ventricular aberrant chordae or 'web' seen in an apical four-chamber view in a normal echocardiogram. D) Mitral annular calcification may be taken for a cardiac mass.

observed in patients with mechanical prosthesis, where it appears as very small, discrete echogenic targets that are located in different parts of the heart during successive cycles.

Extracardiac masses may compress the heart and create a mass effect. Examples of such masses include mediastinal tumours, coronary aneurysms, or hiatal hernias.

Artefacts

Echocardiographic artefacts may present as intracardiac configurations that may lead the clinician to misdiagnosis of cardiac masses. Various causes of echocardiographic artefacts have been described. The generation of artefacts may be attributed to technical issues such as a poor acoustic window and/or the physical nature of the ultrasound beam (beam width artefact). Reverberations may also appear to represent abnormal structures. Strong reflectors such as areas of atelectasis or pleural effusion may lead to the generation of echocardiographic artefacts, especially in the critical patient in the intensive care unit. Appropriate transducer selection and evaluation from multiple windows is crucial to differentiate artefacts from real anatomical structures. Artefacts should be suspected if there are no distinct borders, no clear attachment, lack of visualization of the structure in multiple view or its visualization as a multiple of other structures, or if contrast or colour Doppler does not respect the boundaries of the structure. Whenever doubts arise from TTE, multiple acoustic windows and views obtained by TOE, facilitates the differential diagnosis of intracardiac artefact from true cardiac anomalies.

Cardiac source of emboli

Patients with suspected cardiac origin of systemic embolic events should be investigated, in order to identify:

♦ Abnormal intracardiac masses, such as LV and LA thrombus, vegetation, cardiac tumours, especially LA myxomas.

♦ Predisposing conditions to develop intracardiac masses, such as LV aneurysm, mitral stenosis, and atrial blood flow stasis.

♦ Cardiac abnormalities that may represent a potential conduit for systemic embolization.

♦ Aortic atheroma with superimposed protruding thrombus.

A definite cardiac source of emboli can be identified by TTE in only 10–15% of cases. Often, echocardiographic examination *after* an embolic event may fail in detecting intracardiac embolic masses, because at that time eventual thrombus is not longer in the heart. In such conditions, a careful search for predisposing conditions to systemic embolization is recommended, in order to confirm or definitively rule out the suspicion.

Predisposing conditions

Intracardiac thrombi may occur in patients with LV aneurysm and severe impairment of contractile function, as well as in the presence of LV pseudoaneurysm which is always associated with thrombus lining the pseudoaneurysm cavity. In patients with rheumatic mitral stenosis and paroxysmal or persistent atrial fibrillation, intracardiac thrombus formation is frequent, even though it is not documented by TOE. Also congenital heart disease may predispose to intracardiac masses development, particularly LV dysfunction, atrial dilation, or intracardiac shunts. Indeed, often atrial septal defect is associated with LA-to-RA shunt, but transient reverse of pressure gradients, as occurs during Valsalva manoeuvre, may determine a paradoxical embolization from peripheral veins to systemic arterial circulation. Eisenmenger's syndrome in the presence of ventricular septal defect frequently causes systemic embolic events, whereas small defects in IVS have low probability to embolize due to unidirectional LV-to-RV pressure gradients. In cases of potential embolization from prosthetic valves, identification of thrombi is very difficult even by TOE, due to shadowing and reverberations from prosthetic leaflets and sewing ring. The clinical suspicion may be stronger in the presence of inadequate anticoagulation levels and recommendation of echocardiographic examination are directed toward evaluation of prosthetic function and exclusion of other potential intracardiac sources of emboli.

Among cardiac abnormalities that may serve as a conduit for systemic embolization, a PFO is the most common. It has been found in 25–35% of patients referred for autopsy and is caused by incomplete closure of interatrial septal shunt during the first few days after birth. In adult age, RA-to-LA passage of emboli may be facilitated by transient or chronic increase of RA pressure, as occurs during cough, Valsalva manoeuvre, or in pulmonary hypertension, respectively. Echocardiographic detection of PFO is based on imaging by TTE and mostly by TOE. Often, correct diagnosis requires infusion of ultrasound contrast agents, such as air gas microbubbles (see ❥ Chapter 7). By using contrast agents, identification of PFO is achieved at rest in about 5% of the patients; when Valsalva manoeuvre is performed, such detection increases up to 25%. A PFO is frequently detected in young people (< 45 years), suffering from transient ischaemic attacks or cerebrovascular events: in patients with systemic embolic events, the prevalence of PFO is about 30%, as compared with the prevalence of 10% in control subjects. Percutaneous device closure of such interatrial septal defect is spreading, even by TOE or intracardiac monitoring (see ❥ Chapters 4 and 23).

A possible association between increased risk of systemic embolization and cardiac predisposing conditions has been also found for interatrial septal aneurysm. Interatrial septal aneurysm is defined as a transient bulging of the fossa ovalis region of the interatrial septum, greater than 15mm in the absence of chronically elevated LA or RA pressure. TOE use is widely raising recognition of this anatomical variant.

Indication for echocardiography in patients with suspected cardiac source of emboli

According to current guidelines, echocardiographic assessment of potential cardiac sources of emboli in patients with cerebral or peripheral vascular events should be performed:

◆ When there is abrupt occlusion of a major peripheral or visceral artery.

◆ In young patients (<45 years) with known cerebrovascular embolic events.

◆ In older patients with cerebrovascular embolic events, after exclusion of other more common causes.

◆ In patients in whom the clinical therapeutic management may substantially differ on the basis of echocardiographic examination results.

Personal perspective

Nowadays, most of the knowledge regarding cardiac tumours is still mainly based on postmortem studies, and the neoplastic nature and histotype of a cardiac mass can be established only by histology. Intracardiac masses are more and more frequently detected by chance during routine imaging examinations. Therefore, it is very important for the echocardiographer to be prepared to gather and properly interpret the full range of data provided by cardiac ultrasound, and to investigate the achievements that technological advances such as 3D and contrast echocardiography may grant in this context. Because of its rarity, an effort of centralization and collaboration among different professionals and specialties who deal with these patients would be welcome, in order to explore and establish the strengths and weaknesses of echocardiography and other new imaging modalities (CMR, CT, and PET) for the diagnosis, therapy, and prognosis of this specific pathology.

References

1 Thiene G, Valente M, Lombardi M, Basso C. Tumours of the heart. In: Camm AJ, Luscher TF, Serruys PW (eds). *The ESC Textbook of Cardiovascular Medicine*, 2nd ed. Oxford: Oxford University Press, 2009, pp.735–61.

2 Butany J, Nair V, Naseemuddin A, Nair GM, Catton C, Yau T. Cardiac tumours: diagnosis and management. *Lancet Oncol* 2005; 6:219-28.

3 Goswami, KC, Shrivastava S, Bahl VK, Saxena A, Manchanda SC, Wasir HS. Cardiac myxomas: clinical and echocardiographic profile. *Int J Cardiol* 1997; 63:251–9.

4 Yuan S-M, Shinfeld A, Lavee J, Kuperstein R, Haizler R, Raanani E. Imaging morphology of cardiac tumours. *Cardiol J* 2009; 16:26–35.

5 Truscelli G, Torromeo C, Miraldi F, Vittori C, Silenzi PF, Caso A, *et al*. The role of intraoperative transoesophageal echocardiography in the diagnosis and management of a rare multiple fibroelastoma of aortic valve: a case report and review of literature. *Eur J Echocardiogr* 2009; 10:884–6.

6 Uzun O, Wilson DG, Vujanic GM, Parsons JM, De Giovanni JV. Cardiac tumours in children. *Orphanet J Rare Dis* 2007; 2:11.

7 Andrés AS, Albert BI, Moreno JI, Sánchez AC, Bonora AM, Palacios JM. Primary cardiac tumours in infancy. *An Pediatr (Barc)* 2008; 69(1):15-22.

8 Neragi-Miandoab S, Kim J, Vlahakes GJ. Malignant tumours of the heart: a review of tumour type, diagnosis and therapy. *Clin Oncol* 2007; 19:748–56.

9 Shanmugam G. Primary cardiac sarcoma. *Eur J Cardiothorac Surg* 2006; 29:925–32.

10 Aqel R, Dobbs J Lau Y, Lloyd S, Gupta H, Zoghbi GJ. Transjugular biopsy of a right atrial mass under intracardiac echocardiographic guidance. *J Am Soc Echocardiogr* 2006; 19:1072.e5–e8.

11 Rabbani LE, Waksmonski C, Iqbal S, Stant J, Sciacca R, Apfelbaum M, *et al*. Determinants of left ventricular thrombus formation after primary percutaneous coronary intervention for anterior wall myocardial infarction. *J Thromb Thrombolysis* 2008; 25:141–5.

12 Srichai MB, Junor C, MD, Rodriguez L, Stillman AE, Grimm RA, Lieber ML, *et al*. Clinical, imaging, and pathological characteristics of left ventricular thrombus: a comparison of contrast-enhanced magnetic resonance imaging, transthoracic echocardiography, and transesophageal echocardiography with surgical or pathological validation. *Am Heart J* 2006; 152:75–84.

13 Osherov A, Borovik-Raz M, Aronson D, Agmon Y, Kapeliovich M, Kerner A, *et al*. Incidence of early left ventricular thrombus after acute anterior wall myocardial infarction in the primary coronary intervention era. *Am Heart J* 2009; 157:1074–80.

14 Fauveau E, Cohen A, Bonnet N, Gacem K, Lardoux H. Surgical or medical treatment for thrombus straddling the patent foramen ovale: Impending paradoxical embolism? Report of four clinical cases and literature review. *Arch Cardiovasc Dis* 2008; 101:637–44.

15 Sohail M, Uslan DZ, Khan AH, Friedman PA, Hayes DL, Wilson WR, *et al*. Infective endocarditis complicating permanent pacemaker and implantable cardioverter-defibrillator infection. *Mayo Clin Proc* 2008; 83(1):46–53.

16 Mansencal N, Revault-d'Allonnes L, Pelage J-P, Farcot J-C, Lacombe P, Dubourg O. Usefulness of contrast echocardiography

for assessment of intracardiac masses. *Arch Cardiovas Dis* 2009; **102**:177–83.

17 Mulvagh SL, Rakowski H, Vannan MA, Abdelmoneim SS, Becher H, Bierig M. American Society of Echocardiography consensus statement on the clinical applications of ultrasonic contrast agents in echocardiography. *J Am Soc Echocardiogr* 2008; **21**:1179–201.

18 Uenishi EK, Caldas M, Saroute AN, Tsutsui JM, Piotto GH, Falcão SN, *et al*. Contrast echocardiography for the evaluation of tumours and thrombi. *Arq Bras Cardiol* 2008; **91**(5):e56–e60.

19 Kirkpatrick JN, Wong T, Bednarz JE, Spencer KT, Sugeng L, Ward RP, *et al*. Differential diagnosis of cardiac masses using contrast echocardiographic perfusion imaging. *J Am Coll Cardiol* 2004; **43**:1412–19.

20 Yelamanchili P, Wanat FE, Knezevic D, Nanda NC, Patel V. Two-dimensional transthoracic contrast echocardiographic assessment of metastatic left ventricular tumours. *Echocardiography* 2006; **23**:248–50.

21 Moustafa, SE, Sauvé C, Amyot R. Assessment of a right atrial metastasis using contrast echocardiography perfusion imaging. *Eur J Echocardiogr* 2008; **9**:326–8.

22 Plana JC. Added value of real-time three-dimensional echocardiography in assessing cardiac masses. *Echocardiography* 2009; **11**:205–9.

23 Muller S, Feuchtner G, Bonatti J, Muller L, Laufer G, Hiemetzberger R, *et al*. Value of transesophageal 3D echocardiography as an adjunct to conventional 2D imaging in preoperative evaluation of cardiac masses. *Echocardiography* 2008; **25**:624–31.

24 Anwar AM, Nosir YF, Ajam A, Chamsi-Pasha H. Central role of real-time three-dimensional echocardiography in the assessment of intracardiac thrombi. *Int J Cardiovasc Imaging* 2010; **26**:519–26.

25 George A, Parameswaran A, Nekkanti R, Lurito K, Movahed A. Normal anatomic variants on transthoracic echocardiogram. *Echocardiography* 2009; **26**:1109–17.

26 Xanthos T, Giannakopoulos N, Papadimitriou L. Lipomatous hypertrophy of the interatrial septum: a pathological and clinical approach. *Int J Cardiol* 2007; **121**:4–8.

27 O'Connor S, Recavarren R, Nichols LC, Parwani AV. Lipomatous hypertrophy of the interatrial septum: an overview. *Arch Pathol Lab Med* 2006; **130**:397–9.

28 Agmon Y, Khandheria BK, Gentile F, Seward JB. Echocardiographic assessment of the left atrial appendage. *J Am Coll Cardiol* 1999; **34**:1867–77.

29 Aziz F, Baciewicz FA. Lambl's excrescences. Review and recommendations. *Tex Heart J* 2007; **34**:366–8.

Further reading

Butany J, Nair V, Naseemuddin A, Nair GM, Catton C, Yau T. Cardiac tumours: diagnosis and management. *Lancet Oncol* 2005; **6**:219–28.

George A, Parameswaran A, Nekkanti R, Lurito K, Movahed A. Normal anatomic variants on transthoracic echocardiogram. *Echocardiography* 2009; **26**:1109–17.

Neragi-Miandoab S, Kim J, Vlahakes GJ. Malignant tumours of the heart: a review of tumour type, diagnosis and therapy. *Clin Oncol* 2007; **19**:748–56.

Oh JK, Seward JB, Tajik AS (eds). *The Echo Manual*, 3rd ed. Philadelphia, PA: Lippincott Williams and Wilkins, 2007, pp.310–21.

Otto, CM (ed). *Textbook of Clinical Echocardiography*, 3rd ed. Philadelphia, PA: Elsevier/Saunders, 2007, pp.377–96

Plana JC. Added value of real-time three-dimensional echo-cardiography in assessing cardiac masses. *Echocardiography* 2009; **11**:205–9.

Thiene G, Valente M, Lombardi M, Basso C. Tumours of the heart. In: Camm AJ, Luscher TF, Serruys PW (eds). *The ESC Textbook of Cardiovascular Medicine*, 2nd ed. Oxford: Oxford University Press, 2009, pp.735–61.

Yuan S-M, Shinfeld A, Lavee J, Kuperstein R, Haizler R, Raanani E. Imaging morphology of cardiac tumours. *Cardiol J* 2009; **16**:26–35.

Additional DVD and online material

20.1–20.4 Large left atrial myxoma recorded from the parasternal long-axis (= 20.1), parasternal short-axis at the level of the mitral valve (= 20.2), apical four-chamber (= 20.3), and from the sub-costal (= 20.4) views. During diastole, the tumour prolapses into the left ventricle (LV), completely obstructing the mitral valve orifice. Note the site of tumour attachment in the interatrial septum.

20.5–20.7 Transoesophageal views from a large left atrial myxoma. Note the high mobility, the irregular and friable contours, the inhomogeneous echogenicity, and the location of the stalk in the interatrial septum.

20.8 Transoesophageal view showing a papillary fibroelastoma of the mitral valve. Note its small size, high mobility, its frond-like appearance, and the attachment site on the ventricular surface of the anterior mitral leaflet.

20.9 and 20.10 Longitudinal (⊞ 20.9) and transverse (⊞ 20.10) transoesophageal views of a small papillary fibroelastoma attached to the arterial surface of the aortic valve.

20.11 Fetal echocardiogram showing multiple cardiac tumours in both ventricles. This is a typical example of multiple rhabdomyoma. (Courtesy of Ana Teixeira, MD.)

20.12 Parasternal long-axis view from a young boy showing multiple intracardiac rhabdomiyomas in the interventricular septum. (Courtesy of Ana Teixeira, MD.)

20.13–20.15 Parasternal long-axis (⊞ 20.13), apical four-chamber (⊞ 20.14), and parasternal short-axis (⊞ 20.15) views from a patient with a primary germ cell tumour, which presented with syncope. Note the bulky right-sided metastases causing right ventricular outflow obstruction.

20.16 Transverse transoesophageal view from a right atrial mass attached to the junction of the inferior vena cava with the right atrium. The patient had a pelvic tumour that reached the heart through the venous system.

■ 20.17 Transverse transoesophageal view showing a free-floating thrombus in the left atrium. Note the left atrial abundant left atrial spontaneous echo contrast.

■ 20.18 Transthoracic four-chamber view from a patient with a device-related infective endocarditis. Vegetations are seen attached both to the tricuspid septal leaflet and to the pacemaker wire.

■ 20.19 Transthoracic four-chamber view from a patient with mitral valve bacterial endocarditis. Note the attachment site of the vegetation in the atrial side of the valve.

■ 20.20 Two-dimensional (left), and 2D colour Doppler (right) transthoracic long-axis view from a patient with

bacterial endocarditis. An aortic valve vegetation is seen in the ventricular side of the aortic cusps. Note its movement through systole (into the aorta) and diastole (into LVOT). Note also that there is a perforation on the anterior mitral leaflet (ruptured abscess) where now and then the aortic vegetation penetrates. An eccentric jet of mitral regurgitation (throughout the perforation) is also shown.

■ 20.21 Transthoracic right ventricular inflow view from a patient with tricuspid valve endocarditis that completely destroyed the valve. Note the huge size of the vegetation. (Courtesy of António Freitas, MD.)

⮡ For additional multimedia materials please visit the online version of the book (http://escecho.oxfordmedicine.com).

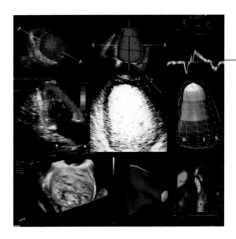

CHAPTER 21

Diseases of the aorta

Arturo Evangelista and T. González-Alujas

Contents

Summary

Evaluation of the aorta is a routine part of the standard echocardiographic examination, because echocardiography plays an important role both in the diagnosis and follow-up of aortic diseases. In particular, echocardiography is useful for assessing aorta size, biophysical properties, and atherosclerotic involvement of the thoracic aorta.

Transthoracic echocardiography (TTE) permits adequate assessment of several aortic segments, particularly the aortic root and proximal ascending aorta. Transoesophageal echocardiography (TOE) overcomes the limitations of TTE in thoracic aorta assessment, so TTE and TOE should be used in a complementary manner.

Although TOE is the technique of choice in the diagnosis of aortic dissection, TTE may be used as the initial modality in the emergency setting. Intimal flap in proximal ascending aorta, pericardial effusion/tamponade, and left ventricular function can be easily visualized by TTE. However, a negative TTE does not rule out aortic dissection and other imaging techniques must be considered. TOE should define entry tear location, mechanisms of aortic regurgitation, and true lumen compression.

In addition, echocardiography is essential in selecting and monitoring surgical and endovascular treatment and in detecting possible complications. Although other imaging techniques have a greater field of view, echocardiography is portable, rapid, accurate, and cost-effective in the diagnosis and follow-up of most aortic diseases.

Introduction

Echocardiography has become the most used imaging test in the evaluation of cardiovascular disease and plays an important role in the diagnosis and follow-up of aortic diseases.

Transthoracic echocardiography

Evaluation of the aorta is a routine part of the standard echocardiographic examination.[1] Transthoracic echocardiography (TTE) permits adequate assessment of several aortic segments, particularly the aortic root and proximal ascending aorta. All scanning planes should be used to obtain information on most aortic segments including the left and right parasternal long-axis (PLAX) views, the suprasternal view, the apical three-chamber (A3C) view and the subcostal view. Although TTE is not the ideal tool for visualizing all aortic segments, important information can always be gained by careful use of all echo-windows (➲ Figs. 21.1 and 21.2).

Transoesophageal echocardiography

Proximity of the oesophagus to the thoracic aorta permits high-resolution images from higher-frequency transoesophageal echocardiography (TOE). Furthermore, the availability of multiplane imaging permits improved incremental assessment of the aorta from its root to the descending aorta.[2] The most important transoesophageal views of the ascending aorta, aortic root, and aortic valve (AoV) are the high transoesophageal long-axis (at 120–150 degrees) and short-axis (at 30–60 degrees) views. A short segment of the distal ascending aorta, just before the innominate artery, remains unvisualized owing to interposition of the right bronchus and trachea (blind spot). The descending aorta is easily visualized in short-axis (0 degrees) and long-axis (90 degrees) views from the cocliac trunk to the left subclavian artery. Further withdrawal of the probe shows the aortic arch. In the distal part of the arch, the origin of the subclavian artery is easily visualized. However, in awake patients, the origin of innominate and left carotid arteries is not clearly visualized, although in anaesthetized patients it is possible to identify the origin of these supra-aortic arteries.[3] The proximal part of the coeliac trunk is visualized in most cases.[4] TOE overcomes limitations encountered by TTE. TTE and TOE should be used in a complementary manner (➲ Fig. 21.3).

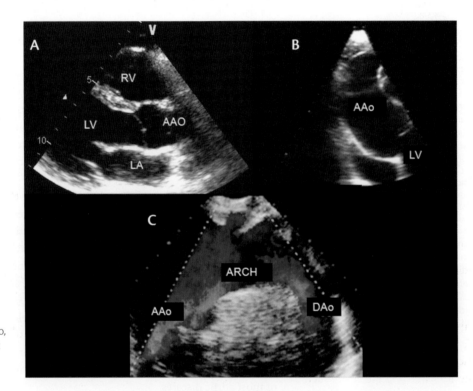

Figure 21.1 Aortic imaging by transthoracic echocardiography. A) Parasternal long-axis view showing aortic root. B) Mean and distal parts of ascending aorta may be visualized by upper right parasternal long-axis view. C) Suprasternal view showing aortic arch and supra-aortic great arteries. AAo, ascending aorta; Dao, descending thoracic aorta; LA, left atrium; LV, left ventricle; RV, right ventricle.

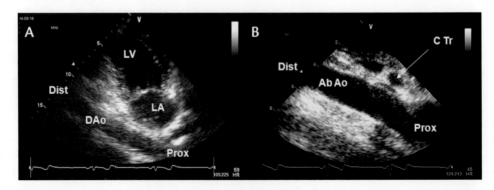

Figure 21.2 Aortic imaging by transthoracic echocardiography. A) Posteriorly angulated apical two-chamber view showing the median part of the descending thoracic aorta. B) By subcostal view, suprarenal abdominal aorta is easily visualized in non-obese patients. Arrow shows coeliac trunk. Ab Ao, abdominal aorta; C Tr, coeliac trunk; Dist, distal: Prox: proximal.

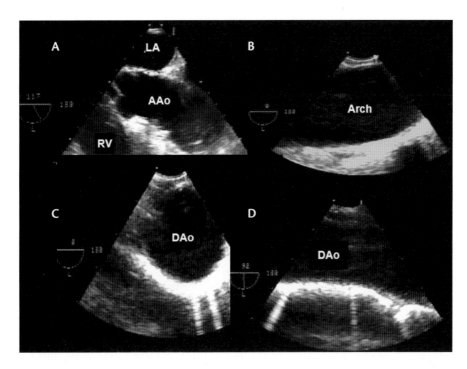

Figure 21.3 Aortic imaging by transoesophageal echocardiography. A) Ascending aorta in long-axis view at 120 degrees. B) Aortic arch in transverse view. C) Descending aorta visualised by transverse view. D) Descending aorta visualized by longitudinal view.

Aortic size and biophysical properties

Assessment of aortic size

Measurements of aortic diameter by echocardiography are accurate and reproducible when care is taken to obtain a true perpendicular dimension and gain settings are appropriate. Two-dimensional (2D) aortic measurements are preferable to M-mode owing to cyclic motion of the heart and changes in M-mode cursor location. Standard measurement conventions established the leading edge-to-leading edge diameter in end diastole,[5] and the normative data published in the literature were obtained using the leading edge technique.[6,7] Some experts[8,9] favour inner edge-to-inner edge diameter measurements to increase reproducibility and match those obtained by other methods of imaging the aorta, such as cardiac magnetic resonance (CMR) and computed tomography (CT) scanning. However, recent improvements in echocardiographic image quality and resolution minimize the differences between these measurement methods. Aortic annular diameter is measured between the hinge points of the AoV leaflets (inner edge-inner edge) in the left PLAX view, during systole, which reveal the largest aortic annular diameter. In a normal ascending aorta, the diameter at sinus level is the largest, followed by the sinotubular junction and the aortic annulus. If aortic dilation is detected at any level, its maximum diameter should be measured and reported (◆ Fig. 21.4).

Aorta size is related most strongly to BSA and age.[6,7] Therefore, BSA may be used to predict aortic root diameter in

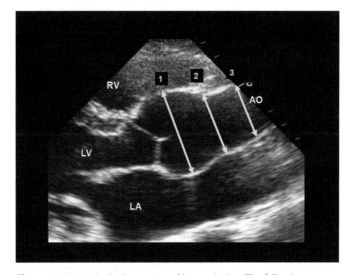

Figure 21.4 Aortic size in parasternal long-axis view. The following diameters are shown: sinuses of Valsalva (1), sinotubular junction (2), and tubular ascending aorta (3).

several age intervals. Roman et al.[6] considered three age strata. These normal values have been accepted to date as the reference values. In adults, a diameter of 2.1cm/m^2 has been considered the upper normal range in ascending aorta.[10] TTE suffices to quantify maximum aortic root and proximal ascending aorta diameters when the acoustic window is adequate. Nevertheless, the technique is more limited for measuring the remaining aortic segments. TOE overcomes part of these TTE limitations by affording better measurement of aortic arch and descending thoracic aorta size. TOE may make oblique measurements when the descending aorta is elongated or tortuous.

Measurements of descending thoracic aorta in short axis and of the aortic arch in long axis are recommended.

Assessment of aortic biophysical properties

Assessment of aortic biophysical properties includes:

- **Distensibility** This is evaluated by aortic pressure-dimensions relationship. Changes in arterial diameter can be measured at the level of ascending aorta, approximately 3cm above the AoV in 2D guided M-mode of PLAX view, with the diastolic aortic diameter measured at the peak of the QRS complex (AoD) and systolic aortic diameter (AoS) measured at the maximal anterior motion of the aorta and the pulse pressure (PP) measured at the right arm by cuff sphygmomanometer as the difference between systolic and diastolic arterial pressure.

$$\text{Distensibility} = [2(AoS - AoD)/AoD] \, PP \qquad (21.1)$$

- **Arterial stiffness** Aorta stiffness may be assessed by pulsed-wave velocity (PWV), defined as the travel speed throughout the aorta of the pulsed wave of aorta flow. Normal PWV values increase from 4–5m/s in the ascending aorta to 5–6m/s in the abdominal aorta.[11]

Aortic atherosclerosis

Atheroma prevalence increases with age, smoking, and pulse pressure. In patients with known significant carotid artery disease, the prevalence of aortic atheromas was 92% in those with significant coronary artery disease. Aortic atheroma is a major factor in determining outcome. The risk of stroke has been shown to be significantly higher in patients with atherosclerotic disease of the aorta. The appearance of aortic atheroma may be variable, and this in turn may be related to its prognostic impact.

Aortic atheromas are characterized by irregular intimal thickening of at least 2mm, with increased echogenicity. They often have superimposed mobile components, mainly thrombi. TOE is the imaging modality of choice for diagnosing aortic atheromas. It provides higher-resolution images than TTE and has good interobserver reproducibility.[12,13] However, suprasternal harmonic imaging by TTE also permits the visualization of protruding arch atheromas in many cases.[14] TOE imaging may identify atheroma as bright spots due either to the thickness of the plaque or to calcification. Plaque thickness should be measured from the intimal surface perpendicularly to the outer edge of the vessel wall. Atheroma may be stratified by five grades, starting at normal and progressing to simple intimal thickening, then sessile atheroma (attached throughout its base, not mobile and not attached by a *stalk*) of varying thickness, to protruding atheroma with mobile elements visible (◆ Table 21.1).

Table 21.1 Grading the severity of atheroma

Grade	Severity	Description
1	Normal	No intimal thickening
2	Mild	Intimal thickening ≥ 3mm without irregularities
3	Moderate	Sessile atheroma < 5mm
4	Severe	Sessile atheroma ≥ 5mm
5	Severe	Atheroma with mobile components or ulceration

Atherosclerotic plaques are defined as *complex* in the presence of protruding atheromas of more than 4mm in thickness, mobile debris, or presence of plaque ulceration, and defined as *simple* if the plaques lack these morphological features[15] (◆ Fig. 21.5; ◼ 21.1)

Large mobile aortic thrombi are possible causes of systemic emboli[16] and appear to be a complication of atherosclerosis. TOE is the best technique for diagnosing and monitoring the evolution of these large thrombi. Another echocardiographic modality is intraoperative epi-aortic ultrasound which facilitates the selection of a suitable aortic clamping site by avoiding calcifications with an increased risk of embolization (◆ Fig. 21.6; ◼ 21.2).

Aortic aneurysm

The aetiology of a true aortic aneurysm has much in common with aortic dissection. Atherosclerosis, often associated with hypertension and aging, and connective tissue and inflammatory conditions have all been implicated. Coarctation and bicuspid AoV are recognized as associated conditions. Aortic aneurysm in patients with Marfan syndrome frequently has a characteristic appearance of a widely dilated aortic root and tapering aneurismal dilation of the ascending aorta—the so-called *inverted pear* appearance.

TTE is an excellent modality for imaging aortic root dilation,[6,8,9] which is important for patients with annuloaortic ectasia, Marfan syndrome, or bicuspid AoV. Since the predominant sites of dilation area is the proximal aorta, TTE often suffices for screening (◆ Fig. 21.7A). In ascending aorta dilation, TOE may provide better visualization of the upper part of sinotubular junction (◆ Fig. 21.7B).

Some echocardiographic features play an important role in the assessment of the mechanisms of functional AR. Functional classification of aortic root abnormalities responsible for aortic insufficiency has been suggested.[17,18] This classification is based on assessment of leaflet function and aortic root size and provides important information for surgical management strategies.

TOE is clearly superior to TTE for assessing aneurysms located in the aortic arch and descending thoracic aorta (◆ Fig. 21.7C). In proximal aneurysms involving the aortic root, the diameter

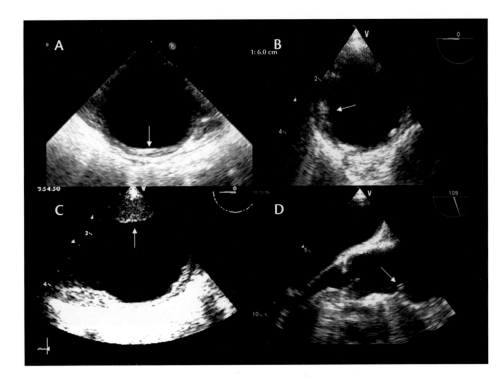

Figure 21.5 Aortic atherosclerosis. TOE showing different aortic atherosclerosis severity. A) Minimal thickening of atherosclerosis. B) Atherosclerosis with thickening of 5mm. C) Atheroma of 9mm and D) mobile atheroma in ascending aorta (arrow).

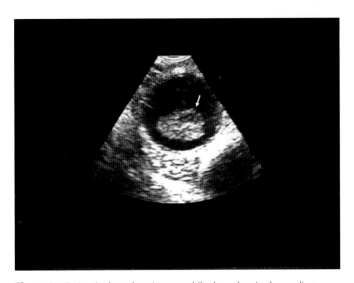

Figure 21.6 Aortic thrombus. Large mobile thrombus in descending thoracic aorta visualized by TOE in a patient with acute leg ischemia secondary to right femoral embolism.

of the aortic annulus, sinuses of Valsalva, and sinotubular junction should be assessed from the mid-oesophageal aortic long axis view, and the short-axis view may also be useful if there is annular dilation and regurgitation. However, TOE is limited in tortuous aortas since in these cases the aorta may be separated from the oesophagus, resulting in inability to image these aorta segments. Assessment and follow-up of descending aorta and arch aneurysm usually require other imaging techniques, such as CT or CMR, with greater field of view and measurement reproducibility.

Although TTE transducers are not optimal for assessing the abdominal aorta, the segment of the aorta between the coeliac trunk and renal arteries is frequently well visualized. The presence of abdominal aorta aneurysms in patients with atherosclerosis or aortic diseases is not uncommon and assessment of the abdominal aorta may be useful (➲ Fig. 21.7D).

Sinus of Valsalva aneurysms

Sinus of Valsalva aneurysms can consist in congenital abnormalities or occur after an acute infection (usually endocarditis) or inflammatory process. On both TTE and TOE, they appear as dilated and distorted sinuses in PLAX and parasternal short-axis (PSAX) view at the aortic valve level. Congenital forms have a *wind sock* shape, as an irregular mass protruding from aortic sinuses into adjacent cardiac chamber: specifically, an aneurysm of the right coronary sinus protrudes into the right ventricular (RV) outflow tract, while the left coronary sinus protrudes into the left atrium (LA) and non-coronary sinus into the right atrium (RA). Often, they can be fenestrated, particularly when an infective process damages a congenital sinus of Valsalva aneurysm: Doppler examination by continuous wave (CW), pulsed wave (PW) Doppler and colour Doppler (CD) show passage of blood flow from a high-pressure cavity, such as aortic root, to an adjacent low-pressure chamber. In Marfan syndrome, sinus of Valsalva aneurysms may involve all three aortic sinuses and appear rounded: in these patients, replacement of ascending aorta and aortic root with reimplantation of coronary arteries is performed.

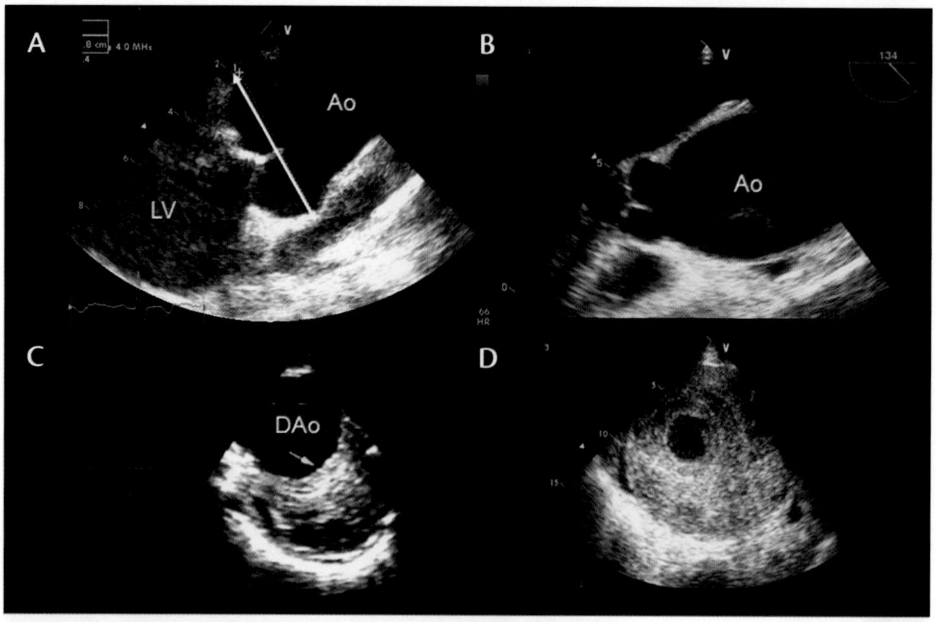

Figure 21.7 Anuloaortic ectasia. A) Parasternal long-axis view by TTE showing annuloaortic ectasia with typical pyriform morphology. Arrows show maximum aortic diameter. B) Ascending aorta aneurysm located in the upper part of the sinotubular junction on TOE in long-axis view. C) Thrombosed saccular aneurysm located in aortic arch on TOE by longitudinal-axis view. D) Abdominal view showing a large abdominal aneurysm (10cm) with massive circular thrombosis.

Acute aortic syndrome

Acute aortic syndrome has a high mortality rate and early medical and surgical treatment is crucial. Therefore, rapid and accurate diagnostic techniques, which can be applied in critically-ill patients, are essential. The diagnosis of acute aortic syndrome can be made with similar accuracy using different imaging techniques.[19]

However, the decision to use a specific technique depends on two major factors:

♦ Availability of the techniques.

♦ Experience of the imaging staff.

Echocardiography has the advantage of being applicable in any hospital setting (emergency, intensive care, operating theatre), without the need to transfer the patient who is often in an unstable haemodynamic situation, monitored, and with intravenous drugs.

Diagnosis of aortic dissection

Aortic dissection is a surgical emergency. Patients may present with a variety of features but severe chest pain is usually a symptom. Back pain may also be present. Involvement of the innominate and/or carotid arteries may lead to focal neurological signs which may be transient or permanent. Loss of consciousness is not uncommon. Involvement of the aortic valve may produce severe aortic regurgitation, and rupture at the level of the sinuses of Valsalva will produce cardiac tamponade; compression or hypo-perfusion of the coronary arteries may lead to myocardial ischaemia. The dissection occurs as an initial tear in the aortic intima, which may penetrate the partial or full circumference of the aorta, in the latter case leading to a

double-barrelled aorta. This may rarely lead to intussusception of the intimal flap into the vessel lumen. If the adventitia, is breached, then massive blood loss may occur causing sudden cardiac tamponade if the tear is proximal, or hypotension and massive blood loss if the tear occurs more distally, i.e. outside the pericardiac sac, which extends to approximately the first 4cm of the ascending aorta. Diseases which cause degradation of the aortic media will be important causative factors. Age, systemic hypertension and atherosclerosis may be contributory. Aortic dissection usually occurs within 10cm of the aortic valve or immediately distal to the left subclavian artery, associated with the high shearing forces in these areas. However, in fact the dissection may occur anywhere in the aorta.

Different classifications of aortic dissection are shown in ➲ Fig. 21.8. The most commonly used is the Stanford classification, especially since this is easily associated with surgical decision making. Aortic dissection and its variants[20] can be correctly diagnosed by echocardiography. The sensitivity of TOE has been shown to be significantly greater than angiography. Whilst CMR has been shown to have greatest sensitivity and specificity for diagnosis, the test itself is time-consuming particularly for an ill patient and may not be available in the referring community or general hospital. However, contrast-enhanced CT particularly using a 64-slice machine or greater, will be able to demonstrate an aortic dissection almost as effectively as CMR and is an investigation that is more commonly available and perhaps more appropriate also in the emergency setting. A useful management protocol is to perform contrast-enhanced CT either at the referring hospital or at the surgical unit to establish the presence and extent of the vascular dissection, followed by TOE to assess the involvement of the AoV. In these circumstances, TOE is undertaken with the patient anaesthetized and immediately before surgery in order to prevent a

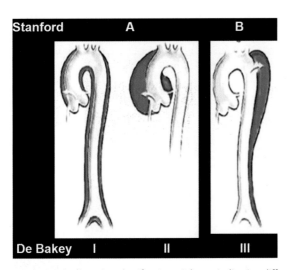

Figure 21.8 Aortic dissection classifications. Schema indicating different types of aortic dissections, according to two commonly used classifications:

De Bakey classification:
 I. Involving the ascending and descending aorta and the arch (60%);
 II. Involving the ascending aorta but not descending aorta (10%);
 III. Involving only the descending aorta (30%).
Stanford classification:
 A. De Bakey types I and II: involves the ascending aorta;
 B. De Bakey type III: involves the descending aortav

potentially dangerous burst of hypertension developing during the passage of the probe. The surgical team thence has TOE images available in real time.

The echocardiographic diagnosis of classical aortic dissection is based on the demonstration of the presence of an intimal flap that divides the aorta into two, true and false, lumina (➲ Fig. 21.9A). In most cases, false lumen flow is detectable by CD but may be absent in totally thrombosed and retrograde dissections[21] (➲ Fig. 21.9B, ◳ 21.3 and 21.4)

Intramural haematoma is characterized by circular or crescentic thickening of the aortic wall more than 5mm (➲ Fig. 21.10), and *penetrating aortic ulcer* presents as an image of crater-like outpouching with jagged edges in the aortic wall, generally associated with extensive aortic atheromas (➲ Fig. 21.11).

Transthoracic echocardiography

Classically, TTE has been considered limited in the diagnosis of aortic dissection. However, harmonic imaging and the use of contrast enhancement have been shown to improve the sensitivity and specificity of TTE in the diagnosis of aortic dissection[22] (➲ Figs. 21.12 and 21.13; ◳ 21.5 and 21.6)

Contrast TTE has similar accuracy to TOE in the diagnosis of type A aortic dissection (sensitivity 93% and specificity 97%), although it is more limited in type B involvement (sensitivity 84% and specificity 94%), mainly in the presence of non-extended dissection, intramural haematoma and aortic ulcers.[22] However, given its availability, rapidity, and additional information on cardiac status, TTE may be used as the initial imaging modality when aortic dissection is clinically suspected in the emergency room.[23] The low negative predictive value of TTE does not permit dissection to be ruled out, and further tests will be required if the TTE exam is negative (➲ Fig. 21.14; ◳ 21.7 and 21.8)

Transoesophageal echocardiography

Several studies have demonstrated the accuracy of TOE in the diagnosis of aortic dissection with sensitivity of 86–100%, specificity 90–100%, and negative predictive value 86–100%.[21,22,24–26] The low specificity of the technique described in some series[24] is explained by the fact that the majority of intraluminal images in the ascending aorta were considered diagnostic of dissected intima. In the ascending aorta, particularly when dilated, linear reverberation images are very common.[25] Assessment of location and movement of these intraluminal images by M-mode echocardiography is the best way to differentiate between intimal flap and imaging reverberations (➲ Fig. 21.15; ◳ 21.9 and 21.10)

TOE is clearly superior to TTE in the diagnosis of intramural haematoma and aortic ulcers. TOE is semi-invasive, requires sedation and may cause a rise in systemic blood pressure from retching and gagging. Therefore, adequate sedation with strict blood pressure control is mandatory. When therapeutic decision-making is definitive by other techniques, TOE should be performed in the operating room before surgery or when the

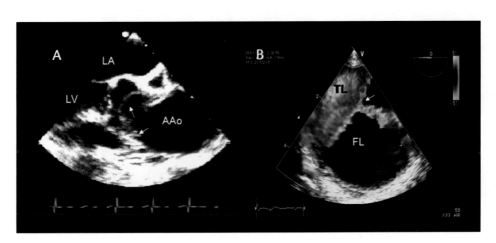

Figure 21.9 TOE in aortic dissection. A) Ascending aorta dissection by long-axis view. Arrows show the intimal flap. B) Descending thoracic aorta dissection by transverse view. Arrow shows a jet from true lumen to false lumen owing to the presence of a secondary communication.

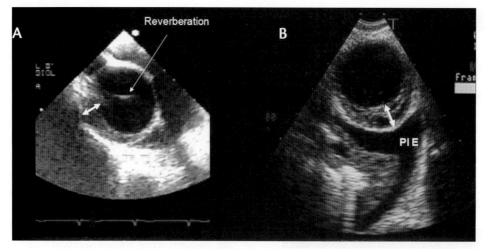

Figure 21.10 Intramural haematoma. TOE. A) Crescentic intramural haematoma in ascending aorta (double-head arrow). A reverberation from the posterior aorta wall is observed in ascending aorta lumen. (arrow). B) Intramural haematoma in descending aorta (double-head arrow) and left pleural effusion. Pl E, pleural effusion.

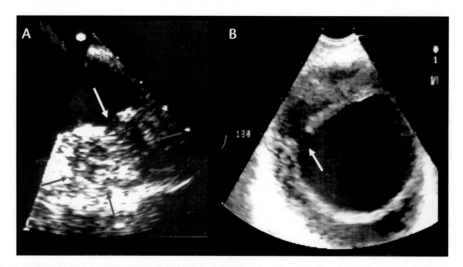

Figure 21.11 Aortic ulcers by TOE. A) Penetrating atherosclerotic ulcer deforming the adventitia (large arrow) surrounded by intramural haematoma (small arrows). B) Ulcer-like image secondary to localized dissection in intramural haematoma evolution.

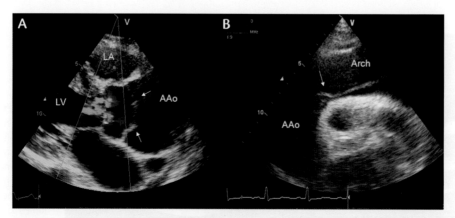

Figure 21.12 Aortic dissection diagnosis by TTE with harmonic imaging. Intimal flap (arrows) and two lumina are visualized in: A) aortic root; B) distal ascending aorta and aortic arch.

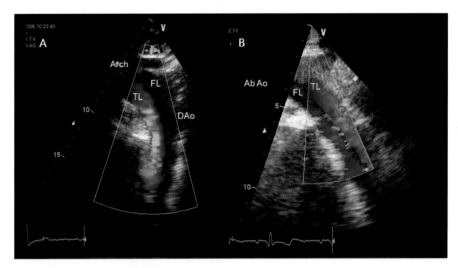

Figure 21.13 Descending aorta dissection. A) Suprasternal long-axis view showing a descending thoracic aorta dissection. Colour Doppler helps to identify true lumen flow (blue colour). B) Subcostal long-axis view showing abdominal aorta dissection.

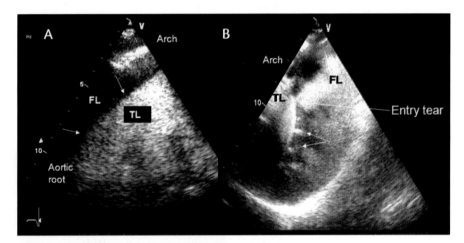

Figure 21.14 Contrast-enhanced transthoracic echocardiography. A) Upper right parasternal view showing intimal flap (arrow) and the different density of contrast in true lumen (TL) and false lumen (FL). B) Suprasternal view in type B dissection: the entry tear is located in the upper part of descending aorta (arrow) and secondary tears are visualized (small arrows). Absence of contrast in the proximal part of the false lumen indicates that no other proximal tear is present.

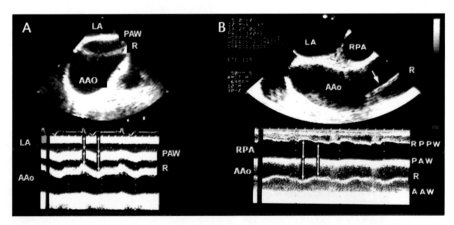

Figure 21.15 Reverberation mimicking intimal flap. TOE showing reverberations mimicking intimal flap in ascending aorta: A) Reverberation in aortic root (yellow arrow) by transverse view. M-mode image shows the reverberation (yellow arrow) located at twice the distance from the transducer as from the posterior aortic wall (red arrow) and with twice the amplitude of displacement. B) Reverberation in the middle third of ascending aorta by longitudinal view. M-mode: the reverberation (yellow arrow) is located at twice the distance from the right pulmonary artery posterior wall (red arrow) as from the posterior aortic wall. Reverberation movement is inverse to that of the pulmonary artery wall.

patient is in stable haemodynamic conditions with no chest pain. Given its accuracy in the diagnosis of aortic dissection, intramural haematoma, and aortic ulcers, TOE is a technique of choice in acute aortic syndrome diagnosis when an expert echocardiographer is available.

Assessment of morphological and haemodynamic findings in aortic dissection

TOE permits assessment of the main anatomical and functional aspects of interest for the management of aortic dissection.

Intimal tear

The intimal tear appears as a discontinuity of the intimal flap. TOE provides a direct image of the tear and permits its measurement. TOE permits identification of the tear in 78–100% of cases.[27] CD can reveal the presence of multiple small communications between the two lumina, especially in descending aorta (→ Fig. 21.16). Anatomical controls showed that most of these communications might correspond to the origin of intercostal or visceral arteries. It is important to differentiate these secondary communications from the main intimal tear which usually has a diameter over 5mm and is frequently located in the proximal part of the ascending aorta in type A dissections and immediately below the origin of the left subclavian artery in type B dissections. Three-dimensional (3D) TOE may be highly useful in entry tear size measurement particularly when entry tear is not circular (→ Fig. 21.17; ▪ 21.11). On occasions, 2D or 3D TOE does not permit visualization of the intimal tear in the proximal part of the arch. In these cases, contrast echocardiography may help by showing how contrast flows in the false lumen from the more proximal part of the aortic arch dissection.[22]

True lumen identification

Identification of the true lumen is of special clinical interest. When the aortic arch is involved, the surgeon needs to know whether the supra-aortic vessels originate from the false lumen. Similarly, when the descending aorta dissection affects visceral arteries and ischaemic complications arise, it may be important to identify the false lumen prior to surgery or endovascular

treatment such as intima fenestration or graft stent implantation.

Echocardiographic signs for differentiating the true lumen from the false lumen are (→ Fig. 21.18):

- True lumen systolic expansion by M-mode
- Early and fast flow of true lumen assessed by CD or contrast echo.

Diagnosis of aortic dissection complications

Appropriate diagnosis of dissection complications during the initial study may affect therapeutic decisions in the acute phase:

Pericardial effusion and periaortic bleeding

Pericardial effusion is not always due to extravasation of blood from the aorta and may be secondary to irritation of the adventitia produced by the aortic haematoma or small effusion from the wall. In any event, the presence of pericardial effusion in an ascending aorta dissection is an indicator of poor prognosis and suggests rupture of the false lumen in the pericardium (→ Fig. 21.19A). Echocardiography is the best diagnostic technique for estimating the presence and severity of tamponade. Periaortic haematoma and pleural effusion may be visualized by TOE but are best diagnosed by CT.

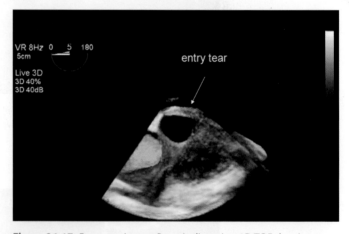

Figure 21.17 Entry tear in type B aortic dissection. 3D TOE showing a large entry tear in type B aortic dissection

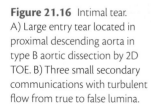

Figure 21.16 Intimal tear. A) Large entry tear located in proximal descending aorta in type B aortic dissection by 2D TOE. B) Three small secondary communications with turbulent flow from true to false lumina.

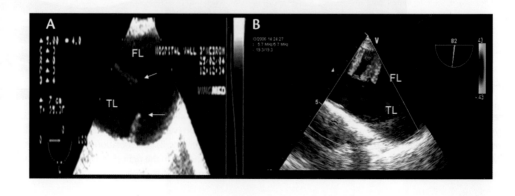

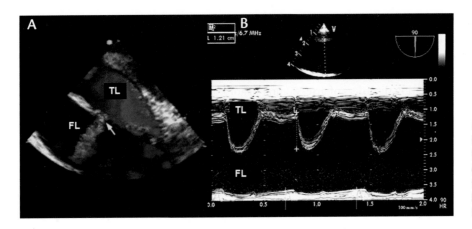

Figure 21.18 True lumen identification. A) Colour Doppler helps to identify the true lumen (TL); arrow shows secondary tear flow from true lumen to false lumen. B) True lumen is identified by systolic expansion in M-mode.

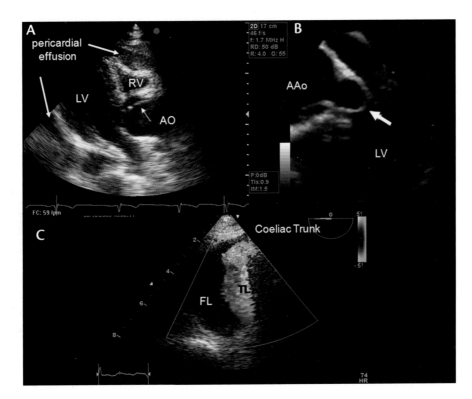

Figure 21.19 Aortic dissection complications. A) Case of type A dissection (arrow) with pericardial tamponade (large arrows) with right ventricle compression. B) TOE shows prolapse of the intima in left ventricular outflow tract to be the aetiology of severe aortic regurgitation. C) Coeliac trunk dissection visualized by colour TOE in transversal view.

Aortic regurgitation

AR is a frequent complication, occurring in approximately 40–76% of patients. The diagnosis andp quantification of AR severity can be correctly made with Doppler echocardiography, both TTE and TOE.

Furthermore, TOE provides information on possible mechanisms that influence AR, which may greatly aid the surgeon in deciding whether to replace the AoV[27] (➲ Fig. 21.19B):

◆ Dilation of the aortic annular support.

◆ Rupture of the aortic annular support.

◆ Asymmetrical displacement of sigmoid coaptation level.

◆ Prolapse of the intima through the AoV.

Arterial vessel involvement

Diagnosis of involvement of the main arterial vessels of the aorta is important as it may explain some of the symptoms or visceral complications that accompany the dissection and permit selection of an appropriate therapeutic strategy. TOE shows the most proximal segment of the coronary arteries; thus, it can be verified whether the coronary ostium originates in the false lumen or whether coronary dissection is present. TOE is not a good technique for assessing supra-aortic branch involvement, although the origin of the left subclavian artery is easily observed. TOE permits the diagnosis of coeliac trunk involvement, dissection or compression in most cases (➲ Fig. 21.19C).

Visceral or peripheral malperfusion syndrome is a complication with high morbidity and mortality.

TOE can diagnose two types of circulation disorders of arterial branches:

◆ Dissection.

◆ Dynamic obstruction of the ostium of the arterial branches leaving the aorta by intimal dissection.

Differentiating the two mechanisms has important therapeutic implications.[4]

Aortic rupture

Aortic rupture represents one of the most important life-threatening conditions which usually occur at the level of aortic isthmus as consequence of trauma, particularly deceleration injury during motor vehicle accident. Indeed, up to 15% of deaths following motor vehicle collisions are due to complete aortic transection. Although all segments of thoracic aorta can be affected by a blunt injury, the proximal thoracic aorta is frequently interested because the relatively mobile aortic arch usually moves against the descending aorta which is fixed by ligamentum arteriosum. Patients who survive up to the emergency department usually show an aortic pseudoaneurysm.

Prompted diagnosis, achieved by TOE, aortography, CT or CMR, and surgical treatment are required to save patient life. Because of its capability to visualize entire thoracic aorta, TOE may initially be performed, without complications, in all patients with suspected aortic rupture to confirm diagnosis; aortography should represent the second procedure of choice if TOE is not diagnostic. Correct diagnosis requires differentiation of aortic rupture from other conditions that may mimic its echocardiographic findings: aortic debris or atheromatous plaque.

Pseudoaneurysms resulting from trauma or infections develop by leakage of blood throughout an aortic wall tear or perforation into a contained aneurysmal cavity. Contrary to true aneurysms, aortic pseudoaneurysm are characterized by a visible rupture site of aortic wall, where lumen communicates with pseudoaneurysm cavity. In order to avoid rupture, pseudoaneurysm repair is strongly recommended.

Prognosis and follow-up

Prognostic and therapeutic implications of TOE in aortic dissection are well established. Antegrade or retrograde false lumen flow, false lumen thrombosis and the presence of communications have prognostic implications and are easily detected by TOE.[27] TOE has an important role in the follow-up of patients with aortic dissection as it shows the structure of the dissection, surgical repair, healing of the dissection and obliteration of the false lumen, or blood flow dynamics in true and false lumina.

The intramural haematoma can heal or evolve to aneurysm formation or even dissection.[29] In addition to maximum aortic diameter, some TOE information such as echolucent areas has been related to dissection and enlargement evolution. The natural history of penetrating aortic ulcer is unknown. Like intramural haematomas, several evolutive possibilities have been proposed. As in other acute aortic syndromes, ascending aorta involvement carries a higher risk of severe complications than type B involvement.

Intraoperative and postoperative echocardiography

Echocardiography plays a crucial role in the preoperative, intraoperative, and postoperative assessment of aortic diseases. Knowledge of aortic root dimensions, AR severity and its mechanisms would enable preoperative selection of the best surgical strategy and preparation of an adequately-sized graft tube, repair or replacement of AoV and shorten surgical ischaemic time. Previous studies have demonstrated that preoperative measurement of aortic annular diameter by TTE and multiplane TOE is accurate and clinically feasible.[30]

The important role of echocardiography in AoV repair lies in the recognition of the exact lesions that may be responsible for the insufficiency, and the selection of adequate operative manoeuvres to correct these abnormalities. The combination of functional evaluation by TOE and anatomical inspection at surgery is therefore paramount when assessing the suitability of the conditions for repair. By echocardiography, the tethering indices might have the potential to guide the planning of AoV-sparing surgery. Accurate echocardiographic measurements of aortic root diameters are also essential in other types of surgery such as the Ross procedure, homograft aortic valves, or in percutaneous AoV implantation.[31]

Preoperative or intraoperative TOE is essential for planning the surgical treatment of acute aortic syndrome and in deciding whether to replace the AoV,[28] and may help to avoid early reoperations by showing the correct connection of the distal part of the graft tube to the true lumen, arch and supra-aortic vessel involvement and the severity of residual AR. Finally, intraoperative TOE may detect complications such as pseudoaneurysm formation (➲ Fig. 21.20; ◼ 21.12), most of which are secondary to a leak in coronary artery reimplantation to the graft tube, communication of the distal part of the tube to the false lumen, significant AR, periaortic haemorrhage, or segmental abnormalities in LV contraction (➲ Fig. 21.20).

Intraoperative TOE is also highly useful during endovascular therapy, especially in type B aortic dissection. It permits correct guidewire entrance by identifying the true lumen in aortic dissections, provides additional information helpful for guiding correct stent-graft positioning, and identifies suboptimal results and the presence of leaks and/or small re-entry tears, with much higher sensitivity than angiography[32] (➲ Fig. 21.21).

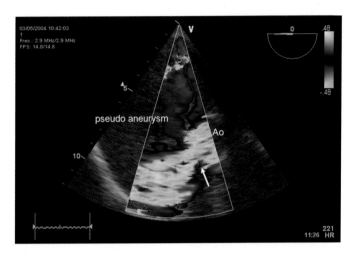

Figure 21.20 Postoperative pseudoaneurysm. Pseudoaneurysm secondary to right coronary ostium reimplantation in a Bentall procedure. Colour Doppler shows the jet flow from the aorta to the pseudoaneurysm cavity.

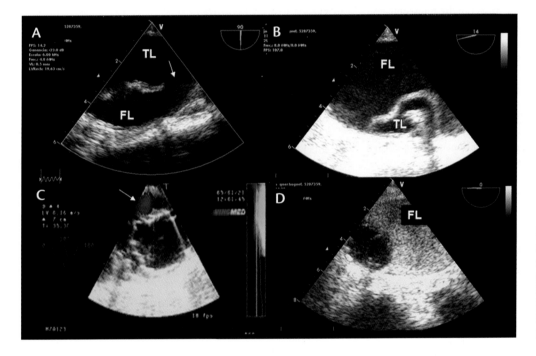

Figure 21.21 Role of TOE in endovascular therapy. A) Entry tear identification. B) Correct guidewire entrance in true lumen. C) Diagnosis of the endovascular leak by colour Doppler (arrow). D) Progressive thrombosis of false lumen.

Personal perspective

Echocardiography is a reference imaging technique in the diagnosis and follow-up of aortic diseases. Its main advantages are that is portable, rapid, and does not require irradiation. Complementary TTE and TOE should be used according to indications. TTE appears to suffice for aortic root assessment and may be useful to establish a rapid diagnosis of aortic dissection, mainly using contrast. TOE is a gold standard in thoracic aorta assessment. It provides excellent morphological information on aortic dissection and is superior to TTE in the diagnosis of intramural haematomas and aortic ulcers. Contrast enhancement substantially improves haemodynamic information of aortic dissection which may improve prognostic assessment and adequate patient management. 3D TOE may be highly useful in entry tear size evaluation and maximum aortic diameter measurement, particularly in tortuous aortas. TOE is also useful in aortic atherosclerosis assessment and should be used in intraoperative monitoring of surgical and endovascular treatment of aortic disease.

References

1 Evangelista A, Flachskampf F, Erbel R, Antonini-Canterin F, Vlachopoulos C, Rocchi G, Sicari R, Nihoyannopoulos P, Zamorano J. Echocardiography in aortic diseases. EAE recommendations for clinical practice. *Eur J Echocardiogr* (in press).

2 Flachskampf FA, Decoodt P, Fraser AG, Daniel WG, Roelandt JR; Subgroup on Transoesophageal Echocardiography and Valvular Heart Disease; Working Group on Echocardiography of the European Society of Cardiology. Guidelines from the Working Group. Recommendations for performing transoesophageal echocardiography. *Eur J Echocardiogr* 2001; **2**:8–21.

3 Orihashi K, Matsuura Y, Sueda T, Watari M, Okada K, Sugawara Y, et al. Aortic arch branches are no longer a blind zone for transesophageal echocardiography: a new eye for aortic surgeons. *J Thorac Cardiovasc Surg* 2000; **120**:466–72.

4 Orihashi K, Sueda T, Okada K, Imai K. Perioperative diagnosis of mesenteric ischemia in acute aortic dissection by transeophageal echocardiography. *Eur J Cardiothorac Surg* 2005; **28**:871–6.

5 Lang R, Bierig M, Devereux R, Flachskampf FA, Foster E, Pellikka P, et al. Recommendations for Chamber Quantification. A report from the American Society of Echocardiography's Nomenclature and Standards Committee, the Task Force on Chamber Quantification, and the European Association of Echocardiography. *Eur J Echocardiogr* 2006; **7**:79–108.

6 Roman MJ, Devereux RB, Kramer-Fox R, O'Loghlin J. Two-dimensional echocardiographic aortic root dimensions in normal children and adults. *Am J Cardiol* 1989; **64**:507–12.

7 Vasan RS, Larson MG, Levy D. Determinants of echocardiographic aortic root size. The Framingham heart study. *Circulation* 1995; **91**:734–40.

8 Brooke BS, Habashi JP, Judge DP, Patel N, Loeys B, Dietz HC 3rd. Angiotensin II blockade and aortic-root dilation in Marfan's syndrome. *N Engl J Med* 2008; **358**:2787–95.

9 Schaefer BM, Lewin MB, Stout KK, Gill E, Prueitt A, Byers PH, et al. The bicuspid aortic valve: an integrated phenotypic classification of leaflet morphology and aortic root shape. *Heart* 2008; **94**:1634–8.

10 Drexler M, Erbel R, Müller U, Wittlich N, Mohr-Kahaly S, Meyer J. Measurement of intracardiac dimensions and structures in normal young adult subjects by transesophageal echocardiography. *Am J Cardiol* 1990; **65**:1491–6.

11 Antonini-Canterin F, Carerj S, Di Bello V, Di Salvo G, La Carrubba S, Vriz O, et al.; Research Group of the Italian Society of Cardiovascular Echography (SIEC). Arterial stiffness and ventricular stiffness: a couple of diseases or a coupling disease? A review from the cardiologist's point of view. *Eur J Echocardiogr* 2009; **10**:36–43.

12 Montgomery DH, Ververis JJ, McGorisk G, Frohwein S, Martin RP, Taylor WR. Natural history of severe atheromatous disease of the thoracic aorta: A transesophageal echocardiographic study. *J Am Coll Cardiol* 1996; **27**:95–101.

13 Zaidat OO, Suarez JI, Hedrick D, Redline S, Schluchter M, Landis DM, et al. Reproducibility of transesophageal echocardiography in evaluating aortic atheroma in stroke patients. *Echocardiography* 2005; **22**:326–30.

14 Schwammenthal E, Schwammenthal Y, Tanne D, Tenenbaum A, Garniek A, Motro M, et al. Transcutaneous detection of aortic arch atheromas by suprasternal harmonic imaging. *J Am Coll Cardiol* 2002; **39**:1127–32.

15 The French study of aortic plaques in stroke group: atherosclerotic disease of the aortic arch as a risk factor for recurrent ischemic stroke. *N Engl J Med* 1996; **334**:1216–2170.

16 Avegliano G, Evangelista A, Elorz C, González-Alujas MT, García del Castillo H, Soler-Soler J. Acute peripheral arterial ischemia and suspected aortic dissection. usefulness of transesophageal echocardiography in differential diagnosis with aortic thrombosis. *Am J Cardiol* 2002; **90**:674–7.

17 de Waroux JB, Pouleur AC, Goffinet C, Vancraeynest, Van Dyck M, Robbert A, et al. Functional anatomy of aortic regurgitation. Accuracy, prediction of surgical repairability, and outcome implications of transesophageal echocardiography. *Circulation* 2007; **116**(11 Suppl):I264–9.

18 La Canna G, Maisano F, De Michele L, Grimaldi A, Grassi F, Capritti E, et al. Determinants of the degree of functional aortic regurgitation in patients with anatomically normal aortic valve and ascending thoracic aorta aneurysm. Transesophageal Doppler echocardiography study. *Heart* 2009; **95**:130–6.

19 Shiga T, Wajima Z, Apfel C, Inoue T, Ohe Y. Diagnostic accuracy of transesophageal echocardiography, helical computed tomography and magnetic resonance imaging for suspected thoracic aortic dissection. Systematic review and meta-analysis. *Arch Intern Med* 2006; **166**:1350–6.

20 Erbel R, Alfonso F, Boileau C, Dirsch O, Eber B, Haverich A. Diagnosis and management of aortic dissection. Recommendations of the task force on aortic dissection. European Society of Cardiology. *Eur Heart J* 2001; **22**:1642–81.

21 Erbel R, Engberding R, Daniel W, Roelandt J, Visser C, Rennollet H. Echocardiography in diagnosis of aortic dissection. *Lancet* 1989; **1**:457–61.

22 Evangelista A, Avegliano G, Aguilar R, Cuellar H, Igual A, González-Alujas T, et al. Impact of contrast-enhanced echocardiography on the diagnostic algorithm of acute aortic dissection. *Eur Heart J* 2010; **31**:472–80.

23 Meredith EL, Masani ND. Echocardiography in the emergency assessment of acute aortic syndromes. *Eur J Echocardiogr* 2009; **10**:131–9.

24 Nienaber CA, von Kodolitsch Y, Nicolas V, Siglow V, Piepho A, Brockhoff C, et al. The diagnosis of thoracic aortic dissection by noninvasive imaging procedures. *N Engl J Med* 1993; **328**:1–9.

25 Evangelista A, García-del-Castillo H, González-Alujas T, Domínguez-Oronoz R, Salas A, Permanyer-Miralda G, et al. Diagnosis of ascending aortic dissection by transesophageal echocardiography: utility of M-mode in recognizing artifacts. *J Am Coll Cardiol* 1996; **27**:102–7.

26 Pepi M, Campodonico J, Galli C, Tamborini G, Barbier P, Doria E. Rapid diagnosis and management of thoracic aortic dissection and intramural haematoma: a prospective study of advantages of multiplane vs biplane transoesophageal echocardiography. *Eur J Echocardiogr* 2000; **1**:72–9 89.

27 Erbel R, Oelert H, Meyer J, Puth M, Mohr-Kahaly S, Hausmann D, et al. Effect of medical and surgical therapy on aortic dissection evaluated by transesophageal echocardiography. Implications for prognosis and therapy. *Circulation* 1993; **87**:1604–15.

28 Movsowitz HD, Levine RA, Hilgenberg AD, Isselbacher EM. Transesophageal echocardiography description of the mechanisms of aortic regurgitation in acute type A aortic dissection: Implications for aortic valve repair. *J Am Coll Cardiol* 2000; **36**:884–890.

29 Evangelista A, Domínguez R, Sebastia C, Salas A, Permanyer-Miralda G, Avegliano G. Long-term follow-up of aortic intramural hematoma. Predictors of outcome. *Circulation* 2003; **108**:583–9.

30 Weinert L, Karp R, Vignon P, Bales A, Lang RM. Feasibility of aortic diameter measurement by multiplane transesophageal echocardiography for preoperative selection and prepararation of homograft aortic velves. *J Thorac Cardiovasc Surg* 1996; **112**: 954–61.

31 Moss RR, Ivens E, Pasupati S, Humphries K, Thompson CR, Munt B, et al. Role of echocardiography in percutaneous aortic valve implantation. *J Am Coll Cardiol Imag* 2008; **1**:15–24.

32 Koschyk DH, Nienaber CA, Knap M, Hofmann T, Kodolitsch YV, Skriabina V, et al. How to guide stent-graft implantation in type B aortic dissection? Comparison of angiography, transesophageal echocardiography and intravascular ultrasound. *Circulation* 2005; **112**(9 Suppl):I260–4.

Further reading

Bansal RC, Chandrasekaran K, Ayala K, Smith DC. Frequency and explanation of false negative diagnosis of aortic dissection by aortography and transesophageal echocardiography. *J Am Coll Cardiol* 1995; **25**:1393–401.

Chughtai A, Kazerooni EA. CT and MRI of acute thoracic cardiovascular emergencies. *Crit Care Clin* 2007; **23**:835–53.

Erbel R, Alfonso F, Boileau C, Dirsch O, Eber B, Haverich A, Diagnosis and management of aortic dissection. Recommendations of the task force on aortic dissection. European Society of Cardiology. *Eur Heart J* 2001; **22**:1642–81.

Evangelista A, Flachskampf F, Erbel R, Antonini-Canterin F, Vlachopoulos C, Rocchi G, Sicari R, Nihoyannopoulos P, Zamorano J. Echocardiography in aortic diseases. EAE recommendations for clinical practice. *Eur J Echocardiogr* (in press).

Goldberg SP, Sanders C, Nanda NC, Holman WL. Aortic dissection with intimal intussusception: diagnosis and management. *J Cardiovasc Surg (Torino)* 2000; **41**:613–5.

Kronzon I, Tunick PA. Atheromatous disease of the thoracic aorta: pathologic and clinical implications. *Ann Intern Med* 1997; **126**:629–37.

La Canna G, Maisano F, De Michele L, Grimaldi A, Grassi F, Capritti E et al. Determinants of the degree of functional aortic regurgitation in patients with anatomically normal aortic valve and ascending thoracic aorta aneurysm. Transesophageal Doppler echocardiography study. *Heart* 2009; **95**:130–6.

Nienaber CA, von Kodolitsch Y, Nicolas V et al. The diagnosis of thoracic aortic dissection by noninvasive imaging procedures. *N Engl J Med* 1993; **328**:1–9.

Rocchi G, Lofiego C, Bigini E, Pica T, Lovato L, Parlapiano M, Ferito M, Rapezzi C, Branzi A, Fattori R. Transesophageal echocardiography-guided algorithm for stent-graft implantation in aortic dissection. *J Vasc Surg* 2004; **40**:880–5.

Roman MJ, Devereux RB, Kramer-Fox R, O'Loghlin J. Two-dimensional echocardiographic aortic root dimensions in normal children and adults. Am J Cardiol 1989; **64**:507–12.

Smith AD, Schoenhagen P. CT imaging for acute aortic syndrome. *Cleve Clin J Med* 2008; **75**:7–9.

Additional DVD and online material

- 21.1 TTE. Mobile atheroma in ascending aorta
- 21.2 TOE showing a large mobile thrombus in descending aorta.
- 21.3 Longitudinal view in TOE showing ascending aorta dissection.
- 21.4 Transverse view in TOE showing a type B dissection with secondary communication.
- 21.5 Type A dissection visualized by TTE in left parasternal view.
- 21.6 Type B aortic dissection visualized by TTE in suprasternal view.
- 21.7 Contrast-enhanced TTE in type A aortic dissection.
- 21.8 Contrast-enhanced TTE in type B aortic dissection.
- 21.9 Aortic root reverberation mimicking an intimal flap by TOE in transverse view.
- 21.10 Ascending aorta reverberation mimicking an intimal flap by TOE in longitudinal view.
- 21.11 Large entry tear by TOE in type B aortic dissection.
- 21.12 Large pseudoaneurysm secondary to right coronary ostium reimplantation in a Bentall procedure.

⮌ For additional multimedia materials please visit the online version of the book (http://escecho.oxfordmedicine.com).

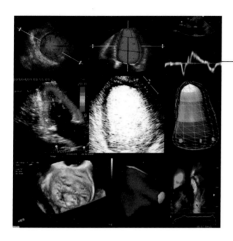

CHAPTER 22

Adult congenital heart disease

G.P. Diller, A. Kempny, and H. Baumgartner

Contents

Summary

The heterogeneity of adult congenital heart disease requires a thorough understanding of cardiac anatomy as well as common surgical and interventional techniques. Echocardiographic studies should be comprehensive and performed in a structured fashion, to avoid missing important anatomical or functional information. The majority of clinical questions can be answered based on the results of echocardiographic studies, but the echocardiographer should be aware of the inherent limitations of the technique and additional image modalities such as cardiac magnetic resonance and computed tomography should be used when appropriate. Assessment of pulmonary artery pressure and pulmonary vascular resistance may be essential and still requires cardiac catheterization.

Introduction

Echocardiography has emerged as the main imaging modality for assessing adults with congenital heart disease. Some lesions such as atrial septal defect (ASD), congenitally corrected transposition of the great arteries (ccTGA), or Ebstein's anomaly may not uncommonly be encountered undiagnosed in adult life. The majority of cardiac defects, however, are diagnosed in infancy and childhood in industrialized countries. Therefore, the adult cardiologist is mainly faced with a patient known to have congenital heart disease. Nevertheless, the diagnosis may, for historical reasons, be incomplete or sometimes incorrect and has to be established in adulthood. Hence, a thorough understanding of cardiac anatomy is required and especially for describing complex malformations a structured approach (sequential segmental analysis) is recommended. In addition, as many patients have undergone surgical or interventional treatment, anatomy and physiology are different from that encountered in paediatric cardiology. Beyond the echocardiographic characteristics, we provide a description of the anatomy and pathophysiology of the most common malformations, reference to further imaging modalities, and highlight information required for clinical decision making based on current European Society of Cardiology guidelines. The orientation of echo images in congenital heart disease is currently controversial. Paediatric echo labs have, in part, moved to an anatomical orientation. When congenital heart disease is practised in the adult setting, conventional image orientation—as is standard in adult echocardiography—is generally used. Due to the wide variety of congenital heart disease and the complexity of its imaging only an overview of the defects most frequently seen in adults can be provided here.

Shunt lesions

Atrial septal defect

ASD represents one of the most common lesions in adult congenital heart disease patients (accounting for approximately 8% of congenital heart defects). Due to a lack in early symptoms and subtlety of physical findings, ASDs are often undiagnosed until adulthood. Depending on the location of the communication between the atria, several types of ASDs can be distinguished.

The secundum ASD is by far the most common type accounting for approximately 80% of ASDs. It is located within the region of the fossa ovalis (⊃ Fig. 22.1). In contrast to a persistent foramen ovale (PFO) with its valve-like morphology, an ASD even if it is small, is always characterized by a deficiency of atrial septal tissue. This distinction between PFO and small ASD may not be clear on transthoracic echocardiography (TTE) and may require transoesophageal echocardiography (TOE).

The primum ASD is located near the crux of the heart and accounts for approximately 15% of ASDs. Anatomically, it belongs to the group of atrioventricular septal defects (AVSD), also called partial AVSD or partial atrioventricular (AV) canal, in which there is fusion between the bridging leaflets of the common AV valve and the crest of the interventricular septum (IVS), as is discussed in detail later.

The sinus venosus defects are located in the region of the mouths of the caval veins. The superior sinus venosus defect is much more common (approximately 5% of ASDs) than the inferior one (<1%) and is typically associated with partial (sometimes complete) connection of right pulmonary veins to the superior caval vein.

The unroofed coronary sinus is a rare form of ASD, characterized by a communication between the coronary sinus and the left atrium (LA). It is almost always associated with a persistent left caval vein draining to the roof of the LA. Most ASDs occur sporadically and the aetiology is likely multifactorial. Secundum ASDs may be associated with the so-called Holt–Oram syndrome (heart–hand syndrome) characterized by skeletal abnormalities of the upper limb (an autosomal dominant disease).[1]

Pathophysiology

ASD typically results in left-to-right shunting with the extent depending on right ventricular (RV) or left ventricular (LV) compliance, defect size, and LA or right atrial (RA) pressure. In a simple ASD, the left-to-right shunt is primarily due to the higher compliance of the RV compared to the LV. Relevant shunt generally occurs with defect sizes greater than or equal to 10mm. RV volume overload and pulmonary overcirculation are the consequences. Reduction in LV compliance or any condition with elevation of LA pressure (hypertension, ischaemic heart disease, cardiomyopathy, aortic and mitral valve disease) increases the left-to-right shunt. Reduced RV compliance (pulmonary stenosis [PS], pulmonary arterial hypertension [PAH], other RV disease) or tricuspid valve (TV) disease may decrease left-to-right shunt or eventually cause shunt reversal resulting in cyanosis. With advancing age, LV compliance decreases and shunt volume increases. Clinically, the majority of patients with a secundum ASD present in their 40s or 50s with increasing exercise intolerance, shortness of breath, atrial fibrillation, or right heart failure (HF).[2] Although pulmonary artery pressure (PAP) may be normal, some degree of pulmonary hypertension is expected due to increased pulmonary blood flow. Severe pulmonary vascular disease is rare and Eisenmenger syndrome occurs in less than 5% of patients (arguably those with a coexisting genetic predisposition). In addition to supraventricular arrhythmias and right HF, ASDs may cause paradoxical embolism.

Echocardiographic assessment

Current guidelines highlight the central role of echocardiography in establishing the diagnosis and the haemodynamic relevance of the defect. Shunting at the atrial level should be suspected in the presence of unexplained RV dilation (⊃ Fig. 22.2 and Fig. 22.3). Direct defect visualization should be attempted from a parasternal short-axis (PSAX) view, a modified apical four-chamber (A4C) view (with the probe displaced medially and tilted to align the atrial septum at an angle with the ultrasound beam), and a subcostal view. A suspected defect should be confirmed with colour Doppler (CD) echocardiography, as small signal drop-outs can represent artefacts (especially if atrial septum and ultrasound

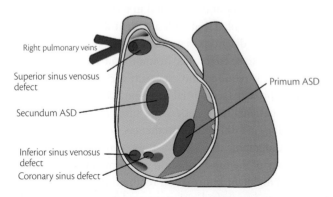

Figure 22.1 Diagram illustrating different types of atrial septal defects (ASD). Note that sinus venosus defects are located posterior close to the mouth of the superior or inferior caval vein, while primum ASDs (partial AVSD) are located at the bottom of the atrial septum in the area of the atrioventricular valves.

Right pulmonary veins

Superior sinus venosus defect

Secundum ASD

Inferior sinus venosus defect

Coronary sinus defect

Primum ASD

beam are in parallel). In some patients the defect cannot be visualized by TTE (especially in the setting of sinus venosus defects) and TOE should be performed. TOE allows for improved visualization of the atrial septum (especially useful if interventional ASD closure is contemplated) and assessment of pulmonary venous return (anomalous pulmonary venous drainage is common in the setting of sinus venosus defects). TOE is superior to TTE with respect to measurement of defect size, assessment of residual septum morphology, and rim size. The defect should not be assumed to be circular and measurement from different views is recommended. Three-dimensional (3D) echocardiography allows appreciation the defect's shape. Shunt ratio calculations can be attempted from the time-velocity integral of pulmonary and aortic flow and the according cross-sectional flow areas (➲ Fig. 22.2; ➲ Chapter 5, Equations 5.23 and 5.24), but accuracy is hampered by measurement errors, particularly of the pulmonary dimension. Assessment of the RV volume overload (enlargement of the RV with normal or hyperdynamic function) is preferred to estimate the haemodynamic relevance of an ASD. PAP should be estimated from the tricuspid regurgitation (TR) velocity. In the elderly, prior to ASD closure, particular attention should be paid to the LV systolic and diastolic function. Examples are shown in ➲ Figs. 22.3 and 22.4.

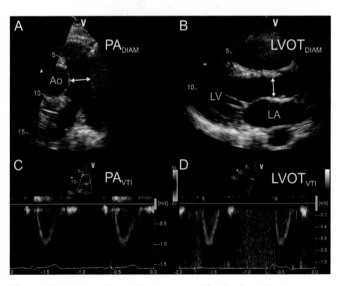

Figure 22.2 Echocardiographic shunt quantification by estimating pulmonary to systemic flow ratio (Qp/Qs). Pulmonary (Qp) and systemic (Qs) blood flow equal the product of stroke volume and heart rate. Stroke volume, in turn, can be calculated as the product of the time velocity integral across the right and left ventricular outflow tract (here demonstrated at the level of the pulmonary artery and left ventricular outflow tract) and the cross-sectional area ([diameter/2]$^2 \times \pi$) at the site of velocity measurement (see ➲ Chapter 5, 'Study of valvular stenosis'). The main limitation of this method is inaccurate measurement of the outflow tract and PA diameter. This measurement error is subsequently squared and leads to incorrect Qp/Qs estimates. If this method is used, the results should be checked for plausibility (signs of RV volume overload and increase of flow in the PA). LVOT, left ventricular outflow tract; PA, pulmonary artery, VTI, velocity time integral.

Echocardiography and treatment decision

Current guidelines recommend ASD closure in patients with a significant shunt defined by signs of RV volume overload irrespective of symptoms. Thus, the decision is generally based on echocardiographic assessment. However, in the few patients in whom echo detects high PAP (>50% of systemic pressure) cardiac catheterization with pulmonary vascular resistance calculation is indispensable for further decision making. If resistance exceeds 5 Wood units (but less than two-thirds of systemic vascular resistance), closure should only be performed if vasoreactivity can be demonstrated after vasodilator challenge or with specific pulmonary hypertension therapy. According to current guidelines ASD closure is also reasonable in patients with previous paradoxical embolism. In the current era, secundum ASDs are generally closed interventionally if TOE demonstrates suitability (ASD with stretched diameter below 38mm and adequate rim of approximately 5mm, although no such rim may be required towards the aorta). TOE and intracardiac echocardiography (ICE) are also particularly helpful for monitoring the catheter intervention. Interventional closure is not an option for patients with sinus venosus or primum ASD (AVSD) and these patients must be referred for surgical closure.

Ventricular septal defect

VSD represents the most common congenital cardiac malformation (accounting for approximately 30% of congenital heart defects). It may be isolated or associated with other conditions, such as tetralogy of Fallot (see later).

Depending on the location of the defect within the IVS (➲ Fig. 22.5) and the relationship to the so-called membranous septum, VSDs are classified as:

◆ Perimembranous defects (also named *paramembranous* or *conoventricular* VSDs).

◆ Muscular defects.

◆ Doubly committed VSD (also called supracristal, subarterial, conal, or infundibular VSD).

Perimembranous defects border the membranous septum (hence the name) and represent the most common form of VSD (accounting for approximately 80% of defects). The membranous septum forms part of the fibrous body of the heart and borders, both the aortic valve (AoV) and the TV. Perimembranous VSDs, thus, are subaortic and subtriscupid and characterized by fibrous continuity between the AoV and the TV. The defect, however, can extend into the inlet or outlet part of the IVS.

Muscular VSDs account for approximately 15–20% of VSDs and are completely surrounded by ventricular musculature. They can occur within the inlet, apical (trabecular), or outlet portion of the RV. Muscular VSDs can be multiple and if present in large numbers produce the so-called *Swiss-cheese septum.*

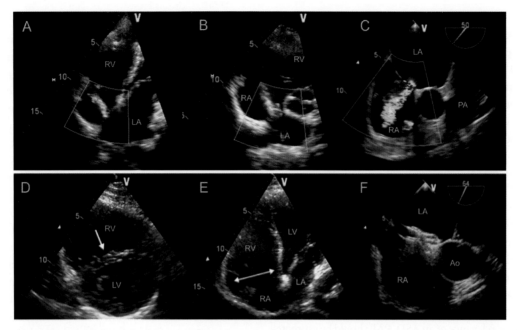

Figure 22.3 Secundum atrial septal defect. Colour Doppler echocardiography showing a secundum ASD with a diameter of approximately 10mm. A) and B) Apical four-chamber view and parasternal short-axis view on TTE. C) Short axis view on TOE. D) and E) Dilation of the RV as illustrated on a short-axis and apical four-chamber view is a hallmark of a haemodynamically relevant interatrial communication and should prompt the search for an ASD. (D) This also illustrates a flattened interventricular septum ('D-sign') in addition to RV enlargement. F) Short-axis view on TOE after closure with an Amplatzer ASD occluder (corresponds to C). Ao, aorta; LA, left atrium; LV, left ventricle; PA, pulmonary artery; RA, right atrium; RV, right ventricle.

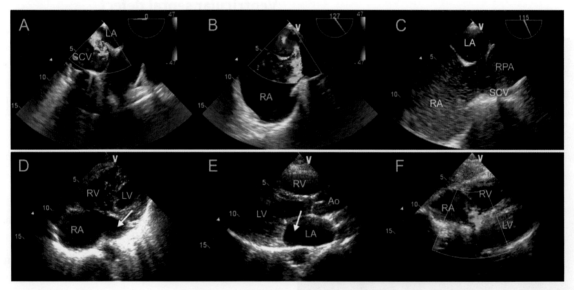

Figure 22.4 Superior sinus venosus and coronary sinus defects. A) Transoesophageal transverse and (B) longitudinal plane (bicaval view) showing a superior sinus venosus defect with left-to-right shunt, evident also as contrast medium washout (C). Coronary sinus defect with a completely unroofed coronary sinus and persistent left superior caval vein draining into the coronary sinus. D) A modified apical four-chamber view demonstrates a severely dilated coronary sinus (24mm). E) The parasternal long-axis view reveals that the coronary sinus is not separated from the left atrium. The arrow points at the absent roof of the coronary sinus. F) Colour Doppler imaging from a subcostal view demonstrates shunting from the left atrium via the coronary sinus into the right atrium. LA, left atrium; RA, right atrium; RPA, right pulmonary artery; SCV, superior caval vein.

Doubly committed VSDs are characterized by fibrous continuity between the AoV and pulmonary valve (PV) and are located directly beneath the semilunar valves. In normal hearts the PV is supported by a sleeve of free-standing infundibular muscle and is located above the level of the other valves. Therefore, such defects can only occur if there is intrinsic malformation of the RV infundibulum. These defects are relatively rare in Europe (only approximately 5% of VSDs) but are reported to be relatively common in southeast Asia (approximately 30% of VSDs). These defects are typically associated with aortic cusp prolapse (usually the right) and aortic regurgitation (AR) which may be progressive. A deficiency of the AV

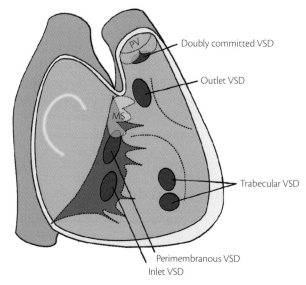

Figure 22.5 Different locations of ventricular septal defects (VSD) as viewed from the right ventricle (see ➲ text). MS; membranous septum; PV; pulmonary valve.

component of the membranous septum, the so-called *Gerbode defect*, is a communication between the LV and RA.

The type of VSD has implications for the cardiac surgeon as the location of the conduction system is different between defects, and muscular defects are more likely to close spontaneously.

AR due to prolapsing of the right or non-coronary cusp of the AoV is a recognized complication of doubly committed VSDs and less common in perimembranous VSDs. A double chambered RV represents a rare complication that may develop over time especially in perimembranous VSDs. In this condition, hypertrophy of muscular bundles divides the ventricle into a high-pressure inflow and low-pressure outflow chamber.

Pathophysiology

The direction and magnitude of the shunt depends on the size of the defect and the pulmonary vascular resistance. Small restrictive VSDs are occasionally associated with endocarditis; however, survival of patients has been demonstrated to be comparable to that of the general population. If not operated upon, patients with a large left-to-right shunt may die of intractable HF early in life. Patients who survive this period gradually become less symptomatic because pulmonary blood flow decreases, a consequence of pulmonary vascular disease that has developed because of excessive pulmonary blood flow and pressure overload. Eventually, Eisenmenger physiology will develop.

Echocardiographic assessment

Except in patients with very limited acoustic windows, TTE almost always permits accurate identification of the defect(s) and the haemodynamic impact. Different planes should be used to image the defect. Useful image planes include the parasternal

long-axis (PLAX) view (for perimembranous defects with outlet extension, muscular and doubly committed VSDs), the PSAX view at LVOT level (perimembranous, outlet and doubly committed VSDs), short-axis planes (muscular VSDs), the A4C view (inlet VSD and muscular VSDs), and A5C view (perimembranous and muscular). In addition, subcostal views may be useful in identifying defects. As illustrated in ➲ Fig. 22.6, perimembranous and outlet including doubly committed VSDs are difficult to distinguish in the PLAX view. However, in the PSAX view, a perimembranous VSD projects to the area of the TV (10 o'clock position), while a doubly committed VSD is located adjacent to the PV (2 o'clock position). Special attention should be given to identify apically located muscular VSDs as these can be difficult to visualize. Indirect (non-specific) signs for the presence of a haemodynamically significant VSD are LV and LA dilation and an elevated RV pressure. As a consequence Doppler peak velocity of tricuspid or pulmonary regurgitation should be recorded in patients with a VSD. The VSD jet may interfere with TR jet and may make it difficult to measure TR velocity. VSD velocity has been proposed for the

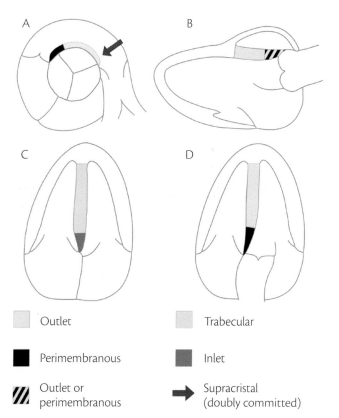

Figure 22.6 Ventricular septal defect. Different segments of the ventricular septum in standard TTE views. Note that both, perimembranous and doubly committed VSDs are seen beneath the aortic valve on a parasternal long-axis view. In a parasternal short-axis view, the perimembranous VSD is located at approximately 10 o'clock in relation to vthe aortic valve in proximity to the tricuspid valve, whereas a doubly committed VSD is seen at approximately 2 o'clock in proximity to the pulmonary valve. A) Parasternal short-axis view. B) Parasternal long-axis view. C) Apical four-chamber view. D) Apical five-chamber view.

estimation of RV pressure by calculating the LV–RV gradient and subtracting it from the systolic systemic pressure. However, VSD velocity often significantly overestimates the LV–RV pressure difference and such calculations may be misleading.

The size of the VSD should be assessed in different planes (as the defect should not be assumed to be circular) on two-dimensional (2D) echocardiography. A high velocity turbulent flow is suggestive of a restrictive VSD and this should be confirmed by continuous wave (CW) Doppler sampling (velocity > 4m/s). In contrast, large non-restrictive VSDs are characterized by laminar or bidirectional flow, with low velocities. Aneurysmatic accessory TV tissue or, rarely, true aneurysms of the ventricular septum may partially or completely cover perimembranous VSDs and flow within this aneurysm may mimic residual VSDs.[3,4] In perimembranous defects and especially doubly committed VSDs, the defect may be partly covered by aortic cusp tissue and this may lead to significant AR. TOE plays a minor role in the assessment of VSDs and may be useful in assessing patients with very poor acoustic windows or to distinguish between a suspected VSD and a ruptured sinus of Valsalva. Examples of VSDs are shown in ⦾ Fig. 22.7.

Echocardiography and treatment decision

Current guidelines recommend VSD closure in patients with significant left-to-right shunt and signs of LV volume overload (with or without symptoms). Patients with progressive AR due to prolapsing of aortic cusps into the defect should be considered

for surgery to prevent a need for AoV replacement. All this information can basically be provided by echo. However, in patients with Doppler-estimated PAP greater than 50% of systemic pressure, invasive assessment of PAP and vascular resistance are indispensable. It has been suggested that patients with VSD and established pulmonary hypertension should be considered for closure if there is preserved net left-to-right shunting and pulmonary pressures or pulmonary vascular resistance do not exceed two-thirds of the systemic value.

Atrioventricular septal defects

AVSDs are characterized by a common AV junction with deficient AV septation. The prevalence of the condition among patients with congenital heart disease is reported to range from 2.9–7.4 %.[5] In contrast, the prevalence of AVSDs in patients with Down syndrome is around 30%.[6]

The main anatomical features of the condition are a common ovoid-shaped AV junction, a defect of the inlet ventricular septum, a five-leaflet common valve (left and right mural leaflet, right anterosuperior leaflet, and superior and inferior bridging leaflet), and an unwedged aorta with an elongated LVOT (i.e. *gooseneck deformity*). Traditionally, AVSDs have been classified into partial (also called *primum ASD* or *partial AV-canal*) and complete forms. It is now recognized that partial AVSDs represent AVSDs with fused superior and inferior-bridging leaflets and attachment of these bridging leaflets to the scooped

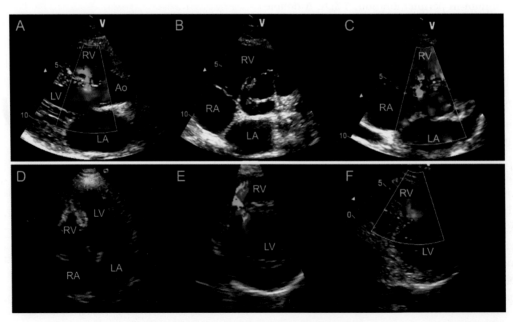

Figure 22.7 Haemodynamic characterization of ventricular septal defect (VSD). A) Parasternal long-axis view in a patient with restrictive ventricular septal defect (VSD) in the supracristal portion of the outlet septum (doubly committed VSD). Note, that in this view the outlet septum defect cannot be distinguished from a perimembranous VSD. B) Parasternal short-axis view provides the correct diagnosis. Note the lack of the support of the aortic valve, being one of the factors that can lead to aortic valve prolapse and progressive regurgitation. C) Parasternal short-axis view showing a restrictive perimembranous VSD. D) Apical four-chamber view showing a large non-restrictive inlet VSD. E) Parasternal short-axis view showing a restrictive trabecular (muscular) VSD. F) Parasternal short-axis view showing a non-restrictive trabecular VSD. Ao, aorta; LA, left atrium; LV, left ventricle; PA, pulmonary artery; RA, right atrium; RV, right ventricle.

out crest of the ventricular septum. These patients, therefore, have two valve orifices (albeit with a common AV junction) and present with atrial shunting, only. There is, however, a continuum between partial and complete forms. There may be a VSD that is completely or partially covered by valve tissue forming an aneurysmatic basal inlet ventricular septum with or without a restrictive VSD. This is called intermediate AVSD and may—as is a partial AVSD—be encountered unrepaired in adults.

Pathophysiology

The pathophysiology of the condition is largely dependent on the magnitude of atrial and ventricular left-to-right shunting (size of the ASD and the inlet VSD) and severity of AV valve regurgitation. Whereas a patient with predominant atrial shunting will present with RV enlargement (*ASD like*), LV and atrial enlargement is a hallmark of predominant shunting at ventricular level. In patients with a common AV valve, biventricular enlargement is to be expected. The left-to-right shunt results in increased pulmonary blood flow. Significant shunt at ventricular level typically leads to pulmonary vascular disease with a high likelihood of eventually developing suprasystemic PAP resulting in shunt reversal and cyanosis (i.e. Eisenmenger syndrome). This is particularly common in patients with Down syndrome. Cyanosis can occasionally also occur independently of Eisenmenger syndrome due to streaming effects of venous blood across the defect leading to systemic desaturation.

Echocardiographic assessment

Adults with complete AVSD will, in general, present after repair. If not repaired they are likely to present with Eisenmenger syndrome. The AVSD should be assessed in different views. In the A4C view the defects of the atrial and ventricular septum can normally be clearly visualized. In addition, this view is helpful in quantifying AV valve regurgitation and in assessing ventricular and atrial dimensions. In this view the loss of offset between the TV and MV (in normal hearts the TV inserts more apically compared to the MV) can be displayed and the common AV valve may be apparent. Septal malalignment with straddling and overriding valves should be assessed. Parasternal and subcostal views should be used to visualize the elongation and curvature of the LVOT (obstruction should be excluded). Visualization of the common AV junction and the five-leaflet AV valve should be attempted in the PSAX view. It should be noted that unlike in the normal heart, the LV papillary muscles are abnormally arranged (located in anteroinferior and posterosuperior positions). In some patients chordae converge into one major papillary muscle and this is often called a parachute MV. Further possible anomalies include a double orifice left AV valve. The parasternal and possibly subcostal short-axis views demonstrate the three zones of apposition of the left AV valve and this has been referred to as cleft MV. However, in the

setting of AVSD the terms MV and TV should be avoided as this represents a common valve and bears little resemblance to normal AV valves.

In the setting of right AV valve regurgitation, the RV systolic pressure should be estimated. In patients with cyanosis, where abnormal streaming of blood is suspected, a contrast study should be considered. Examples are shown in ➲ Fig. 22.8.

Echocardiography and treatment decisions

Surgery is indicated in most patients with AVSD and significant shunts. Echocardiography provides the essential anatomical and functional information. However, in patients with Doppler-estimated PAP greater than 50% of systemic pressure invasive assessment of PAP and vascular resistance are indispensable. Surgical repair should not be attempted in patients with established Eisenmenger physiology.

Re-intervention primarily for residual AV-valve regurgitation, less commonly residual shunting is also primarily guided by echocardiography.

Persistent ductus arteriosus

The arterial duct represents an essential structure of the fetal circulation connecting the left PA with the descending aorta and allowing blood to bypass the lungs. Postnatal functional duct closure occurs within hours after birth, and the duct is normally converted to a fibrous ligament within the first year of life. A persistent ductus arteriosus has been reported to account for approximately 2.4% of patients with congenital heart disease. It represents a vessel with various configurations between the left PA and the descending aorta, distal to the left subclavian artery.

Pathophysiology

Failure of the duct to close results in shunting from the aorta to the pulmonary circulation. The pathophysiology varies depending on PDA size. Small ducts remain generally asymptomatic, while moderate and large PDAs lead to LA and LV volume overload as well as pulmonary hypertension, eventually culminating in shunt reversal and development of Eisenmenger syndrome in patients with large ducts. Further complications include an elevated risk of endarteritis and the potential for aneurysm formation (rare).

Echocardiographic assessment

The PDA should be visualized in a PSAX view (➲ Fig. 22.9). In addition, a high left parasternal view can be attempted. This shows the characteristic diastolic flow in the PAs on CD echocardiography. The Doppler signal normally reveals a systolic-diastolic flow, however in patients with elevated PAPs the diastolic component may be missing. The diagnosis of a PDA in patients with established Eisenmenger syndrome and slow bidirectional flow can be challenging. Beyond the direct assessment of the duct,

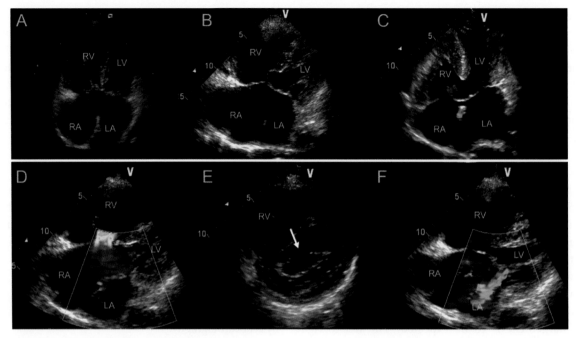

Figure 22.8 Atrioventricular septal defect (AVSD). A) Apical four-chamber view in a patient with incomplete (partial) AVSD. Note that the two atrioventricular valves are set in one plane. B) Modified four-chamber view of an intermediate AVSD. Note that the VSD in the inlet septum is covered by aneurysmatic tissue and that the two atrioventricular valves are set in one plane. C) Apical four-chamber view of a patient with a complete AVSD. Note the presence of a defect, both, in the interventricular and interatrial septum. D) Colour Doppler shows left–right shunting through the atrial septal defect of patient with partial AVSD. E) Short-axis view in a patient with partial AVSD showing the cleft (arrow), the gap between the two parts of the anterior leaflet of the left-sided valve that can cause regurgitation. F) Regurgitation of the left-sided atrioventricular valve as shown on colour Doppler in a modified apical four-chamber view. LA, left atrium; LV, left ventricle; PA, pulmonary artery; RA, right atrium; RV, right ventricle.

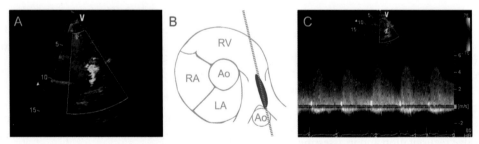

Figure 22.9 Persistent arterial duct. A) Parasternal short-axis view in an adult patient with persistent arterial duct. Colour Doppler echocardiography shows a turbulent jet from the descending aorta into the pulmonary artery. B) Diagram illustrates the typical localization of the lesion. Note the high velocities on the continuous–wave Doppler suggesting that there is no significant elevation of pulmonary artery pressure (C). Ao, aorta; LA, left atrium; RA, right atrium; RV, right ventricle.

the echocardiographic study should focus on assessing LV dimensions and function as well as estimating PAP (using TR velocity and PDA velocity). PA dilation is typically seen. Pulmonary hypertension and Eisenmenger syndrome may lead to RV hypertrophy, dilation, and ultimately failure. Adults with a small PDA typically present with normal ventricles and PAP. Patients with a moderate PDA may present either with predominant LV volume overload (when they develop HF they may be misdiagnosed as cardiomyopathy) or with predominant PAH and the signs of RV pressure overload (may be misdiagnosed as idiopathic PAH).

Echocardiography and treatment decision

Closure is indicated in patients with a PDA and LV volume overload and can be considered in patients with a small PDA and a continuous murmur with device closure being the method of choice. Echocardiography provides the required information. However, if PAP is estimated to be greater than 50% of systemic, invasive measurement of PAP and pulmonary vascular resistance should be performed. Closure is indicated if PAP and resistance are below two-thirds of systemic levels and should be considered in patients with higher PAP but still left-to-right shunt or demonstrated vasoreactivity. In patients with a small silent duct (visible on echo but without murmur) and those with established Eisenmenger syndrome, PDA closure is not recommended.

Obstructive lesions

Left ventricular outflow tract obstruction

Left ventricular outflow tract obstruction (LVOTO) is most commonly due to valvular aortic stenosis (AS) (accounting for approximately 75% of cases); however, it can also occur at sub- or supravalvular levels and at multiple levels simultaneously (e.g. in Shone syndrome).

Valvular aortic stenosis

The normal AoV is tricuspid. Bicuspid aortic valves are relatively common (the reported prevalence in the normal population ranges from 1–2%) and accounts for the vast majority of congenital cases of valvular AS. Unicuspid or quadricuspid valves are very rare, but when present, may also be associated with congenital AS. Genetic abnormalities have been related to bicuspid aortic valves, and biscupid aortic valves are associated with abnormalities of the aortic wall and are linked to aortic coarctation.[7,8] The progression of AS in this setting may be related to mechanical changes due to abnormal valvular shear stress; however, it is nowadays appreciated that pathophysiology of calcific AS represents an active process related to inflammation and fibrosis.[9,10]

Echocardiographic assessment

Qualitative and quantitative echocardiographic assessment of AS is described in ➲ Chapter 14a. The diagnosis of a primary bicuspid valve is often difficult to establish, once secondary calcification and severe stenosis have occurred. TOE is helpful for morphological assessment of the AoV. While highest transvalvular velocities in acquired AS are most frequently obtained from an apical or right parasternal approach, the suprasternal approach is, however, frequently best in congenital AS.

Echocardiography and treatment decision

Diagnostic criteria and therapeutic options for severe AS are largely identical to those used in patients with acquired heart disease (see ➲ Chapter 14a). Unlike in elderly patients with calcific AS, however, balloon valvuloplasty may represent a treatment option in selected patients with valvular stenosis and without significant calcification or relevant regurgitation.

Subaortic stenosis

The spectrum of subaortic stenosis ranges from isolated subvalvar fibrous ridges or diaphragms to a diffuse tunnel-like narrowing of the LVOT associated with a hypoplastic aortic root. In addition, subaortic stenosis can occur in patients with an AVSD, a VSD, or Shone syndrome, or may develop after previous surgical repair of these lesions.

Echocardiographic assessment

The subaortic stenosis can usually be well visualized from the PLAX and the A5C view. CD is helpful to recognize the level of velocity increase below the valve. If TTE is inconclusive, TOE should be performed (➲ Fig. 22.10). In addition to the morphology and the location of the stenosis, Doppler echocardiography should be used to measure peak and mean gradients across the stenosis. Aortic valve morphology and the degree of AR should be assessed as well as LV function and LV hypertrophy which may be out of proportion considering the LVOT gradient.

Echocardiography and treatment decision

Indications for surgical resection of the membrane are based on symptoms, the severity of the obstruction (mean gradient >50mmHg), the presence of AR and its progression, and the presence of LV hypertrophy. Since no prosthetic material is required, surgery may be considered even in asymptomatic patients without LV hypertrophy and with a normal exercise test when the mean gradient is more than 50mmHg. Although diagnostic information required for the treatment decision can be provided by echo, Doppler may in this setting not uncommonly overestimate the LVOT gradient and confirmation by invasive measurement may be required.

Supravalvular aortic stenosis

Compared to valvular or subvalvular AS, supravalvular stenosis is relatively rare. The lesion is typically localized above the aortic sinuses at the level of the sinotubular junction. Most commonly, the lesion occurs as an hourglass deformity with dilation of the distal aorta, although it can also be localized or diaphragmatic. Most often it is seen in patients with Williams–Beuren syndrome, a syndrome characterized by various vascular stenoses associated with typical facial characteristics, although it can also occur sporadically.

Echocardiographic assessment

The supravalvular stenosis can usually be visualized in a PLAX view with focus on the ascending aorta. Doppler echocardiography should be used to measure peak and mean gradients across the stenosis; however, it should be noted that Doppler gradients tend to overestimate the degree of obstruction and they may require invasive confirmation before treatment is contemplated. CD imaging is also helpful in assessing the origin of flow acceleration in relation to the AoV. LV function, degree of hypertrophy, and dimensions should be assessed. Given the generalized nature of the disease a detailed assessment of the aorta (including abdominal aorta) and pulmonary arteries is

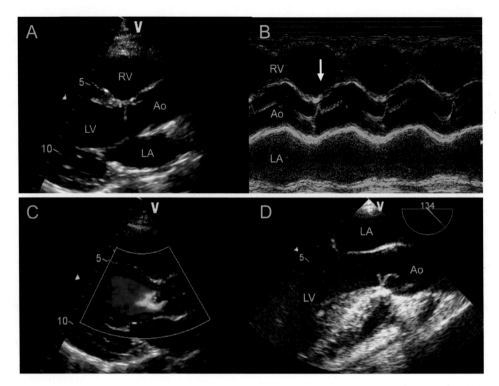

Figure 22.10 Membranous subaortic stenosis. Long-axis views, on TTE (A) and TOE (D) showing a membrane below the aortic valve. Turbulent flow is seen to originate from the level of the membrane, i.e. below the aortic valve (C). The jet alters the mechanics of the aortic valve causing a premature closure (arrow) and subsequent discrete fluttering (B). Ao, aorta; LA, left atrium; LV, left ventricle.PA, pulmonary artery; RA, right atrium; RV, right ventricle.

recommended which requires additional imaging modalities such as cardiac magnetic resonance (CMR) and computed tomography (CT).

Echocardiography and treatment decision

Treatment indications include symptoms in the presence of a mean gradient above 50mmHg, LV dysfunction, and severe hypertrophy. Asymptomatic patients with gradients higher than 50mmHg and no other criteria for intervention may be considered for surgery when the expected risk is very low. Echocardiography can commonly provide the diagnosis. However, prior to surgery additional imaging modalities and invasive evaluation are generally required.

Aortic coarctation

Aortic coarctation is characterized by a narrowing of the aorta close to the area where the arterial duct inserts (distal to the origin of the left subclavian artery) and accounts for approximately 5–8% of all congenital heart defects. Morphologically the lesion can occur either as a localized obstruction (the more common form, ranging in severity from a discrete shelf to a fibrous diaphragm with a pin-hole orifice) or as a hypoplastic aortic segment. Traditionally, aortic coarctation has been classified into pre-, para-, and postductal forms. This is, however, of limited relevance in adults, where the duct is almost always closed and ligamentous. It has been emphasized that the condition is part of a generalized arteriopathy and is commonly associated with other lesions of the aorta, such as a bicuspid AoV (up to 85%), hypoplasia of the arch, additional stenotic areas

within the aorta, and anomalies of the head and neck vessels including intracranial aneurysms. Aortic coarctation is more common in patients with Turner or Williams syndrome, congenital rubella syndrome, neurofibromatosis, and Takayasu disease.

Pathophysiology

Severe aortic coarctation will manifest in infancy, while patients with less severe forms or significant collateral circulation may only be diagnosed in adulthood. Signs and symptoms of aortic coarctation in these patients include upper body arterial hypertension, reduced lower body perfusion (cold feet, leg claudication), HF (as a consequence of increased afterload, ventricular hypertrophy and LV failure), aortic dissection (due to increased blood pressure and intrinsic aortic wall abnormalities such as cystic media necrosis[11]), endocarditis and intracranial haemorrhage (as a consequence of hypertension and due to associated intracranial aneurysms[12]). The severity of these second organ complications depends on the degree of narrowing and upper body blood pressure.

In the presence of a significant collateral circulation, the gradient across the stenosis may be reduced. Even after surgical or interventional therapy, significant coarctation may recur and signs and symptoms are similar to those discussed for native coarctation. Aortic aneurysms may develop after surgical correction (especially after patch aortoplasty). Upper body arterial hypertension is frequent even after repair without significant re- or residual coarctation. It has been suggested that this is due to abnormal aortic compliance and wave reflection at the site of coarctation repair (and use of prosthetic material) as well as intrinsic endothelial dysfunction in this setting.[13,14]

Echocardiographic assessment

Echocardiographic assessment should focus on the site of coarctation as well as on possible associated lesions and complications. The aortic coarctation can be visualized from a high PLAX view or a suprasternal view. Depending on the quality of the acoustic window it may provide important anatomic information (localized fibrous shelf or hypoplastic aortic arch), demonstrate turbulent flow at the site of coarctation, and allow the measurement of vessel dimensions. While high systolic velocities are commonly found on CW Doppler, this does not represent a reliable sign of significant coarctation. More characteristic of severe coarctation are high Doppler velocities that continue throughout the cardiac cycle, resulting in a diastolic *run-off* or *diastolic tail* phenomenon (→ Fig. 22.11). Although a recent study suggested that measurements based on this phenomenon may have nearly ideal diagnostic performance in distinguishing patients with or without significant coarctation, this sign requires preserved proximal aortic compliance (i.e. aortic Windkessel effect) to produce sufficient diastolic forward flow and thus may be false negative in patients with very stiff or hypoplastic proximal vessels.[15] In addition, the presence of extensive collaterals makes Doppler signs of coarctation generally unreliable.

Assessment of the LV with quantification of LV hypertrophy is of particular importance. Evaluation of the AoV (bicuspid), the ascending aorta, and the aortic arch are essential part of the echocardiographic work-up.

Echocardiography and treatment decision

In the current era, interventional angioplasty with or without stent implantation has become the treatment of choice for adults with native or re-coarctation at most centres if anatomically suitable.[10,16] If morphology appears not suitable for catheter intervention, surgical repair (including ascending-to-descending aorta conduits in complex cases) should be considered.

Intervention is recommended in patients with arterial hypertension and a non-invasive pressure difference greater than 20mmHg between upper and lower limbs. Hypertensive patients should be considered for intervention independently of the gradient if there is more than 50% aortic narrowing relative to the aortic diameter at the diaphragm (on CT, CMR). Whether such patients should be treated without hypertension remains more controversial. Although echocardiography may provide the diagnosis in most patients, the information for treatment decision requires additional imaging with CMR and/ or CT as well as assessment of the pressure difference between upper and lower limbs.

Right ventricular outflow tract obstruction

Right ventricular outflow tract obstruction (RVOTO) can occur at subvalvular, valvular, or supravalvular levels. Subvalvular stenosis is frequently associated with other conditions such as

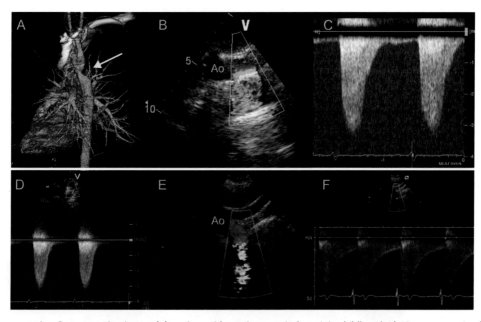

Figure 22.11 Aortic coarctation. Re-coarctation in an adult patient with previous surgical repair in childhood. A) 3D reconstruction based on computed tomography shows a marked reduction of the aortic diameter just below the left subclavian artery (arrow). B) Colour Doppler echocardiography from a suprasternal view shows turbulent flow in the descending aorta. C) Continuous wave Doppler across the coarctation in the suprasternal view shows only discrete diastolic tailing. The patient had a pressure difference of 40mmHg between left arm and legs. D) Doppler spectrum of a patient after coarctation repair without tailing. E) Colour Doppler image from a suprasternal approach in a patient with severe native coarctation and the corresponding Doppler spectrum with diastolic tailing (F). Ao, aorta.

double-chambered RV or tetralogy of Fallot. Double-chambered RV represents a rare complication (3–10%) in patients with a (a mainly perimembranous) VSD. Due to hypertrophy of muscle bundles in the direction of the VSD jet, the RV is separated into a low and high pressure chamber. Infundibular stenosis is part of tetralogy of Fallot but may also occur in patients with valvular PS.

Valvular PS is by far the most common type of RVOTO (80–90%) accounting for approximately 9% of congenital heart defects.[2] In the majority of cases there is a preserved mobile valve with fused commissures and an obstructed central opening. In this setting the valve leaflets are thin and there is doming of the valve in systole. A dysplastic pulmonary valve, with myxomatous and poorly mobile leaflets is less common (15–20%). Very rarely, valvular PS may be due to a bicuspid pulmonary valve. Valvular PS is frequently associated with post-stenotic dilation of the pulmonary trunk or the pulmonary arteries (mainly in the doming form of PS).

Supravalvular PS or PA stenosis is caused by narrowing of the main pulmonary trunk, PA bifurcation, or pulmonary branches. It is commonly associated with tetralogy of Fallot, Williams–Beuren syndrome, or Noonan syndrome. Stenosis of the main PA may be secondary to previous placement of a pulmonary band.

Pathophysiology

Significant RVOTO leads to increased RV afterload causing RV hypertrophy and this may induce an additional component of subvalvular (dynamic) RVOTO. Symptoms include angina, dyspnoea, dizziness, or syncope, although patients with mild or moderate stenosis usually remain asymptomatic.

Echocardiographic assessment

Echocardiography can visualize the level of RVOTO, delineate PV anatomy, assess RV hypertrophy, and identify coexisting lesions (◗ Fig. 22.12). Visualization of RVOTO should be initially attempted from a PSAX view, although modified views such as subcostal short-axis views or an A5C view with anterior angulation may be helpful. On 2D echocardiography the morphology of the PV (doming, dysplastic, etc.) should be assessed. In addition, post-stenotic pulmonary dilation should be visualized. If echocardiography cannot provide all morphological

details—which is not uncommon—CMR is used to complement the information. CD flow demonstrates narrow turbulent flow across the stenosis and can be used to delineate the level of stenosis. CW Doppler measurements allow assessment of the severity of the stenosis. According to current guidelines RVOTO is considered mild when the peak gradient across the valve is less than 36mm Hg (peak velocity <3m/s), moderate from 36–64mmHg (peak velocity 3–4m/s), and severe when the gradient is greater than 64mm Hg (peak velocity >4m/s). Doppler measurements may be unreliable particularly in patients with tubular lesions, stenoses in series (overestimation of gradient), and in double-chambered RV where it is in general not possible to align jet and Doppler beam (underestimation of gradient). The severity of obstruction should therefore always be confirmed by estimating the RV pressure from TR velocity. RV hypertrophy should be visually quantified and RV systolic function assessed. In patients with previous pulmonary valvotomy the degree of pulmonary regurgitation should be assessed.

Echocardiography and treatment decision

Balloon valvotomy is recommended for patients with significant valvular PS (doming form). In patients with peripheral PS balloon dilation and stent implantation are usually advocated. Surgery represents the mainstay of therapy for all other forms of RVOTO and patients with dysplastic or hypoplastic PVs.

Intervention is recommended with a Doppler gradient higher than 64mmHg regardless of symptoms as long as no valve replacement is required. Asymptomatic patients who require valve replacement should have a RV pressure greater than 80mmHg (i.e. TR velocity >4.3m/s). A Doppler gradient less tan 64mmHg may justify intervention in the presence of symptoms related to RVOTO or decreased RV function or relevant arrhythmias. A more aggressive approach is advocated for patients with a double-chambered RV (due to the progressive nature of the disease). In many patients this information can be provided by echocardiography. If morphology is insufficiently demonstrated, CMR (or CT) may be required. If severity is uncertain invasive confirmation is required (particularly in asymptomatic patients).

It has been suggested that treatment of peripheral PA stenosis should be considered, if diameter narrowing exceeds 50%,

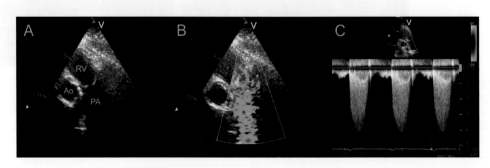

Figure 22.12 Valvular pulmonary stenosis (PS). Short-axis view of a patient with valvular PS and doming valve (A). Corresponding view with Colour Doppler (B) and continuous-wave Doppler spectrum (C).

RV systolic pressure is above 50mmHg and/or lung perfusion abnormalities are present. Echo can only provide part of this information and additional diagnostic modalities are required.

Complex congenital heart disease

The segmental approach

Although isolated congenital heart defects (such as simple shunt lesions and obstructive lesions) can be characterized by describing their anatomical position within the normal heart, this approach fails in complex congenital heart disease. Some complex cardiac malformations tend to occur in combination and can be described as a syndrome or using eponymous titles. However, a systematic approach is required to unequivocally describe all individual lesions that can coexist in a malformed heart and all their possible combinations. The *sequential segmental analysis* provides such a framework for describing complex malformation in a systematic fashion. It is equally applicable to patients with simple isolated defects and those with the most unusual complex malformations. In clinical practice it is often avoided in patients with simple defects (such as secundum ASD), though this is only acceptable if a rigorous analysis has been performed, to exclude associated malformations and to ascertain that the arrangement of the cardiac chambers and their connection is normal (i.e. there is—as described later—situs solitus as well as atrioventricular and ventriculoarterial concordance).

For the sequential segmental analysis, the heart is divided in three segments: the atrial chambers, the ventricles, and the great arteries. First, the position of the (morphological) atrial chambers is examined. The most constant feature to distinguish the morphologically right from the morphologically left atrium is the atrial appendage. The LA appendage is long and tubular, whereas the right appendage is triangular in shape with a broad base and a terminal crest. In addition, the coronary sinus is a specific feature of the morphologically LA. Fortunately, the arrangement of the atria is generally consistent with the arrangement of thoracic and abdominal organs. Therefore, radiological assessment of the morphology of the bronchi and imaging of the abdominal organs helps to determine atrial arrangement. There are four possible combinations:

- Situs solitus (morphologically LA on the left, morphologically RA on the right).
- Situs inversus (morphologically RA on the left, morphologically LA on the right).
- Situs ambiguous (isomerism): LA isomerism (two morphologically LAs) and RA isomerism (two morphologically RAs).

As discussed earlier this normally coincides with the arrangement of the bronchi (the left bronchus being long, whereas the right main bronchus short) and the abdominal organs (liver and stomach) (➲ Fig. 22.13). Mirror imaged arrangement of the bronchi and the abdominal organs would suggest situs inversus, whereas two morphologically left bronchi with a central liver would suggest LA isomerism. Furthermore, the location of the aorta and inferior vena cava (IVC) below the diaphragm (relative to each other and the spine) is generally related to atrial situs. Normally, the aorta is located posterior

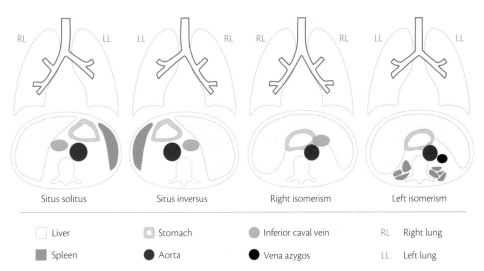

| Liver | Stomach | Inferior caval vein | RL Right lung |
| Spleen | Aorta | Vena azygos | LL Left lung |

Figure 22.13 Abdominal and thoracic situs. In general, atrial situs correlates with the bronchial arrangement and to a lesser degree the abdominal situs. The left main bronchus (LB) is usually at least twice as long as the right main bronchus (RB), when measured to the first branching. A length ratio of less than 1.5:1 suggests isomerism. The LB is usually more horizontal than the RB. The RB subdivides into three lobar bronchi while the LB divides into two. Note the different relationship between abdominal aorta and caval vein as well as the position of liver and stomach. Left atrial isomerism is commonly associated with polysplenia and azygos continuation (located posterior to the aorta), while right atrial isomerism is commonly associated with asplenia (see ➲ text).

and to the left of the IVC. In atrial situs inversus these positions tend to be inversed (aorta to the right). In patients with isomerism, the great vessels lie to the same side of the spine. In patients with RA isomerism, the aorta is located posterior and to the right of the IVC, whereas in patients with LA isomerism, the IVC is generally interrupted and continued via an azygos vein. As a consequence, the aorta lies anterior to the vein. As a general rule (with exceptions), RA isomerism is associated with asplenia and LA isomerism with polysplenia. Also, patients with RA isomerism have total anomalous pulmonary venous connection, whereas LA isomerism is associated with interruption of the IVC and venous return passing via the azygos or hemiazygos veins (a persistent left superior vena cava is frequently found).

Next, the position of the (morphological) ventricular chambers is examined. Various features may distinguish the morphologically right from the morphologically LV. These include:

♦ The RV is characterized by a grossly trabeculated apex and moderator band while the LV is rather smooth.

♦ The hinge point of the septal leaflet of the TV (indicating the RV) is more apically positioned than the hinge point of the MV (echocardiographically recognisable from an A4C view) (see ➲ Fig. 22.18 in 'Congenitally corrected transposition of the great arteries' section).

♦ There is septal attachment of the tricuspid but not of the MV.

♦ There is fibrous continuity between the anterior leaflet of the MV and the AoV, whereas the PV is elevated by muscular infundibulum above the levels of the other cardiac valves (although the presence of an infundibulum is not necessarily linked to ventricular morphology).

Having identified the ventricular chambers, the connection between the atria and the ventricles is described. In patients with a morphologically left and right atrium and a morphologically left and right ventricle the connection can be *concordant* (normal) or *discordant* (abnormal). In patients with isomeric atria, the connections cannot be described as concordant or discordant. Instead connection is mixed and the ventricular topology—the spatial relationship of one ventricle to the other—needs to be described. This is based on the concept of *chirality* (*handedness*). If the palm of the right hand could be placed on the septal surface of the RV with the wrist is at the apex, thumb in the inlet and the fingers in the outlet, this is described as *right-hand pattern*. In patients with a univentricular heart, the connection between the atria and the dominant ventricle can be described as double inlet ventricle, absent right AV, or absent left AV connection. In this setting the morphology of the dominant ventricle needs to be delineated.

Next the junctions between the atria and ventricles should be described. This includes presence of two distinct valves or a common valve, valve morphology, imperforate valves where appropriate as well as straddling and overriding of valves.

As a last step, the ventriculoarterial junctions are analysed and the arterial relationship is described. The ventriculoarterial connection can be *concordant*, *discordant*, or *double-outlet* (with the greater part of both valves supported by one ventricle). The aorta is identified as the vessel giving rise to the coronary arteries and usually the three arch arteries, the PA as the vessel bifurcating into the right and left PA. If one of the vessels occurs in isolation, this is described as single aortic or pulmonary trunk. Alternatively, a common trunk can exist, giving rise to the aorta, the coronaries and at least on pulmonary vessel. The arterial relationship should be described in anterior–posterior and right–left coordinates (e.g. aorta anterior and to the right of the pulmonary artery).

Finally, although not part of the morphology of the heart, its position within the chest should be described (heart located in the left or right chest or midline = *laevocardia*, *dextrocardia* or *mesocardia*), and the location of the apex specified (directed to the left, right, or the midline).

Tetralogy of Fallot and pulmonary atresia with ventricular septal defect

Tetralogy of Fallot represents the most common cyanotic congenital cardiac defect and accounts for approximately 6.8% of congenital heart defects. The defect consists of a non-restrictive VSD (approximating in size the diameter of the aortic root and in 80% perimembranous), overriding aorta, RVOTO and secondary RV hypertrophy. Anatomically, the hallmark of the defect is the anterocephalad deviation of the outlet septum. This abnormal position of the outlet septum accounts for the overriding aorta, and together with the hypertrophy of the septoparietal trabeculations, for the commonly present subpulmonary stenosis. The RVOTO, however, is usually a combination of subpulmonary and valvular obstruction, occasionally also associated with supravalvular PS. The malformation is part of a spectrum that ranges from non-restrictive VSD with overriding aorta but without relevant outflow tract obstruction (so-called Eisenmenger complex) to pulmonary atresia with VSD. In addition, as the degree of aortic overriding varies, the defect forms part of a spectrum with double outlet RV (aortic overriding >50%). Tetralogy of Fallot can be associated with right aortic arch, anomalous coronary arteries, and additional ASD (pentalogy of Fallot) or VSDs. It is increasingly recognized that 15–20% of cases[17] are linked to a microdeletion of a region on chromosome 22 (22q11, previously called Di George syndrome) which generally occurs sporadically but carries a 50% of transmission risk to the offspring and is frequently associated with psychiatric disease.

Pulmonary atresia with VSD shares the intracardiac anatomy with tetralogy of Fallot but the RV and the PAs are not directly connected. In the presence of a non-restrictive VSD, these patients generally have a good sized RV and are candidates for biventricular repair. The PAs can be unifocal with confluent good sized PAs supplied by a patent arterial duct; multifocal, with confluent but hypoplastic PAs, supplied by multiple aortic-pulmonary collaterals (MAPCAS); or (at the worst end of the spectrum) multifocal with non-confluent arteries supplied by MAPCAS. Depending on the pulmonary anatomy establishing a connection between the RV and the pulmonary vascular bed is sometimes a challenge.

Pathophysiology

Patients with uncorrected tetralogy of Fallot are cyanotic. Although the non-restrictive VSD and overriding aorta predispose to cyanosis, its severity mainly depends on the degree of infundibular stenosis. Infants with severe infundibular stenosis develop cyanosis hours after birth. In children with less severe infundibular stenosis at birth, development of cyanosis may be delayed to childhood or occasionally patients continue to have only mild cyanosis (so-called *pink tetralogy*). In the current era patients generally undergo reparative surgery at presentation or when they become symptomatic. Attacks of severe cyanosis are a feature of tetralogy of Fallot, commonly occurring between the age of 6–24 months. Such cyanotic attacks would prompt reparative surgery. Longstanding cyanosis and increased RV afterload also impact on RV function and may predispose to higher incidence of ventricular dysfunction, RV failure and sudden cardiac death, supporting the current practice of early reparative surgery. The patients with tetralogy of Fallot repaired a few decades ago—and now attending adult congenital heart disease services—may have undergone palliative surgery previous to any reparative operations (if any). These early palliations, aimed at increasing pulmonary blood flow, include Blalock–Taussig (BT), Waterston and Potts shunts (for explanation, see later). Palliative procedures may cause PA stenosis or kinking. They lead to LV volume overload and if sized too large to pulmonary vascular disease. As a consequence these procedures have been largely abandoned and primary repair between 6–18 months of age is the rule nowadays, performed with very low perioperative mortality. Reparative surgery consists of VSD closure and relief of the RVOTO and is currently generally performed via a transatrial–transpulmonary approach. In contrast, repair was previously done via a right ventriculotomy and commonly a transannular patch was placed for *complete relief* of RVOTO. This approach generates an arrhythmogenic substrate in the infundibulum and leads to severe PR.

Long-term outcome after repair is excellent (35-year survival of approximately 85%). Sequelae and complications, however, are not uncommon and include:

◆ Pulmonary regurgitation (PR): previously considered a benign lesion, it is now recognized that, over time, significant PR induces RV dilation, impaired RV function, represents a substrate for (potentially malignant) arrhythmias, and is accompanied by symptoms of HF. Severe PR is the rule in patients after transannular patch repair. The severity of PR also depends on the compliance (Windkessel function) of the

pulmonary circulation and is aggravated by PA stenoses. Echocardiographic quantification of PR is described later. CMR allows quantification of PR based on the regurgitant fraction, with a regurgitant fraction of more than 30–45% generally considered severe to free PR.

◆ RV dilation and dysfunction: this is generally related to severe PR. Due to the multipartite anatomy of the RV, CMR is superior to echocardiography in quantifying RV volumes and function (based on EF) and current guidelines for PV replacement rely on CMR measurements.

◆ Residual VSD: it may occur and the haemodynamic relevance should be assessed (signs of LV volume overload and pulmonary hypertension).

◆ LV dysfunction: it may occur as a consequence of RV dysfunction (ventriculoventricular interaction) and may in itself represent an adverse prognostic marker.

◆ Aortic root dilation with AR: it has been described due to intrinsic aortic wall abnormalities associated with tetralogy of Fallot.

◆ Arrhythmias and sudden cardiac death: approximately 50% of patients die suddenly. The propensity for (malignant) arrhythmias is related to haemodynamic substrates, surgical scars and myocardial fibrosis.

Early management in patients with pulmonary atresia and VSD depends on PA size and anatomy. Patients with confluent, good size PAs and a pulmonary trunk are candidates for a Fallot-like repair using a transannular patch. Patients with good size PAs but without pulmonary trunk undergo repair with a RV to PA conduit. Patients with confluent but hypoplastic PAs generally require an arterial shunt or reconstruction of the RVOT (without VSD closure). This should augment PA growth and be assessed at a later stage for repair using a valved conduit. Patients with non-confluent PAs with adequate, but not excessive, pulmonary blood flow in infancy can survive into adulthood without surgery. Some groups advocate a staged unifocalization approach for this challenging group of patients, eventually aiming for a conduit repair.

Echocardiographic assessment

In patients with uncorrected or palliated tetralogy of Fallot, echocardiography demonstrates the anatomical features described earlier. PLAX and PSAX views demonstrate the perimembranous VSD with overriding aorta, the narrowed RVOT, and valvar stenosis (◆ Fig. 22.14). The size of the PAs should be assessed. The A4C and A5C views allow assessment of the inflow part of the ventricles and should be used to exclude the presence of an associated AVSD and malformations of the AV valves.

In patients with repaired tetralogy of Fallot, echocardiographic assessment should focus on haemodynamic sequelae, the severity of PR, RV dilation and function (for RV function

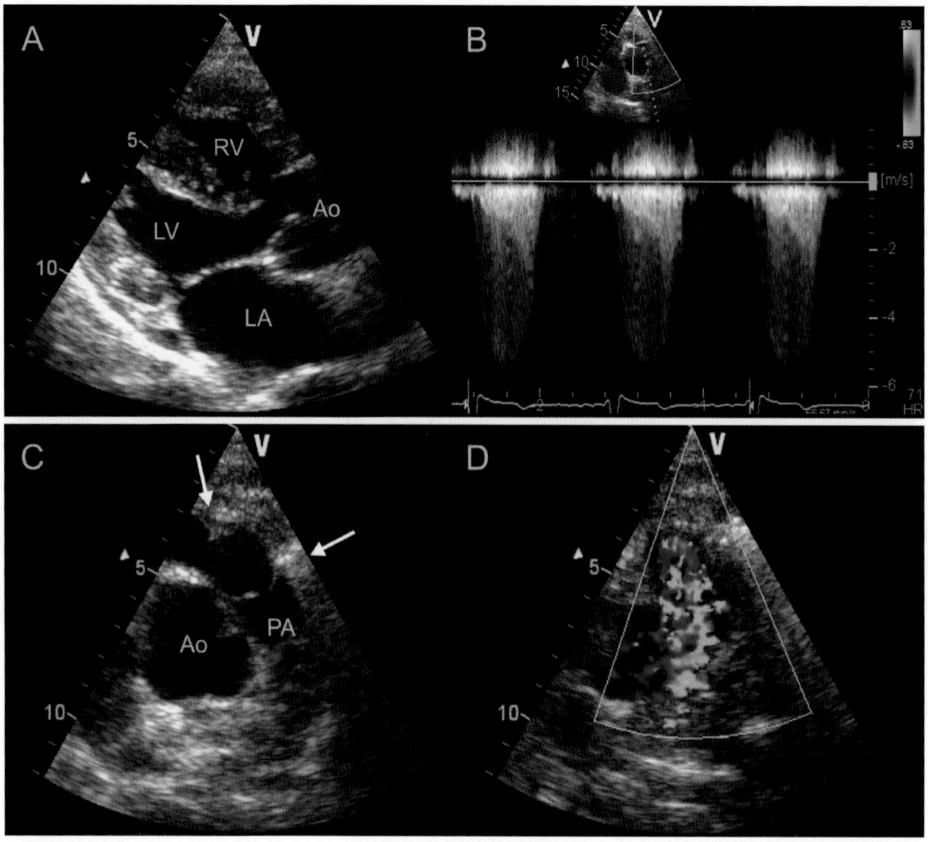

Figure 22.14 Uncorrected tetralogy of Fallot. A) Parasternal long-axis view reveals the presence of a perimembranous ventricular septal defect and an overriding aorta. B) Continuous wave Doppler across the right ventricular outflow tract and pulmonary valve shows high flow velocities (Vmax 5.6m/s) due to severe stenosis. C) Parasternal short axis view demonstrating the infundibular and valvular right outflow tract obstruction (arrows). D) Corresponding colour Doppler image. Ao, aorta; LA, left atrium; LV, left ventricle; PA, pulmonary artery; RA, right atrium; RV, right ventricle.

assessment see ➲ 'Transposition of the great arteries'). The degree of PR is generally best assessed in a PSAX view. Criteria suggesting severe PR include diastolic flow reversal in the branch pulmonary arteries, a dense PR Doppler spectrum with steep decay, termination of the PR spectrum well before the end of diastole, and a broad regurgitant jet at PV level (➲ Fig. 22.15). In addition, the degree of residual PS should be quantified, a possible residual VSD should be excluded, RV and LV size and function, the degree of TR, aortic root size, and AR should be assessed.

Some patients have undergone homograft implantation for PR and these should be assessed for homograft degeneration (stenosis or regurgitation) employing modified echocardiographic views as appropriate. Patients after transcatheter PV implantation represent an evolving cohort requiring periodic echocardiographic follow-up.

MAPCAs can be recognized as vessels with continuous turbulent flow by CD imaging.

Echocardiography and treatment decision

Current guidelines recommend PV replacement in symptomatic patients with severe PR and/or PS (defined as a peak gradient ≥64mmHg or a TR velocity >3.5m/s). PV replacement should be considered in asymptomatic patients with severe PR and/or PS and additional criteria such as decreasing objective exercise

capacity, progressive RV dilation, progressive RV dysfunction, progressive TR, very severe RVOTO (RV systolic pressure >80mmHg; TR velocity >4.3m/s), or sustained arrhythmias. AoV replacement should be performed in patients with severe AR with symptoms or signs of LV dysfunction or dilation. VSD closure is reasonable in patients with residual VSD and signs of significant LV volume overload. Cut-off values for RV volumes to consider elective PV replacement are based on CMR measures and generally range between 150–170mL/m^2 for RV end-diastolic volumes and >80mL/m^2 end-systolic volumes. Although echocardiography may, in clear-cut cases, provide sufficient information for the decision to intervene, diagnostic work-up should in general include CMR and, depending on the non-invasive findings, cardiac catheterization may be indicated.

Transposition of the great arteries

Transposition of the great arteries (TGA) is characterized by the origin of the great arteries from morphologically inappropriate ventricles (*ventriculoarterial discordance*), while there is a normal connection between the atria and the ventricles (*atrioventricular concordance*). The term TGA should not been used in patients with atrial isomerism, as atrioventricular con- or discordance implies the presence of two different morphological atria. Equally, the term should not be used to simply describe

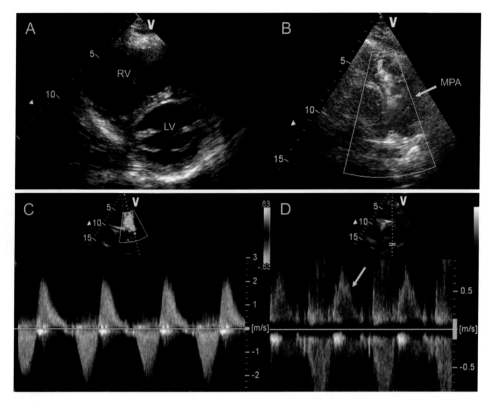

Figure 22.15 Tetralogy of Fallot after repair. Echocardiography in an adult patient after surgical repair with a transannular patch performed in the childhood. A) There is a marked dilation of the right ventricle (RV) in the parasternal short-axis view with flattened interventricular septum. B) Colour Doppler echocardiography in a parasternal short-axis view demonstrates retrograde flow in the main pulmonary artery (MPA) and the proximal part of the right and left pulmonary artery. C) Continuous wave Doppler echocardiography across the right ventricular outflow tract shows marked retrograde flow with steep decay of regurgitation velocity and slightly enhanced antegrade transvalvular velocity, resulting from the regurgitant volume. D) Pulsed wave Doppler in the right pulmonary artery shows holodiastolic retrograde flow (arrow). Severe pulmonary regurgitation was confirmed with cardiac magnetic resonance imaging (regurgitant fraction of 57%). LV, left ventricle; MPA, main pulmonary artery; RV, right ventricle.

ventriculoarterial discordance or arterial malposition in patients with complex intracardiac anatomy (such as functionally univentricular hearts). In this setting the sequential segmental analysis should be employed and the position of the great vessels described. Owing to the arrangement of the ventricles (*d-loop*) the condition is sometimes called *d-TGA* (→ Fig. 22.16).

Clinically, TGA is frequently classified as *simple* (two-thirds of cases) or *complex*, based on the presence or absence of significant associated malformations. These commonly include a VSD (approximately 45% of cases), significant LVOTO (approximately 25%) and occasionally aortic coarctation.

Most commonly the aorta is located anterior and to the right of the PA (approximately 95% of cases), although, sometimes it may also be located directly anterior or to the left and in very rare cases even posterior to the PA. Unlike in the normal heart (with cross-over arrangement of the vessels), the great vessels run in parallel (side-by-side arrangement) and this helps to make the echocardiographic diagnosis of the condition. Generally the aorta (arising from the morphological RV) is supported by a muscular infundibulum and the PA is in fibrous continuity with the MV. However, infundibular morphology is variable and there may be bilateral muscular infundibula,

especially in the presence of a VSD. The anatomy of the coronary arteries is abnormal and variable.

Pathophysiology and early management

The pulmonary and systemic circulations are arranged in parallel and early survival depends on the presence of associated lesions allowing adequate mixing of blood. In patients without significant intracardiac shunt lesions, a balloon atrioseptostomy is generally performed in the first days of life to allow for shunting after the arterial duct closes. Other palliative measures include the creation of a (modified) Blalock–Taussig shunt to improve pulmonary perfusion. Further management depends on the presence of associated lesions (VSD and PS). In the current era, patients with simple TGA undergo arterial switch operation within the first weeks of life. In the era of atrial redirection operations, repair was generally performed later, but within the first year of life. In patients with complex TGA the Rastelli procedure (or alternatives such as the Réparation à l' Etage Ventriculaire [REV] or the Nikaidoh Procedure) is commonly performed.

◆ *Arterial switch operation:* this is the preferred option for patients with simple TGA in the current era. It involves

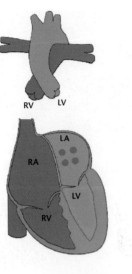

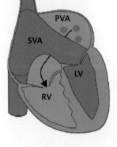

Figure 22.16 Anatomy in transposition of the great arteries. Diagram illustrating normal anatomy (left panel), the anatomy in complete transposition of the great arteries (TGA) after atrial (Mustard type) switch operation (middle panel) as well as congenitally corrected transposition of the great arteries (ccTGA; right panel). LA, left atrium; LV, left ventricle; RA, right atrium; RV, right ventricle.

Normal heart

Complete transposition of the great arteries after atrial switch operation

Congenitally corrected transposition of the great arteries

transecting the great vessels above the valve sinus. The arteries are subsequently *switched*, with the bifurcation of the PAs translocated anteriorly to the aorta (Lecompte manoeuvre). The procedure requires re-implantation of the coronary arteries. The morphologically LV becomes the systemic ventricle, avoiding long-term problems associated with a morphologically right systemic ventricle (see later). Although operative survival is good (>95%) and short- to mid-term results are encouraging, long-term complications include supravalvular PS and PA stenoses, requiring reintervention in as many as 10–25% in some series, aortic root dilation and neoaortic valve regurgitation (generally not more than moderate) as well as coronary artery abnormalities with uncertain long-term impact.

♦ *Atrial switch operation:* two main variations exist, the Senning and the Mustard operation. Both redirect the blood on atrial level, rerouting the systemic venous blood into the LV and the pulmonary venous blood to the RV (◆ Fig. 22.17). The Senning operation utilizes autologous tissue from the interatrial septum and atrial wall to redirect the blood, while the Mustard operation involves placing a baffle made of synthetic material or pericardium to reroute the blood. Both operations have been largely abandoned in the current era, but were routinely used before the arterial switch became the procedure of choice in the 1990s. Therefore, the majority of adults with TGA currently seen still underwent an atrial-switch operation. Long-term problems associated with the atrial switch operation are related to the baffle creation, surgical manipulation within the atria as well as the fact that the morphological RV becomes the systemic pumping chamber. Complications include baffle-stenosis (mostly located within the superior limb of the systemic venous baffle), baffle leaks, sinus node dysfunction, atrial arrhythmias, RV dysfunction

and dilation, (functional) TR, ventricular arrhythmias and sudden cardiac death.

♦ *Rastelli procedure in patients with complex TGA:* the Rastelli procedure utilizes the VSD as part of the LVOT by placing a synthetic patch or baffle within the RV. Thus, the morphologically LV is connected to the aorta and acts as the systemic ventricle. The PV is oversewn and a valved conduit is implanted to connect the RV to the pulmonary trunk. As the lifetime of the conduit is limited and the patients require re-interventions such as surgical replacement or more recently transcatheter valve implantation.

Echocardiographic assessment

Echocardiographic finding vary with the type of surgical procedures described previously:

♦ *Atrial switch operation (Mustard or Senning operation):* the atrial cavity is divided into a systemic and pulmonary-venous chamber. Obstruction of the superior caval vein pathway is relatively frequent. It can be asymptomatic if the blood drains to the IVC via the azygos system. It may be difficult to visualize on TTE (subcostal view) and establishing the diagnosis frequently requires TOE or CMR/CT. Obstruction of the IVC can in general be evaluated by TTE but is less common. Obstruction or narrowing of the venous channels should be excluded, as they are nowadays commonly amenable to percutaneous stent implantation. The venous chambers should be imaged by 2D echocardiography; however, Doppler echocardiography is usually required to fully assess baffle patency as well as leaks. A4C view adjusted and tilted to follow the systemic and pulmonary venous flow to the AV valves, subcostal views and tilted PLAX and PSAX views are helpful. Flow disturbance on CD with non-phasic flow and

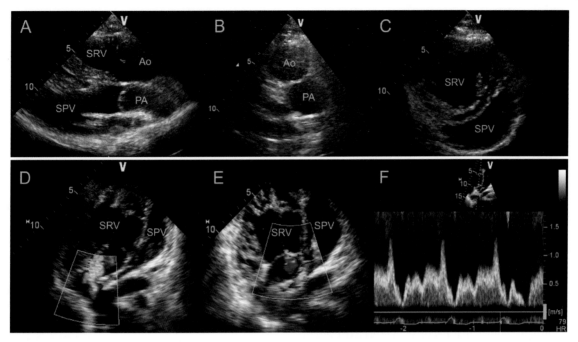

Figure 22.17 Transposition of the great arteries (TGA) after atrial switch operation. A) and B) Parasternal long-axis and short-axis views, respectively. Note the parallel arrangement of the great vessels with the aorta anterior and to the right of the pulmonary artery. C) Short-axis view illustrating the hypertrophied and enlarged systemic right ventricle (SRV) anterior and the small subpulmonary left ventricle posteriorly with bulging of the septum towards the subpulmonary ventricle (SPV). D) Colour Doppler imaging of the pulmonary venous flow. E) Colour Doppler echocardiography illustrating flow in the systemic venous baffle. F) Pulsed Doppler study showing phasic flow in the baffle of a patient after Mustard type repair. Ao, aorta; PA, pulmonary artery.

Doppler velocities greater than 1.5m/s are generally suggestive of an obstruction. Flow velocities in the inferior and superior vena cava should be similar. Pronounced discrepancy in flow velocities, therefore represent an indirect sign of stenosis. Obstructions of the pulmonary venous channel are rare. This should be suspected when there is flow disturbance on CD with non-phasic flow, dilated pulmonary veins and narrowing of the pulmonary venous channel.[18,19] A recent study suggested, that routine echocardiographic assessment fails to detect systemic venous baffle obstruction in approximately 50% of patients when compared to invasive haemodynamics and venograms.[20] Therefore, additional imaging, primarily CMR, should be used to evaluate venous pathways. Contrast echocardiography may assist in the diagnosis of baffle stenoses; however, its main role is in the assessment of baffle leaks. In the absence of a significant stenoses of the superior baffle, the systemic venous atrium should be contrasted within a few heartbeats after injection of echocontrast in a cubital vein. If contrast appearance is delayed, and contrast enters the atrium through the inferior baffle, this is suggestive of superior baffle obstruction. If contrast appears in the pulmonary venous chamber and the systemic ventricle within seconds this is suggestive of a baffle leak. TOE is a useful adjunct in identifying pulmonary venous limb stenosis.[21] Echocardiography confirms ventricular arrangement. Size and function of the systemic right (subaortic) ventricle should be assessed. Quantification of RV function is usually performed as described in ➲ Chapter 11. Especially in the setting of RV dilation, functional TR is common. It complicates assessment of RV function as afterload is reduced and even minor reduction in RV function may represent significant myocardial dysfunction. In addition, residual VSDs and sub-pulmonary LVOTO (due to leftward bulging of the IVS and systolic anterior movement of the MV) should be excluded. The malposition of the great arteries, with the aorta and PA running in parallel is generally evident on TTE (➲ Fig. 22.17).

◆ *Arterial switch operation:* echocardiographic evaluation focuses on evaluation of aortic root dimensions, presence and severity of AR, and narrowing of the PA at the anastomotic site or in the branches. Doppler measurements may be useful in assessing the severity of stenosis, but should be crosschecked with systolic RV pressure estimated from TR velocity. In addition, LV function, ostia of the coronary arteries, and their proximal course should be assessed. Stress echocardiography may detect inducible myocardial ischaemia.

◆ *Rastelli operation:* biventricular function should be assessed. Residual VSDs are often difficult to assess, due to the unusual course of the conduit or patch used to connect the LV to the AoV. Doppler gradients across the conduit may be difficult to measure and may be unreliable. Therefore, RV pressure estimation from TR velocity is of particular importance for assessment of conduit stenosis.

Echocardiography and treatment decision

After atrial switch operation, surgical therapy is recommended for severe TR in symptomatic patients with preserved systolic systemic ventricular function. Stenting should be performed in symptomatic patients with significant baffle obstruction and should be considered in asymptomatic patients. Occlusion of baffle leaks should be performed in symptomatic patients with relevant right-to-left (cyanosis) or left-to-right shunt (HF) and should be considered in asymptomatic patients. Subpulmonary outflow tract obstruction should only be addressed surgically when patients are symptomatic or subpulmonary ventricular function deteriorates. In patients post arterial switch operation, complications such as relevant PS or AR should be addressed according to current guidelines. In patients with previous Rastelli repair, conduit stenosis requires intervention in symptomatic patients with RV pressure greater than 60mmHg (TR velocity >3.5m/s). Intervention should be considered in asymptomatic patients with severe stenosis or regurgitation, if additional criteria are present such as decrease in objective exercise capacity, progressive RV dilation, progressive RV dysfunction, progressive TR, severe RVOTO (RV systolic pressure >80mmHg; TR velocity >4.3m/s) or sustained arrhythmias. Although echocardiography will in many patients provide the first hint that reintervention may need to be considered, final decisions will, in general, require additional diagnostic work-up including CMR (CT) and invasive study.

Congenitally corrected transposition of the great arteries

Congenitally corrected transposition of the great arteries (ccTGA) is a rare condition (approximately 1% of congenital cardiac malformations) characterized by a combination of atrioventricular and ventriculoarterial discordance (➲ Fig. 22.16).

As a consequence, the morphological RV supports the systemic circulation. The great arteries are parallel to each other with the aorta commonly located anterior and to the left of the PA. The majority of patients (approximately 90%) have associated cardiac defects such as VSDs (50%, usually perimembranous), PS (30–50%), malformations of the TV (90% at autopsy, including Ebstein-like malformation), and conduction system abnormalities.

Pathophysiology

The systemic and pulmonary circulations are arranged in series. Early symptoms and haemodynamic problems are due to associated malformations. With time, increasing TR, systemic RV failure and arrhythmias develop even in patients without significant associated malformations.

Echocardiographic assessment

Echocardiography demonstrates the RA, receiving the systemic venous return, draining into the morphologically LV. Usually there is fibrous continuity between the MV and the PV. The LV drains into the PA. The morphological RV has a left hand topology (thus the lesion is commonly called *l-TGA*) and drains into the aorta (usually anterior and to the left of the PA), which is usually supported by a muscular infundibulum. Echocardiography normally reveals these features. The malformation is easiest recognized in the A4C view when looking at the characteristics of a left versus right ventricle (see ➲ 'Segmental approach' and ➲ Fig. 22.18). Evaluation of the systemic TV is of particular importance. Secondary regurgitation (due to systemic RV failure) may be difficult to separate from organic TR unless Ebstein-like malformation is obvious. Associated lesions including VSD, ASD and RVOTO can be identified. Evaluation of systemic RV size and function should be attempted but remains challenging (see ➲ 'Transposition of the great arteries').

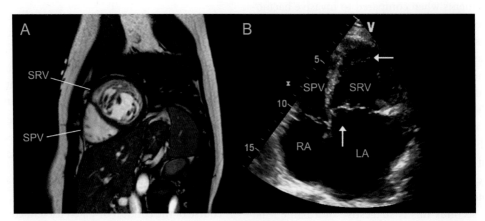

Figure 22.18 Congenitally corrected transposition of the great arteries (ccTGA). A) Short-axis view on cardiac magnetic resonance imaging. The systemic right ventricle (SRV)—characterized by coarse trabeculations—is located posteriorly and is markedly hypertrophied. B) Apical four-chamber view on TTE. The right ventricle is identified by the tricuspid valve—which is characterized by a more apical position compared to the mitral valve (vertical arrow)—and the moderator band (horizontal arrow), a thick muscular band running across the ventricle near to the apex. LA, left atrium; RA, right atrium; SPV, subpulmonary ventricle (morphological left ventricle).

Echocardiography and treatment considerations

Surgical therapy should be considered for severe TR before systemic ventricular function deteriorates (ejection fraction >45%). Haemodynamically-relevant associated lesions should be addressed. Cardiac resynchronization therapy is experimental. Although echocardiography will in many patients provide the first hint that intervention may need to be considered, final decisions will, in general, require additional diagnostic work-up including in particular CMR.

Ebstein's anomaly

Ebstein's anomaly is a malformation of the right heart, characterized by rotation and apical displacement of the tricuspid orifice into the RV. The leaflets are markedly abnormal. The anterior leaflet is frequently large and sail-like with abnormal chordal attachments to the RV wall, whereas septal and posterior leaflets are displaced towards the RV apex and often tethered to the endocardium. This commonly leads to TR (of variable degree), but may occasionally also be associated with tricuspid stenosis (TS). The apical displacement of the functional valve annulus results in an atrialized portion of the RV and variable reduction in the size of the functional right RV. Associated lesions include abnormalities of the mitral valve, shunts at atrial level (ASD or PFO in >50% of patients) and accessory conduction pathways (approximately 25%), as well RVOTO, VSD and coarctation.

Pathophysiology

The pathophysiology is mainly determined by the degree of TR, the degree of atrialization of the RV, contractility of the remaining functional RV and LV, the magnitude of atrial left-to-right or right-to-left shunting, and the presence of relevant arrhythmias. Overall, the haemodynamic and clinical spectrum is broad.

Echocardiographic assessment

The level of insertion of the septal leaflet of the TV should be recorded from an A4C view (➔ Fig. 22.19). An apical displacement—measured as the distance between the hinge points of the septal leaflet of the tricuspid and anterior leaflet of the MV—greater han or equal to $0.8cm/m^2$ body surface area (BSA) is suggestive of Ebstein's anomaly. In addition, the size of the anterior leaflet, possible fenestrations, tethering of the septal and posterior leaflet on the septum and ventricular wall should be evaluated in apical, modified (medially angulated) PLAX, and subcostal views. The size of the atrialized and functional RV should be assessed from different views. An area of the functional RV less than one-third of the total RV area is related to worse prognosis and may preclude surgical repair. The severity of TR should be evaluated based on morphology and CD imaging. Systolic flow reversal in the superior and inferior vena cava and hepatic veins can confirm the diagnosis of severe TR. Occasionally redundant anterior leaflet tissue leads to dynamic obstruction of the RVOT and this should be excluded on Doppler echocardiography. Particular attention should be paid to LV size and function, as Ebstein's anomaly may be associated with LV dysfunction (due to interventricular interaction or intrinsic LV abnormalities, such as non-compaction myocardium). Atrial shunt lesions are common in Ebstein's anomaly and may cause cyanosis or desaturation on exercise. TOE and/or contrast echocardiography with Valsalva manoeuvre should be used for evaluation.

Echocardiography and treatment decision

TV repair should be performed in symptomatic patients with severe TR if anatomy is suitable and the functional RV is adequate. Repair should be considered independently of symptoms in patients with progressive right heart dilation or reduction of RV systolic function. Generally surgical repair is challenging

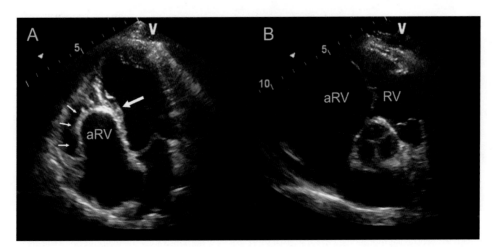

Figure 22.19 Ebstein's anomaly. A) Apical four-chamber view showing apical displacement of the septal hinge point of the septal tricuspid valve leaflet (large arrow). Note also the sail-like shape of the anterior tricuspid leaflet (small arrows). Both the parasternal short axis view (B) and apical four-chamber view (A) show the reduced size of the functional right ventricle (RV) and the large atrialized portion of the right ventricle (aRV).

and should only be performed in centres with specific experience with this complex lesion. Echocardiography in general provides the diagnosis and morphologic characteristics for treatment decision. CMR may be helpful particularly when echo image quality is poor.

Univentricular heart

A wide spectrum of conditions may be associated with a functionally univentricular heart. Although there is only one dominant functional pumping chamber, a second rudimentary chamber is nearly always present. In patients with a functionally univentricular heart, a sequential segmental analysis should be performed due to the complex anatomy and the multitude of associated malformations. Examples of conditions with a functionally univentricular heart include double inlet LV and RV, tricuspid atresia, hypoplastic left heart syndrome, hypoplastic right heart syndrome (e.g. pulmonary atresia with intact ventricular septum variants), and unbalanced AVSDs. These conditions are always associated with additional cardiac lesions including ASD and VSDs, PDA, LVOTO, RVOTO, aortic coarctation, discordant ventriculoarterial connections, atrial isomerism (with associated abnormal systemic venous and pulmonary venous return), and abnormal lung perfusion (such as MAPCAs). The morphology of the dominant chamber should be assessed based on the criteria discussed previously.

Although beyond the scope of the sequential segmental analysis, the location of the chambers may provide clues to chamber morphology. The ventricle located anterior and superior is generally a morphological RV, whereas the LV is located posterior. Features of pathophysiological and prognostic importance include the degree of AV valve regurgitation and the presence of a restriction to pulmonary blood flow. Generally, unrestrictive pulmonary blood flow may lead to overt HF due to ventricular volume overload and is associated with the development of severe pulmonary vascular disease which may be prevented by PA banding. Restrictive pulmonary blood flow is generally preferable, but if pulmonary blood flow is too low and cyanosis is severe, a surgical systemic-to-PA shunt (such as a Blalock–Taussig shunt) may have been required.

The double inlet left ventricle (DILV) is the most common form of univentricular heart in adults and is discussed to illustrate some of the principles and pitfalls of echocardiographic evaluation (➲ Fig. 22.20). The diagnosis implies that more than 50% of the circumference of both AV valves is related to the morphologically LV. The atrial situs should be determined based on morphological features (see earlier), bronchial and abdominal situs. The morphology and function of the AV valve (there can be two valves or one common valve) requires attention. AV valve regurgitation is common and if severe it is prognostically adverse. The rudimentary (morphological right)

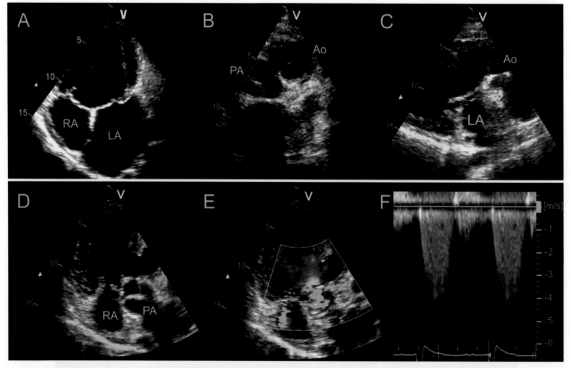

Figure 22.20 Double inlet left ventricle. A) Apical four-chamber view showing two atria with intact atrial septum and the two atrioventricular valves connecting to a ventricle with left ventricular morphology. B) Parasternal short-axis view demonstrating the malposition of the great arteries with the aorta (Ao) anterior and to the left to the pulmonary artery (PA). C) Parasternal long-axis view showing the aorta arising from an outlet chamber. D) Tilted apical view demonstrating subvalvular and valvular pulmonary stenosis. E) Corresponding colour image. F) Continuous wave Doppler recording of the flow across the subvalvular and valvular stenosis. LA, left atrium; RA, right atrium.

chamber is usually located anteriorly and superiorly. The size of the VSD (also called *foramen bulboventriculare*) connecting the dominant and the rudimentary chamber should be assessed. Most commonly the ventriculoarterial connections are discordant with the aorta arising anteriorly from the rudimentary RV, also called *outflow chamber*, and the PA from the dominant LV (posteriorly). A non-restrictive bulboventricular foramen is, therefore, required for unobstructed blood flow into the aorta. The degree of PS should be assessed as this has pathophysiologic and prognostic implications.

Patients with functionally univentricular hearts are unsuitable for biventricular repair and a number of palliative procedures have been introduced.

Palliative procedure to reduce pulmonary blood flow

Pulmonary artery banding: *a surgically created stenosis of the main PA* to protect the pulmonary circulation from pulmonary vascular disease due to high blood flow and pressure. This palliative procedure is used when definitive correction of the underlying anomaly is not possible or not immediately advisable.

Palliative procedures to increase pulmonary perfusion

◆ *Blalock–Taussig (BT) shunt:* the classic BT shunt represents an end-to-side anastomosis between the subclavian artery and the ipsilateral PA. The modified BT shunt uses interposition of a graft between the subclavian artery and the PA.

◆ Waterston shunt: side-to-side anastomosis between the ascending aorta and the right PA. Due to the high incidence of pulmonary hypertension this procedure has been largely abandoned.

◆ Potts shunt: side-to-side anastomosis between the descending aorta and the left PA. Due to the high incidence of pulmonary hypertension this procedure has been largely abandoned.

◆ Glenn shunt: palliative procedure to increase pulmonary blood flow, and systemic oxygen saturation. A direct anastomosis is created between the superior vena cava and a PA.

Modifications include the classic Glenn shunt with end-to-end anastomosis of the superior vena cava to the distal end of the divided right PA and the later modified bidirectional Glenn shunt (or partial cavopulmonary connection) with end-to-side anastomosis of the divided superior vena cava to the undivided PA. A Glenn procedure is nowadays commonly performed as part of a staged palliation for univentricular heart, culminating in a Fontan type palliation. In contrast to arterial shunts, a Glenn shunt avoids systemic ventricular volume overload and is therefore preferable. It requires, however, a low PAP.

Fontan type operations

The essence of Fontan type operations is to divert the systemic venous return to the PA, without the interposition of a subpulmonary ventricle. Modifications include:

◆ Classic Fontan: direct anastomosis between RA and PA.

◆ Lateral tunnel Fontan: IVC flow is directed by a baffle within the RA into the lower portion of the divided superior vena cava or the right atrial appendage, which is connected to the PA. The upper part of the superior vena cava is connected to the superior aspect of the PA as in the bidirectional Glenn procedure (⮞ Fig. 22.21). Frequently, a fenestration is created to allow right-to-left shunting to reduce pressure in the systemic venous circuit, at the expense of systemic hypoxaemia. If haemodynamically suitable, the fenestration can be closed later by catheter intervention.

◆ Extracardiac Fontan: IVC blood is directed to the PA via an extracardiac conduit. The superior vena cava is anastomosed to the PA as in the bidirectional Glenn shunt.

Echocardiographic assessment

Depending on thoracic situs, the heart may be located abnormally (e.g. right hemithorax) and this may affect acoustic windows and image views requiring CMR. It is recommended to first assess the cardiac anatomy systematically using a segmental approach (see earlier). The morphology and systolic function of the dominant ventricle should be assessed. The degree of AV

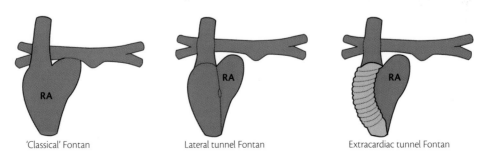

'Classical' Fontan   Lateral tunnel Fontan   Extracardiac tunnel Fontan

Figure 22.21 Modifications of the Fontan operation. Diagram illustrating the so-called classical Fontan operation (atriopulmonary Fontan) with direct connection of the right atrial appendage to the right pulmonary artery (A), the lateral tunnel Fontan (B), where a patch is used to form a tunnel within the right atrium (which can be fenestrated to unload the systemic venous pathway), and an extracardiac tunnel Fontan (C), using a tube graft to connect the inferior caval vein with the pulmonary circulation. RA, right atrium.

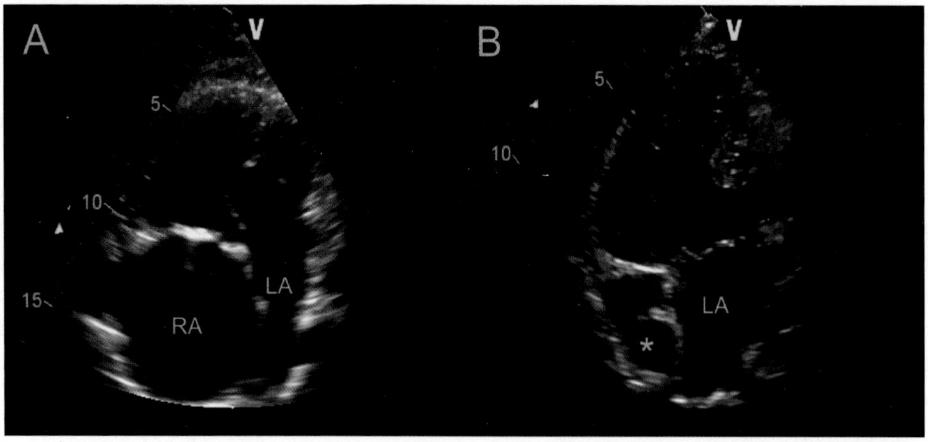

Figure 22.22 Fontan circulation. Apical four-chamber views in a patient with an atriopulmonary Fontan connection (A), showing an enlarged right atrium (RA) in a patient with classical Fontan and (B) the lateral tunnel in a patient with lateral tunnel Fontan. The tunnel is labelled with an asterisk. LA, left atrium; RA, right atrium.

valve regurgitation should be estimated. In addition, significant regurgitation or stenosis of the arterial valves should be assessed. The size and haemodynamic characteristics of VSDs should be estimated based on CD imaging and Doppler gradients.

In patients with PA banding, the gradient should be estimated to provide information on its efficacy or presence of pulmonary hypertension. Arterial shunt flow can be interrogated (supraclavicular for BT, parasternal for central shunts) but velocity measurements are unreliable for estimation of PAP.

In patients after Fontan palliation the patency of cavopulmonary pathways should be evaluated (although this frequently requires TOE and CMR) and the size of fenestrations should be assessed. In patients with classic Fontan the size of the RA may be considerable (Fig. 22.22) and may lead to mechanical obstruction of pulmonary venous flow.

Echocardiography and treatment decision

Although in some patients with univentricular heart echocardiography may provide a comprehensive evaluation, the frequently limited image quality in adults and missing information on PAP and pulmonary vascular resistance make additional CMR or CT and invasive evaluation necessary for treatment decision.

Personal perspective

Due to advances in surgical and interventional treatment over the last six decades, the majority of children born with congenital heart disease now survive to adulthood. As a consequence, the number of adult patients with congenital heart disease is constantly increasing and currently exceeds the number of children with the condition. The majority of patients requires lifelong follow-up at specialized centres and echocardiography has emerged as the main modality for regular assessment of cardiac and valvular function in this setting. Although patients may require additional invasive and non-invasive investigations (such as CMR and CT), many clinical decisions can be based on the results of echocardiographic studies. With improving image quality, new modalities that assess ventricular function (such as strain and strain rate based on tissue Doppler and speckle-tracking imaging), and the advent of 3D echocardiography (offering new ways to assess valvular lesions and to measure ventricular volumes), the role of echocardiography in this evolving population is expected to increase further.

References

1 Li QY, Newbury-Ecob RA, Terrett JA, Wilson DI, Curtis ARJ, Yi CH, et al. Holt-Oram syndrome is caused by mutations in TBX5, a member of the Brachyury (T) gene family. *Nat Genet* 1997; **15**: 21–9.

2 Craig RJ, Selzer A. Natural history and prognosis of atrial septal defect. *Circulation* 1968; **37**:805–15.

3 Anderson RH, Lenox CC, Zuberbuhler JR. Mechanisms of closure of perimembranous ventricular septal defect. *Am J Cardiol* 1983; **52**:341–5.

4 Ramaciotti C, Keren A, Silverman NH. Importance of (perimembranous) ventricular septal aneurysm in the natural history of isolated perimembranous ventricular septal defect. *Am J Cardiol* 1986; **57**:268–72.

5 Samanek M, Goetzova J, Benesova D. Distribution of congenital heart malformations in an autopsied child population. *Int J Cardiol* 1985; **8**:235–50.

6 Rowe RD, Uchida IA. Cardiac malformation in mongolism: a prospective study of 184 mongoloid children. *Am J Med* 1961; **31**:726–35.

7 Aboulhosn J, Child JS. Left ventricular outflow obstruction: subaortic stenosis, bicuspid aortic valve, supravalvar aortic stenosis, and coarctation of the aorta. *Circulation* 2006; **114**:2412–22.

8 Garg V, Muth AN, Ransom JF, Schluterman MK, Barnes R, King IN, *et al*. Mutations in NOTCH1 cause aortic valve disease. *Nature* 2005; **437**:270–4.

9 Chan KL, Ghani M, Woodend K, Burwash IG. Case-controlled study to assess risk factors for aortic stenosis in congenitally bicuspid aortic valve. *Am J Cardiol* 2001; **88**:690–3.

10 Robicsek F, Thubrikar MJ, Cook JW, Fowler B. The congenitally bicuspid aortic valve: how does it function? Why does it fail?. *Ann Thorac Surg* 2004; **77**:177–85.

11 Niwa K, Perloff JK, Bhuta SM, Laks H, Drinkwater DC, Child JS, *et al*. Structural abnormalities of great arterial walls in congenital heart disease: light and electron microscopic analyses. *Circulation* 2001; **103**:393–400.

12 Connolly HM, Huston J, 3rd, Brown RD, Jr., Warnes CA, Ammash NM, Tajik AJ. Intracranial aneurysms in patients with coarctation of the aorta: a prospective magnetic resonance angiographic study of 100 patients. *Mayo Clin Proc* 2003; **78**:1491–9.

13 Brili S, Tousoulis D, Antoniades C, Aggeli C, Roubelakis A, Papathanasiu S, *et al*. Evidence of vascular dysfunction in young patients with successfully repaired coarctation of aorta. *Atherosclerosis* 2005; **182**:97–103.

14 Eicken A, Pensl U, Sebening W, Hager A, Genz T, Schreiber C, *et al*. The fate of systemic blood pressure in patients after effectively stented coarctation. *Eur Heart J* 2006; **27**:1100–5.

15 DeGroff C. Doppler echocardiographic profile and indexes. *J Am Coll Cardiol* 2006; **48**:419; author reply 419–20.

16 Forbes TJ, Garekar S, Amin Z, Zahn EM, Nykanen D, Moore P, *et al*. Procedural results and acute complications in stenting native and recurrent coarctation of the aorta in patients over 4 years of age: a multi-institutional study. *Catheter Cardiovasc Interv* 2007; **70**:276–85.

17 Webber SA, Hatchwell E, Barber JC, Daubeney PE, Crolla JA, Salmon AP, *et al*. Importance of microdeletions of chromosomal region 22q11 as a cause of selected malformations of the ventricular outflow tracts and aortic arch: a three-year prospective study. *J Pediatr* 1996; **129**:26–32.

18 Cromme-Dijkhuis AH, Schasfoort-van Leeuwen M, Bink-Boekens MT, Talsma M. The value of 2-D Doppler echocardiography in the evaluation of asymptomatic patients with Mustard operation for transposition of the great arteries. *Eur Heart J* 1991; **12**:1308–10.

19 Stevenson JG, Kawabori I, Guntheroth WG, Dooley TK, Dillard D. Pulsed Doppler echocardiographic detection of obstruction of systemic venous return after repair of transposition of the great arteries. *Circulation* 1979; **60**:1091–6.

20 Shah D, Patel S, Chintala K, Karpawich PP. Abstract 1974: Pre-electrophysiology catheterization recognition of venous baffle problems in young adults post-mustard repair of transposition of the great arteries. *Circulation* 2009; **120**:S580b.

21 Kaulitz R, Stumper OF, Geuskens R, Sreeram N, Elzenga NJ, Chan CK, *et al*. Comparative values of the precordial and transesophageal approaches in the echocardiographic evaluation of atrial baffle function after an atrial correction procedure. *J Am Coll Cardiol* 1990; **16**:686–94.

Further reading

Anderson RH, Becker AE, Freedom RM, Macartney FJ, Quero-Jimenez M, Shinebourne EA, *et al*. Sequential segmental analysis of congenital heart disease. *Pediatr Cardiol* 1984; **5**:281–7.

Anderson RH, Baker EJ, Redington A, Rigby ML, Penny D, Wernovsky G. *Paediatric Cardiology: Expert Consult – Online and Print*, 3rd ed. Edinburgh: Churchill Livingstone, 2009.

Baumgartner H. ESC guidelines for the management of grown-up congenital heart disease. The Task Force on the Management of Grown-up Congenital Heart Disease of the European Society of Cardiology (ESC). *Eur Heart J* 2010 Aug 27 [Epub ahead of print].

Campbell M. Natural history of atrial septal defect. *Br Heart J* 1970; **32**:820–6.

Ferencz C RJ, Loffredo CA, Magee CM. The Epidemiology of Congenital Heart Disease, The Baltimore-Washington Infant Study (1981–1989). In: *Perspectives in Pediatric Cardiology*, vol .4. MountKisco, NY: Futura Publishing Co. Inc, 1993.

Gerbode F, Hultgren H, Melrose D, Osborn J. Syndrome of left ventricular-right atrial shunt; successful surgical repair of defect in five cases, with observation of bradycardia on closure. *Ann Surg* 1958; **148**:433–46.

Hager A, Kanz S, Kaemmerer H, Schreiber C, Hess J. Coarctation Long-term Assessment (COALA): significance of arterial hypertension in a cohort of 404 patients up to 27 years after surgical repair of isolated coarctation of the aorta, even in the absence of restenosis and prosthetic material. *J Thorac Cardiovasc Surg* 2007; **134**:738–45.

Ho S, McCarthy KP, Josen M, Rigby ML. Anatomic-echocardiographic correlates: an introduction to normal and congenitally malformed hearts. *Heart* 2001; **86**(Suppl 2):II3–11.

Houston A, Hillis S, Lilley S, Richens T, Swan L. Echocardiography in adult congenital heart disease. *Heart* 1998; **80**(Suppl 1):S12–26.

Inglessis I, Landzberg MJ. Interventional catheterization in adult congenital heart disease. *Circulation* 2007; **115**:1622–33.

Kidd L, Driscoll DJ, Gersony WM, Hayes CJ, Keane JF, O'Fallon WM, et al. Second natural history study of congenital heart defects. Results of treatment of patients with ventricular septal defects. *Circulation* 1993; **87**:I38–51.

Lindqvist P, Calcuttea A, Henein M. Echocardiography in the assessment of right heart function. *Eur J Echocardiogr* 2008; **9**: 225–34.

Tan JL, Babu-Narayan SV, Henein MY, Mullen M, Li W. Doppler echocardiographic profile and indexes in the evaluation of aortic coarctation in patients before and after stenting. *J Am Coll* Cardiol 2005; **46**:1045–53.

Webb G, Gatzoulis MA. Atrial septal defects in the adult: recent progress and overview. *Circulation* 2006; **114**:1645–53.

⮑ For additional multimedia materials please visit the online version of the book (🖰 http://escecho.oxfordmedicine.com).

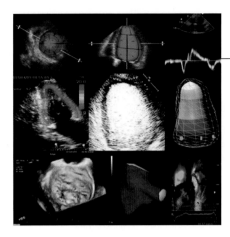

CHAPTER 23

Perioperative echocardiography

R. Feneck and F. Guarracino

Contents

Summary

Perioperative echocardiography is one of the fastest growing areas of echocardiography. Although transthoracic imaging has a role, intraoperative imaging is mostly undertaken using transoesophageal echocardiography (TOE).

The indications for perioperative echo have recently been re-evaluated, resulting in recognition of the ubiquitous benefit in patients undergoing cardiac surgery, and recognition of the value in non-cardiac surgery and critical care also.

Although TOE is safe, it should be remembered that there may be a greater risk of traumatic damage to the soft tissues in anaesthetized patients who cannot complain of pain during probe insertion.

Perioperative imaging should be used to confirm and refine the preoperative diagnosis, detect new or unsuspected pathology, adjust the anaesthetic and surgical plan, and assess the results of surgical intervention. Using imaging to optimize myocardial function is a constantly developing technique, and one which may ensure that patients leave the operating room in the best possible condition. The use of perioperative echo in some procedures, for example, in mitral repair, is now regarded as so valuable that it is arguable that perioperative TOE should be mandatory in these cases.

Indications for perioperative transoesophageal echocardiography

Modern perioperative echocardiography has developed largely as a result of the development of transoesophageal echocardiography (TOE). The value of TOE was established in the 1980s both as an outpatient diagnostic tool, and for intraoperative monitoring of left ventricular (LV) function and air embolism. Further development was accelerated by the value of TOE in establishing the diagnosis of aortic dissection,[1,2] and the development of a high resolution TOE probe with pulsed and colour flow Doppler technology.

In 2010, new recommendations were published in Europe and North America. These reflect contemporary surgical practice where both the age and clinical state of patients undergoing cardiac surgery represents a greater risk than in earlier years. In the light of this changing clinical environment and the continuing publication of

Table 23.1 Provided appropriate personnel, skills and technology are available; it is recommended that:

- **TOE should be used** in adult patients undergoing cardiac surgery or surgery to the thoracic aorta under general anaesthesia

- **TOE may be used** in patients undergoing specific types of major surgery where its value has been repeatedly documented. These include neurosurgery at risk from venous thromboembolism, liver transplantation, lung transplantation, and major vascular surgery, including vascular trauma

- **TOE may be used** in patients undergoing major non-cardiac surgery in whom severe or life-threatening haemodynamic disturbance is either present or threatened

- **TOE may be used** in major non-cardiac surgery in patients who are at a high cardiac risk, including severe cardiac valve disease, severe coronary heart disease, or heart failure

- **TOE may be used** in the critical care patient in whom severe or life-threatening haemodynamic disturbance is present and unresponsive to treatment, or in patients in whom new or ongoing cardiac disease is suspected

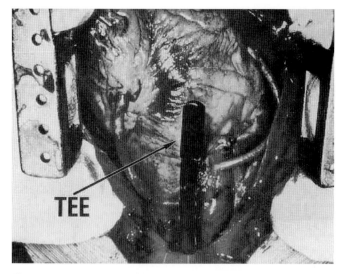

Figure 23.1 Direct trauma following insertion of the probe. TOE probe following perforation of the left side of the hypopharynx, with the probe in the upper anterior mediastinum. The patient was a female aged 75 years undergoing emergency CABG surgery. The probe was passed during surgery after difficulty in weaning from cardiopulmonary bypass. The perforation was identified and repaired, and the patient discharged from hospital. Reproduced with permission from Spahn DR, Schmid S, Carrel T, Pasch T, Schmid ER. Hypopharynx perforation by a transesophageal echocardiography probe. *Anesthesiology* 1995; **82**:581–3.

evidence outlining the value of intraoperative TOE for adult cardiac surgery, both sets of guidelines take a broader approach, recommending perioperative TOE in all adult patients undergoing cardiac surgery and surgery to the thoracic aorta[3,4] (⊃ Table 23.1).

Safety and complications of perioperative transoesophageal echocardiography

In an analysis of intraoperative complications associated with TOE, Kallmeyer et al. found an overall complication rate of 0.2%.[5] More recent data suggests a rate of major complications of less than 0.1%[6] to 0.4%[7] and a mortality from 0.01–0.02%.[8]

In a perioperative setting, TOE will usually be undertaken under general anaesthesia or deep sedation. In both situations, the airway will need to be secured, usually with an endotracheal tube, and anaesthesia (e.g. during surgery) or deep sedation (e.g. in the intensive care unit) will in any case be required for purposes other than TOE. There may be safety issues related to the passage of the probe in anaesthetized patients. Care should be taken to avoid trauma to the lips, teeth, and soft tissues of the oropharynx. It is preferable if the probe can be passed under controlled conditions before surgery, rather than after the patient has been *prepped and draped*.

Although the routine use of antibiotic prophylaxis in patients undergoing TOE is not recommended,[9–12] in perioperative TOE antibiotic prophylaxis is always given for surgical cover.

Perioperative TOE may be associated with both minor and severe complications. Gastrointestinal injury and perforation are rare but serious complications, and may be associated with direct and indirect trauma.[7,8,13–15] Direct trauma may be more

common following blind insertion of the probe, and it is always prudent to insert the probe at the beginning of the surgical procedure and under controlled conditions (⊃ Fig. 23.1). Poor matching of the probe size to the patient (i.e. the use of a large probe in a small patient), excessive flexion of the probe tip, and pre-existing oesophageal pathology have also been implicated in causing oesophageal trauma and perforation.

Trauma and perforation are the major risks at the cricopharyngeal constriction (C6) and at the lower oesophageal sphincter (T10/11), whereas there is a risk of vascular damage to the aortic arch (T4/5) in the case of an aneurysm. There are over 15 cases of oesophageal perforation reported in the literature, almost all occurring in patients undergoing cardiac surgery. Pharyngeal or oesophageal perforation carries a 10–25% mortality, and late onset of symptoms (>24h) may be more common than early onset (<24h). Pre-existing gastrointestinal pathology may be contributive, but it should be noted that difficulty in advancing the probe and poor image quality are not invariable findings in patients with oesophageal perforation.

Although haemorrhage may occur as a result of lacerations near the gastro-oesophageal junction or in the gastric cardia,[16,17] the risk of gastrointestinal haemorrhage in cardiac surgery patients is approximately 2% independent of the use of TOE.[18] Dysphagia (difficulty) and odynophagia (pain) are less serious and more difficult to predict in cardiac surgery patients. Failure to pass the probe may occur even in anaesthetized patients, and traumatic passage of the probe appears more likely in the anaesthetized than the awake patient.

In view of the new wider indications for perioperative TOE, close attention should be given to those situations and patients in whom the procedure is contraindicated. Absolute contraindications to TOE include previous oesophageal surgery, major oesophageal disease (stricture, diverticula, tumour, oesophagitis, Mallory–Weiss tear, oesophageal varices) and external vascular compression by a thoracic aortic aneurysm. However, the issue of contraindication to TOE probe insertion should be seen as a risk–benefit ratio, and in some specific circumstances, for example, liver transplantation, TOE may be used even in presence of oesophageal varices since the benefits of the procedure may outweigh the risks.[19]

The perioperative transoesophageal echocardiography exam

Aims of the exam

Recent guidelines and recommendations for performing perioperative TOE [3,4] and the increasing availability of both suitable equipment and trained personnel, have meant that in many institutions perioperative TOE is a routine procedure undertaken in the majority of adult cardiac surgical patients. It is essential to gain the most benefit out of each examination, and to that end recent publications have made recommendations as to the purpose of perioperative TOE.[3] These are described next.

Confirm and refine the preoperative diagnosis

A perioperative TOE exam should not be the first or only echo exam undertaken on a cardiac patient before surgery. In certain emergency situations, for example, in aortic dissection, it may be the most important echo exam used not only to identify the entry point of the dissection but also to identify involvement of the aortic valve (AoV). In many cases the preoperative echo exam will have provided the diagnosis for surgery, and in others, most notably in CABG patients, a preoperative echo will have been undertaken to grade left ventricular (LV) function and exclude any other relevant pathology. Confirmation of the preoperative diagnosis may be useful in patients undergoing mitral valve (MV) surgery, where the exact nature of the lesion may affect the detail of the surgical plan. It is important to recognize that general anaesthesia may alter the severity of mitral regurgitation (MR), which in turn may lead to an erroneous reappraisal of the severity of MR and the need for operative repair.[20] The state of LV function may also have altered from the time of the initial diagnostic angiogram, and this information may be important also for surgical planning. Patients who are scheduled for AoV surgery may have little need of confirmation of the diagnosis in the immediate preoperative period. However, abnormalities of AoV function may have relevance to patients undergoing surgery for other reasons, and once again this information may affect surgical planning.

Detect new or unsuspected pathology

Although a preoperative echo exam should have excluded other pathology, it is clear that new or unsuspected significant pathology may be revealed. Klein et al.[21] reviewed 2473 cases undertaken over a 3-year period. A change in the planned surgical procedure was documented in 312 (15%) cases. In one-third of these (96; 31%) the change was unpredictable; that is, the intraoperative TOE identified a new and unsuspected finding that changed the surgical plan. The number of predictable changes increased in the latter stages of the study as TOE was increasingly used to guide the operative intervention (2004–5, 8%; vs. 2006–7 13%; p = 0.025). Previous studies have alluded to the value of intraoperative TOE to detect new pathology in a small percentage of cases.[22]

The problem for the patient who is scheduled for coronary artery bypass graft (CABG) surgery and is found to have significant, but not severe, valve dysfunction has recently been highlighted.[23] By established criteria, valve surgery in such a patient would not be justified as a primary procedure. However, in the situation where a patient is already undergoing CABG surgery, the dilemma is whether to undertake valve surgery at the same time as the CABG, or to wait for the valve dysfunction to deteriorate further and bring the patient back for re-do surgery some years later. This is a complex problem calling both for accurate diagnostic information and experienced clinical judgement.

Adjust the anaesthetic and surgical plan

Any new or refined information gleaned from the perioperative echo exam should be communicated throughout the surgical team and appropriate decisions made accordingly. Whilst this may involve changes to the surgical plan, more frequently it will involve altering loading conditions and optimizing contractility during the procedure and thus increasing the chances of a good surgical outcome.[22] One clear benefit of perioperative echo lies in its use as a functional monitor throughout surgery. This can only be achieved if there is a member of the operating room team, usually the anaesthesiologist, with appropriate echo skills who is constantly present during surgery.

Assess the results of surgical intervention

Following cardiac surgery under cardioplegic arrest, LV function may be unstable for some time afterwards. Patients undergoing valve surgery may also need some time to stabilize, and valve gradients and the nature and severity of apparent valve leaks may also change. For these reasons, a perioperative echo exam immediately following surgery has been undervalued in the past. However, modern cardiac surgery, experience in dealing with cardiac surgery patients over many years, and a clear understanding of the early postoperative echo appearances of countless cardiac surgery patients should have eliminated these concerns. Although it is clear that the echocardiographic findings at the time of chest closure may change later, much can be gained from an examination at this time, both to identify the early results of surgery and to establish a baseline that should be consulted postoperatively. In each case the examination should be directed towards the results of the surgical intervention and the overall state of cardiac function.

The conduct of a perioperative transoesophageal echocardiography exam

Guidelines for performing a comprehensive intraoperative multiplane TOE examination were first published in 1999. These guidelines include a set of 20 cross-sectional views of the heart and great vessels[24] and they have since formed the basis of perioperative TOE. Since they are based on patients with relatively normal anatomy, the recommendations for acquiring the views may not be accurate in the presence of severe structural heart disease. In complex cases a series of non-standard views may be necessary. Even in normal patients, some minor adjustments to the probe depth and positioning, and the transducer angulation are frequently necessary. Despite these limitations, the standard views will be sufficient for a comprehensive examination in the majority of adult patients, and form the basis of any modified views that may be necessary in complex cases. An overview of the 20 standard views described by Shanewise et al.[24] is shown in ➲ Fig. 23.2.

The title of each view, and their echo-anatomical correlation is part of a standard nomenclature. The details for acquiring each view are described in ➲ Chapter 4. A perioperative TOE exam may differ in important respects from a TOE exam in the cardiac laboratory. In the latter situation, a TTE exam will usually have been performed very recently, and the TOE exam may be undertaken to answer a single question, or to further examine one area of cardiac anatomy. Often the need for a comprehensive TOE exam is absent, and a comprehensive exam is undertaken by combining the observation so of the TTE and the TOE exam, which may often be reported as a single study.

The abbreviated transoesophageal echocardiography exam in the operating room

The operating room is not an echo-friendly environment. Pressure for both space and time is at a premium.

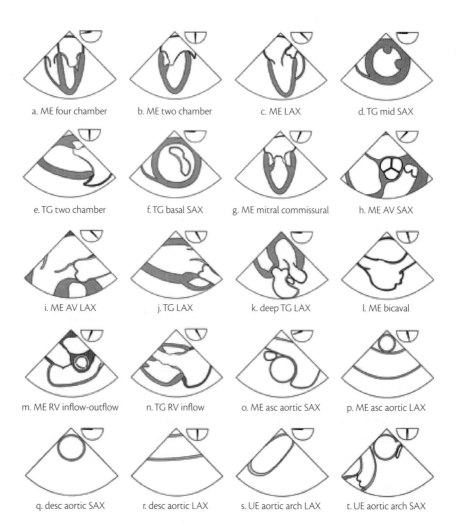

Figure 23.2 Recommended TOE views. Twenty standard cross-sectional views comprising the recommended comprehensive transoesophageal examination.

a. ME four chamber b. ME two chamber c. ME LAX d. TG mid SAX

e. TG two chamber f. TG basal SAX g. ME mitral commissural h. ME AV SAX

i. ME AV LAX j. TG LAX k. deep TG LAX l. ME bicaval

m. ME RV inflow-outflow n. TG RV inflow o. ME asc aortic SAX p. ME asc aortic LAX

q. desc aortic SAX r. desc aortic LAX s. UE aortic arch LAX t. UE aortic arch SAX

Although recent guidelines on continuous quality improvement have recommended that a full TOE exam be undertaken whenever possible,[25] an abbreviated study may be indicated and useful. Such a study should yield the maximum amount of information in the least possible time. One example is shown in ➲ Fig. 23.3,[26] although a patient-centred approach will be necessary to ensure that each study is appropriate to the individual patient.

The concept of an abbreviated study has spawned many others. Valuable additions to the initial approach include transgastric long-axis views to enable accurate calculation of LV stroke output and AoV area, and views of the descending aorta. These alternatives are included in ➲ Table 23.2[27] which represents a routine examination which we frequently use in the absence of any further pathology. It should be noted that again the sequence described is by no means mandatory.

Every study should be recorded, archived, and reported. Modern echo machines may record echo clips digitally, and these clips may be used to make measurements and calculations off line once the study is completed. This is very useful, since the perioperative echocardiographer can initially devote themselves to acquiring the best images without the need to hurry through the calculations.

The abbreviated study described previously has not concentrated on any single pathology or anatomical structure, but it clearly is able to fulfil the criteria of a basic study—that is, to detect markedly abnormal ventricular filling or function, to identify extensive myocardial ischaemia or infarction, to detect severe valve dysfunction, identify cardiac masses or thrombi, to detect large air embolism, large pericardial effusions, and major abnormalities of the great vessels.[24] Interpatient variability will always be a factor on acquiring the necessary views speedily, and experts have underlined the need for concentrating on the most pressing problem first.[24] But we usually find it possible to examine and record the images as described before the onset of surgical diathermy damages the image quality.

Reporting perioperative echo studies

Every perioperative echo study should be accompanied by a written report. The aims of the report, and recommendations

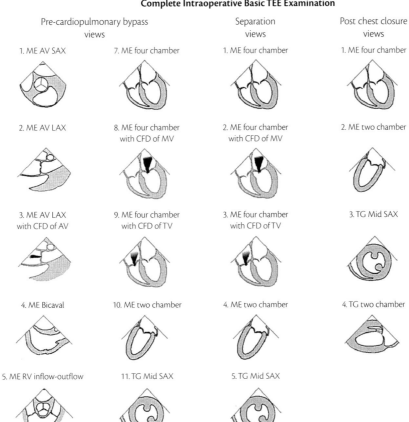

Figure 23.3 Example of TOE abbreviated study. Recommended abbreviated intraoperative TOE study.[26] Reproduced with permission from Miller JP, Lambert AS, Shapiro WA, et al. The adequacy of basic intraoperative transesophageal echocardiography performed by experienced anaesthesiologists. *Anesth Analg* 2001; **92**: 1103–10.

Table 23.2 Abbreviated study for patients undergoing cardiac surgery

View	Modality	Structures	
1. ME 4-chamber	2D	LV: inferoseptal and lateral walls, LV, LA, RV, RA dimensions, atrial septum, mitral and tricuspid valves	Pre - & post- surgery
	CFD	Mitral and tricuspid valves	Pre- & post- surgery
	PWD	Mitral and tricuspid blood flow	Pre-surgery
2. ME 2-chamber	2D	LV: inferior and anterior walls, mitral valve, LA appendage	Pre-post-surgery
3. ME LAX	2D	LV: anteroseptal and inferolateral walls Mitral valve esp. prolapse, aortic valve	Pre-& post-surgery
4. Bicaval view	2D	Superior and inferior vena cavae, RA, TV, atrial septum.	Pre-surgery
	CWD	TV	Pre-surgery
5. MO AV SAX	2D	AV, coronary arteries, LA, RA	Pre-surgery
6. MO RV inflow-outflow	2D	TV,RA, RV, PV, PA	Pre-surgery
	CFD	TV, PV	Pre-surgery
7. MO AV LAX	2D	AV, aortic root, LVOT	Pre-surgery
	M-mode	LVOT dimension (where possible)	Pre-surgery
	CFD	AV	Pre-surgery
8. Descending aorta S/LAX	2D	Descending aorta	Pre-surgery
9. Transgastric mid cavity SAX	2D	LV wall segments (mid-cavity anterior, anteroseptal, inferoseptal, inferior, inferolateral, lateral)	Pre-& post surgery
	M-mode	LV mid-cavity dimension wall thickness	Pre-surgery
10. Transgastric LAX (deep transgastric for CWD)	2D	LV anterior and inferior walls, MV papillary muscles and chordae	Pre-& post surgery
	CWD	AV blood flow	Pre-surgery
	PWD	LVOT blood flow	Pre-surgery

CWD, continuous wave Doppler; ME, mid-(o)esophageal; SAX, short-axis; LAX, long-axis; PWD, pulsed wave Doppler.

to the content and structure of the report have recently been published.[28]

Specific issues in perioperative echo

The right heart

TOE imaging of the structures of the right heart is dealt with in detail elsewhere in this book (see Chapter 4) Perioperative imaging of the right heart may be useful in order to detect the following:

Identify intravascular devices and exclude thrombus and vegetations

All cardiac surgery patients have central venous catheters placed, and many also have pulmonary artery (PA) catheters. The correct positioning of these devices can be easily checked by echocardiography, particularly using the bicaval view. Chronically sick patients may have longstanding devices in situ, including transvenous pacing wires. Both the correct positioning of the catheters and their freedom from thrombus or vegetation should be checked.

Exclude a patent foramen ovale or atrial septal defect

In a study of over 13 000 patients a review of perioperative TOE studies revealed an incidence of 17% of PFO in the adult population.[29] Although the incidence of secundum atrial septal defect (ASD) is considerably less, it is the most common of the remaining ASDs. In the absence of symptoms, the need for surgically closing a PFO is highly debatable. However, in the cardiac surgery context, any open chamber procedure in the presence of even a PFO may lead to the development of an air lock during cardiopulmonary bypass unless a bicaval cannulation technique is used to ensure secure venous drainage from the vena cavae.

Measure right atrial size and exclude masses

A baseline estimate of right atrial size may be useful for comparison in the later postoperative period. However, this is not an easy measurement to make with TOE and measurements of right atrial area are usually made by TTE.

Identify the coronary sinus

Although not easily visualized by a standard TOE view, the coronary sinus may be seen by advancing the TOE probe 3–5cm from the mid-oesophageal four-chamber view. The tricuspid valve (TV) should remain in focus, and the coronary sinus is visible just above the LV wall which is seen in short or oblique axis on the right of the display.

The coronary sinus may be dilated in rare conditions including a left-sided SVC, but more practically identification of the coronary sinus is more important in perioperative practice in order to facilitate cannulation and the delivery of retrograde cardioplegia solution.

Identify the leaflets of the tricuspid valve and the size of the tricuspid annulus

Clearly in patients undergoing surgery to the TV, a detailed evaluation will already have taken place. However, all patients undergoing surgery for left-sided endocarditis should have their TV screened perioperatively, in order to exclude vegetations on the TV. The presence and severity of tricuspid regurgitation (TR) may be assessed using the standard views for viewing the TV. Colour Doppler (CD) may help to identify the direction of the jet, and pulse wave (PW) Doppler may be useful in identifying the peak velocity. Estimation of TR, and also the tricuspid annular size, may also be useful information in surgery of the MV. Recent evidence suggests that a more aggressive approach to TR in patients with left sided valve surgery may be required.[30]

Measure the size of the right ventricle, and identify right ventricular contractility including motion abnormalities of the right ventricular free wall

RV size and function may give important insights into the severity of left-sided contractile and valve dysfunction. Enlargement of the RV with tricuspid annular dilation, flattening, and eventual leftward displacement of the interventricular septum (IVS) are all useful indicators which are easily identifiable.

Although LV dysfunction is rightly recognized as important following cardiopulmonary bypass, in fact RV dysfunction is also highly important and, when sustained, may seriously compromise outcome. The RV is susceptible both to poor cardioplegic protection, and also to early post-bypass air embolus in intracavity procedures, due to the right coronary ostium being located superiorly and therefore a potential conduit for air bubbles. Monitoring of RV size and function is an important part of early post bypass monitoring in every adult cardiac surgery patient.

Estimate systolic pulmonary artery pressure

Measurement of the velocity of a regurgitant jet across the TV will enable the calculation of the pressure gradient across the valve (see ⊃ Chapters 5 and 11). The most useful view to measure the velocity of the regurgitant jet will be determined by its direction, but frequently a modified mid-oesophageal four-chamber view, or the bicaval view will be useful.

The mitral valve

TOE is particularly useful for examining the mitral valve. A protocol for examining the mitral valve using TOE is given in ⊃ Chapter 4.

Intraoperative TOE of the mitral valve

MV dysfunction may occur either as a result of primary pathological processes involving the mitral apparatus, or secondary to alterations in LV structure and function, or both. As a result, intraoperative evaluation of the mitral valve is important in all adult cardiac surgical patients. MV function is often an important guide to LV function before and after surgery. Many patients who are scheduled for CABG surgery may also, on the basis of a preoperative evaluation, be scheduled for MV repair. Care should be taken therefore when re-evaluating such patients intraoperatively; the degree of MR is often underestimated during intraoperative evaluation, and at the very least the haemodynamic parameters should be ensured to reflect the preoperative awake state.[20]

Mitral valve repair

TOE examination of mitral valve apparatus

Intraoperative TOE is aimed at elucidating the mechanism of valve dysfunction, and therefore aiding surgical planning.

Intraoperative evaluation of the regurgitant MV apparatus is performed twice; once before cardiopulmonary bypass, and again after weaning from cardiopulmonary bypass (⊃ Table 23.3).

A systematic examination of the entire MV apparatus should always be performed. This comprises mitral leaflets, the annulus, the subvalvular apparatus (including cordae and papillary muscles), and the LV.[31] Then the regurgitant jet(s) should be examined, by CD evaluation.[32,33] The examination is performed using standard views.[24]

Leaflet mobility may be described using the terminology introduced by Carpentier[34] (see ⊃ Chapter 14b). The two-dimensional (2D) functional evaluation should pay attention to

Table 23.3 Perioperative echocardiography in mitral valve disease

The pre-bypass examination should aim to:
Confirm preoperative diagnosis
Evaluate morphology and function of the mitral valve apparatus
Determine the mechanism of regurgitation
Assess the severity of regurgitation
Assess the feasibility of repair
Check for other cardiac structural and functional abnormalities

The objectives of post-bypass examination are:
Assessment the result of the surgical procedure
Evaluation of ventricular function
Detection of complications

both apposition and coaptation. In normal apposition, both leaflets lie on the same plane at annular level. A coaptation length greater than 6mm is necessary for valvular competence. The precise origin of the regurgitant jet from the closure line and the direction of the jet itself, add useful information to understanding the mechanism of the dysfunction (◑ Fig. 23.4). Measurement of the leaflet dimensions is helpful in the pre-bypass assessment. In a normal valve the ratio of anterior to posterior leaflet height is 3:1 and the ratio of the anterior leaflet length to the anteroposterior annulus diameter is 2:3.

The anteroposterior diameter of the annulus is the most important measurement for the surgeon approaching a repair. Annular shape and motion should also be evaluated, including the presence of calcification, which is more frequently seen in the posterior part of the annulus.

The measurement of the anteroposterior diameter is best performed in views which interrogate the anteroposterior axis of the valve (usually the mid-oesophageal long axis view at about 120 degrees). The commissural diameter can be measured in the two chamber long axis view at around 60 degrees. By comparing the anteroposterior diameter to the commissural it is possible to demonstrate the annular shape. Under normal conditions the annulus is oval and the two diameters are in a ratio of 2:3 with the shortest diameter in the anteroposterior plane (◑ Fig. 23.5). When posterior annulus dilation occurs, both diameters show the same value, the annulus becoming circular in shape. The annulus shortens by about 30% of its length during systole, mainly in the posterior part, contributing to mitral competence during the systolic phase of the cardiac cycle. This systolic change can be evaluated by measuring the diameter both in systole and diastole, or by sampling the annulus with tissue Doppler (TD). This evaluation is helpful in the setting of ischaemic MR, and may help to decide if moderate MR will benefit from annuloplasty combined with revascularization, or from revascularization alone.

Mid-oesophageal views and the transgastric long-axis view allow good visualization and evaluation of chordae tendinae. These views may demonstrate elongated, shortened, or ruptured cordae. Elongated cordae or ruptured secondary cordae may result in leaflet prolapse or billowing. Rupture of a primary cord may result in a flail lesion (◑ Fig. 23.6); a shortened cord may cause restricted leaflet excursion. The same views allow visualization and evaluation of any abnormality of the papillary muscles, including fibrosis, calcification or rupture.

Evaluation of the LV should always complete the systematic perioperative assessment of the mitral apparatus. Wall motion abnormalities (WMAs) or aneurysm may cause MR due to altered ventricular geometry in ischaemic disease.[35]

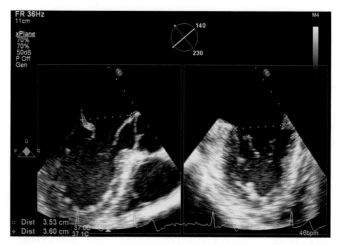

Figure 23.5 Annular diameter of the mitral valve. Anteroposterior and commissural diameter measurement, respectively in long axis view at 140 degrees and in commissural view at 60 degrees.

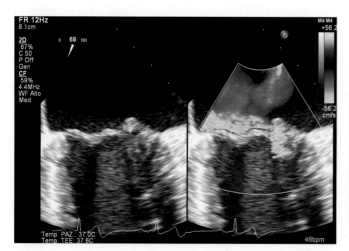

Figure 23.4 Mitral valve regurgitation. Mid-oesophageal two-chamber view. The colour Doppler evaluation reveals a regurgitant jet in the anterior commissural area confirming the P1 prolapse.

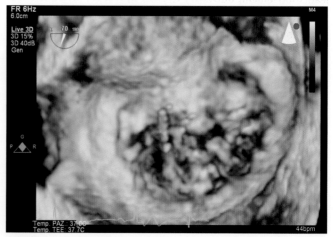

Figure 23.6 Rupture of a mitral valve primary cord. 3D short-axis view of the MV showing a ruptured cordae.

Ischaemic mitral regurgitation

In patients with coronary artery disease (CAD) and MR the valve itself is usually morphologically normal. The regurgitation is caused by ventricular dysfunction often associated with changes in LV geometry.[34]

The role of intraoperative TOE is:

◆ To measure the anteroposterior annular diameter in the appropriate view.

◆ To assess annular motion.

◆ To demonstrate outward papillary muscle displacement with increased interpapillary distance, increased tethering forces on the edges of the leaflets, and apical displacement of the coaptation point.

◆ To distinguish between symmetric and asymmetric tethering.

Application of TOE information to surgical repair

Annular contractility may be assessed by measuring anteroposterior diameter, by TD imaging sampling of posterior annulus velocities, and also by using low-dose dobutamine or atrial pacing with epicardial electrodes.[36] Under such stress conditions, annular systolic shortening and myocardial velocities in the annular region are assessed. Annular shortening by one-third and an increase in systolic velocity indicate the presence of viable myocardium and predict recovery after revascularization.[37] In this case the patient may be treated by revascularization without annuloplasty.[37] If no systolic shortening and no increase of systolic velocity is produced by dobutamine or atrial pacing, a negative predictive value can be attributed to the echo information. This suggests the need for revascularization plus annuloplasty. In ischaemic MR a basal anteroposterior annular diameter greater than 34mm has a similar negative predictive value, and stress testing is unnecessary.

In chronic ischaemic cardiomyopathy, TOE shows restricted leaflet movement, outward displacement of the papillary muscles, and the downward displacement of the coaptation point. It is possible to measure the tenting area and the coaptation depth (the distance from the annular plane to the coaptation point), thus facilitating grading of the severity of the tethering pattern. A tenting area greater than 4cm^2, and a coaptation depth greater than 1.1cm are considered to be severe, and in many centres these are contraindications to annuloplasty and may indicate a need for surgical LV reconstruction.

In symmetric tethering it is often possible to detect an akinetic anterior wall or global LV dysfunction, and CD interrogation shows a centrally originating and centrally directed regurgitant jet. It is important not to mistake the central jet of symmetric tethering for one caused by annular dilation in a Carpentier's class I lesion. In asymmetric tethering a WMA of the inferior wall is usually seen, and thus the regurgitant jet is usually posteriorly directed.

These data help to understand the mechanism of the ischaemic MR, and guide surgical decision making.[38,39]

Feasibility of repair

The feasibility of MV repair depends on valve function and morphology, as assessed by TOE before cardiopulmonary bypass. In modern practice the only contraindication to repair of a MV with organic disease is extensive calcification of the annulus and/or leaflets. In the setting of ischaemic/functional regurgitation, the limiting factor is severe LV dysfunction with inadequate viable myocardium.

Post-bypass assessment of the repair

After the repair, a systematic evaluation of the MV should be undertaken to detect any residual regurgitant jet. The examination is performed after complete weaning from cardiopulmonary bypass, and only after preload, afterload and systolic function have been stabilized (➲ Fig. 23.7). If there is any residual MR after the repair, the severity and the mechanism of the residual regurgitation need to be assessed. Any residual jet should be compared with the pre-bypass evaluation to evaluate its severity. The haemodynamic conditions immediately after cardiopulmonary bypass should be corrected before any decision on grading of the severity of regurgitation is undertaken,[40,41] in order to avoid underestimating the severity of regurgitation. A trivial or mild residual jet is acceptable. If the residual regurgitation is greater, a decision has to be taken to either accept the albeit inadequate result, to go for a second pump run to perform a second repair, or to replace the valve.

A systematic exam should detect the mechanism of a failing repair. For example, in a case of fibroelastic deficiency with leaflet flail repaired with artificial cords, residual prolapse with regurgitation may be due to the artificial cords being too long; or in a valve with degenerative disease treated with quadrangular resection and annuloplasty, a residual jet could be due to an

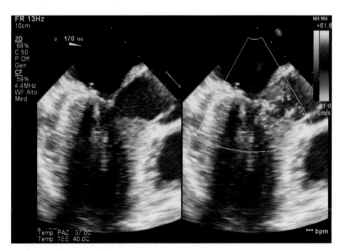

Figure 23.7 Post-bypass assessment of the repair. Post-bypass control of mitral valve repair showing no residual regurgitation.

incomplete annuloplasty. When a complex repair has been performed and moderate residual regurgitation is detected, it is important to consider the risk of a second pump run, for example, in the presence of advanced age and severe LV dysfunction.

Complications of mitral valve repair

The post bypass TOE may identify such complications and guide in treating them:

◆ Residual regurgitation.

◆ Systolic anterior motion (SAM) of the leaflets with dynamic LV outflow tract (LVOT) obstruction.

◆ Mitral stenosis.

◆ Coronary artery damage.

◆ Annular avulsion.

◆ Aortic valve damage.

Limitations

The effect of the relative vasodilation and hypotension produced in the anaesthetized and mechanically ventilated supine patient makes accurate assessment of the severity of MR more difficult. The degree of regurgitation is always reduced by anaesthesia and this must be taken into account when grading the severity of MR.[41] Steps should always be taken to ensure that the haemodynamic conditions during assessment mimic those of the awake state.

Left ventricular assessment

Perioperative evaluation of LV function enables us to obtain baseline information on ventricular function, detect acute changes of systolic and diastolic function, and guide treatment. Intraoperative TOE is recommended in both cardiac and some non-cardiac surgery patients, and particularly in case of haemodynamic instability.[42] In the case of patients undergoing surgery for ischaemic heart disease, perioperative TOE may be invaluable as shown in ➲ Table 23.4.

As an intraoperative monitor, TOE is unique in providing high-quality real-time imaging, thereby monitoring regional and global systolic LV function, and diastolic function also. A systematic study of the LV can be accomplished by M-mode, 2D, Doppler flow and TD investigation, as described in ➲ Chapter 8. In perioperative practice, wall motion abnormalities (WMAs) are not uncommon and may be related to preload,[43] but a significant change may be an indication for considering either further coronary revascularization, or improving coronary blood flow with an intra-aortic balloon pump or relevant pharmacologic therapy.

Study of systolic function

The intraoperative assessment of systolic function is mainly based on the detection and quantification of changes in LV

Table 23.4 Role of perioperative echo in patients undergoing surgery for ischaemic heart disease

Patients undergoing CABG surgery
Evaluate regional and global performance before surgery
Monitor the LV in the pre-bypass phase and identify any WMA due to ischaemia
Monitor the effects of treatment
Evaluate the effects of surgery after weaning from cardiopulmonary bypass
Patients undergoing OPCAB surgery
Evaluate regional and global performance before surgery
Identify the need for intracoronary shunting during grafting
Where possible monitor regional LV wall motion during grafting
Identify recovery of wall motion at the end of each period of grafting and cardiac dislocation
Evaluate the effects of surgery at the end of the procedure
LV reconstruction
Identify preoperative LV function, including the presence of associated conditions, i.e. mitral regurgitation, LV thrombus
Confirm LV dimensions to aid reconstruction.
Optimize LV performance following surgery.

CABG, coronary artery bypass graft; OPCAB, off-pump coronary artery by-pass.

chamber diameters, areas and volumes both in systole and diastole (see ➲ Chapter 8).

Fractional shortening can be obtained using the transgastric short-axis view of the LV at mid-papillary level, by M-mode measurement of the difference between end-diastolic and end-systolic diameters normalized for end-diastolic diameter (➲ Fig. 23.8).

Fractional area change (FAC) is obtained in the transgastric short-axis view at mid-papillary level by 2D measurement of

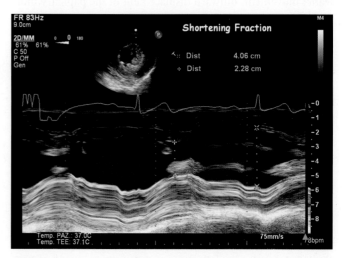

Figure 23.8 Fractional shortening assessment. Transgastric short axis M-mode study showing the calculation of shortening fraction

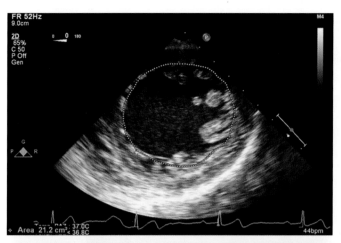

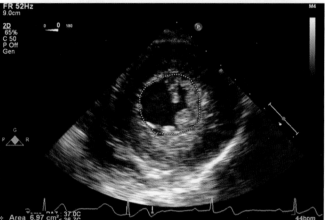

Figure 23.9 Fractional area change assessment. Transgastric short-axis views at end systole and end diastole for calculation of fractional area of change.

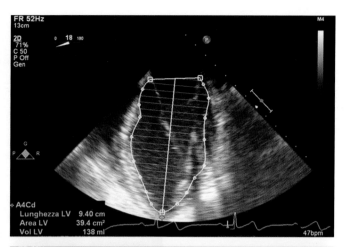

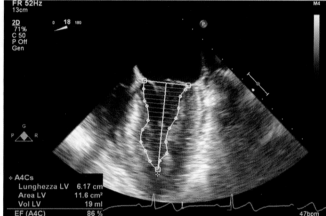

Figure 23.10 Ejection fraction calculation. Mid-oesophageal long-axis view showing calculation of ejection fraction.

end-diastolic and end-systolic areas normalized for end-diastolic area (➲ Fig. 23.9). FAC is influenced by acute changes in loading conditions, which may occur in the intraoperative period.

Ejection fraction (EF) calculation usually requires long-axis views of the LV to be obtained (➲ Fig. 23.10). The calculation of stroke volume (SV) can be obtained with 2D TOE as part of the EF calculation (➲ Fig. 23.11). In the intraoperative setting, where the LVOT diameter and AoV area (AVA) are relatively unchanging, changes in LVOT or AoV velocity time integral (TVI) can rapidly detect changes in cardiac output,[44] which in turn can be used as a method of monitoring a response to treatment.

Other indices of LV function including isovolumic contraction time, maximal LV power, or peak aortic flow acceleration at early systole can also be determined by TOE, but their intraoperative application is limited by their complexity, time consuming nature, and dependence on loading conditions and changes in inotropic state. Similarly, LV dP/dt calculation is not routinely used since MR needs to be present.

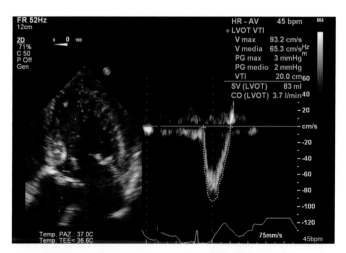

Figure 23.11 Calculation of stroke volume. Deep transgastric view showing pulsed wave Doppler signal from the left ventricular outflow tract. This measurement and LVOT diameter will allow calculation of stroke volume.

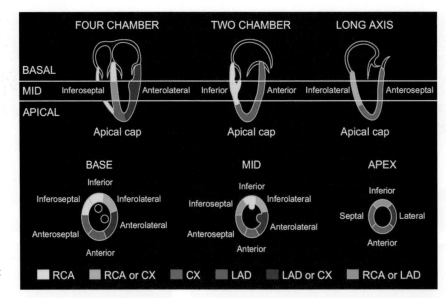

Figure 23.12 Left ventricular segmentation. Schema showing left ventricular walls and segments

Study of left ventricular regional contractility

Intraoperative episodes of myocardial ischaemia may cause abnormal myocardial contractility. For perioperative assessment of WMAs, the 17 segments can be investigated through the mid-oesophageal long-axis views, and the transgastric basal and mid-papillary short-axis views (➲ Fig. 23.12). For routine monitoring of myocardial ischaemia, the transgastric short-axis view at mid-papillary level is the most useful. In this view, good visualization of the myocardial regions supplied by all three main coronary arteries can be obtained (➲ Fig. 23.13).

Automatic detection of the endocardial border, known as acoustic quantification, is also used in TOE to get continuous, real-time determination of areas and volumes (➲ Fig. 23.14). Colour kinesis, representing an extension of acoustic quantification technology, tracks the motion of the endocardium in systole and provides colour-encoded images which reflect the magnitude and timing of endocardial motion (➲ Fig. 23.15). The evaluation of regional myocardial contractility intraoperatively during off-pump coronary artery bypass, on-pump procedures, and non-cardiac procedures in patients at risk for myocardial ischaemia may be performed whenever myocardial ischaemia is suspected by TD imaging. The systolic strain curve is positive when the explored segment expands. There is thickening in the mid-oesophageal short-axis view, and lengthening in the apical views. The systolic strain curve is negative

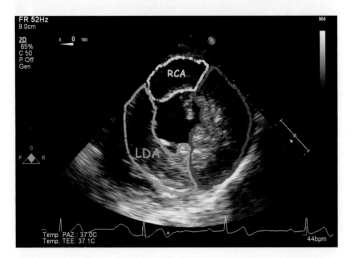

Figure 23.13 Coronary blood flow distribution. Transgastric mid-cavity short-axis view showing blood flow distribution from the coronary arteries

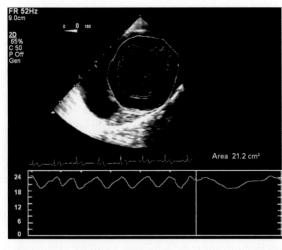

Figure 23.14 Automatic border detection. Transgastric mid cavity short-axis view showing automatic border detection

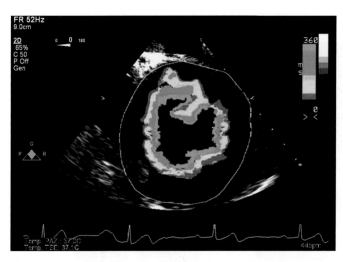

Figure 23.15 Colour kinesis. Transgastric mid-cavity short-axis view showing colour kinesis.

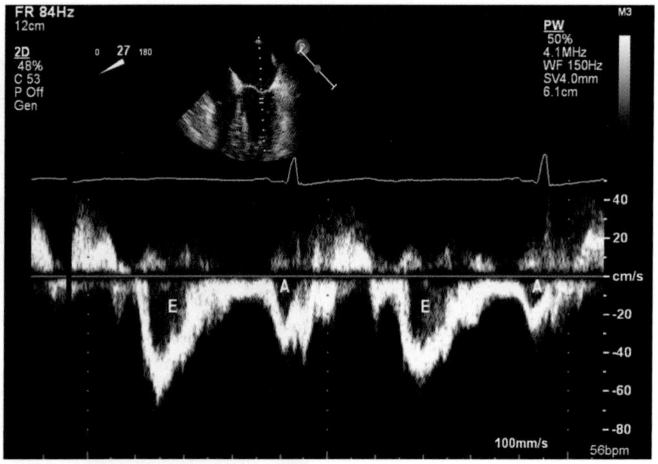

Figure 23.16 Transmitral PW Doppler flow during diastole. Mid-oesophageal long-axis four-chamber view showing transmitral Doppler flow signal.

when the explored segment shows compression, which is thinning in short-axis view and shortening in apical views. The combined use of regional strain indices and the timing of specific regional systolic or diastolic events offer a new non-invasive approach to the quantification and monitoring of myocardial dysfunction by intraoperative TOE, although specific experience in this setting is still limited. A TD segmental analysis allows evaluation of recovery after coronary revascularization, to identify ischaemia in a previously normal segment, and also to identify myocardial segments during ischaemia for off-pump surgery. This last setting is particularly useful. Analysis of myocardial velocities during coronary occlusion by the surgeon facilitates an echo-guided policy of coronary shunting, using the shunt catheter only in those cases in which a reduction of velocities is registered after 1min of coronary artery occlusion.[45–47]

Diastolic function

TOE allows intraoperative evaluation of diastolic phases through measurement of transmitral (➲ Fig. 23.16) and pulmonary vein flow velocities (➲ Fig. 23.17), and the application of CD M-mode (➲ Fig. 23.18) and TD imaging from the mitral annulus (➲ Fig. 23.19).

The aortic valve

A protocol for examining the AoV and the aortic root using TOE is given in ➲ Chapter 4.

Assessment of aortic valve stenosis

Patients who present for surgical AoV replacement will have already been investigated in detail, and the AoV morphology, flow velocity, pressure gradient, and AVA should all have been identified prior to surgery. Whilst confirmation of the diagnosis

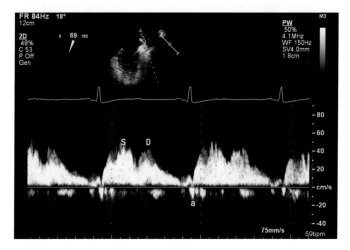

Figure 23.17 Transpulmonary PW Doppler flow during diastole. Mid-oesophageal long-axis view showing Doppler flow signal from the left pulmonary vein.

is valuable, verification of the exact degree of stenosis may be difficult. Estimation of the AVA by planimetry is unreliable in patients with severe aortic stenosis (AS), and calculation of the AVA by Doppler may be difficult due to malalignment of the Doppler beam with the direction of blood flow. The intraoperative examination may help to identify the dimensions of the aortic annulus, the LVOT, the diameter across the sinuses of Valsalva, the sinotubular junction and the ascending aorta. These details may aid surgical planning; the sinotubular junction diameter is important in patients undergoing valve replacement with a stentless prosthesis. Similarly, the nature of the valve stenosis (true bicuspid, functionally bicuspid, tricuspid) may be identified.

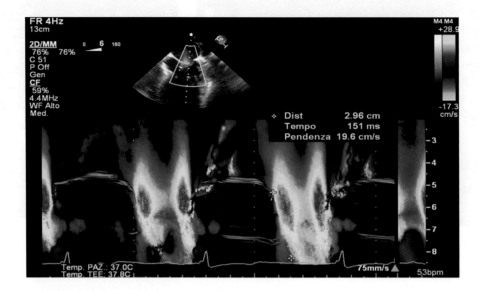

Figure 23.18 Colour Doppler M-mode. Transmitral colour M mode signal.

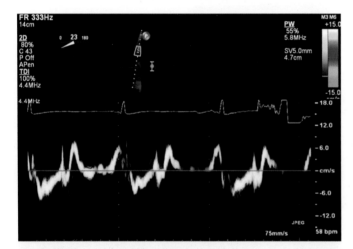

Figure 23.19 Tissue Doppler imaging. Tissue Doppler signal from the mitral annulus.

Assessment of aortic valve regurgitation

Patients with severe AR requiring AoV surgery will have been assessed in detail preoperatively. The intraoperative exam may serve not only to confirm the severity of regurgitation, but also to provide dimension data particularly of the aortic annulus and aortic root. Since the pressure half-time (PHT) decay of the aortic regurgitant (AR) flow rate is susceptible to alterations in haemodynamics, the AR index is more commonly used to assess the severity of AR intraoperatively. Such AR index consists of five echocardiographic parameters: jet width ratio, vena contracta width, PHT, jet density, and diastolic flow reversal in the descending aorta. Each parameter is scored on a 3-point scale from 1–3. The AR index is calculated as the sum of each score divided by the number of parameters. This technique, though valuable, is less useful in patients with eccentric regurgitant jets

and multiple jets. The presence of holodiastolic flow in the descending aorta is another useful indicator of severe AR.

The presence of a lesser degree of regurgitation may be an important finding for the surgical team in any cardiac surgical patient. The delivery of cardioplegia solution into the aortic root may be compromised by even mild AR, and care must be taken to prevent LV distension and ensure adequate distribution of cardioplegia. This may be achieved using retrograde cardioplegia via the coronary sinus, which can also be guided by intraoperative TOE (see earlier).

AR will eventually cause LV dilation. Dilation of the mitral annulus may ensue, with a central jet of MR being a classical feature. Thus any patient with AoV disease should have a detailed examination of the LV and MV function perioperatively.

The thoracic aorta

Perioperative evaluation of the thoracic aorta is valuable in a variety of settings. In patients with known aortic disease, including aortic dissection and aortic aneurysm, it may play a vital role in surgical planning. In other adult cardiac surgery patients, evaluation for aortic atheroma may give important information to guide surgical cannulation and device placement, and may also be useful for prognostic reasons. A protocol for examining the thoracic aorta using TOE is given in ⊃ Chapter 4.

TOE imaging of the thoracic aorta is subject to the same considerations of safety and risk assessment as TOE imaging of any other structure. However, two considerations should be especially borne in mind. Firstly, passage of a TOE probe can be a strong cardiovascular stimulus even in an anaesthetized patient, resulting in a burst of severe hypertension. This may be dangerous for a patient with either an aneurysm or a dissection and who is at risk from aortic rupture. Secondly, the aorta and the oesophagus are in close proximity, and the aortic arch and oesophagus cross at the level of T4/5. Weakness of the aorta due to aneurysmal dilation at this point may increase the risk of aortic rupture on passage of the probe. These considerations should be borne in mind whenever a TOE is performed for disease of the thoracic aorta.

TOE may be used to monitor device placement, including endovascular stents in the thoracic aorta and intra-aortic balloon catheters. In cardiac surgery patients, the aortic cannula and the antegrade cardioplegia cannula may be seen, and endoaortic clamps may be seen also. It may also be used for the newer techniques of transcatheter and transapical AoV replacement.

Aortic dissection

The two methods of classifying aortic dissection are shown in ➲ Fig. 23.20. The most commonly used classification is the Stanford classification, especially since this is most easily associated with surgical decision making. TOE has long been recognized as having an important role.[48] Image quality is usually excellent, particularly in the most important area for the surgeon—that is, at the level of the aortic root and proximal ascending aorta. Difficulty in imaging the ascending aorta and aortic arch is a drawback. Although TOE usually produces striking images of the dissection, this is not invariable. TOE examination protocol in case of aortic dissection is described in ➲ Chapter 21.

Accurate TOE imaging of aortic dissection may be confounded by a number of artefacts. These include reverberation or side lobe artefacts masquerading as an intimal flap, and reverberation artefacts within the aortic lumen. Intravascular catheters and other devices may generate artefacts also, but these can usually simply be moved or removed.

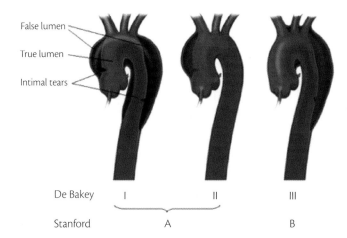

Figure 23.20 Classification of aortic dissection. Schema indicating the two most common methods of classifying aortic dissection.

Aortic aneurysm

The TOE exam should be directed to assessing the location and size of the aneurysm, although the size may differ slightly from an assessment by CT or CMR (see also ➲ Chapter 21). The involvement of any other structures should be sought, particularly the AoV. This may enable surgical planning to consider the need for either replacing, repairing, or resuspending the AoV.

Aortic atherosclerosis

Intraoperative detection of atheroma by TOE has been associated with a higher incidence of early and late cerebral and peripheral embolic events.[49,50] Identification of atheroma in the descending aorta during cardiac surgery is important, not simply because it may lead to peripheral embolization if it becomes detached for any reason, but also because it predicts atheroma both elsewhere in the aorta and in other vessels[51] and correlates with an increased incidence of stroke.[52,53]

Ultrasound imaging has been shown to be superior to surgical digital palpation at detecting all types of atheroma apart from hard calcified plaque.[54,55] However, the distal ascending aorta and aortic arch are not routinely visible during TOE. An obturator has been described to circumvent this problem,[56] but alternatively epivascular scanning has been shown to be more effective than TOE for imaging these areas.[57]

Aortic trauma

Rapid deceleration may produce a transverse injury to the aorta, usually at the level of the aortic isthmus.[58] This area is immediately proximal to the immobile descending aorta, and immediately distal to the mobile aortic arch. It may occur as a full or partial thickness injury, involving the media and intima, or all three layers. Most of these injuries prove immediately lethal, and early surgery may be indicated in many of the survivors.

TOE may provide an effective and rapid imaging technique for diagnosing traumatic injury to the aorta, and also has the benefit of providing a comprehensive imaging assessment of the heart and other vessels.

Localization of devices

Perioperative TOE may guide appropriate placement of endovascular devices, including endovascular stents and intra-aortic balloon pump (IABP) catheters. Endovascular stenting is frequently undertaken under X-ray screening, but TOE may have a role in assessing the aorta pre-procedure and in follow-up.

Accurate IABP catheter placement is important to ensure optimum counter-pulsation. The catheter tip should ideally be located 2cm distal to the left subclavian artery, or several centimetres distal to the junction of the aortic arch and descending aorta. If imaging these structures is difficult, an alternative is to image the AoV, identify the level of the AoV leaflets, and then rotate the probe through 180 degrees to image the descending aorta, and position the IABP catheter tip at the level of the aortic leaflets.

Intraoperative TOE is valuable in locating and positioning devices for minimally invasive cardiac surgery, for example in positioning the endo-aortic balloon clamp. The development of minimally invasive valve surgery has been facilitated by the TOE-aided positioning of the prosthetic AoV.

Other conditions

Atrial myxoma

Although the provisional diagnosis of myxoma will have been made before surgery, intraoperative TOE is valuable to identify any residual tumour and assess damage to the valve apparatus or inter-atrial septum that might have occurred either before or during surgery and need subsequent repair.

Thrombus

Thrombus in the left atrium is easily seen with TOE due to the close proximity between the oesophagus and the left atrium.

Factors promoting left atrial thrombus are associated with blood stasis, and include atrial fibrillation, significant left atrial enlargement which may be associated with LV dysfunction, mitral stenosis, and mitral prosthesis. The presence of spontaneous echo contrast is also an indicator of sluggish blood flow. Screening the LV for thrombus should be undertaken in high risk cases, as the presence of LV thrombus in patients undergoing CABG surgery will alter the surgical plan.

Pericardial effusion

Surgical drainage of a pericardial effusion may be performed under TOE guidance. This may be useful, particularly for posterior loculated effusions, and has the advantage of being able to identify when drainage is complete.

Personal perspective

Perioperative echocardiography has shown enormous growth in recent years. Whilst it should not be used for primary diagnosis, it is invaluable for confirming and refining the preoperative diagnosis, detecting new or unsuspected pathology, adjusting the anaesthetic and surgical plan accordingly, and assessing the results of surgical intervention.

It is now routinely performed in the setting of most cardiac operations and in many non-cardiovascular operations. Often, it is the first imaging approach in conditions of clinical instability after surgery. The possibility to assess both morphology and function provide an immediate overview on the most critical conditions occurring before, during, or after surgery.

References

1 Erbel R, Borner N Stellar D, Brunier], Thelen M, Pfeiffer C, et al. Detection of aortic dissection by transoesophageal echocardiography. Br Heart J 1987; 58:45–51.

2 Erbel R, Engberding R, Daniel W, Roelandt J, Visser C, Rennollet H. Echocardiography in diagnosis of aortic dissection. Lancet 1989; 1:457–61.

3 Practice Guidelines for Perioperative Transesophageal Echocardiography. An Updated Report by the American Society of Anesthesiologists and the Society of Cardiovascular Anesthesiologists Task Force on Transesophageal Echocardiography. Anesthesiology 2010; 112:1084–96.

4 Flachskampf FA, Badano L, Daniel WG, Feneck RO, Fox GF, Fraser AG, et al.; Recommendations for transoesophageal echocardiography – update 2010. Eur J Echocardiogr 2010; 11:557–76.

5 Kallmeyer IJ, Collard CD, Fox JA, Body SC, Shernan SK. The safety of intraoperative transesophageal echocardiography: a case series of 7200 cardiac surgical patients. Anesth Analg 2001; 92:1126–30.

6 Piercy M, McNicol L, Dinh DT, Story DA, Smith JA. Major complications related to the use of transesophageal echocardiography in cardiac surgery. J Cardiothorac Vasc Anesth 2009; 23:62–5.

7 Huang CH, Lu CW, Lin TY, Cheng YJ, Wang MJ. Complications of intraoperative transesophageal echocardiography in adult cardiac surgical patients – experience of two institutions in Taiwan. J Formos Med Assoc 2007; 106:92–5.

8 Côté G, Denault A. Transesophageal echocardiography-related complications. Can J Anaesth 2008; 55:622–47.

9 Flachskampf FA, Decoodt P, Fraser AG, Daniel WG, Roelandt JR; Working Group on Echocardiography of the European Society of Cardiology. Guidelines from the Working Group. Recommendations for performing transesophageal echocardiography. Eur J Echocardiogr 2001; 2:8–21.

10 Chambers JB, Klein JL, Bennett SR, Monaghan MJ, Roxburgh JC. Is antibiotic prophylaxis ever necessary before transoesophageal echocardiography? Heart 2006; 92:435–6.

11 Statement on antibiotic prophylaxis before transoesophageal echocardiography. Approved by the Councils of British Society

of Echocardiography, Association of Cardiothoracic Anaesthetists and the Society of Cardiothoracic Surgeons, Working group. ℘ http://www.bse.org (accessed August 2008).

12 Dajani AS, Bisno AL, Durack DT, Freed M, Gerber MA, Karchmer AW, *et al.* Prevention of bacterial endocarditis. Recommenda tions by the American Heart Association. *JAMA* 1990; **264**:2919–22.

13 Badaoui R, Choufane S, Riboulot M, Bachelet Y, Ossart M. Esophageal perforation after transesophageal echocardiography. *Ann Fr Anesth Reanim* 1994; **13**:850–2.

14 Jougon J, Gallon P, Dubrez J, Velly JF. Esophageal perforation during transesophageal echocardiography. *Arch Mal Coeur Vaiss* 2000; **93**:1235–7.

15 Massey SR, Pitsis A, Mehta D, Callaway M. Oesophageal perforation following perioperative transoesophageal echocardiography. *Br J Anaesth* 2000; **84**:643–6.

16 St-Pierre J, Fortier LP, Couture P, Hebert Y. Massive gastrointestinal hemorrage after transoesophageal echocardiography probe insertion. *Can J Anaesth* 1998; **54**:1196-9.

17 Kihara S, Mizutani T, Shimizu T, Toyooka H. Bleeding from a tear in the gastric mucosa caused by transoesophageal echocardiography during cardiac surgery: effective haemostasis by endoscopic argon plasma coagulation. *Br J Anaesth* 1999; **82**:948–50.

18 Hulyalkar AR, Ayd JD. Low risk of gastrointestinal injury associated with transoesophageal echocardiography during cardiac surgery. *J Cardiothorac Vasc Anesth* 1993; **7**:175–7.

19 Wax DB, Torres A, Scher C, Leibowitz AB. Transesophageal echocardiography utilization in high-volume liver transplantation centers in the United States. *J Cardiothorac Vasc Anesth* 2008; **22**:811–13.

20 Cohn LH, Rizzo RJ, Adams DH, Couper GS, Sullivan TE, Collins JJ, *et al.* The effect of pathophysiology on the surgical treatment of ischaemic mitral regurgitation: operative and late risks of repair versus replacement. *Eur J Cardiothorac Surg* 1995; **9**:568–74.

21 Klein AA, Snell A, Nashef SA, Hall RM, Kneeshaw JD, Arrowsmith JE. The impact of intra-operative transoesophageal echocardiography on cardiac surgical practice. *Anaesthesia* 2009; **64**:947–52.

22 Savage RM, Lytle BW, Aronson S, Navia JL, Licina M, Stewart WJ, *et al.* Intraoperative echocardiography is indicated in high-risk coronary artery bypass grafting. *Ann Thorac Surg* 1997; **64**:368–73.

23 Bonow RO, Carabello BA, Chatterjee K, de Leon AC Jr, Faxon DP, Freed MD, *et al.* 2008 Focused update incorporated into the ACC/AHA 2006 guidelines for the management of patients with valvular heart disease: a report of the American College of Cardiology/American Heart Association Task Force on Practice Guidelines. *Circulation.* 2008; **118**:523–661.

24 Shanewise JS, Cheung AT, Aronson S, Stewart WJ, Weiss RL, Mark JB, *et al.* ASE/SCA Guidelines for Performing a Comprehensive Intraoperative Multiplane Transesophageal Echocardiography Examination: Recommendations of the American Society of Echocardiography Council for Intraoperative Echocardiography and the Society of Cardiovascular Anesthesiologists Task Force for Certification in Perioperative Transesophageal Echocardiography. *Anesth Analg* 1999; **89**:870–4.

25 Mathew JP, Glas K, Troianos CA, Sears-Rogan P, Savage R, Shanewise J, *et al.* American Society of Echocardiography/Society of Cardiovascular Anesthesiologists recommendations and guidelines for continuous quality improvement in perioperative echocardiography. *J Am Soc Echocardiogr* 2006; **19**:1303–13.

26 Miller JP, Lambert AS, Shapiro WA, Russell IA, Schiller NB, Cahalan MK. The adequacy of basic intraoperative transesophageal echocardiography performed by experienced anesthesiologists. *Anesth Analg* 2001; **92**:1103–10.

27 Feneck RO Lorini L. The Transesophageal echo exam. In: Feneck RO, Kneeshaw J, Ranucci M (eds) *Core Topics in Transesophageal Echocardiography.* Cambridge: Cambridge University Press; 2010, pp. 43–58.

28 Feneck RO, Kneeshaw J, Fox K, *et al.* Recommendations for reporting perioperative transesophageal echo studies. *Eur J Echocard* 2010; in press.

29 Krasuski RA, Hart SA, Allen D, Qureshi A, Pettersson G, Houghtaling PL, *et al.* Prevalence and repair of intraoperatively diagnosed patent foramen ovale and association with perioperative outcomes and long-term survival. *JAMA* 2009; **302**:290–7.

30 Song H, Kim MJ, Chung CH, Choo SJ, Song MG, Song JM, *et al.* Factors associated with development of late significant tricuspid regurgitation after successful left-sided valve surgery. *Heart* 2009; **95**:931–6.

31 Lambert AS, Miller JP, Merrick SH, Schiller NB, Foster E, Muhiudeen-Russell I, *et al.* Improved evaluation of the location and mechanism of mitral valve regurgitation with a systematic transoesophageal echocardiography examination. *Anesth Analg* 1999; **88**:1205–12.

32 Colombo PC, Wu RH, Weiner S, Marinaccio M, Brofferio A, Banchs J, *et al.* Value of quantitative analysis of mitral regurgitation jet eccentricity by color flow Doppler for identification of flail leaflet. *Am J Cardiol* 2001; **88**:534–40.

33 Aikat S, Lewis JF. Role of echocardiography in the diagnosis and prognosis of patients with mitral regurgitation. *Curr Opin Cardiol* 2003; **18**:334–9.

34 Radermecker MA, Limet R. Carpentier's functional classification of mitral valve dysfunction. *Rev Med Liege* 1995; **50**:292–4.

35 Agricola E, Oppizzi M, Pisani M, Meris A, Maisano F, Margonato A. Ischemic mitral regurgitation: mechanisms and echocardiographic classification. *Eur J Echocardiogr* 2008; **9**:207–21.

36 Roshanali F, Mandegar MH, Yousefnia MA, Alaeddini F, Wann S. Low-dose dobutamine stress echocardiography to predict reversibility of mitral regurgitation with CABG. *Echocardiography* 2006; **23**:31–7.

37 Aklog L, Filsoufi F, Flores KQ, Chen RH, Cohn LH, Nathan NS, *et al.* Does coronary artery bypass grafting alone correct moderate ischemic mitral regurgitation? *Circulation* 2001; **104** (12 Suppl. 1): I68–75.

38 Kim YH, Czer LS, Soukiasian HJ, De Robertis M, Magliato KE, Blanche C, *et al.* Ischemic mitral regurgitation: revascularization alone versus revascularization and mitral valve repair. *Ann Thorac Surg* 2005; **79**:1895 –901.

39 Tibayan FA, Rodriguez F, Zasio MK, Bailey L, Liang D, Daughters GT, *et al.* Geometric distortions of the mitral valvular-ventricular complex in chronic ischemic mitral regurgitation. *Circulation* 2003; **108**(Suppl. 1):II116–21.

40 Shiran A, Merdler A, Ismir E, Ammar R, Zlotnick AY, Aravot D, *et al.* Intraoperative transesophageal echocardiography using a quantitative dynamic loading test for the evaluation of ischemic mitral regurgitation. *Am Soc Echocardiogr* 2007; **20**:690–7.

41 Grewal KS, Malkowski MJ, Piracha AR, Astbury JC, Kramer CM, Dianzumba S, *et al.* Effect of general anesthesia on the severity of mitral regurgitation by transesophageal echocardiography. *J Cardiol* 2000; **85**:199–203.

42 Douglas PS, Khandheria B, Stainback RF, Weissman NJ, Peterson ED, Hendel RC, et al. ACCF/ASE/ACEP/ASNC/SCAI/SCCT/SCMR 2007 appropriateness criteria for transthoracic and transesophageal echocardiography. *J Am Soc Echocardiogr* 2007; **20**:787–805.

43 Seeberger MD, Cahalan MK, Rouine-Rapp K, Foster E, Ionescu P, Balea M, et al. Acute hypovolemia may cause segmental wall motion abnormalities in the absence of myocardial ischemia. *Anesth Analg.* 1997; **85**:1252–7.

44 Guarracino F. The role of transesophageal echocardiography in intraoperative hemodynamic monitoring. *Minerva Anestesiol* 2001; **67**:320–4.

45 Hameed AK, Gosal T, Fang T, Ahmadie R, Lytwyn M, Barac I, et al. Clinical utility of tissue Doppler imaging in patients with acute myocardial infarction complicated by cardiogenic shock. *Cardiovasc Ultrasound* 2008; **6**:11.

46 Minhaj M, Patel K, Muzic D, Tung A, Jeevanandam V, Raman J, et al. The effect of routine intraoperative transesophageal echocardiography on surgical management. *J Cardiothorac Vasc Anesth* 2007; **21**:800–4.

47 Swaminathan M, Morris RW, De Meyts DD, Podgoreanu MV, Jollis JG, Grocott H, et al. Deterioration of regional wall motion immediately aft er coronary artery bypass graft surgery is associated with long-term major adverse cardiac events. *Anesthesiology* 2007; **107**:739–45.

48 Adachi H, Omoto R, Kyo S, Matsumura M, Kimura S, Takamoto S, et al. Emergency surgical intervention of acute aortic dissection with the rapid diagnosis by transesophageal echocardiography. *Circulation* 1991; **84**(5 Suppl):III14–9.

49 Katz ES, Tunick PA, Rusinek H, Ribakove G, Spencer FC, Kronzon I. Protruding aortic atheromas predict stroke in elderly patients undergoing cardiopulmonary bypass:experience with intraoperative transesophageal echocardiography. *J Am Coll Cardiol* 1992; **20**:70–7.

50 Tunick PA, Rosenweig BP, Katz ES, Perez JL, Kronzon I. High risk for vascular events in patients with protruding aortic atheromas; a prospective study. *J Am Coll Cardiol* 1994; **23**:1085–90.

51 Konstadt SN, Reich DL, Kahn R, Viggiani RF. Transesophageal echocardiography can be used to screen for ascending aortic atherosclerosis. *Anesth Analg* 1995; **81**:225–8.

52 Mizuno T, Toyama M, Tabuchi N, Kuriu K, Ozaki S, Kawase I, et al. Thickened intima of the aortic arch is a risk factor for stroke with coronary artery bypass grafting. *Ann Thorac Surg* 2000; **70**:1565–70.

53 Kutz SM, Lee VS, Tunick PA, Krinsky GA, Kronzon I. Atheromas of the thoracic aorta; a comparison of transesophageal echocardiography and breath-hold gadolinium-enhanced 3-dimensional magnetic resonance angiography. *J Am Soc Echocardiogr* 1999; **12**:853–8.

54 Machleder HI, Takiff H, Lois JF, Holburt E. Aortic mural thrombus; an occult source of arterial thrombo-embolism. *J Vasc Surg* 1986; **4**:473.

55 Hartman GS, Yao FF, Bruefach M III, Barbut D, Peterson JC, Purcell MH, et al. Severity of aortic atheromatous disease diagnosed by transesophageal echocardiography predicts stroke and other outcomes associated with coronary artery surgery: a prospective study. *Anesth Analg* 1996; **83**:701–8.

56 Li YL, Wong DT, Wei W, Liu J. A novel acoustic window for trans-oesophageal echocardiography by using a saline-filled endotracheal balloon. *Br J Anaesth* 2006; **97**:624–9.

57 Sylivris S,Calafiore P, Matalanis P, Rosalion A, Yuen HP, Buxton BF, et al. The intraoperative assessment of ascending aortic atheroma; epiaortic imaging is superior to both transesophageal echocardiography and direct palpation. *J Cardiothorac Vasc Anesth* 1997; **11**:704–7.

58 Pretre R, Chilcott M. Blunt trauma to the heart and great vessels. *N Engl J Med* 1997; **336**:626–32.

Further reading

Kallmeyer IJ, Collard CD, Fox JA, Body SC, Shernan SK. The safety of intraoperative transesophageal echocardiography: a case series of 7200 cardiac surgical patients. *Anesth Analg* 2001; **92**:1126–30.

Minhaj M, Patel K, Muzic D, Tung A, Jeevanandam V, Raman J, et al. The effect of routine intraoperative transesophageal echocardiography on surgical management. *J Cardiothorac Vasc Anesth* 2007; **21**:800–4.

Practice Guidelines for Perioperative Transesophageal Echocardiography. An Updated Report by the American Society of Anesthesiologists and the Society of Cardiovascular Anesthesiologists Task Force on Transesophageal Echocardiography. *Anesthesiology* 2010; **112**: 1084–96.

➲ For additional multimedia materials please visit the online version of the book (http://escecho.oxfordmedicine.com).

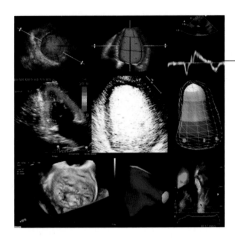

CHAPTER 24

Echocardiography in the emergency room

Aleksandar N. Nešković and
Andreas Hagendorff

Contents

Summary

Echocardiography can provide rapid and accurate assessment of cardiac morphology and haemodynamics under stressful conditions in the emergency room (ER). Using this information, critical decisions regarding management of cardiovascular emergencies and the critically ill are made. To avoid potentially catastrophic errors with medicolegal consequences, adequate education and experience in echocardiography and cardiology are required and teamwork is encouraged. In addition, emergency cases must be well documented and this documentation stored and retrievable. Transthoracic echocardiography is the main source of the information in the emergency setting, while transoesophageal, contrast, and stress echocardiography are used when needed and in special circumstances.

In this chapter, the principles, practice, and specific considerations related to echocardiography in the ER are discussed and a brief overview of echocardiographic assessment in cardiac emergencies is provided. Detailed information regarding echocardiographic features of particular cardiovascular diseases and conditions that may be presented to the emergency physician in the ER can be found elsewhere in this book in the related chapters.

Introduction

The majority of cardiologists would consider echocardiography as the single most valuable technique to assess an unstable cardiovascular patient. There are at least two reasons for this: availability and accuracy. Echocardiographic machines are relatively inexpensive and mobile, which allow examinations to be carried out wherever necessary. Equally important, echocardiography offers rapid and accurate information about the structure and function of the heart and haemodynamics, providing crucial evidence for decision making in cardiovascular emergencies and the critically ill. Consequently, echocardiography is already incorporated into patient management algorithms for the majority of cardiac emergencies. Although its diagnostic power can barely be challenged, recognition of its advantages and limitations in particular clinical situations is essential for correct interpretation, to avoid potential catastrophic diagnostic errors.

Transthoracic echocardiography (TTE) is the main source of information in the emergency setting. However, the roles of special echocardiographic techniques, such as transoesophageal (TOE), contrast, and stress echocardiography, may be important in special circumstances and their advantages should be wisely utilized.

Emergency echocardiography: specific considerations

Emergency setting

Circumstances in the emergency room (ER) are challenging (⊃ Table 24.1). Critical decisions regarding patient management must be made in a situation characterized by constant time constraint, stressful environment, and suboptimal echocardiographic images (often). Thus, the ER is the place where professional medical errors are likely to occur more frequently and where consequences are more serious than anywhere else.

It should be noted that the accuracy of diagnostic information obtained by echocardiography is related not only to local expertise and clinical circumstances, but also to specific patient populations evaluated. Sensitivity, specificity, and accuracy of any diagnostic technique are strongly influenced by the pretest likelihood of the disease (Bayesian theory). Therefore, different results in detection of acute coronary syndromes (ACS) can be expected in the coronary care unit patient population as compared to patients examined in the ER, since they represent a much less selected group of individuals. Successful technique, however, should identify low-risk patients without compromising the detection of those at high risk of coronary events and complications.

Education, training, experience, competence, logistics

Who should perform emergency echo? The answer is probably everyone who knows how to get valuable information: sonographer, fellow, cardiologist, anaesthesiologist, emergency physician. 'Know-how' includes ability to obtain adequate images (imaging technique) and ability to describe and to understand these images (interpretation). Improperly acquired and/or poor

Table 24.1 Emergency room setting

Stressful environment
Critically ill patients
Time constrain
Difficult technical aspects of obtaining the images (often)
Limited time for consultations with other staff
Critical decisions have to be made (surgery, aggressive medical therapy)
Medical errors are likely to occur often

images may result in inaccurate reading, with misleading and potentially dangerous conclusions (⊃ Fig. 24.1; ▪ 24.1).

Adequate cognitive and technical skills (education and training) and clinical experience are mandatory for individuals who perform emergency echocardiography. However, compromises have to be made due to lack of availability of specialized cardiologists at all locations where the critically ill are diagnosed and treated. Therefore, basic and advanced levels of competence must be defined to ensure the best possible quality of echocardiography practice in the emergency settings and optimal patient management.

Basic level of competence enables non-cardiologists (e.g. sonographers, emergency physicians, anaesthesiologists) to perform emergency echocardiography. Even focused echocardiographic examination using hand-held echocardiographic machines might provide key information. This limited approach, however, carries a high risk of failing to detect

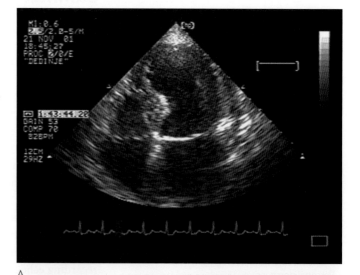

A

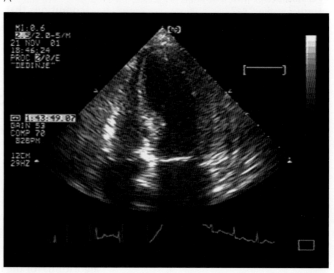

B

Figure 24.1 Poor imaging technique. TTE. Akinesis of the distal septum and LV apex is clearly detectable only when full length of the LV is obtained (B) from the window located one intercostal space lower than for (A).

important findings and the risk of misinterpretation due to deficiency of clinical experience and cardiological competence. Individuals with basic level of competence can function alone (unsupervised images acquisition and initial interpretation) only in potentially life-saving scenarios, where any delay in decision making is likely to be lethal. However, when established, optimal logistics of the echocardiography service should make these situations uncommon. Images acquired by non-cardiologists are always to be re-interpreted simultaneously by the experts. Decision-making process can be considerably improved in hospitals with high-end ultrasound systems, by network and server solutions with a permanent audiovisual connection from the ER to the supervisor laboratory with a cardiologist.

With additional special education, preferably in the accredited echocardiographic laboratory, with defined duration and intensity of the training period under close supervision by experts, an advanced level of competence can be achieved. At this level, TOE should also be included in the training programme. This level of competence guarantees adequate recording and reading in the majority of emergency cases.

The highest level of competence in emergency echocardiography should be reserved for cardiologists specialized and accredited in echocardiography, familiar with all echocardiographic applications and techniques.

An example of recently published standards for training at various levels of clinical competence in adult TTE is provided in ➲ Table 24.2.

An 'ABCD approach' is proposed to be followed while performing emergency echocardiography at all competence levels (➲ Table 24.3).

Finally, other imaging modalities that are frequently used in patients presenting in the ER include computed tomography (CT), multislice CT, cardiac magnetic resonance (CMR) imaging, single photon emission CT (SPECT), and coronary angiography. The emergency physician should have basic knowledge on their advantages and limitations and should use them wisely.

Table 24.2 Minimal training requirements (performance and interpretation) for adult transthoracic echocardiography

	Cumulative duration of training (months)	Minimum total number of examinations performed	Minimum number of examinations interpreted
Level 1	3	75	150
Level 2	6	150	300
Level 3	12	300	750

Modified from Cheitlin MD, Armstrong WF, Aurigemma GP, Beller GA, Bierman FZ, Davis JL, et al. ACC/AHA/ASE 2003 guideline update for the clinical application of echocardiography: a report of the American College of Cardiology/American Heart Association Task Force on Practice Guidelines (ACC/AHA/ASE Committee to Update the 1997 Guidelines for the Clinical Application of Echocardiography). J Am Coll Cardiol 2003; **42**:954–70.

Table 24.3 'ABCD approach' in performing emergency echocardiography

A	**A**wareness	Fight against routine
		Think beyond apparent explanations
B	**B**e Suspicious	Referral diagnosis may be misleading
		Never trust, confirm
C	**C**omprehensiveness	Do as complete examination as suitable
		Careful interpretation
D	**D**ouble R*	The study should be recorded and reviewed
		Team work is crucial

***R**ecord and **R**eview

Medicolegal issues

As diagnostic errors are likely to occur in the ER setting, medicolegal issues should not be ignored and emergency cases should be well documented and this documentation stored and retrievable.

Emergency echocardiography study should be performed using an adequate echocardiographic machine, and must be recorded and stored, preferably in digital (DICOM) data storage format. The stored images/cineloops can be later used for reviewing the case, but also as a document to give evidence of the findings in the acute setting. Reports should always reflect recorded findings which are interpreted, approved, and signed by the individuals with adequate formal education.

Emergency clinical presentations

The most important causes of cardiac and cardiac-like emergencies and their common initial presentations in the ER are shown in ➲ Table 24.4. These conditions are typically serious, often life-threatening if left untreated, and they may be promptly detected and/or assessed in the ER by echocardiography. Of note, the majority of these diseases may have more than one initial clinical presentation, which makes the assessment even more complex and difficult.

Specific issues pertinent to these emergency situations are outlined, because, integrated with certain echocardiographic features, they might be helpful for making a quick and accurate diagnosis. Echocardiographic assessments of specific causes of cardiac emergencies are discussed related mostly to their most frequent presentation in the ER.

Acute chest pain

Patients with acute chest pain account for 20–30% admissions to the ER. The first goal is to identify those with acute coronary syndromes (ACS), notably myocardial infarction. Equally important is to exclude other possible causes without delay (➲ Table 24.5); some of them may be life threatening and need

Table 24.4 Major causes of cardiac and cardiac-like emergencies and their common initial clinical presentations in the emergency room

	ACS	AoD	PE	P	Ptx	ADHF	T	AVR/PVD
Acute chest pain	++++	++++	++	+++	+++	+	+	+
Acute dyspnoea	++	+	++++	0	++	++++	++++	++++
Haemodynamic instability/shock	++	++	+++	+	+	++++	++++	++++
New murmur	+	+	+	+	0	+	0	++++
Cardiac sources of embolism/syncope	+	+	+	0	0	+	0	+
Chest trauma	+	+++	0	+	++	0	+++	+
Cardiac arrest/CPR	++++	+	+++	+	+	+	+++	+

Number of + indicates relative likelihood of association. 0 indicates that association is unlikely

ACS, acute coronary syndrome; ADHF, acute decompensated heart failure; AoD, acute aortic dissection; AVR/PVD, acute valvular regurgitation/prosthetic valve dysfunction; CPR, cardiopulmonary resuscitation; P, acute pericarditis; PE, acute pulmonary embolism; Ptx, pneumothorax; T, cardiac tamponade

Table 24.5 Frequent causes of acute chest pain in patients presenting in the emergency room

Acute coronary syndrome
Aortic dissection
Pulmonary embolism
Pericarditis
Myocarditis
Pneumothorax
Aortic stenosis
Hypertrophic cardiomyopathy
Takotsubo cardiomyopathy
Mitral valve prolapse

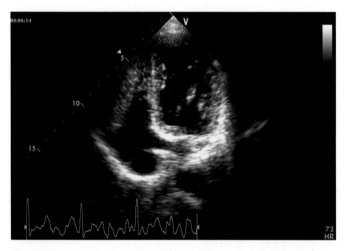

Figure 24.2 2D echo during anginal pain. TTE. Akinesis of the apex in a patient complaining of actual acute chest pain (see also ➲ Fig. 24.3).

a strikingly different therapeutic approach, where misdiagnosis and mistreatment may lead to potentially catastrophic consequences (i.e. acute aortic syndrome vs. ACS). The incremental diagnostic value of echocardiography is highest in patients with suspected ACS presenting with atypical clinical presentation, with normal or non-diagnostic electrocardiogram (ECG), and with normal or marginal increase of cardiac enzymes. In ACS and during transient anginal pain (Figs. 24.2 and 24.3; ▪ 24.2 and 24.3) echocardiography reveals regional dyssynergy (hypokinesis, akinesis, dyskinesis) associated with preserved wall thickness in diastole and normal myocardial reflectivity, while thin, dyssynergic, and bright or highly reflective myocardial wall strongly suggests scar due to old infarction.

The location and the extent of dyssynergy carry important prognostic information. Although it may be difficult to discriminate between ischaemia, stunning, hibernation, and necrosis (infarction) on the basis of the resting echocardiography alone, the actual extent of dysfunctional myocardial region reflects true functional infarct size and directly determines the degree of haemodynamic impairment and the prognosis (➲ Fig. 24.4; ▪ 24.4). An additional problem is that, apart from

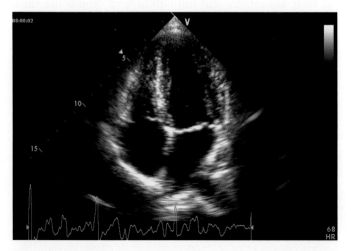

Figure 24.3 2D echo after anginal pain. TTE. The patient is the same as presented in ➲ Fig. 24.2, recorded 2 min later when chest pain was gone. Note normokinesis of the apex.

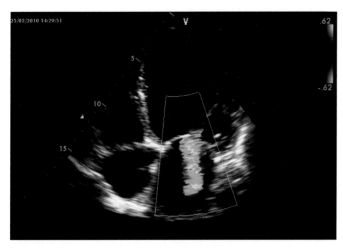

Figure 24.4 Haemodynamically unstable acute myocardial infarction. TTE. The patient presented in the ER in cardiogenic shock. Global LV function was poor (EF measured as 10%) due to large akinetic zone that includes septum, apex and distal two-thirds of the lateral LV wall. Note significant ischemic mitral regurgitation.

being normal or non-diagnostic in significant proportion of patients with suspected ACS, ECG may reveal ST-segment elevation in conditions not necessarily related to ACS, such as left ventricular (LV) hypertrophy, left bundle branch block, hypertrophic cardiomyopathy, acute pericarditis, Brugada syndrome or hyperkalaemia. Also, ST-segment elevation may be typical, but misleading (i.e. due to right coronary artery occlusion as a complication of aortic dissection type A). Echocardiography can be helpful in clarifying these potentially confusing situations in the ER.

On the other hand, dyssynergy detected by echocardiography may be *not due to ischaemia* (➲ Table 24.6) or may be *absent*, if ischaemia/necrosis affects a small amount of myocardium limited to the thin endocardial layer (small non-transmural infarctions).

In the majority of the cases presenting with acute chest pain, standard two-dimensional (2D) and Doppler transthoracic examination are sufficient to give information that may be effectively used for decision making in the ER. It should be emphasized that detection and interpretation of regional wall motion abnormalities is a difficult task to learn and is highly operator-dependent. Excellent technical skills are required to obtain images of good enough quality in suboptimal situations,

Table 24.6 Conditions other than coronary artery disease presenting with regional wall motion abnormalities on the resting echocardiographic study

Acute myocarditis
Cardiomyopathies
Left bundle branch block
Pacemaker
Right ventricular pressure or volume overload
Takotsubo cardiomyopathy

to allow fair interpretation. Overall, sensitivity of the technique is high, over 90%, but specificity and positive predictive value are more variable and less convincing, indicating interpretation challenges in the emergency setting. As a consequence, confusion and frequent overdiagnosis may occur in attempts not to miss those with true ACS. Of note, the absence of dyssynergy in patients without a history of infarction or known coronary artery disease has a negative predictive value as high as 99%, strongly suggesting favourable prognosis in patients with ACS and normal echocardiogram.

Contrast echocardiography can be used to improve delineation of endocardial borders and detection of dyssynergy, as well as to simultaneously assess myocardial perfusion at the bedside. Contrast perfusion echocardiography showed comparable results with SPECT in the ER setting and provided accurate short- and long-term prognostic information, identifying patients with abnormal myocardial perfusion as at highest risk.

Exercise and pharmacological (dobutamine/atropine, dipyridamole/atropine, adenosine) stress echocardiography can also be used in the triage of the chest pain patients in the ER, reported as feasible, safe, and cost-effective, providing good risk stratification in particular through a negative predictive value as high as 97%.

However, both contrast and stress echocardiography require special training and experience and currently they can not be considered as standard care in the ER setting.

Finally, TOE may also be helpful, especially in critically ill patients. In experienced hands, TOE is safe and feasible. It may be of value particularly in differential diagnosis, to exclude other life-threatening conditions with similar clinical presentation, such as aortic dissection or massive pulmonary embolism.

Acute aortic dissection

This must be always considered as a possible cause of acute chest pain in the ER, due to extremely high associated mortality and morbidity if not detected at initial presentation. Clinical characteristics of the typical severe (migrating) chest pain might be helpful, but imaging is mandatory for management decisions. Although echocardiographic signs of aortic dissection (aortic dilation, intimal flap, true/false lumen, entry point, aortic regurgitation, pericardial effusion) can be detected in up to 75% of cases by TTE (➲ Fig. 24.5; ◼ 24.5), with specificity of over 90%, normal findings can not rule out the disease due to difficulties in visualization of distal ascending and descending aorta (➲ Fig. 24.6; ◼ 24.6) and frequent reverberation artefacts responsible for false negative studies. If proximal aortic dissection is detected by initial TTE in the ER, the patient should be immediately transferred to the cardiac surgery operating room and TOE can be performed there. If the diagnosis is uncertain, TOE should be performed in the ER to identify the type and complications of dissection or to exclude the disease. In practice, the presence of (new) aortic regurgitation or pericardial effusion on TTE in a patient with severe chest pain, unclear

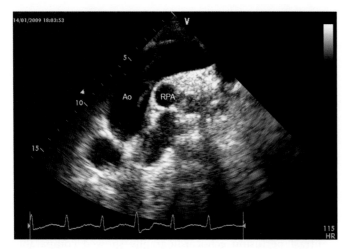

Figure 24.5 Acute proximal aortic dissection. TTE. Note mobile, linear echogenic structure (intimal flap) in the lumen of ascending aorta and arch assessed using suprasternal view. The patient presented in the ER with abrupt, crushing chest pain, radiating towards back. Ao, aorta; RPA, right pulvmonary artery.

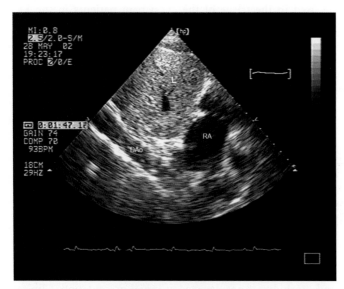

Figure 24.6 Acute aortic dissection. TTE. The image is obtained from the subxyphoid view in a young patient referred to the ER as suspected postinfarction ventricular septal defect. This is one of only two frames with visible flap in the descending aorta, indicating dissection. Images obtained from other views where completely unremarkable. DAo, descending aorta; L, liver; RA, right atrium.

shock, or neurological deficit, should be considered as highly suggestive of proximal aortic dissection, even if an intimal flap is not detectable, and the disease should be ruled out by TOE. In experienced hands, TOE appears to be the first-line choice in the ER for the assessment of patient with suspected dissection. It can be rapidly performed in the ER. Of note, every efforts must be made to avoid significant rise of blood pressure due to discomfort or gagging during TOE in cases of suspected aortic dissection (consider sedation and intubation if necessary).

Since the distal ascending aorta and parts of the aortic arch are frequently blind zones for TOE probe, not every diagnosis

of aortic dissection or intramural haematoma (see later) can confidently be made by TOE alone, even by a highly experienced examiner. Although TOE is practically as good as CT or CMR imaging for the detection of dissection (sensitivity up to 99%, specificity around 90%), in rare cases where the findings are not convincing, additional imaging modalities must be used. Differentiation between proximal and distal aortic dissection directly influence patient management, with the need for immediate referral to cardiac surgery in the first case and more conservative approach in the second.

CMR and CT may be of particular value in detecting two other causes of acute aortic syndrome, *intramural haematoma* and *penetrating aortic ulcers*, that have similar clinical presentation as aortic dissection. While TTE is not particularly useful, TOE may detect both intramural haematoma (aortic wall thickness >7mm and/or an echolucent zone in the aortic wall) and ulcers (more often in the descending aorta). If any doubt exists, CMR should be used.

In rare cases, when the cause of ACS is dissection of coronary vessel wall or obstruction with intimal flap in proximal acute aortic dissection, misdiagnosis of aortic dissection as (primary) myocardial infarction is the rule, leading to mistreatment (fibrinolysis or percutaneous coronary intervention) with serious consequences. Therefore, proximal aortic dissection should be ruled out by TOE if any reasonable suspicion that it can be the underlying cause of the ACS is present.

Acute pulmonary embolism

In patient with unexplained chest pain in the ER, acute pulmonary embolism must be ruled out. Since pulmonary embolism is almost always associated with some degree of dyspnoea, it is discussed in detail later in this chapter.

Takotsubo cardiomyopathy

Patients with takotsubo cardiomyopathy, acute, stress-induced LV dysfunction, seen in (not exclusively) elderly women, can also reach the ER complaining of acute chest pain. Echocardiography in acute phase reveals balloon-like apical wall motion abnormality with hyperkinetic LV base ('apical ballooning'). Typically, wall motion abnormality encompasses vascular territories of more than one coronary vessels and complete recovery occurs within 2 weeks (⮕ Fig. 24.7; ▯ 24.7) (see also ⮕ Chapter 7).

It might be helpful to be aware of relative incidence of conditions that may mimic each other in the ER. Hence, acute aortic dissection is 800–1000 times less frequent than acute myocardial infarction, while around 2% of patients presenting as ACS have, in fact, takotsubo cardiomyopathy.

Acute pericarditis

Acute pericarditis might be confused with ACS due to the presence of chest pain, ECG changes, and slightly elevated troponin level. It can also occur as a complication of acute myocardial

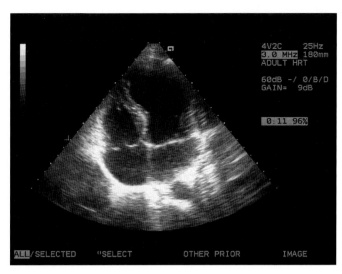

Figure 24.7 Takotsubo cardiomyopathy. TTE. Echocardiogram of 34-year-old female doctor presented in the ER with LV apical ballooning. She was successfully resuscitated at home after cardiac arrest following emotional stress. Coronary angiography was normal. Complete recovery of LV function was noted after 10 days.

infarction. Echocardiography may be helpful in detecting pericardial effusion when present, or sometimes thickened pericardium. Regional dyssynergy can be found in associated myocarditis or infarction. Pericardial effusion seen in acute aortic dissection is the grim sign, associated with impending aortic rupture and cardiac tamponade. Echo-free space around the heart due to pericardial effusion should be distinguished from a pericardial fat pad, which is usually located anteriorly, in front of the right ventricular (RV) free wall, and typically is not accompanied by posterior effusion. In addition, distinction from pleural fluid should be made with the descending thoracic aorta as a marker: pericardial fluid will appear anterior to the descending aorta in the parasternal long-axis view, and left pleural effusion will be located posterolateral to the descending aorta.

Pneumothorax

Pneumothorax may be suspected in patients with chest pain when the echocardiographic window is difficult to find and images could not be obtained due to the presence of air in the pleural space in front of the heart. Lung ultrasound typically reveals the absence of normal lung sliding pattern (if present, negative predictive value is 100%) and lung point sign, indicating the presence of the area of the chest wall where the regular reappearance of the lung sliding replaces the pneumothorax pattern (sensitivity 65%, specificity 100%).

Other conditions

Pleural fluid could be detected in *pleuritis*. Characteristic echocardiographic findings in other possible causes of acute chest pain, including *aortic stenosis, hypertrophic cardiomyopathy* (HCM), and *mitral valve prolapse,* are described elsewhere in this book.

Acute dyspnoea

In addition to causes listed in ➲ Table 24.4, patients with acute dyspnoea may suffer from common respiratory (exacerbation of chronic obstructive pulmonary disease, pneumonia) or psychiatric disorders. Echocardiography may be helpful in some of these situations to rule out serious cardiac cause.

Acute pulmonary embolism

Among many presentations of *acute pulmonary embolism* (PE) dyspnoea appears to be the most common. Since signs and symptoms of PE are non-specific, diagnostic algorithm is complex and not easy to follow. Detection rate before death is still low; overdiagnosis and overtreatment are frequent. If untreated, mortality reaches 30%. Aggressive therapy reduces mortality to 3–8%. Importantly, the majority of preventable deaths due to PE (up to 68% in various autopsy series) can be attributed to missed diagnosis rather than therapeutic failure.

In a patient with haemodynamically significant PE, TTE can easily reveal pathophysiological responses to increased pulmonary artery (PA) pressure: right heart dilation, McConnell's sign (RV free wall hypokinesis with sparing of the apex; non-specific, can be found in RV infarction), flattening and paradoxical motion of the interventricular septum (IVS) which is displaced towards LV, tricuspid regurgitation (TR), dilated inferior vena cava (IVC) without inspiratory collapse, moderately increased PA pressure (<60mmHg) (➲ Fig. 24.8; ▤ 24.8). These (and other) indirect signs strongly suggest PE in a patient at risk for deep vein thrombosis. However, direct visualization of thrombus in the right heart and/or PA is rare (4% in ICOPER registry) by TTE (➲ Fig. 24.9; ▤ 24.9).

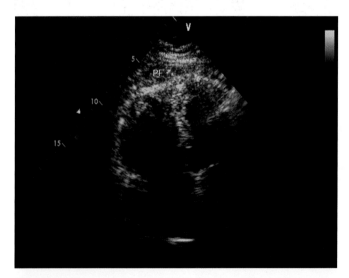

Figure 24.8 Acute pulmonary embolism. TTE. Note dilated right heart (with McConnell's sign and paradoxical septal movements—not detectable on the still image) in a patient referred to the ER from the regional hospital due to suspected unstable angina. Echo-free space in front of the heart represents pericardial fat pad. PF, pericardial fat.

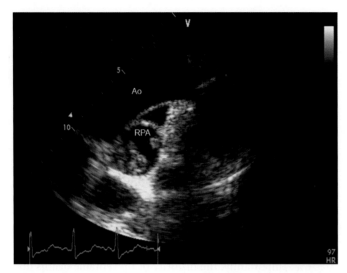

Figure 24.9 Acute pulmonary embolism. TTE. Cross-section of the right pulmonary artery from the suprasternal view reveals masses in the lumen, consistent with thrombi. Patient was presented in the ER with tachypnoea and chest pain. Ao, aorta; RPA, right pulmonary artery.

However, it should be emphasized that due to its low sensitivity (around 50%) in unselected cases (without hypotension, syncope, and other clinical signs of massive PE), TTE should not be used as a single test for diagnosis of PE. Even TOE has quite poor sensitivity in unselected cases. In contrast, in patients with PE associated with RV dysfunction, hypotension/shock, sudden cardiac arrest, or pulseless electrical activity, TOE can detect the presence of thrombus in the main pulmonary trunk or in the right and left (more difficult to visualize) PA in up to 80% of cases, with specificity of 97% (➲ Fig. 24.10; ▯ 24.10). This renders TOE as a first choice diagnostic test in the ER for evaluation selected patients with RV dysfunction, shock, or during cardiopulmonary resuscitation.

Since no single non-invasive diagnostic test is sensitive or specific enough for diagnosis of PE, other non-invasive imaging modalities, including chest CT with intravenous contrast which probably is the most accurate (negative predictive value of 99%), should be used in doubtful situations.

Apart from diagnosis, echocardiography is particularly useful for early risk stratification in patients with PE. Patients with RV dysfunction, right heart thrombi, and/or patent foramen ovale (PFO) detected by echocardiography are considered at high-risk for early and long-term mortality and morbidity and should be treated aggressively (➲ Fig. 24.11; ▯ 24.11).

Acute pulmonary oedema

In patients with *acute decompensated heart failure* and *acute pulmonary oedema,* echocardiography in the ER may help in distinction between mainly systolic (dilated heart chambers, poor global LV systolic function, functional mitral regurgitation (MR) and/or TR) or diastolic (normal ventricular size with normal or near normal global LV function, LV hypertrophy, LA enlargement, Doppler signs of high LV filling pressures) dysfunction. This distinction has direct therapeutic implications. Importantly, in patients with acute hypertensive pulmonary oedema LV systolic function is usually normal, while there is an evidence of acute worsening of diastolic dysfunction.

The presence of a multiple 'ultrasound lung comets' (➲ Fig. 24.12; ▯ 24.12) detected by the ultrasound lung examination (hyperechoic, vertical lines, arising from the pleural line, spreading to the edge of the screen and moving with lung sliding) has been reported as a clinically useful sign of extravascular lung water, that could reliably differentiate cardiogenic pulmonary

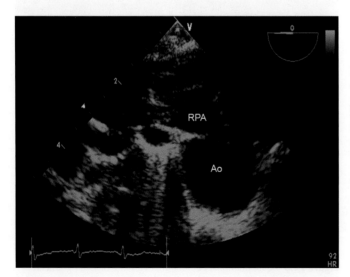

Figure 24.10 Acute massive pulmonary embolism. TEE. Note large packed masses in the lumen of the right pulmonary artery. Patient collapsed at the street and was brought to the ER by the ambulance in shock. Ao, aorta; RPA, right pulmonary artery.

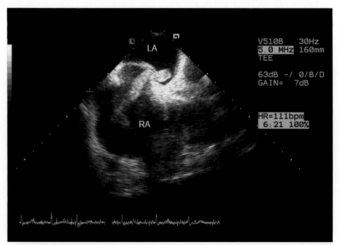

Figure 24.11 Acute pulmonary embolism with paradoxical peripheral embolization. TTE. The patient had a swollen left leg, and presented in the ER with stroke. Note the worm-like mass in the dilated right atrium, stuck in the patent foramen ovale and protruding into the left atrium, which is consistent with right heart thrombus. Note also the of the shape of the interatrial septum, indicating higher pressure on the right side. LA=left atrium, RA=right atrium.

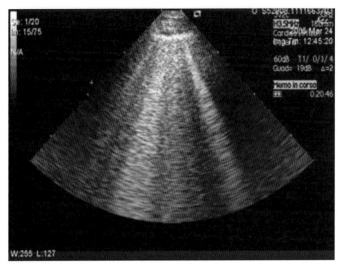

Figure 24.12 Ultrasound lung comets. In a patient with acute decompensated heart failure, lung ultrasound examination reveals hyperechoic vertical lines, consistent with extravascular lung water. (Courtesy of L. Gargani).

oedema from non-cardiogenic acute dyspnoea (i.e. exacerbated COPD), with sensitivity of 100% and a specificity of 92%.

Other common causes of acute pulmonary oedema (such as large myocardial infarction and its mechanical complications, acute valvular regurgitations, critical valvular stenosis, and prosthetic valve dysfunction) could be identified rapidly in the ER by TTE (➲ Fig. 24.13; ■ 24.13) and/or TOE (in intubated patient). Dynamic nature of ischaemic MR has to be considered in attempts to interpret the contribution of relatively mild degrees of regurgitation detected at initial presentation in the development of acute pulmonary oedema. After complete haemodynamic stabilization and before hospital discharge, these patients should undergo exercise-echocardiography to assess stress-induced ischaemia-related increase of the severity of MR.

Haemodynamic instability (shock)

All cardiac emergencies may lead to haemodynamic instability and shock (➲ Table 24.4). Not infrequently, shock is the initial presentation in the ER (➲ Fig. 24.14; ■ 24.4, 24.10, 24.14).

Rapid or excessive accumulation of pericardial fluid can cause increase of intrapericardial pressure above intracardiac pressures and such compression reduces diastolic filling, leading to *cardiac tamponade*. In these cases, echocardiography may provide immediate visualization of pericardial effusion and its haemodynamic consequences, suggesting pending cardiac tamponade (RA and RV diastolic collapse, dilated non-collapsible IVC during inspiration, significant inspiratory increase in right

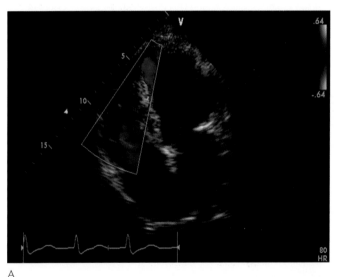

A

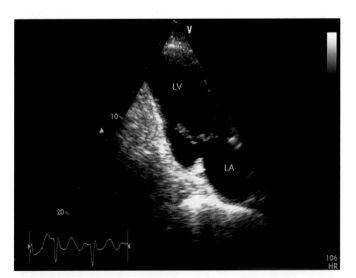

Figure 24.13 Papillary muscle rupture. TTE. Acute pulmonary oedema and cardiogenic shock after uncomplicated inferior myocardial infarction, due to ruptured posteromedial papillary muscle 2 days after early discharge from the hospital. Note the detached papillary muscle. LA, left atrium; LV, left ventricle.

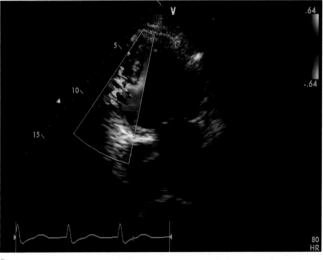

B

Figure 24.14 Postinfarction ventricular septal defect. TTE. Irregular shaped hole at mid portion of the interventricular septum is visible only while scanning in different planes. Colour Doppler reveals turbulent jet directed through the hole and in the right ventricle (B).

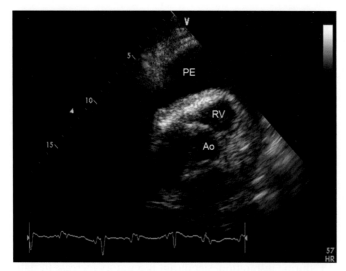

Figure 24.15 Cardiac tamponade. TTE. Note the large amount of pericardial fluid and diastolic right ventricular collapse in the parasternal short-axis view, indicating tamponade physiology. The patient had history of metastatic lung cancer, and was presented in the ER with worsening dyspnoea and profound hypotension. Ao, aorta; PE, pericardial effusion; RV, right ventricle.

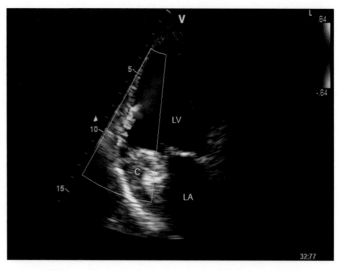

Figure 24.16 Confined rupture of the myocardial free wall. TTE. The patient with recent acute MI was referred to the ER for worsening dyspnoea and a new murmur 5 days after discharge. Significant ischaemic mitral regurgitation was detected (not show here). In addition, unexpected turbulent flow was detected through the infarcted region into pericardial space, with accumulation of echodense content (coagulated blood). C, coagulum; LA, left atrium; LV, left ventricle.

heart and parallel decrease of left heart velocities) (➲ Fig. 24.15; ▣ 24.15). Urgent pericardiocentesis, if indicated, may be safely performed in the ER under echocardiographic guidance, which allows verification of optimal site on the chest for the needle insertion and its position within pericardial space, as well as immediate follow-up after fluid removal. If the acute aortic dissection is suspected as a cause of cardiac tamponade, TOE should be performed to confirm the diagnosis and pericardiocentesis should not be attempted out of the operating room due to excessive mortality.

New murmur

Newly detected murmur in a patient presenting in the ER is almost always the result of acute valvular regurgitations (degenerative, infective endocarditis, ischaemic, trauma), mechanical complications of acute myocardial infarction (IVS rupture, papillary muscle rupture) (➲ Fig. 24.16; ▣ 24.16), rupture of the sinus of Valsalva, or acute aortic dissection. Prosthetic valve obstruction or leak may also be the cause. Rarely, cardiac tumours may generate heart murmurs. The murmur is usually paired with at least one of the other signs or symptoms of cardiac diseases, such as chest pain, dyspnoea, shock, etc. Different valves may be affected in line with actual aetiology. The valve anatomy and the origin and severity of the regurgitation/obstruction could be accurately assessed by TTE and Doppler echocardiography in majority of cases, which is explained in detail in the appropriate chapters of this book. TOE is often needed to detect vegetations or provide better insight into pathophysiology and the severity of valvular (especially mitral) regurgitation in complex cases or in emergencies related to great vessels.

Cardiac sources of embolism

In patient with cerebrovascular (neurological) or peripheral vascular event of unclear aetiology, embolic cause should be considered. The source of emboli is often (up to 20% of cases) cardiac or they may originate from complex aortic atherosclerotic plaques (➲ Fig. 24.17; ▣ 24.17). Echocardiography may reveal findings that are likely related with embolization (poor LV function, LV aneurysm, large akinetic myocardial segment, LA enlargement, atrial septal aneurysm, complex atheromatosis of the aorta), or directly detect intracardiac mass with embolic potential (➲ Fig. 24.18; ▣ 24.18). Of note, the absence of the

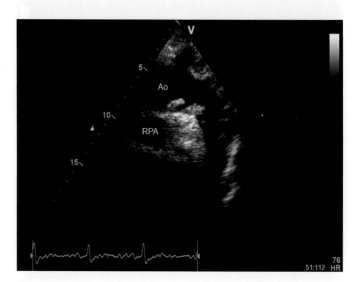

Figure 24.17 Aortic atheromatosis. TTE. From the suprasternal view, two complex aortic arch atheromas can be noted on the posterior aortic wall. Mobile components indicate large embolic potential. Ao, aorta.

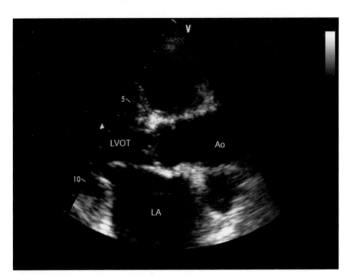

Figure 24.18 Aortic valve vegetations. TTE. Note mobile, thin, linear masses attached to the aortic leaflets, consistent with vegetations. Ao, aorta; LA; left atrium; LVOT, left ventricular outflow tract.

intracardiac masses may simply mean that it has been already embolized and caused the actual event. The exact nature of the identified mass (thrombi, vegetation, tumour) is not possible to determine on the basis of echocardiographic features alone without pathohistological examination, although localization, size, shape, and echocardiographic appearance of the mass have certain predictive value (➲ Fig. 24.19; ▣ 24.19). Paradoxical embolism through the PFO (▣ 24.11) may occur in patients with right heart masses and increased right heart pressure (i.e. pulmonary embolism).

TOE is proven to be superior than TTE in detecting cardiac source of embolism, providing detailed anatomical information (tumours, valve vegetations, prosthetic valve thrombosis) and visualizing areas which are not easily accessible by TTE (LA appendage, PFO).

Echocardiographic findings may be useful to guide acute patient management (anticoagulation), including surgical options.

Chest trauma

Blunt or penetrating chest trauma may cause severe injuries of the heart and great vessels. It is essential that emergency physicians are aware of and understand potential trauma mechanisms suggesting the possibility of myocardial contusion, heart rupture, valve injuries, dissection or injury of the coronary arteries, and traumatic acute aortic syndrome. Depending on affected structures, actual echocardiographic signs may include regional (often non-coronary) distribution of RV and/or LV dyssynergy, increased myocardial wall echogenicity and thickness, signs of myocardial rupture in various locations (atrial, septal, and free-wall rupture) with or without tamponade or pseudoaneurysm formation, acute valve regurgitations, and signs of acute aortic syndrome. TOE is often needed and preferred in patient with polytrauma and/or on mechanical ventilation, or in searching for the acute aortic syndrome (➲ Fig. 24.20; ▣ 24.20).

Cardiac arrest/cardiopulmonary resuscitation

In patient presenting in the ER with cardiac arrest or during ongoing cardiopulmonary resuscitation (CPR), echocardiography can provide key information to direct the resuscitation team. This is the case especially in patients with pulseless electrical activity. In such an extreme emergencies, a highly trained

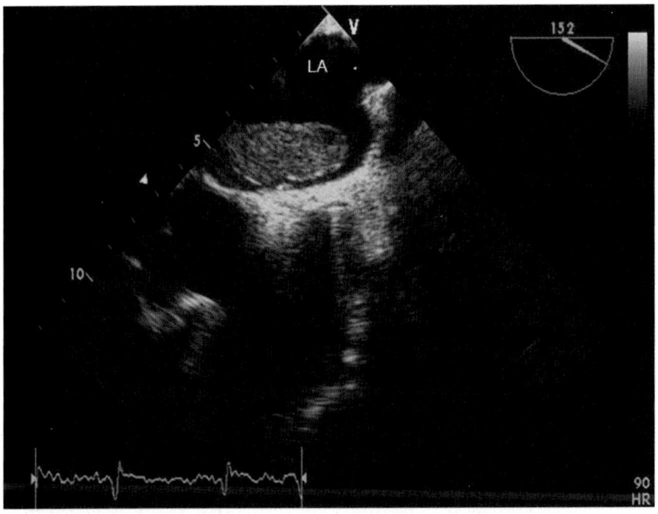

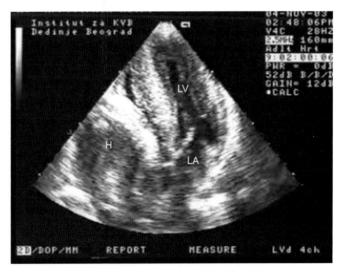

Figure 24.19 Left atrial mass. TEE. Large oval mass in the left atrium, attached to the atrial wall, with hypoechogenic zones. Differential diagnosis between tumour (myxoma?) and thrombus could not be definitively made by the echocardiography alone. LA, left atrium.

Figure 24.20 Cardiovascular collapse after blunt chest trauma. TTE. Note almost complete obliteration of the right ventricular cavity due to compression by the huge mass in the pericardial space (haematoma?). Also note small LV cavity with 'thickened' walls, indicating hypovolaemia (haemorrhagia?). H, haematoma; LA, left atrium; LV, left ventricle.

and experienced echocardiographer is needed, not just to obtain images, but also to interpret often confusing findings and make critical decisions.

TOE is often more useful during CPR to overcome obvious technical difficulties of TTE acquisition in this setting, particularly in intubated patients. Findings, such as cardiac tamponade, acute PE, HCM, hypovolaemic heart (small chambers with LV/RV cavity obliteration during vigorous contractions), etc. might be helpful in choosing adequate, possibly life-saving therapeutic procedures.

Emergency echocardiographic study report

An emergency echocardiographic study report, in general, should stick as much as possible to the basic format recently recommended by the European Association of Echocardiography. However, since time is often extremely limited, the initial report might be focused on critical findings and integrated in the decision-making process. Whenever the result of the study indicates the need for urgent treatment, the responsible physician needs to be informed. Detailed, more complete, the final report should follow soon after the patient is transferred/referred for further diagnostic or therapeutic procedure. It seems wise to prepare this final report after carefully reviewing

the case together with the experienced colleague. The report should end with clear and understandable conclusions regarding the diagnosis and severity of the disease.

Focused peri-resuscitation and critical care echocardiography

Recently a number of protocols for basic focused echo examinations in the emergency or critical care situation have been developed. These protocols aim to enable individuals, after limited training, to identify basic (and only basic) but critical cardiac pathologies, such as catastrophic ventricular dysfunction or tamponade.

Focused Echocardiography in Emergency Life Support (FEEL) is a limited echo protocol that can be performed by operators with minimal training during emergency life support and aims to identify true asystole, tamponade and other catastrophic states. Studies have shown that the findings may alter management including decisions on cessation or prolongation of resuscitation. Training contains 'E' learning, a one day practical course and 50 supervised scans.

Other critical care protocols include Focused Assessed Transthoracic Echocardiography (FATE) which includes also pleural ultrasound and Focused Abdominal Sonography in Trauma (FAST) which uses subxiphoid images to view the heart.[41]

Personal perspective

Echocardiography in the emergency setting is a highly demanding procedure and due to the serious implications of the examination result it should not be attempted by inexperienced personnel without supervision.

In order to solve logistics problems related to the decision-making process, digital echo laboratories with internal network/server and telemedicine solutions will enable immediate/permanent audiovisual connection with the ER, and direct supervision of the interpretation based on acquired images.

Echocardiography appears to be simple to the uninformed, however, it is only simple to apply, but not to perform. In the years to come, we shall observe an increasing trend towards

performance of focused echocardiographic studies by non-cardiologists. A large choice of inexpensive, miniaturized, hand-held, convenient for use echocardiographic machines will be available in the market, and it seems highly likely that many non-cardiologists and cardiologists with insufficient formal training will use it instead of the stethoscope. Although this approach might save a number of lives by straightforward access to cardiac imaging wherever needed, unfortunately, it will be indisputably linked to an increased likelihood of disastrous errors in the emergency setting. This practice will raise key issues regarding education in echocardiography. Precise and strict requirements consisting of a carefully prepared curriculum have to be defined, in order to preserve the quality and the accuracy of the data provided by echocardiography, especially in the emergency setting.

Further reading

Arvan S, Varat MA. Two-dimensional echocardiography versus surface electrocardiography for the diagnosis of acute non-Q wave myocardial infarction. *Am Heart J* 1985; **110**:44–9.

Blatchford O, Capewell S. Emergency medical admissions in Glasgow: general practices vary despite adjustments for age, sex and deprivation. *Br J Gen Pract* 1999; **49**:551–4.

Breitkreutz R, Price S, Steiger HV, Seeger FH, Ilper H, Ackermann H, *et al.* Focused echocardiographic evaluation in life support and peri-resuscitation of emergency patients: A prospective trial, from the Emergency Ultrasound Working Group of the Johann Wolfgang Goethe-University Hospital, Frankfurt am Main. *Resuscitation* 2010; 81(11):1527–33.

Breitkreutz R, Walcher F, Seeger S. Focused echocardiographic evaluation in resuscitation management: concept of an advanced life support–conformed algorithm. *Crit Care Med* 2007; **35**(Suppl.):S150–61.

Cheitlin MD, Armstrong WF, Aurigemma GP, Beller GA, Bierman FZ, Davis JL, *et al.* ACC/AHA/ASE 2003 guideline update for the clinical application of echocardiography: a report of the American College of Cardiology/American Heart Association Task Force on Practice Guidelines (ACC/AHA/ASE Committee to Update the 1997 Guidelines for the Clinical Application of Echocardiography). *J Am Coll Cardiol* 2003; **42**:954–70.

Colon PJ, Cheirif J. Long-term value of stress echocardiography in the triage of patients with atypical chest pain presenting to the emergency department. *Echocardiography* 1999; **16**:171–7.

Douglas PS, Khandheria B, Stainback RF, Weissman NJ. ACCF/ASE/ACEP/ASNC/SCAI/SCCT/SCMR 2007 appropriateness criteria for transthoracic and transesophageal echocardiography. *J Am Coll Cardiol* 2007; **50**:187–204.

Ehler D, Carney D, Dempsey A, Rigling R, Kraft C, Witt S, *et al.* Guidelines for cardiac sonographer education: recommendations of the American Society of Echocardiography Sonographer Training and Education Committee. *J Am Soc Echocardiogr* 2001; **14**:77–84.

Evangelista A, Flachskampf F, Lancelotti P, Badano L, Aguilar R, Monaghan M, *et al.*, on behalf of the European Association of Echocardiography. European Association of Echocardiography recommendations for standardization of performance, digital storage and reporting of echocardiographic studies. *Eur J Echocardiogr* 2008; **9**:438–48.

Feissel M, Maizel J, Robles G, Badie J, Faller JP, Slama M. Clinical relevance of echocardiography in acute severe dyspnea. *J Am Soc Echocardiogr* 2009; **22**:1159–64.

Flachskampf F, Decoodt P, Fraser A, Daniel W, Roeland J, for the Subgroup on Transesophageal Echocardiography and Valvular Heart Disease on behalf of the Working Group on Echocardiography of the European Society of Cardiology. Guidelines from the Working Group – Recommendations for performing transesophageal echocardiography. *Eur J Echocardiography* 2001; **2**:8–21.

Gibler WB, Runyon JP, Levy RC, Sayre M, Kacich R, Hattemer C, *et al.* A rapid diagnostic and treatment center for patients with chest pain in the emergency department. *Ann Emerg Med* 1995; **25**:1–8.

Goldhaber SZ, Visani L, De Rosa M. Acute pulmonary embolism: clinical outcomes in the International Cooperative Pulmonary Embolism Registry (ICOPER). *Lancet* 1999; **353**:1386–9.

Greaves SC. Role of echocardiography in acute coronary syndromes. *Heart* 2002; **88**:419–25.

Hagendorff A. Transthoracic echocardiography in adult patients– a proposal for documenting a standardized investigation. *Eur J Ultrasound* 2008; **29**:2–31.

Heger JJ, Weyman AE, Wann LS, Rogers EW, Dillon JC, Feigenbaum H. Cross-sectional echocardiographic analysis of the extent of left ventricular asynergy in acute myocardial infarction. *Circulation* 1980; **61**:1113–18.

Jaarsma W, Visser CA, Eenige van MJ, Verheugt FW, Kupper AJ, Roos JP. Predictive value of two-dimensional echocardiographic and hemodynamic measurements on admission with acute myocardial infarction. *J Am Soc Echocardiogr* 1988; **1**:187–93.

Jeetley P, Burden L, Senior R. Stress echocardiography is superior to exercise ECG in the risk stratification of patients presenting with acute chest pain with negative troponin. *Eur J Echocardiogr* 2006; **7**:155–64.

Kaul S, Senior R, Firschke C, Wang X, Lindner J, Villanueva F, *et al.* Incremental value of cardiac imaging in patients presenting to the emergency department with chest pain and without ST-segment elevation: a multicenter study. *Am Heart J* 2004; **148**:129–36.

Kucher N, Rossi E, De Rosa M, Goldhaber SZ. Prognostic role of echocardiography among patients with acute pulmonary embolism and a systolic arterial pressure of 90mm Hg or higher. *Arch Intern Med* 2005; **165**:1777–81.

Lichtenstein D, Meziere G, Biderman P, Gepner A. The lung point: an ultrasound sign specific to pneumothorax. *Intensive Care Med* 2000; **26**:1434–40.

Lichtenstein D, Meziere G. A lung ultrasound sign allowing bedside distinction between pulmonary edema and COPD: the comet-tail artifact. *Intensive Care Med* 1998; **24**:1331–4.

Loh IK, Charuzi Y, Beeder C, Marshall LA, Ginsburg JH. Early diagnosis of nontransmural myocardial infarction by two-dimensional echocardiography. *Am Heart J* 1982; **104**:963–8.

Mookadam F, Jiamsripong P, Goel R, Warsame T, Emani U, Khandheria BK. Critical appraisal on the utility of echocardiography in the management of acute pulmonary embolism. *Cardiol Rev* 2010; **18**:29–37.

Neskovic AN, Flachskampf FA, Picard MH (eds). *Emergency Echocardiography.* London: Taylor & Francis; 2005.

Neskovic AN, Popovic AD, Babic R, Otasevic P. Color-Doppler transesophageal echocardiography in detection of massive pulmonary embolism: is pulmonary angiography always the gold standard? *Echocardiography* 1996; **13**:631–3.

Nienaber CA, Sievers HH. Intramural haematoma in acute aortic syndrome: more than one variant of dissection? *Circulation* 2002; **106**:284–5.

Nihoyannopoulos P, Fox K, Fraser A, Pinto F, on behalf of the Laboratory Accreditation Committee of the EAE. EAE laboratory standards and accreditation. *Eur J Echocardiogr* 2007; **8**:80–7.

Pandian NG, Skorton DJ, Collins SM. Myocardial infarct size threshold for two-dimensional echocardiographic detection: sensitivity of systolic wall thickening and endocardial motion abnormalities in small versus large infarcts. *Am J Cardiol* 1985; **55**:551–5.

Peels CH, Visser CA, Kupper AJ, Visser FC, Roos JP. Usefulness of two-dimensional echocardiography for immediate detection of myocardial ischemia in the emergency room. *Am J Cardiol* 1990; **65**:687–91.

Picano E, Frassi F, Agricola E, Gligorova S, Gargani L, Mottola G. Ultrasound lung comets: a clinically useful sign of extravascular lung water. *J Am Soc Echocardiogr* 2006; **19**:356-63.

Picano E, Gargani L, Gheorghiade M. Why, when, and how to assess pulmonary congestion in heart failure: pathophysiological, clinical, and methodological implications. *Heart Fail Rev* 2010; **15**:63–72.

Pierard LA, Lancellotti P. Echocardiography in the emergency room: non-invasive imaging. *Heart* 2009; **95**:164–70.

Pruszczyk P, Torbicki A, Kuch-Wocial A, Chlebus M, Miskiewicz ZC, Jedrusik P. Transoesophageal echocardiography for definitive diagnosis of haemodynamically significant pulmonary embolism. *Eur Heart J* 1995; **16**:534–8.

Quinones M, Douglas P, Foster E, Gorscan J, Lewis J, Pearlman A, *et al.* ACC/AHA Clinical Competence Statement on Echocardiography. A Report of the American College of Cardiology/American Heart Association/American College of Physicians–American Society of Internal Medicine Task Force on clinical competence developed in collaboration with the American Society of Echocardiography, the Society of Cardiovascular Anesthesiologists, and the Society of Pediatric Echocardiography. *J Am Coll Cardiol* 2003; **41**(4): 687–708.

Sabia P, Afrookteh A, Touchstone DA, Keller MW, Esquivel L, Kaul S. Value of regional wall motion abnormality in the emergency room diagnosis of acute myocardial infarction. A prospective study using two-dimensional echocardiography. *Circulation* 1991; **84**(Suppl I):85–92.

Stewart WJ, Douglas PS, Sagar K, Seward JB, Armstrong WF, Zoghbi W, *et al.* Echocardiography in emergency medicine: a policy statement by the American Society of Echocardiography and the American College of Cardiology. The Task Force on Echocardiography in Emergency Medicine of the American Society of Echocardiography and the Echocardiography TPEC Committees of the American College of Cardiology. *J Am Soc Echocardiogr* 1999; **12**:82–4.

Tayal V, Blaivas M, Mandavia D, Blankenship R, Boniface K, Ferre R, *et al.* Emergency ultrasound guidelines. *Ann Emerg Med* 2009; **53**:550–70.

Tong KL, Kaul S, Wang XQ, Rinkevich D, Kalvaitis S, Belcik T, *et al.* Myocardial contrast echocardiography versus thrombolysis in myocardial infarction score in patients presenting to the emergency department with chest pain and a nondiagnostic electrocardiogram. *J Am Coll Cardiol* 2008; **46**:920–27.

Torbicki A, Perrier A, Konstantinides S, Agnelli G, Galiè N, Pruszczyk P, *et al.* Task Force for the Diagnosis and Management of Acute Pulmonary Embolism of the. Guidelines on the diagnosis and management of acute pulmonary embolism: the Task Force for the Diagnosis and Management of Acute Pulmonary Embolism of the European Society of Cardiology (ESC). *Eur Heart J* 2008; **29**:2276–315.

Zabalgoitia M, Ismaeil M. Diagnostic and prognostic use of stress echocardiography in acute coronary syndromes including emergency department imaging. *Echocardiography* 2000; **17**:479–93.

Additional DVD and online material

Important note Videoclips 24.1–24.20 related to this chapter are carefully chosen to reflect the complexity of the echocardiographic assessment in the emergency settings. The intention was not to cover all examples, but to represent true, real-life cases, illustrating a few important messages. Videoclips and figures of many different conditions that are detected in the ER can be found elsewhere in this book, in the related chapters, and online.

■ 24.1 Poor imaging technique. TTE. Note akinesis of the distal septum and LV apex which is clearly detectable only when full length of the LV is obtained (second image in the loop is acquired from the window located one intercostal space lower than the first one).

■ 24.2 2D echo during anginal pain. TTE. Note akinesis of the apex in patient complaining on actual acute chest pain (see also ■ 24.3).

■ 24.3 2D echo after anginal pain. TTE. The patient is the same as presented on ■ 24.2. Note normokinesis of the apex 2 min later, when chest pain was gone.

■ 24.4 Haemodynamically unstable acute myocardial infarction. TTE. The patient was presented in the ER in cardiogenic shock. Note poor global LV function (EF measured as 10%) due to large akinetic zone that includes septum, apex, and distal two-thirds of the lateral LV wall, and significant ischaemic mitral regurgitation.

■ 24.5 Acute proximal aortic dissection. TTE. Note mobile, linear echogenic structure (intimal flap) in the lumen of ascending aorta and arch assessed using suprasternal view. The patient was presented in the ER with abrupt, crushing chest pain, radiating towards back.

■ 24.6 Acute aortic dissection. TTE. The image is obtained from the subcostal view in a young patient referred to the ER as suspected postinfarction ventricular septal defect. There are only two frames with visible flap in the descending aorta, indicating dissection. Images obtained from other views where completely unremarkable.

■ 24.7 Takotsubo cardiomyopathy. TTE. Echocardiogram of a 34-year-old female doctor presented with LV apical ballooning in the ER. She was successfully resuscitated at home after cardiac arrest following emotional stress. Coronary angiography was normal. Complete recovery of LV function was noted after 10 days.

■ 24.8 Acute pulmonary embolism. TTE. Note dilated right heart with McConnell's sign and paradoxical septal movements in a patient referred to the ER from the regional hospital due to suspected unstable angina. Echo-free space in front of the heart represents pericardial fat pad.

■ 24.9 Acute pulmonary embolism. TTE. Cross-section of the right pulmonary artery from the suprasternal view reveals masses in the lumen, consistent with thrombi. Patient was presented in the ER with tachypnoea and chest pain.

■ 24.10 Acute massive pulmonary embolism. TOE. Note large packed masses in the lumen of the right pulmonary artery. Patient collapsed at the street and was brought to the ER by the ambulance in shock.

■ 24.11 Acute pulmonary embolism with paradoxical peripheral embolization. TTE. The patient with swollen left leg, presented in the ER with stroke. Note the worm-like mass in the dilated right atrium, stuck in the patent foramen ovale and protruding into the left atrium, which is consistent with right heart thrombus. Note also the shape of the interatrial septum, indicating higher pressure on the right side.

■ 24.12 Ultrasound lung comets. In patient with acute decompensated heart failure, lung ultrasound examination reveals hyperechoic vertical lines, consistent with extravascular lung water. (Courtesy of L. Gargani)

- 24.13 Papillary muscle rupture. TTE. Acute pulmonary oedema and cardiogenic shock after uncomplicated inferior myocardial infarction, due to ruptured posteromedial papillary muscle 2 days after early discharge from the hospital. Note the flail posterior and prolapsed anterior mitral leaflets and free movements of the detached papillary muscle.

- 24.14 Postinfarction interventricular septal defect. TTE. Note the irregular shaped hole at mid portion of the interventricular septum, visible during scanning in different planes. Colour Doppler reveals turbulent jet directed through the hole and in the right ventricle.

- 24.15 Cardiac tamponade. TTE. Note the large amount of pericardial fluid and diastolic right ventricular collapse in the parasternal short-axis view, indicating tamponade physiology. The patient had a history of metastatic lung cancer, and was presented in the ER with worsening dyspnoea and profound hypotension.

- 24.16 Confined rupture of the myocardial free wall. TTE. The patient with recent acute myocardial infarction was referred to the ER for worsening dyspnoea and a new murmur 5 days after discharge. Significant ischaemic mitral regurgitation was detected (not show here). In addition, unexpected flow was detected through the infarcted region into pericardial space, with accumulation of echodense content (coagulated blood).

- 24.17 Aortic atheromatosis. TTE. From the suprasternal view, two complex aortic arch atheromas can be noted on the posterior aortic wall. Mobile components indicate large embolic potential.

- 24.18 Aortic valve vegetations. TTE. Note mobile, thin, linear masses attached to the aortic leaflets, consistent with vegetations.

- 24.19 Left atrial mass. TOE. Large oval mass in the left atrium, attached to the atrial wall, with hypoechogenic zones. Differential diagnosis between tumour (myxoma?) and thrombus could not be definitively made by the echocardiography alone.

- 24.20 Cardiovascular collapse after blunt chest trauma. TTE. Note almost complete obliteration of the right ventricular cavity due to compression by the huge mass in the pericardial space (haematoma?). Also note small LV cavity with 'thickened' walls, indicating hypovolaemia.

- For additional multimedia materials please visit the online version of the book (￼ http://escecho.oxfordmedicine.com).

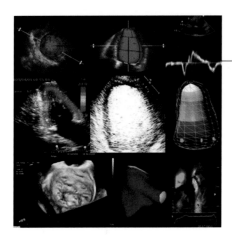

CHAPTER 25

Vascular imaging

Mónica M. Pedro and N. Cardim

Contents

Summary

The use of vascular ultrasonography (alone or combined with newer techniques like angio-magnetic resonance or angio-computed tomography) is an essential tool for the diagnosis and the assessment of vascular diseases. It is also useful for the follow-up after surgical or endovascular interventions (avoiding the need to use angiography in any therapeutic decision in most cases). The integration of two-dimensional echocardiography, colour flow imaging and spectral Doppler makes the morphological and functional assessment of vascular disease possible in almost every territory.

For a long time, vascular ultrasonography was exclusively performed by non-cardiologists. Nowadays, in modern echo laboratories, vascular echography is frequently performed by cardiologists, often in cooperation with vascular surgeons and radiologists.

In this chapter, we review the essential concepts of the use of vascular ultrasound imaging in the study of the territories that are most commonly evaluated:

◆ Cerebrovascular circulation.

◆ Abdominal circulation.

◆ Lower limb circulation (arterial and venous disease).

In each of these sections, we describe the technical details of the ultrasonic examination, the normal recordings, the abnormal findings of specific diseases/syndromes affecting each territory, and the postoperative/post-interventional evaluation and follow-up.

Cerebrovascular circulation

Colour-flow duplex scan

Colour-flow duplex scan (CFDS) is the main ultrasound-based method used in the assessment of extracranial cerebral arteries.[1] Using this technique, it is possible to visualize the carotid and vertebral arteries, to analyse and to quantify the thickness of the arterial wall, to identify and characterize atherosclerotic plaques, and to measure the degree of stenosis by morphological and haemodynamic criteria.

It is a reliable, cheap, and non-invasive method (avoids radiation and contrast) that can obviate the need for angiography in the therapeutic decision in most cases of carotid disease. It may also be combined with newer techniques like angio-magnetic resonance or angio-computed tomography. Nevertheless, it depends on the observer and on the quality of the equipment.

Presently, CFDS is an essential tool for the diagnosis and assessment of carotid disease and it is also useful for the follow-up after surgical or endovascular interventions.

Examination technique

For the performance of a CFDS study, the patient must lie in the supine position, with the supraclavicular and cervical regions exposed. The operator is usually positioned by the patient's right side with the equipment in front. A linear and multifrequency 7–10MHz probe is usually used and the carotid scanning begins at the base of the neck and continues to behind the angle of the mandibular. This permits the identification and assessment of the common carotid artery (CCA), the bifurcation, the origin of the external carotid artery (ECA), and the first portion of the internal carotid artery (ICA) with its proximal dilation (carotid bulb) (➲ Fig. 25.1).

The study should be performed in longitudinal and transversal sections and it is often necessary to change the probe angulation for a better visualization of some vascular segments. It should also include a morphological evaluation as well as the assessment of flow characteristics along the carotid axis with determination of velocities (peak systolic velocity and end diastolic velocity).

The flow in the carotid artery can be assessed by Doppler and colour-flow Doppler. Usually, it is laminar, with upward direction and there may be a small area of turbulence due to different directions of flow in the area of bifurcation. For a correct assessment of flow and velocities the sample volume should be positioned in the area of higher stenosis and the angle of examination should be equal or less than 60 degrees.

The morphology of the flow in the CCA is identical to the one of the ICA, with a peak systolic flow followed by a gentle slope and a slower flow present during diastole, typical of low resistance haemodynamic territories. In the ECA, the morphology of the flow is different, with a higher systolic peak, a rapid decline and virtually absent diastolic flow (➲ Fig. 25.1).

In the ICA the normal peak systolic velocity (PSV) is less than 120cm/s and the normal end-diastolic velocity is less than 40cm/s.

The cervical segment of the vertebral arteries should also be analysed, assessing the waveform between the vertebral processes. The flow direction is similar to that of the CCA, i.e. towards the head. The presence of reverse flow in the vertebral arteries (➲ Fig. 25.2) must raise the suspicion of occlusion or severe stenosis of the pre-vertebral segment of the ipsilateral subclavian artery (subclavian steal syndrome). The vertebral artery on each side can be viewed by angling the probe outwards and backwards from the ipsilateral carotid, and the left one is usually larger than the opposite.

Assessment of early atherosclerotic disease

Atherosclerosis is a systemic disease, affecting several arterial territories. Its prognosis is mainly dependent on the involvement of the coronary and cerebral areas. Thus, treatment of complications of atherosclerosis in a given territory implies the active search for lesions in other sectors. The identification of early atherosclerotic disease appears to have implications in the assessment of global cardiovascular risk and in the strategies of medical treatment aimed at the prevention of atherothrombosis. The detection of subclinical changes at certain sectors of the arterial tree, such as the carotid arteries, has a linear relationship with the future occurrence of coronary and cerebral complications, as well as with mortality due to cardiovascular disease.[2]

These early and subclinical manifestations of carotid atherosclerosis are reflected in a progressive increase in thickness of the intima and the media layers of the carotid artery (intima-media thickness, IMT). The advanced phases correspond to the presence of atheromatous plaques.[2]

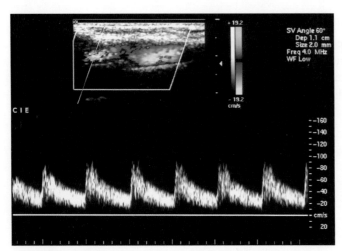

Figure 25.1 Colour-flow image of the carotid bifurcation. Colour-flow image of the carotid bifurcation and the origin of the ICA (above) with a normal Doppler waveform pattern (below).

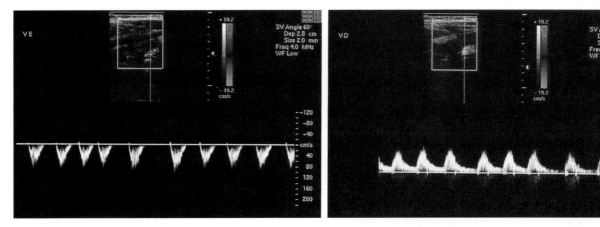

Figure 25.2 Doppler flow image of vertebral arteries. Assessment of Doppler flow pattern in both vertebral arteries with inversion in the left side. The patient had an occlusion of the pre-vertebral portion of the left subclavian artery.

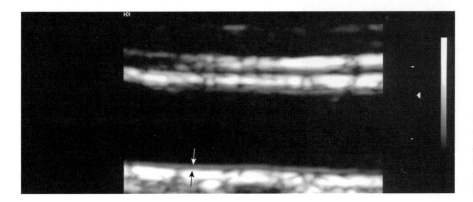

Figure 25.3 Ultrasonographic morphology of the CCA. The arrows mark the quantification of IMT, in a place where the normal three layers of the distal wall can be seen.

IMT is measured by two-dimensional (2D) ultrasonography and corresponds histologically to intima plus media layers: 2D measurement corresponds to the thickness of the first two echogenic lines of the arterial wall. IMT should be measured in the posterior wall of the CCA (where it is best viewed), about 1–2cm upstream to the carotid bifurcation (➲ Fig. 25.3).

Although there is no definite consensus about what is a normal IMT (as the thickness of the intima-media layer increases with age in a linear fashion), several studies suggest that values above 0.9–1cm are abnormal. So, IMT can be considered a new cardiovascular risk factor, important not only in risk stratification but also in the strategy of overall medical treatment.

Assessment of advanced atherosclerotic disease

Atherosclerosis is a progressive disease and in its advanced stages is associated with the development of atheromatous plaques. The carotid bifurcation is a common location for these lesions which are a cause of amaurosis fugax, transitory focal neurological symptoms or stroke.[3] The risk of stroke associated with carotid occlusive disease is related to the degree of stenosis and also to the structure of the plaque. Some lesions are prone to rupture (*vulnerable or unstable*) and to the formation of thrombus on their surface which can embolize to the brain or determine arterial occlusion.

CFDS is an appropriate technique to identify carotid plaques, to determine the degree of stenosis and to assess plaque structure. Two main types of criteria are used to study carotid disease:

- Morphological criteria: assessment of plaques and obstruction using 2D ultrasonography.

- Haemodynamic criteria: assessment of turbulence and acceleration of blood flow with quantification of systolic and diastolic velocities using Doppler effect and its colour codification.

Quantification of the degree of stenosis

Doppler ultrasound allows the morphological quantification of stenosis as diameter in longitudinal section or area in transversal

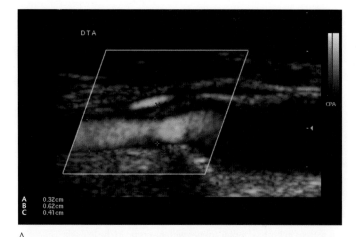

A

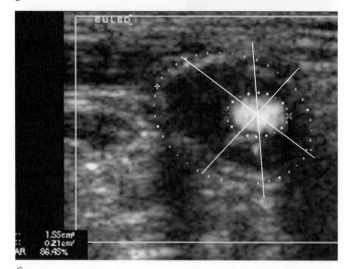

B

C

Figure 25.4 Quantification of carotid stenosis using morphological criteria. A) Longitudinal measurement according to the European method $(1 - (A/B) \times 100 = 48\%)$ and to the American method $(1 - (A/C) \times 100 = 22\%)$. B) Area measurement in a cross-section of the stenosis when the lumen is round and regular. C) Area measurement in a cross-section of the stenosis when the lumen is elliptical. Depending on the assessment plane, very different lumen diameters can be obtained in a longitudinal measurement of the stenosis.

cross section, as well as its haemodynamic repercussion (acceleration of flow):

- *Diameter*: stenosis can be quantified according to the European method (ECST,[4] ACST[5]), which compares the minimum luminal diameter at stenosis level with the diameter of the carotid bulb; or according to the American method (NASCET,[6] ACAS[7]) which compares the minimum luminal diameter at stenosis level with the diameter of the distal internal carotid artery (◗ Fig. 25.4A). This form of measurement is suitable for regular and concentric lesions (◗ Fig. 25.4B). In irregular or elliptical lesions (◗ Fig. 25.4C), it can be difficult to measure the diameter of greatest stenosis (which depends on the selected cross-section zone), resulting in false values.

- *Area*: stenosis can be estimated by the ratio between the luminal area at the stenosis and the entire area of the artery at the same location. This is the most accurate measurement of the morphological degree of carotid stenosis since it is independent of the shape and location of the parietal plaque, and it can even be used in eccentric lesions. It is of the utmost importance to locate correctly the point of maximum stenosis.

- *Haemodynamics:* Doppler ultrasound can also measure the degree of stenosis based on the haemodynamic effect of the plaque on the blood flow (*acceleration*). Beyond measurement of PSV and end diastolic velocity, the assessment of the degree of flow disturbance distal to the stenosis may be of diagnostic value. In fact, distal to the stenosis, blood flow shows a zone of increased velocity (*velocity jet*) and alterations in the overall Doppler tracing. As stenosis degree increases, such downstream flow disturbances cause the Doppler spectrum to be broadened (*spectral broadening*), as red blood cells diverge from the velocity jet and change in direction.

Criteria have been published for determining the cut-off values for stenosis used in multicentre studies concerning symptomatic and asymptomatic carotid disease (◗ Fig. 25.5).

According to these studies, carotid surgery, such as endarterectomy, is of benefit in:

- Symptomatic stenosis >70% by the American[6] and European methods.[4]

- Symptomatic stenosis of 50–70% by the American method,[6] only if the surgical risk is <3%.

- Asymptomatic stenosis >80% by the European method.[5]

- Asymptomatic stenosis >60% by the American method.[7]

◗ Tables 25.1 and 25.2 show the haemodynamic criteria most often used in clinical practice and the cut-off values.

It is sometimes difficult to differentiate between stenosis and occlusion (◗ Fig. 25.6), since in very severe obstruction (99%) the amount of flow can be so small that there is no acceleration and so it is not detectable by spectral Doppler. It is therefore important in these cases to evaluate the lesion with colour

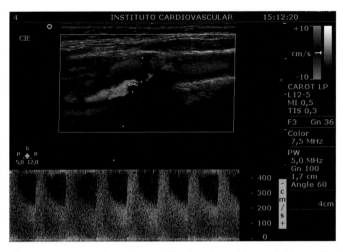

Figure 25.5 Haemodynamic quantification of carotid stenosis. Note a PSV >500cm/s and EDV >200cm/s, corresponding to a >90% stenosis.

Table 25.1 University of Washington criteria for grading ICA stenosis[8] (cut-off 50% and 80%)

% Diameter reduction	Velocity	Spectral characteristics
0	PSV <125cm/s	No spectral broadening
1–15%	PSV <125cm/s	Spectral broadening in systolic deceleration
16–49	PSV >125cm/s	Spectral broadening throughout systole
50–79	PSV >125cm/s	Extensive spectral broadening
80–99	PSV >125cm/s and EDV >140cm/s	Extensive spectral broadening
Occlusion	No ICA flow	Low or no diastolic flow in CCA

CCA, common carotid artery; EDV, end diastolic velocity; ICA, internal carotid artery; PSV, peak systolic velocity.

Doppler (CD) and pulsed wave (PW) Doppler, which has greater sensitivity in low velocity flows. The loss of the diastolic flow in CCA flow wave is an indirect criterion of complete occlusion of the ICA. Another aspect that may hinder the

Table 25.2 Society of Radiologists–Ultrasound Consensus Criteria for Grading Carotid Stenosis[8,9] (cut-off 50% and 70%)

% Diameter reduction	ICA PSV	ICA EDV	ICA/CCA PSV ratio
Normal	<125	<40	<2
<50	<125	<40	<2
50–69	125–230	40–100	2–4
>70	>230	>100	>4
Occlusion	0	0	<1

CCA, common carotid artery; EDV, end diastolic velocity; ICA, internal carotid artery; PSV, peak systolic velocity.

quantification of stenosis is the presence of extensive calcification since the shadowing can hide a severe obstruction. However, if the blind zone is short (<1cm) and the downstream flow is normal, it can be inferred with considerable certainty that there is not a significant stenosis.

In conclusion, Doppler ultrasound examination has unique characteristics that allow the quantification of the degree of stenosis, which should result from a combination of morphological and haemodynamic techniques, which increases their diagnostic accuracy.

Plaque characterization

The CFDS allows direct visualization of atherosclerotic plaques and their ultrasonographic morphological assessment. In general, these lesions can be classified according to the echo structure in homogeneous (they may be echolucent—*type 1*, hyperechoic—*type 4*) (➲ Fig. 25.7A), and heterogeneous (predominantly echolucent—*type 2* or predominantly hyperechoic—*type 3*). One of the most used classifications is the one proposed by Geroulakos[10] which includes, in addition to the previously mentioned types *type 5*, which corresponds to very calcified plaques, with significant shadowing on the imaging, and not suitable for detailed ultrasound examination.

Plaques predominantly echolucent can be difficult to visualize by ultrasound. This can be solved with the use of colour coding to determine their presence and contour (➲ Fig. 25.7B), followed by the application of the quantification methods described earlier.

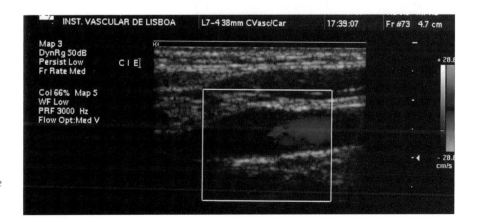

Figure 25.6 Colour flow imaging of carotid occlusion. Carotid CFDS showing complete occlusion of the ICA. There is no progression of the colour-flow inside ICA.

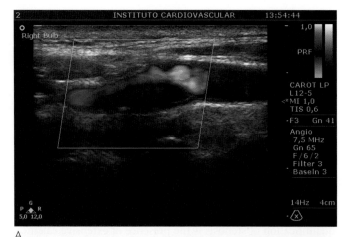

A

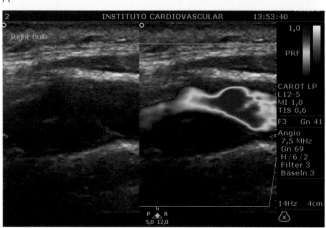

B

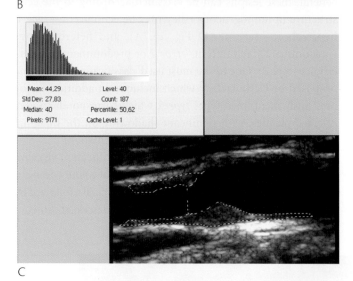

C

Figure 25.7 Plaque characterization. A) Example of a homogenous and echolucent plaque—Geroulakos type 1. B) Echolucent plaque in which colour flow is helpful to visualize its contour. C) computer-assisted plaque characterization of an echogenic plaque (GSM-40).

The typical morphology of the unstable or vulnerable to rupture atherosclerotic plaque is well known. It is mainly characterized by a wide lipid-necrotic centre, thin fibrous cap, juxtaluminal lipid-necrotic centre, high lipid content, intraplaque haemorrhage, increased levels of inflammation, and erosion or rupture of the plaque.[11]

Ultrasonography allows the study of some of these aspect and equivalent ultrasonographic characteristics of those aspects of instability of lesions have been proposed[11] (➲ Table 25.3).

Computer-assisted analysis provides greater accuracy and reproducibility of ultrasound assessment and characterization of the lesions. It is based on previous standardization of the images of the plaques so that they may be comparable. A comparison between symptomatic and asymptomatic plaques revealed that the echomorphological factors associated with increased risk were:[11]

- The degree of stenosis.

- The heterogeneity of the echo structure.

- The echolucency.

- The juxtaluminal location of the echolucent part of heterogenous plaques.

- The evidence of plaque surface disruption.

The echolucency of the plaque is expressed by two parameters obtained from a histogram of the grey-scale distribution of pixels within the entire area of the plaque: the grey-scale median (GSM) and the percentile 40 (P40) which represents the percentage of echolucent pixels.

The combination and the determination of the relative importance of each of these parameters led to the creation of an Activity Index (➲ Fig. 25.8) for each plaque that is correlated with the occurrence of cerebrovascular complications.[12] The cut-off with the best predictive value for the identification of symptomatic plaques is the value of 65.

Evaluation and follow-up after interventions

The carotid CFDS study can also be applied in patients after carotid endarterectomy or stenting, in order to detect the presence of restenosis or other local complications.

Transcranial Doppler ultrasound

Although the description of this technique goes beyond the scope of this chapter, it is important to emphasize that it allows the non-invasive study of intracranial circulation, including the circle of Willis and major intracranial vessels. Using a low-frequency (2MHz) ultrasound probe applied to the temporal bone it is possible to obtain both spectral and CD recordings of blood flow crossing.

Table 25.3 Ultrasonographic equivalents of histological parameters associated with vulnerable and ruptured plaques[11]

Histological parameter	Ultrasonographic equivalent	
	Homogenous	Heterogenous
Wide lipid/necrotic	Echolucency	Echolucency
		Echolucency
Juxtaluminal lipid/necrotic		Juxtaluminal echolucent area
Intraplaque hemorrhage	Echolucency	Echolucency
Thin fibrous cap	Thin or invisible echogenic cap	Thin or invisible echogenic cap
	% echogenic cap	
Plaque disruption	Disruption of plaque surface	Disruption of plaque surface
	Ulceration	Ulceration

One of the most common clinical applications of transcranial Doppler ultrasonography is the assessment of right-to-left shunt in management of patients with patent Foramen Ovale and cryptogenetic stroke, migraine, cluster headache, and obstructive apnoea. By intravenous administration of an ultrasound contrast agent during basal conditions and the Valsalva manoeuvre, the presence and number of microbubbles passing across middle cerebral artery are determined using a Doppler system with high sensitivity and specificity. A semiquantitative classification, taking into account the number of microbubbles recorded within the spectrum, considers:

◆ The test negative when no microbubble is detected on the Doppler spectrum.

◆ The test positive with a low-grade shunt, when 1–10 microbubbles are detected.

◆ The test positive with a medium-grade shunt, when >10 microbubbles are detected.

◆ The test positive with a large-grade shunt, when >10 microbubbles are detected plus a *curtain effect* seen when the microbubbles are in so great a number that they are no longer distinguishable.

Furthermore, the shunt is classified as *permanent* if already present under basal conditions and *latent* when it is detected only during the Valsalva manoeuvre.

Abdominal circulation

Assessment and follow-up of abdominal aorta aneurysms

True aneurysms may be defined as abnormal dilations of arteries in general more than two times the diameter in a non-dilated area.

The abdominal aorta is the commonest location of aneurysms. They are usually considered when the dilation is greater than 3cm. The abdominal aorta aneurysms (AAA) occur in the majority of cases (95%) below the renal arteries (infra-renal aneurysms) and may be fusiform or saccular. Their development has an important familial link and is usually associated with atherosclerosis. (Most aneurysms are degenerative leading to destruction of the elastic fibres in the media causing dilation of the artery), but some of them are inflammatory or infectious (mycotic aneurysms).

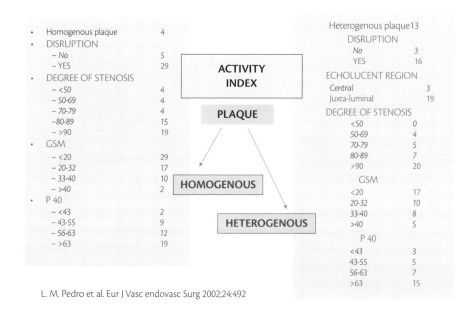

L. M. Pedro et al. Eur J Vasc endovasc Surg 2002;24:492

Figure 25.8 Example of calculation of Activity Index.

The most dramatic complication of AAA is rupture, and the risk of rupture increases with size. Elective surgery is usually recommended for aneurysms with a diameter greater than 55mm (or even 50mm in women).[13]

Clearly there are benefits in detecting aneurysms at an early stage,[14] so that serial follow-up can be carried out and elective surgery performed if the aneurysm becomes too large, because the survival rate of acute rupture is very low (<30%). Aortic aneurysms are treated using straight tube grafts (unless iliac extension exists, in which case bifurcating grafts are used) or percutaneous inserted endovascular grafts, reducing the risks of conventional surgical approaches.

Ultrasound is a simple, non-invasive method of detecting aneurysms and can be used for serial investigations to monitor any changes in size.[15] The purpose of the scan is to detect an aneurysm, its location and dimensions and to monitor its size on a serial basis. A 3.5-MHz curved linear array transducer is the most suitable and a depth setting of 12cm is usually enough (a major pitfall is to set the image depth too deep in thin patients and to misinterpret the lumbar spine as the aorta). Another important role of ultrasonography is in screening programs of AAA, where this technique has been considered ideal because of its non-invasiveness and accuracy. Ultrasound should be combined with CD assessment in order to characterize the blood flow. Scanning also plays a major role in the follow-up after surgical or percutaneous approaches.

Normal recordings

The maximal diameter of the abdominal aorta is usually less than 25mm. Measurements must be performed in the transverse and longitudinal scan plane.

Abnormal recordings

The aorta appears abnormally enlarged, and thrombus may be imaged as concentric layers with different degrees of echogenicity depending on the age and organization, sometimes with hypoechoic areas inside it, corresponding to localized liquefaction or fresh thrombus (➲ Fig. 25.9). It is very important to locate the renal arteries in order to be sure that the AAA is infrarenal and also to measure the distance between these arteries and the beginning of the dilation (*aneurysm neck*). The distance between the superior mesenteric artery and the renal arteries can also be measured.

The examination should also include the visualization of both iliac axes where dilation or aneurysm extension may be identified and measured. Also, visualization of renal and visceral arteries is essential, with characterization of flow pattern and detection of possible concomitant occlusive disease in these trunks.

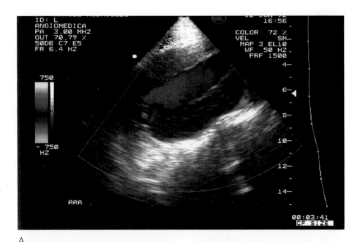

A

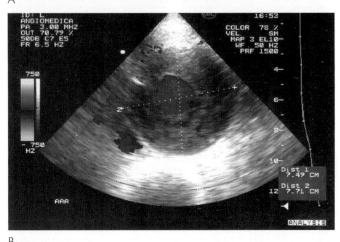

B

Figure 25.9 Assessment of abdominal aortic aneurysm. A) Longitudinally. B) Transversal evaluation and measurement of aortic diameter. Note the presence of a clot adherent to the walls.

Renal and visceral circulation

Renal arteries

Occlusive disease of the renal arteries is responsible for about 1–4%[15] of the total number of cases of arterial hypertension, causing the so-called *renovascular* arterial hypertension (RAH). However, this prevalence may be higher in some groups such as malignant or resistant AH, RAH associated with aneurysms or manifestations of atherosclerosis in other territories, flushing pulmonary oedema, abdominal bruit or chronic renal failure (especially if triggered or aggravated by ACE drugs). The detection of renovascular AH is essential as it may be treated by endovascular or surgical techniques, which favours the treatment and control of AH and reduces the risk of worsening chronic renal failure preventing, in many cases, the need of haemodialysis.

Among the most common causes of RAH, atherosclerosis is responsible for about 80% of the cases. It involves predominantly the origin and the initial segment of the renal artery. Usually, patients are older, with risk factors and show evidence of atherosclerotic involvement in other territories. Medial fibrodysplasia is another common cause of renovascular AH, representing about 10–15% of cases. It involves the middle and distal segments and sometimes also the terminal branches of the renal arteries, typically in younger female patients.

The current main indications for performing a renal artery evaluation are the suspicion of occlusive disease of these arteries, particularly in patients with hypertension and ischaemic nephropathy, and the follow-up of renal revascularization procedures.

CFDS of renal arteries is the method of choice for screening and identification of occlusive lesions, particularly when they involve the initial segment of renal arteries, which is more common in atherosclerosis. In fact, CFDS is the first line screening method of examination when there is clinical suspicion of a renovascular cause for the AH. With an experienced operator and a high definition equipment, in 95% of the cases it is possible to properly visualize the renal arteries in adults,[16] with high diagnostic accuracy.

The examination must be conducted with the patient in supine position, after 6 hours fasting. A multifrequency sectorial probe should be used. The exam begins with the longitudinal viewing of the aorta (to exclude aneurysms and significant occlusive disease), and the finding of the origin of the superior mesenteric artery. Then, placing the probe across the aorta, in a cross-sectional view, it is possible to identify the origin of the renal arteries. A detailed analysis of each of these arteries includes the visualization of its entire length and the acquisition of velocity waveforms at various levels (at least in initial, middle and distal thirds). The normal renal flow pattern[17] has a low resistance profile (i.e. high diastolic velocity) and the mean PSV is 84.7 ± 13.9cm/s, while the mean end diastolic velocity is 31.2 ± 7.8cm/s ($\supset$ Fig. 25.10).

The renal Resistance Index is derived from blood flow velocities according the formula:

$$\text{Resistance Index} = (\text{Peak systolic velocity} - \text{End-diastolic velocity}) / \text{Peak systolic velocity}$$

(25.1)

It is automatically determined and provides information on the state of microcirculation and the haemodynamic resistance to flow. This parameter is considered predictive of the success of revascularization and its normal value is 0.66 ± 0.07.

The diagnostic criteria for renal occlusive disease are haemodynamic. A focal acceleration of flow with PSV of 180cm/s or greater is considered suggestive of stenosis greater than 60%. If the stenosis exceeds 80% the renal-aortic index ($\text{PSV}_{renal}/\text{PSV}_{aorta}$) is greater than 3.5 ($\supset$ Fig. 25.11). The absence of flow in the renal artery is characteristic of occlusion.

These criteria have a sensitivity greater than 90% and a specificity of 95%.[18] The examination should be completed with the determination of kidney length.

Renal CFDS has, however, major limitations:

- It is dependent on the observer, on some underlying conditions and circumstances of the patients and of the examination.
- It may not detect occlusive disease of polar and accessory renal arteries, which can be present in 12–22% of patients.[19]

Visceral arteries

Coeliac trunk, superior mesenteric artery, and inferior mesenteric artery supply most of the abdominal organs and are called *visceral arteries*. Occlusive disease in these vessels is less common but its diagnosis is very important as they may be related to acute, severe and life-threatening clinical situations. The main cause for stenosis or occlusion of these trunks is atherosclerotic disease which involves their origin and initial segment.

Non-invasive diagnosis with CFDS usually allows the assessment of the coeliac trunk and superior mesenteric artery, as the inferior mesenteric artery is difficult to visualize due to its small diameter ($\supset$ Fig. 25.12).

The preparation and principles of the examination are common to the evaluation of renal arteries but the probe should stand longitudinally.

The normal flow pattern of the coeliac trunk is that of a low resistance artery with high diastolic velocity. The normal values are for PSV 100–237cm/s and for end-diastolic velocity 23–58cm/s. The normal waveform in the superior mesenteric artery has a relationship with meals. In fasting period the resistance is higher and the diastolic flow is low or absent; in the post-prandial period it shows the pattern of a low resistance artery. The normal fasting velocities are for PSV 124–218cm/s and for end-diastolic velocity 5–30cm/s.

The diagnostic criteria[17] for significant stenosis are haemodynamic. For the celiac trunk a PSV greater than 220–250cm/s is suggestive of more than 50% stenosis and PSV greater than 280–300cm/s is diagnostic of more than 70% stenosis. In the superior mesenteric artery a PSV greater than 200cm/s is suggestive of more than 50% stenosis and PSV greater than 280cm/s is diagnostic of more than 75% stenosis.

Lower limb circulation

Duplex scanning is the most commonly performed procedure to assess arterial and venous lower limb circulation. This section provides an overview of these topics and offers practical advice on the B-mode and Doppler evaluation of peripheral arteries and veins.

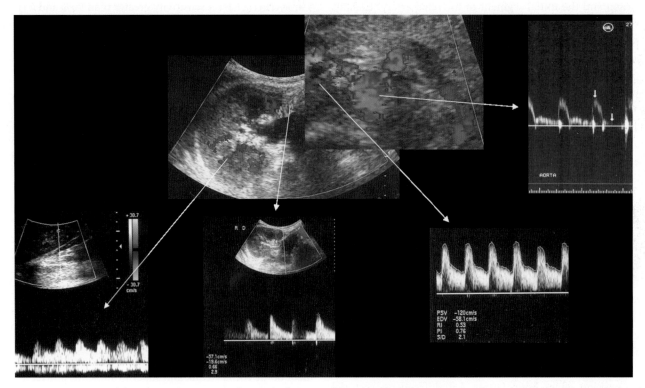

Figure 25.10 Assessment of the right renal artery. Waveform and velocities at different levels of the trunk and at the cortical renal arteries are displayed. The peak systolic velocity at the aorta should also be recorded to permit the calculation of the renal–aortic index.

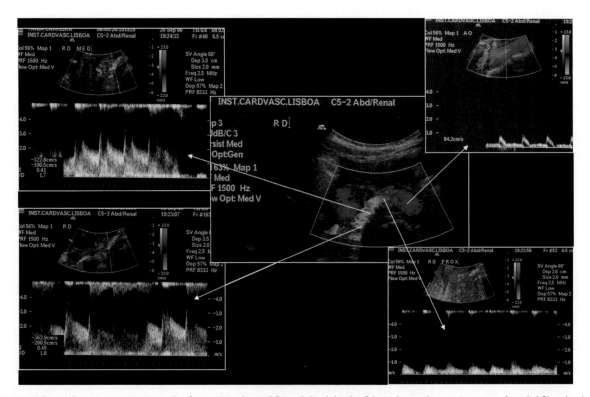

Figure 25.11 Right renal artery stenosis. Example of stenosis in the middle and distal thirds of the right renal artery in a case of medial fibrodysplasia. Note the acceleration of flow (PSV 362cm/s and the renal-aortic index of 4.3) typical of a >80% stenosis.

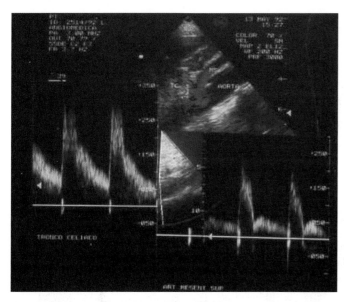

Figure 25.12 Coeliac trunk and superior mesenteric artery. Evaluation of the origin of coeliac axis and superior mesenteric artery with CFDS and acquisition of normal waveform and velocity curves.

Lower limb arterial disease

Occlusive disease

The objective of the examination is to locate and grade the severity of arterial disease in the lower limb arterial system. A 5-MHz flat linear array transducer is suitable for scanning most arteries, but the aortoiliac segment is better assessed with a 3.5-MHz curved linear array probe. A combination of B-mode imaging, CD, and spectral Doppler should be used throughout the examination.

The ankle–brachial pressure index

This is one of the most common methods of grading arterial disease and it is defined as the ratio between the systolic pressure in the ankle and in the arm (measured by continuous wave Doppler using a blood pressure cuff). The normal value of this ratio is usually equal to or greater than 1 (⊃ Fig. 25.13), and is considered abnormal if below 0.95, reflecting mild (0.85–0.95), moderate (0.4–0.85), or severe (<0.4) arterial disease. In mild to moderate disease, it may be normal at rest becoming abnormal during exercise.[20]

Normal recordings

The lumen of a normal artery should appear free of echoes and the walls uniform along each segment. CD imaging normally shows a pulsatile flow with red alternating with blue due to flow reversal during the diastolic phase. Spectral Doppler assessment typically shows a triphasic flow pattern.

Chronic ischaemia

Its major cause is atherosclerosis, which may cause both macro- and microvascular disease. Plaques of atheroma, particularly

if they are calcified, may be seen within the vessel lumen (⊃ Fig. 25.14). When they are echolucent, the use of CD is very important because it may show a filling defect in the arterial lumen. If a significant stenosis is present, the flow is turbulent when assessed by CD and aliasing is demonstrated by spectral Doppler. Haemodynamic changes are an essential tool in grading stenosis severity through parameters like the PSV, the end-diastolic velocity and the *PSV ratio*.[20] The PSV ratio is calculated by:

$$\text{PSV ratio} = \text{maximum PSV across the stenosis/} \atop \text{PSV just proximal to stenosis} \qquad (25.2)$$

A PSV ratio greater than 2 is used to define a significant stenosis:

- PSV >2 corresponds to 50–74% diameter reduction, with waveform usually bi- or monophasic with increased end-diastolic velocity.

- PSV ratio >3 corresponds to 75–99% diameter reduction, with waveform usually monophasic with a significant increase in end diastolic velocity.[20]

Complete occlusion is present when no flow is seen in an artery. In younger patients microvascular disorders such as Buerguer's disease lead to low flow and high resistance wave forms in distal calf vessels with normal flow in large proximal arteries.

Acute ischaemia

Acute ischaemia usually occurs by sudden occlusion of an artery as a consequence of thrombosis (acute thrombosis of an existing arterial lesion) or embolism coming from a proximal part of the arterial system. The lumen of an occluded artery by fresh thrombus will appear clear or anechoic on the image, because thrombus has a similar echogenicity to blood. The addition of CD mode reveals absence of flow in the vessel. Spectral Doppler waveforms proximal to an occlusion often demonstrate a high resistance flow pattern.

Popliteal and femoral aneurysms and false aneurysms

Approximately 4% of patients with aortic aneurysms have another aneurysm elsewhere and 6% of patients with popliteal aneurysms have aortic aneurysms. Ultrasound is the primary technique for assessing popliteal aneurysms and a 5-MHz flat linear array transducer must be used. B-mode is used to assess the size, length and amount of thrombus inside it and CD imaging to confirm the size of the lumen. Care must be taken not to confuse Baker's cysts with popliteal aneurysms.

True femoral aneurysms are uncommon but false or pseudoaneurysms are more frequent, occurring after arterial puncture for catheter access. Blood travels back and forth through a hole in the arterial wall into the surrounding tissue, forming a flow cavity in the tissue adjacent to the artery, sometimes with

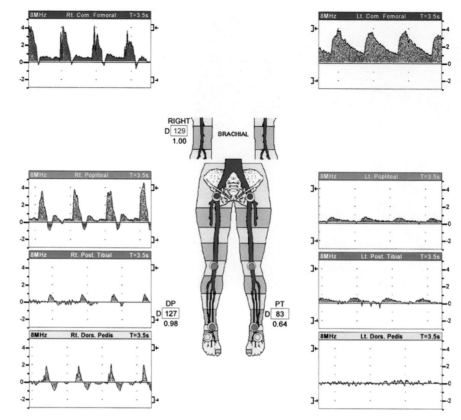

Figure 25.13 Lower limbs Doppler assessment. Doppler assessment of waveforms and velocities in the femoral, popliteal, and distal arteries in both limbs. The right lower limb is normal with ankle–brachial index (ABI) of 0.98. In the left lower limb there is evidence of iliac occlusion with low resistance curves along the limb and a decreased ABI of 0.6.

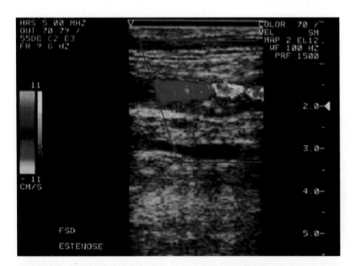

Figure 25.14 Doppler assessment of the superficial femoral artery. Direct visualization of a calcified plaque in the superficial femoral artery using CFDS.

thrombus (➲ Fig. 25.15). CD imaging shows a high-velocity jet originating in the artery and a swirling pattern inside the false lumen. PW Doppler demonstrates the forward and reverse flow as the arterial jet enters and exits the false lumen.

Postoperative/postinterventional evaluation and follow-up

Arterial bypass operations are widely used to restore arterial circulation to the lower extremities. Bypass grafts can be made of synthetic materials or constructed from native veins. Bypass stenosis or occlusion is a serious complication threatening graft patency and regular surveillance (essentially of venous grafts) is a common and cost-effective practice.

Vein graft stenosis occurs in about one-third of venous grafts, 77% of them in the first year after surgery. Patients are usually scanned at 1, 3, 6, 9, and 12 months after surgery and in some centres indefinitely once or twice a year. The implementation of surveillance protocols of synthetic grafts is still a controversial issue because many occlusions occur due to spontaneous graft thrombosis. Most cases of graft stenosis are successfully treated with angioplasty but sometimes surgical therapy is required.

Lower limb venous disease

In comparison with arterial ultrasonography, venous investigations can be technically challenging due to the wide range of anatomical variations in the superficial and deep venous system.

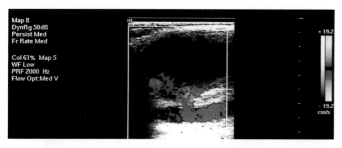

Figure 25.15 Femoral pseudoaneurysm post-catheterization. The flow runs freely to and from the pseudoaneurysm.

Venous insufficiency

The basic purpose of the scan is to characterize the origin of varicose veins and to assess the patency of the superficial and deep veins. A venous preset should be selected (PRF 1000Hz, low level colour wall filter). A 5–10-MHz multifrequency transducer is suitable for scanning superficial and deep veins and junctions. A combination of B-mode imaging, CD, and spectral Doppler should be used throughout the examination.

Varicose veins

Varicose veins are relatively easy to identify on the B-mode image, appearing as single or multiple tortuous vessels that vary randomly in diameter as the probe is swept across the varicose area. Perforators are identified running the transducer steadily along the trunk of the superficial vein in transverse-section.

The most commonly employed methods to assess venous valve competency, during the assessment with CFDS, are:

- Calf compression: this consists of producing flow augmentation towards the heart with transitory squeezing of the calf region. Flow augmentation must be strong enough to produce

a transient peak flow velocity of >30cm/s in the main superficial trunks so that valve closure is rapid on releasing the squeeze.

- The Valsalva manoeuvre: with this manoeuvre, the competence of the proximal deep veins and saphenous-femoral junction is assessed, but in some cases competent valves in the iliac veins preclude the usefulness of this manoeuvre.

Using CD mode, if the valves are competent, there should be no important venous reflux after calf release or during the Valsalva manoeuvre. Significant reflux will be demonstrated by a sustained period of retrograde flow following calf release or during the Valsalva manoeuvre (◑ Fig. 25.16).

Deep venous thrombosis

Duplex scanning is the primary non-invasive technique for the diagnosis of deep venous thrombosis (DVT). The objective of the scan is to detect DVT and to locate its proximal position because it may influence subsequent treatment. Most DVTs are located in the calf veins and can extend to proximal veins. Isolated thrombosis of proximal veins is less common but may also occur.

A 5-MHz flat linear array transducer should be used (except for the iliac veins that are best assessed with a 3.5-MHz curved linear array transducer), the colour PRF must be set very low to detect low velocity flow, colour wall filters should be set at a low level, and the spectral Doppler sample volume should cover all the lumen. The investigation of DVT can be very difficult in some areas like the internal iliac veins, the profunda femoral territory and also in calf veins. It is important to know that other diseases, such as superficial thrombophlebitis, haematoma, lymphoedema, cellulitis, Baker's cysts or enlarged lymph nodes may mimic DVT and must not be confused with it.

The normal appearance of deep veins should be free of echoes or they may contain just speckles and reverberation artefacts,

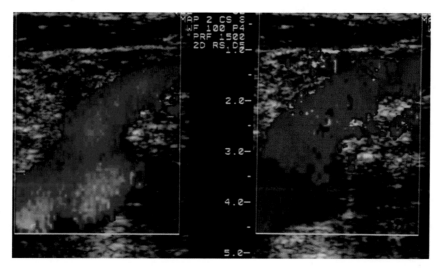

Figure 25.16 Assessment of saphenous-femoral junction for reflux. When calf compression is relieved there can be seen retrograde flow (reflux) to the saphenous vein.

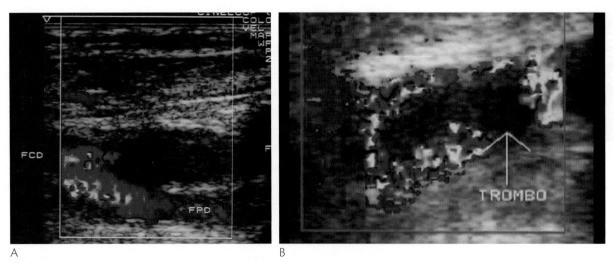

Figure 25.17 Deep venous thrombosis. A) Recent venous occlusion of the superficial femoral vein, where no flow can be seen and the lumen is relatively echo-free. B) Free-floating thrombus in the popliteal vein.

with spontaneous phasic flow with CD and normal venous flow pattern with spectral Doppler.

The main diagnostic criterion for excluding DVT is complete collapse of the vein under transducer pressure. Deformation but not collapse of the vein during firm transducer compression should raise the suspicion of DVT. In very early stages, the clot has an echogenicity identical to blood (echolucent) (➲ Fig. 25.17A). Within several days it becomes echogenic, which will increase with time (allowing the evaluation of DVT evolution time). Sometimes a free-floating thrombus may be present (➲ Fig. 25.17B). CD mode is very important in

the examination and shows absence of flow in occluded veins or reduced flow around the thrombus, if the occlusion is partial.

Acknowledgements

We thank L Mendes Pedro, MD, PhD and J Fernandes e Fernandes, MD, PhD, from Instituto Cardiovascular, Lisbon, Portugal, for all their help and support and for providing all the images presented in this chapter.

Personal perspective

Vascular ultrasound plays a central role in the diagnosis of both arterial and venous diseases. It allows the study of almost all vascular territories in a safe, non-invasive, easily accessible (even at the bedside), repeatable, and inexpensive

way. It permits the diagnosis from the earliest stages of the disease, the characterization and determination of its severity, and the follow-up of patients. Nowadays, it can almost be considered as part of the physical examination of the vascular system, and has become an essential tool in the evaluation of patients in our daily clinical practice.

References

1 Daffertshofer M, Karasch, T, Meairs S. *Vascular Diagnosis with Ultrasound*, 2nd ed. New York: Thieme, 2006.

2 O'Leary DH, Polak JF, Kronmal RA, Manolio TA, Burke GL, Wolfson SK Jr. Carotid-artery intima and media thickness as a risk factor for myocardial infarction and stroke in older adults. Cardiovascular Health Study Collaborative Research Group. *N Engl J Med* 1999; **340**:14–22.

3 Fernandes e Fernandes J, Pedro LM. Extracranial carotid artery disease. In: Liapis C, Balzer K, Beneditti-Valenti F, Fernandes e Fernandes J (eds) *European Manual of Vascular Surgery*. New York: Springer, 2007, pp. 137–53.

4 European Carotid Surgery Trialists' Collaborative Group. MRC European Carotid Surgery Trial. Interim results for symptomatic patients with severe (70-99%) and with mild (0–29%) stenosis. *Lancet* 1991; **337**:1235–43.

5 Halliday A, Mansfield A, Marro J, Peto C, Peto R, Potter J, et al. MRC Asymptomatic Carotid Surgery Trial (ACST) Collaborative Group. Prevention of disabling and fatal strokes by successful carotid endarterectomy in patients without recent neurological symptoms: randomised controlled trial. *Lancet* 2004; **363**:1491–502.

6 North American Symptomatic Carotid Endarterectomy Trial Collaborators. Beneficial effect of carotid endarterectomy in symptomatic patients with high grade carotid stenosis. *N Engl J Med* 1991; **325**:445–63.

7 Executive Committee for the Asymptomatic Carotid Atherosclerosis Study. Endarterectomy for asymptomatic carotid artery stenosis. *JAMA* 1995; **273**:1421–8.

8 Moneta GL, Mitchell EL, Esmonde N, *et al.* Extracranial carotid and vertebral arteries. In: Zierler RE (ed) *Strandness's Duplex Scanning in Vascular Disorders*, 4th ed. Philadelphia, PA: Lippincott Wiliams and Wilkins, 2010, p.85.

9 Grant EG, Benson CB, Moneta GL, Alexandrov AV, Baker JD, Bluth EI, *et al.* Carotid artery stenosis: gray-scale and Doppler US diagnosis. Society of Radiologists Consensus Conference. *Radiology* 2003; **229**:340–6.

10 Geroulakos G, Ramaswami G, Nicolaides AN, James K, Labropoulos N, Belcaro G, *et al.* Characterization of symptomatic and asymptomatic carotid plaques using high-resolution real-time ultrasonography. *Br J Surg* 1993; **80**:1274–7.

11 Pedro LM, Pedro MM, Gonçalves I, Carneiro TF, Balsinha C, Fernandes e Fernandes R, *et al.* Computer-assisted carotid plaque analysis: characteristics of plaques associated with cerebrovascular symptoms and cerebral infarction. *Eur J Vasc Endovasc Surg* 2000; **19**:118–23.

12 Pedro LM, Fernandes e Fernandes J, Pedro MM, Gonçalves I, Dias NV, Fernandes e Fernandes R, *et al.* Ultrasonographic risk score of carotid plaques. *Eur J Vasc Endovasc Surg* 2002; **24**:492–8.

13 Powell JT, Greenhalgh RM. Small abdominal aortic aneurysms. *N Engl J Med* 2003; **348**:1895–901.

14 Thompson SG, Gao L, Scott R, on behalf of the Multicentre Aneurysm Screening Study Group. Screening men for abdominal aortic aneurysm: 10 year mortality and cost effectiveness results from the randomised Multicentre Aneurysm Screening Study. *BMJ* 2009; **338**:b2307.

15 Neumyer MM. Duplex evaluation of the renal arteries. In: AbuRahama AF, Bergan JJ (eds) *Non Invasive Vascular Diagnosis*. New York: Springer; 2000, p.379.

16 Pellerito JS, Zwiebel WJ. Ultrasound assessment of native renal vessels and renal allografts. In: Pellerito JS, Zwiebel WJ (eds) *Introduction to Vascular Ultrasonography*, 5th ed. Philadelphia, PA: Elsevier Saunders; 2005, p.611.

17 Schäberle W. *Ultrasonography in Vascular Diagnosis*. New York: Springer, 2004.

18 Pedro LM, Freire JP, Machado AS, Cunha e Sá D, Martins C, Pedro MM, *et al.* [Assessment of arterial occlusive disease with Duplex sonography. Prospective study.] *Rev Port Cardiol* 1993; **12**(11):905–11.

19 Bakker J, Beek FJ, Beutler JJ, Hene RJ, de Kort GA, de Lange EE, *et al.* Renal artery stenosis and accessory renal arteries: accuracy of detection and visualization with gadolinium-enhanced breath-hold MR angiography. *Radiology* 1998; **207**:497–504.

20 Needham T. Physiologic testing of lower extremity arterial disease: segmental pressures, plethysmography and velocity waveforms. In: Mansour MA, Labropoulos N (eds) *Vascular Diagnosis*. Philadelphia, PA: Elsevier Saunders, 2005, p.215.

Further reading

⊃ For additional multimedia materials please visit the online version of the book (http://escecho.oxfordmedicine.com).

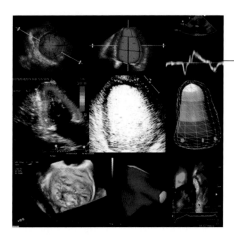

CHAPTER 26

Quality assurance in echocardiography

K.F. Fox and B.A. Popescu

Contents

Summary

Quality assurance (QA) in echocardiography is the systematic process of ensuring that information sent out by echo laboratories is timely, appropriate, and accurate. All aspects of a service need to be continuously monitored and optimized if quality is to be maintained and furthermore improved.

Particular focus is needed on reporting and measurement with continuous checking for reporting errors and assessment of measurement variability.

A systematic QA programme needs to be an essential part of any echo laboratory. Life-determining clinical decisions may depend on it. In this chapter we describe the background to QA, current evidence and guidelines, and a systematic approach to QA.

Introduction

The intention of every echocardiographer and every echocardiography laboratory is to provide timely, accurate, clinically relevant information. Quality assurance (QA) is the systematic process by which one ensures this aim is fulfilled.

Knowledge of all the information within this textbook is just one part of fulfilling this aim. QA requires attention to all elements of echocardiography, patient selection, workflow organization, equipment maintenance, knowledge and skill of practitioners, and systematic audit of studies undertaken. A QA programme is an inextricable part of quality improvement (QI).

What is quality assurance?

The definition of QA includes the planned, systematic activities that are necessary to ensure that a product or service fulfils its requirements. Echocardiography certainly falls within the category of a *product or service*.

QA programmes can be intermittent (e.g. an audit) or continuous (e.g. regular re-reporting of a proportion of studies). In general the best schemes are continuous and fully integrated with the work of the echo laboratory.

QA may be both an internal and an external process. QA relates to all aspects of a service, so not only should reports be timely, accurate, and useful but the patient's experience should be a safe and positive one.

Why should we undertake quality assurance?

It is intuitive that an accurate report is better than an inaccurate one. However, objectively demonstrating the adverse effects of poor quality echocardiography is challenging. Studies of patient adverse events secondary to inaccurate echo reports are unlikely publications. In clinical practice an echo should be as accurate as possible. Some specific clinical decisions may depend on a discrete measurement, for example, treatments for left ventricular (LV) dysfunction may depend on the presence of an ejection fraction (EF) of less than 35%.

In oncology, trastuzumab is used for management of breast cancer but can cause LV impairment. Guidelines apply to its use such that a 10% fall in EF leads to cessation of therapy. It is therefore imperative that a measured fall in EF of 10% is a true change and not a measurement error.[1]

A further area where inaccurate echocardiography does impact is in research studies. Measurement errors will dilute and mask true changes in echo parameters and lead to the misinterpretation of trial outcomes. A recent study to find echo parameters useful to identify responders to biventricular pacemaker insertion was hampered by inter- and intraobserver variability in the measurement of the echo parameters under investigation.[2]

Therefore beyond the intuitive desire for accuracy, there are objective clinical and research situations where one must be assured of the quality of an echo study.

Current recommendations

QA is increasingly integrated into recommendations for the operation of echocardiography services. This is typically included in the requirements of accreditation schemes.

The EAE requirements for Accreditation of Echocardiography Laboratories include the need for a *system for review of studies in place* for Standard Level accreditation. Laboratories awarded Advanced Accreditation must provide evidence of more *formal and systematic quality control* and particularly for stress echo *audit of results against angiography or other independent standard.*[3]

In the USA, Laboratory accreditation is increasingly linked to reimbursement. The National scheme for Echo Lab Accreditation is run by the Intersocietal Commission for the Accreditation of Echocardiography Laboratories (ICAEL) whose requirements include the need for QA.

The American Society of Echocardiography and partner organizations have also produced guidelines for quality assurance and the closely linked quality improvement in clinical practice and trials.[4] Various countries in Europe and across the world also include recommendations for QA. However, the requirements often contain few details of exactly what is required. Currently accreditation is generally not a mandatory or statutory requirement to provide echo services but this may change over the next few years.

Very general, although exacting, standards for QA programmes within industry and commerce are covered by an international standard (ISO 9000) and these could be applied to echo laboratories.

Training in echocardiography

A prerequisite for providing a quality service is adequately trained staff. The EAE has published documents relating to the training required to achieve competence in echocardiography. These include a curriculum and a document on training.[5] In addition, the EAE runs a certification* programme for echocardiographers. Certifications are offered in Adult Transthoracic Echocardiography, in collaboration with the European Association of Cardiothoracic Anaesthesiology in Transesophageal Echocardiography and in collaboration with the Association of European Paediatric Cardiologists in Echocardiography for Congenital Disease.

To achieve certification individuals must undertake a programme of training and then pass a Knowledge Based Assessment (exam) and submit evidence of practical training in the form of a log book including images obtained, or in the case of congenital disease assessed by directly observed practical skills (DOPS).

While numbers of studies performed do not guarantee competence, and are not evidence based, they are commonly used as part of a package of recommendations for training. The supervised *hands-on* experience needs to be combined with attendance at local review meetings, national and international educational conferences, and courses together with personal study. Competence must be maintained and therefore the EAE certifications include a requirement for 5-yearly renewal (recertification) based on continued clinical practice and learning. The EAE accreditation principles are shared with other national and international certifications including the USA where they are known as credentialing programmes.

At present, individual echocardiographer certification programmes do not include a requirement for QA. However, by participating in QA programmes trainees may gain useful insight into their position on the learning curve.

---

* previously accreditation

Quality assurance as applied to echo: equipment, people, patient selection and triage, study performance, study quality

A comprehensive QA programme will address all aspects of a service.

The infrastructure, process, and personnel

Laboratories should have indications for echocardiography and audit regularly against those standards.

Waiting times for performing and reporting studies should be audited and reasonable targets established. Typically it is useful to divide reporting into *initial reports* which generally should be available in less than 24 hours and *final reports* which may reasonably have to wait, although not excessively, for a meeting of expert echocardiographers.

The environment must be clean, adequately sized and preserve the dignity of patients. Recommendations for room sizes and facilities are listed in the EAE guidelines for laboratory accreditation.[3]

While there are few data linking length of study to quality, it is reasonable to state that staff should not be overburdened and studies given adequate time. The staff should be adequately skilled and be maintaining their skill through a programme of CME.

Particularly for stress and transoesophageal echocardiography (TOE), safety aspects should be addressed through the use of protocols, safety checks, and audit.

Equipment should be systematically and regularly maintained and updated, not just the echo machines but monitoring equipment and infusion devices where appropriate. The EAE requirements for laboratory accreditation give guidance on equipment specifications and renewal frequency requiring that equipment is renewed or replaced at least every 7 years.

The echo study

The largest part of a QA programme concerns the performance and reporting of the echo study. Before embarking on QA it is important that all echo examinations are performed correctly. Consistent methodology using parameters shown to have maximum accuracy and minimum variability are essential and the EAE have published such recommendations.[6]

The two broad aspects that need to be assessed are the *accuracy* of the studies and their *variability*. Accuracy reflects comparison against an absolute or gold standard while variability describes differences in repeat measurements of identical parameters. This is a key distinction. For example, while data suggest that the E/E′ ratio is the least variable measure of diastolic function, it may not necessarily be the best measure (particularly in isolation) of diastolic function.

In comparing studies and measurements, different statistical methods can be applied. Comparing values against an absolute standard can be done using McNemar's test. If there is uncertainty about the true reading, agreement between observers on dichotomous categories (i.e. normal vs abnormal) can be measured using Cohen's kappa. A kappa statistic greater than 0.61 suggests substantial agreement.

Bland Altman plots provide a helpful and very visual description of the spread of measurements. Modern statistical software packages typically have some or all of these tests included. In fact, the plethora of statistical methods makes comparisons of data and therefore identifying appropriate benchmarks for measurement variability challenging.

The *accuracy* of the echo implies comparison to a gold standard but typically it means in relation to other data, i.e. from other imaging modalities. There may be controversy over what is the *true* reading. For EF, cardiac magnetic resonance (CMR) may be currently regarded as the gold standard and comparison with the echo measured EF in patients having both investigations gives an example of this element of QA. While caution must be used when comparing modalities measuring different parameters (i.e. stress echo which measures perfusion vs coronary angiography demonstrating anatomy), such comparisons are useful audit tools for an echo service. Operative findings provide another gold standard. A study by Faletra et al. published in 2000 identified a 12% error rate in identifying prosthetic valve pathology when comparing the echo report with subsequent operative findings.[7]

Systematic re-reporting of studies is a key part of QA and is separate from regular discussion and review of interesting and difficult cases which should also be part of the work of an echo laboratory. The gold standard for accuracy of reporting is usually taken to be that of a panel of experts. Therefore comparing reports against a panel decision is an effective part of QA. However, a final panel decision may mask considerable disagreement within a panel. A study of the reporting of MR gave information about the variability of grading of MR amongst a large group of experienced echocardiographers.[8] Substantial variation in grading even amongst experts was noted but the paper does give an indication of what variation might be expected. Less than 10% of cases were classified by individuals as greater than one grade away from the modal classification (where a change from mild to moderate to moderate = one grade).

A number of methods can be used to measure differences in reporting between echocardiographers or between an echocardiographer and a panel. The UK Royal College of Radiology established a classification[9] that can be applied to echocardiography (➲ Table 26.1)

The categories can be compressed into Green errors (4 and 5), Amber errors (3), and Red errors (1 and 2). However, there are few data or standards on acceptable proportions for each category. For category 1 and 2 the target should intuitively

Table 26.1 Classification of reporting differences

5	No difference
4	Minor difference of wording or style or non-inclusion of clinically insignificant features
3	Debatable but possible difference in reporting but with low likelihood of harm
2	Difference in reporting that is likely to have an adverse clinical, but non-life threatening effect
1	Definite difference in reporting with unequivocal potentially serious or life threatening effect

be 0%. Categories 4 and 5 are acceptable and inevitable variations. In defining a target for category 3 (amber) errors audit data from high volume service suggest that between experienced echocardiographers a category 3 error rate may be up to 7% (UK Department of Health personal communication).

The number of cases that require re-reporting to ensure an adequate sample size is not defined. About 10% of studies may be appropriate but this is a formidable logistical undertaking for busy laboratories. The proportion will depend on the total number of studies performed and also the number of studies done by each operator and their seniority.[10]

Despite the fact that the majority of the workload of echo laboratories is represented by transthoracic studies there is a more substantial literature on the reporting of stress echo, transoesophageal, and even intraoperative studies. A number of studies have looked at interobserver (between echocardiographers) and intraobserver (consistency of repeat reporting by the same echocardiographer) variability of stress echos. Results for reproducibility of stress echo reports have often been disappointing with kappa values of 0.37 (fair agreement only) but have also shown training effects and a clear links with quality of the imaging and the effectiveness of the haemodynamic stress.[11,12]

The second main focus of QA is in measurement of individual echo parameters. Reproducibility (consistency of repeat measurements) subdivided into interobserver and intraobserver variability should be measured and minimized. Since a substantial part of the work of echo laboratories is the longitudinal monitoring of patients with cardiac disease an understanding of measurement error is essential to differentiate true changes from artefactual changes due to measurement variability.

However, just like reporting variation, there is little guidance on reasonable standards for measurement variability. Reported data on measurement variability are derived mainly from research studies or selected series which may not be realistic in clinical practice. EF is one of the parameters most frequently studied. Optimal conduct of the echo examination is particularly relevant as studies have clearly shown that the accuracy and reproducibility of EF can be improved by use of contrast and 3D scanning.

Few specific requirement exists although the British Society of Echocardiography have published that when measuring EF for patients receiving trastuzumab chemotherapy, echo laboratories performing such studies should have evidence (i.e. through audit or other quality control processes), not more than 12 months old, that they can reproducibly measure EF to the requirements of the guidelines. This means that they can identify a 10% change in EF as a true change.[1]

This therefore represents one target for a QA programme but is based on the needs of a clinical guideline rather than an analysis of benchmark practice. In a large study of measurement of EF using real-time 3D echocardiography, correlation coefficients of 0.9 were obtained.[13]

Ideally interobserver variability should be measured by different echocardiographers repeating studies but more typically this is assessed by repeat measurements by different echocardiographers based on stored images. Similarly, intraobserver variability is ideally measured through repeat studies but using stored images is a surrogate.

In research studies *core labs* often provide a dual function of re-reporting of studies and re-measuring particular parameters and such data do give an insight into variability in current practice. In the Val-HeFT trial, investigating the value of Valsartan in Heart Failure, only 50% of participating centres were felt to be of sufficient quality (measured on a 16-point scale) to provide echo data at the start of the study. However, with training, this proportion improved.[14]

One intriguing yet effective method of quality assessment is to assume that all echocardiographers in a busy laboratory scan echo patients from the same pool. One would therefore expect that, on average, the mean EF (and its standard deviation) of all the studies performed by each echocardiographer would be the same. Differences in mean EF between echocardiographers are likely to represent differences in technique.[15] With electronic reporting such an analysis can often be produced relatively easily and is a useful adjunct to a QA programme.

The difficulty in finding absolute standards for reporting and measurement variability should not be seen as a barrier to developing QA programmes (⊃ Table 26.2). Rather, laboratories can

Table 26.2 Examples of tolerances for Echo QA programmes [1,16,17]

Parameter	Target
Ejection fraction	Inter- and intraobserver variability <10%
Aortic valve area (planimetry)	Inter- and intraobserver variability <10%
Stress echo reporting (abnormal/normal)	Kappa >0.37
Category 3 reporting errors	<7%

use the opportunity to identify their own standards and preferred measures. More importantly the focus should not simply be on achieving an absolute level but on a philosophy of continuous improvement.

A quality assurance programme as part of continuous quality improvement

Combining the elements previously described together is the basis of a comprehensive QA programme. The complexity of a QA programme will vary. It will depend on the size and output of the laboratory and will, in any individual laboratory, evolve over time. An example of a comprehensive QA programme, and how one might develop it, is described in ➲ Table 26.3.

For echo laboratories trying to introduce QA, a stepwise introduction may be appropriate. For example:

1) Establish a regular review meeting of difficult or interesting cases.

2) Develop equipment and echocardiographer training log.

3) Introduce random cases into the Review Meeting for re-reporting.

4) Develop indications, triage, and study protocols.

5) Undertake audits of practice against protocols.

6) Develop systematic re-reporting programmes.

7) Add measurement variability exercises based on re-measurement from stored images.

Introducing a quality assurance programme

The essentials of introducing a QA programme are: preparation, planning, communication, and adequate resource.

◆ **Preparation** There should be a shared wish to undertake QA. While leadership is required, the whole team must be involved and committed.

◆ **Planning** Thinking through the exact logistics of the QA programme is necessary, particularly identifying time and resource for the work.

Table 26.3 Elements of a QA programme

1. Regular (at least annual) assessment of environment and equipment
2. Regular review of protocols for patient selection, patient information, indications for studies, triage, and study performance
3. Regular (annual) audit of parameters of process of care: waiting times for studies, waiting times for reports, proportion of studies fulfilling appropriateness criteria/indications, number of studies performed, patient satisfaction
4. Regular (monthly) clinical governance review of safety (especially stress echo and TOE)
5. Documented programme of staff training including internal and external CME
6. Regular (weekly) meeting to discuss complex or interesting cases
7. Regular re-reporting of a randomly selected percentage of studies performed. Percentage depending on laboratory and individual echocardiographer workload and experience. Up to 10% for low volume/less experienced operators. Feedback mechanism for reporting differences and alert system for high difference rates
8. Regular programme of measurement variability assessment exercises

◆ **Communication** Regular and wide communication with all stakeholders is necessary. It is important to be aware of sensitivities around QA where identification of errors can be seen as a criticism of individuals rather than a non-judgemental QI opportunity. Feedback of the positive aspects of the QA programme and evidence of QI will maintain enthusiasm.

◆ **Adequate resource** A QA programme will fail if inadequately resourced. Similarly an over ambitious programme will also fail and a graduated approach may be more successful.

In general, the introduction of QA should be seen as a positive development, building the team through demonstration and continuous improvement of the quality of the service.

Continuous quality improvement

The aim of a QA programme is not just to maintain quality but also, on the basis that no service is as good as we would wish, to develop the central part of a continuous QI strategy. In addition to a QA programme, QI requires that where deficiencies are identified, solutions are designed and implemented and the impact on quality measured. A cycle of measurement, change, and re-measurement is established.

Personal perspective

QA tends to be at the bottom of the priority list for echo laboratories, and yet in many ways it should be the top. Working furiously to undertake ever larger numbers of studies is of no value if the information generated is unreliable.

QA can be challenging. It asks uncomfortable questions of us and requires time that seemingly could be spent on doing more studies. Success requires leadership and teamwork and often works best when built up steadily over time. But a successful QA programme brings credit to the laboratory, job satisfaction for all staff, and clinical benefit for the patients.

References

1 Fox KF. The evaluation of left ventricular function for patients being considered for or receiving trastuzumab (Herceptin) therapy. *Br J Cancer* 2006; **95**:1454.

2 Chung ES, Leon AR, Tavazzi L, Sun JP, Nihoyannopoulos P, Merlino J, *et al*. Results of the predictors of response to CRT (PROSPECT) trial. *Circulation* 2008; **117**:2608–16.

3 Nihoyannopoulos P, Fox KF, Fraser AG, Pinto FJ, on behalf of the Laboratory Accreditation Committee of the EAE. EAE laboratory standards and accreditation. *Eur J Echocardiogr* 2007; **8**:79–87.

4 Douglas PS, Decara JM, Devereux RB, Duckworth S, Gardin JM, Jaber WA, *et al*. Echocardiographic Imaging in Clinical Trials: American Society of Echocardiography Standards for Echocardiography Core Laboratories Endorsed by the American College of Cardiology Foundation. *J Am Soc Echocardiogr* 2009; **22**:755–65.

5 Popescu BA, Andrade MJ, Badano LP, Fox KF, Flachskampf FA, Lancellotti P, *et al*. European Association of Echocardiography recommendations for training, competence, and quality improvement in echocardiography. *Eur J Echocardiogr* 2009; **10**:893–905.

6 Evangelista A, Flachskampf F, Lancellotti P, Badano L, Aguilar R, Monaghan M, *et al*. European Association of Echocardiography recommendations for standardization of performance, digital storage and reporting of echocardiographic studies. *Eur J Echocardiogr* 2008; **9**:438–48.

7 Faletra F, Constantin C, De Chiara F, Masciocco G, Santambrogio G, Moreo A, *et al*. Incorrect echocardiographic diagnosis in patients with mechanical prosthetic valve dysfunction: Correlation with surgical findings. *Am J Med* 2000; **108**:531–7.

8 Fox KF, Porter A, Unsworth B, Collier T, Leech G, and Mayet J. Report on a National Quality Control Excercise. *Eur J Echocardiogr* 2009; **10**:314–18.

9 Jolly BC, Ayers B, MacDonald MM, Armstrong P, Chalmers AH, Roberts G, *et al*. The reproducibility of assessing radiological reporting: studies from the development of the General Medical Council's Performance Procedures. *Med Educ* 2001; **35** (Suppl 1):36–44.

10 Mathew JP, Glas K, Troianos CA, Sears-Rogan P, Savage R, Shanewise J, *et al*. American Society of Echocardiography/Society of Cardiovascular Anesthesiologists Recommendations and Guidelines for Continuous Quality Improvement in Perioperative Echocardiography. *J Am Soc Echocardiogr* 2006; **19**:1303–13.

11 Hoffmann R, Lethen H, Marwick T, Arnese M, Fioretti P, Pingitore A, *et al*. Analysis of interinstitutional observer agreement in interpretation of dobutamine stress echocardiograms. *J Am Coll Cardiol* 1996; **27**:330–6.

12 Picano E, Lattanzi F, Orlandini A, Marini C, Labbate A. Stress echocardiography and the human factor - the importance of being expert. *J Am Coll Cardiol* 1991; **17**:666–9.

13 Cosyns B, Haberman D, Droogmans S, Warzee S, Mahieu P, Laurent E, *et al*. Comparison of contrast enhanced three dimensional echocardiography with MIBI gated SPECT for the evaluation of left ventricular function. *Cardiovasc Ultrasound* 2009; **7**:27.

14 Wong M, Staszewsky L, Volpi A, Latini R, Barlera S, Hoglund C. Quality assessment and quality control of echocardiographic performance in a large multicenter international study: Valsartan in Heart Failure Trial (Val-HeFT). *J Am Soc Echocardiogr* 2002; **15**:293–301.

15 Berger AK, Gottdiener JS, Yohe MA, Guerrero JL. Epidemiological approach to quality assessment in echocardiographic diagnosis. *J Am Coll Cardiol* 1999; **34**:1831–6.

16 Goland S, Trento A, Iida K, Czer LSC, De Robertis M, Naqvi TZ, *et al*. Assessment of aortic stenosis by three-dimensional echocardiography: an accurate and novel approach. *Heart* 2007; **93**:801–7.

17 Hoffman RM, Lethen H, Marwick T, Arnese M, Fioretti P, Pingitore A, *et al*. Analysis of interinstitutional observer agreement in interpretation of dobutamine stress echocardiograms. *J Am Coll Cardiol* 1996; **27**(2):330–6.

Further reading

Mathew JP, Glas K, Troianos CA, Sears-Rogan P, Savage R, Shanewise J, *et al*. American Society of Echocardiography/Society of Cardiovascular Anesthesiologists recommendations and guidelines for continuous quality improvement in perioperative echocardiography. *J Am Soc Echocardiogr* 2006; **19**:1303–13. [An excellent systematic approach to QA.]

Online resources

- EAEL laboratory Accreditation: http://www.escardio.org/communities/EAE/accreditation/Pages/laboratory.aspx

- EAE Individual Accreditation: http://www.escardio.org/communities/eae/accreditation/Pages/welcome.aspx

- ICAEL Echo Laboratory Accreditation Guidelines: http://www.icael.org/icael/news/articles/board0406.htm

- ISO 9000: http://www.iso.org/iso/home.htm

- For additional multimedia materials please visit the online version of the book (http://escecho.oxfordmedicine.com).

Index

Page numbers in *italic* indicate figures and tables.